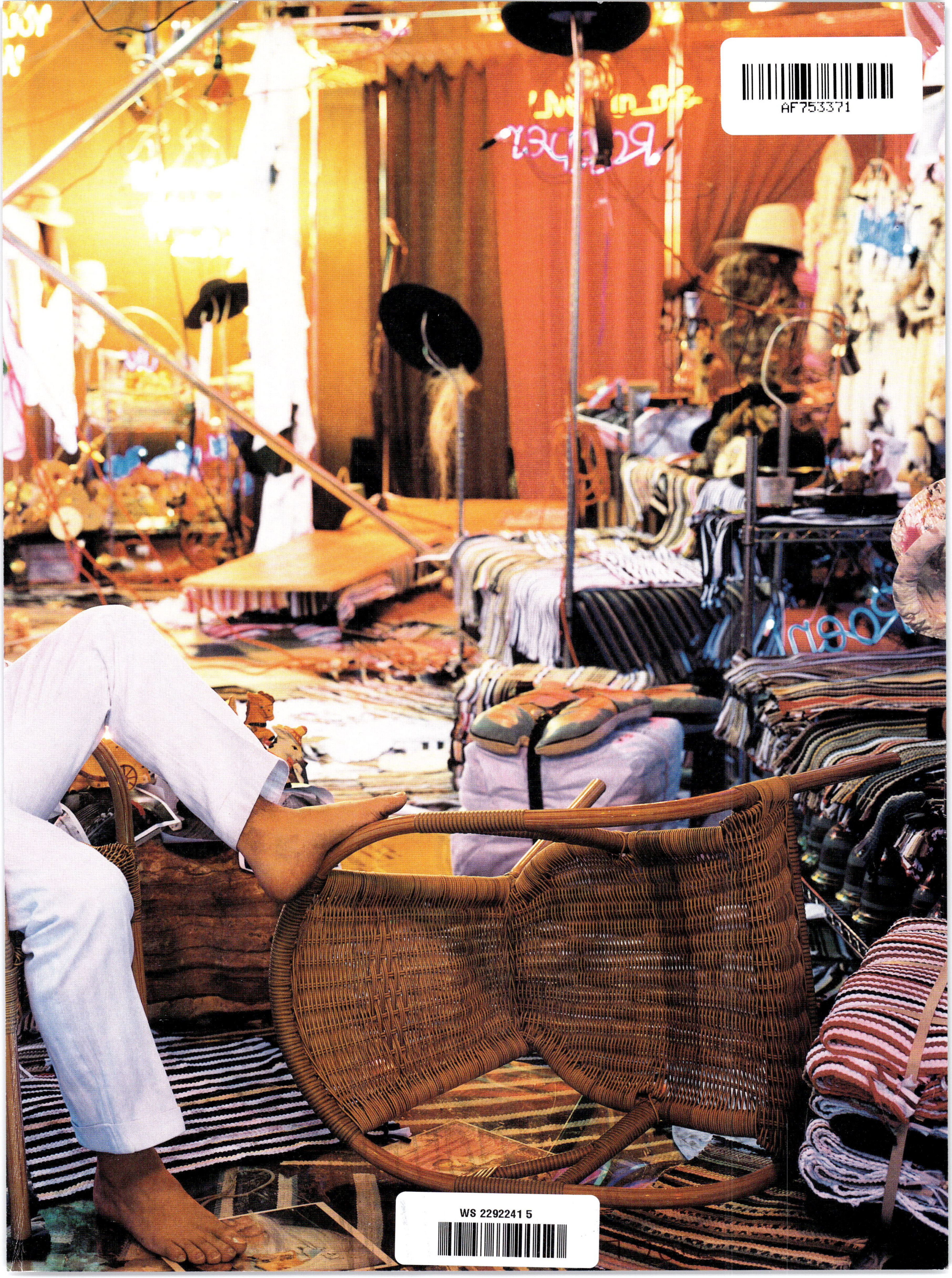

AF753371
WS 2292241 5

Jason Rhoades' Black Pussy Cocktail Coffee Table Book © 2006

Black Pussy Soirée Cabaret Macramé was held officially in 2006 on January 26, February 2, 9, 15, 23, March 1, 16, April 1, May 19, and July 2.

First edition 2007

© 2007 Jason Rhoades for the images
© 2007 Steidl Publishers for this edition

All rights reserved. No part of this publication may be reproduced or transmitted in any form or by any means, including photocopy, recording, or any other information storage and retrieval system, without prior permission in writing from the publisher.

Designed by Brian Roettinger, www.handheldheart.com
Fonts: *Haircrimes One* by Andrea Tinnes, *Latienne* by Mark Jamra, *Dalliance Flourishes* by Frank Heine, and *Swift* by Gerard Unger.

Dust jacket designed by Brian Roettinger and Jason Rhoades.

Additional photography by our many guests who have generously contributed their charisma to the making of this book.

This book was made possible by generous contributions from Hauser & Wirth, Zürich and London, and David Zwirner, New York.

Scans by Steidl's digital darkroom
Production and printing: Steidl, Göttingen

Steidl
Düstere Str. 4 / D–37073 Göttingen
Phone +49 551-49 60 60 / Fax +49 551-49 60 649
E-mail: mail@steidl.de
www.steidlville.com / www.steidl.de

ISBN 978-3-86521-631-1
Printed in Germany

Jason Rhoades' Black Pussy Cocktail

Coffee Table Book

Edited by Alex Israel
Foreword by Kevin West

Photography by
Alexia Pilat and Joshua White

UNIVERSITY OF CHICHESTER

Introduction by Alex Israel

0
709.
2
RHO

Welcome to *Black Pussy.* Thank you for coming, for wearing bright white, and for arriving on time. I hope that you enjoy yourself while you are here. Make yourself at home, and let us know if we can get you anything to make your stay more comfortable.

We have done our best to capture the spirit of the ten planned events, held *Live in the Black Pussy,* in these pages. However, if you speak to someone who witnessed *Black Pussy* first hand, I'm sure that you will hear a different story.

Black Pussy Soirée Cabaret Macramé was held officially in 2006 on January 26, February 2, 9, 15, 23, March 1, 16, April 1, May 19, and July 2.

Black Pussy Soirée Cabaret Macramé has been an amazing team effort. It couldn't have happened without the support and hard work of many individuals. I'd like to take this opportunity to thank many of the people who helped to make this not only possible, but also very special. To everyone at Hauser & Wirth, Zürich and London, and David Zwirner, New York, we send you our deepest gratitude for all of your support for this project, which has happened so far away from home.

To the Rhoades studio team, whose tireless efforts have made the daily creative process both functional and rewarding, Rick Baker, Paco Marcial and Sarah Clothier, thank you.

Thank you Kevin West for your illuminating foreword.

Alexia Pilat and Josh White, your photographs are fantastic, and we are so proud to have had you both take part in this lengthy and involved project. Nathan Danilowicz, thank you for playing your role as nude black and white developer so well. To the many other photographic contributors, thank you for taking the time to send us your pictures. To our guests, thank you for putting our cameras to good use, many of your pictures have been included in this book, and the ones that didn't make it in certainly entertained us. A special thanks to Jason Schmidt for granting us permission to use the fantastic photograph he took of Jason, posed as Jean-Michel Basquiat as photographed for the cover of *The New York Times Magazine*, February 10, 1985.

Thank you Ezra Woods, for inspiring us with your nose; the scents that you created for Black Pussy are remarkable. And to Bettina Korek, our amazing planted guest, thank you for everything. Brian Roettinger, it has been a pleasure working with you on the design of this book. We are so happy with all you have put into it, and of course, we are so happy with the result.

Anita, your voice filled *Black Pussy* with heart and soul at every event. Thank you Jelvis, for lending us your drum.

To our Musical guests, huge thanks for all of your energy, your enthusiasm and your celebrity sets. Ed Hudecek, we wouldn't have heard a thing without you, thank you.

To all of our guests, thank you for your charisma. Hopefully, we have been a successful dreamcatcher, catching bits and pieces of all of you. You have each contributed something, helping Jason to finish the piece, and for that, we are eternally appreciative. While not all of you are pictured in this book, please know that your charisma is an essential part of the sculpture, and will be forever.

Black Pussy Soirée Cabaret Macramé was made possible through the generous contributions of many of our friends and loved ones, who provided links and bricks in our chain-letter-pyramid-scheme method of inviting guests, finding music, and casting out the *Black Pussy* aura. Thank you all, you know who you are.

We hope you've had a memorable experience. Please drive safely. Goodnight.

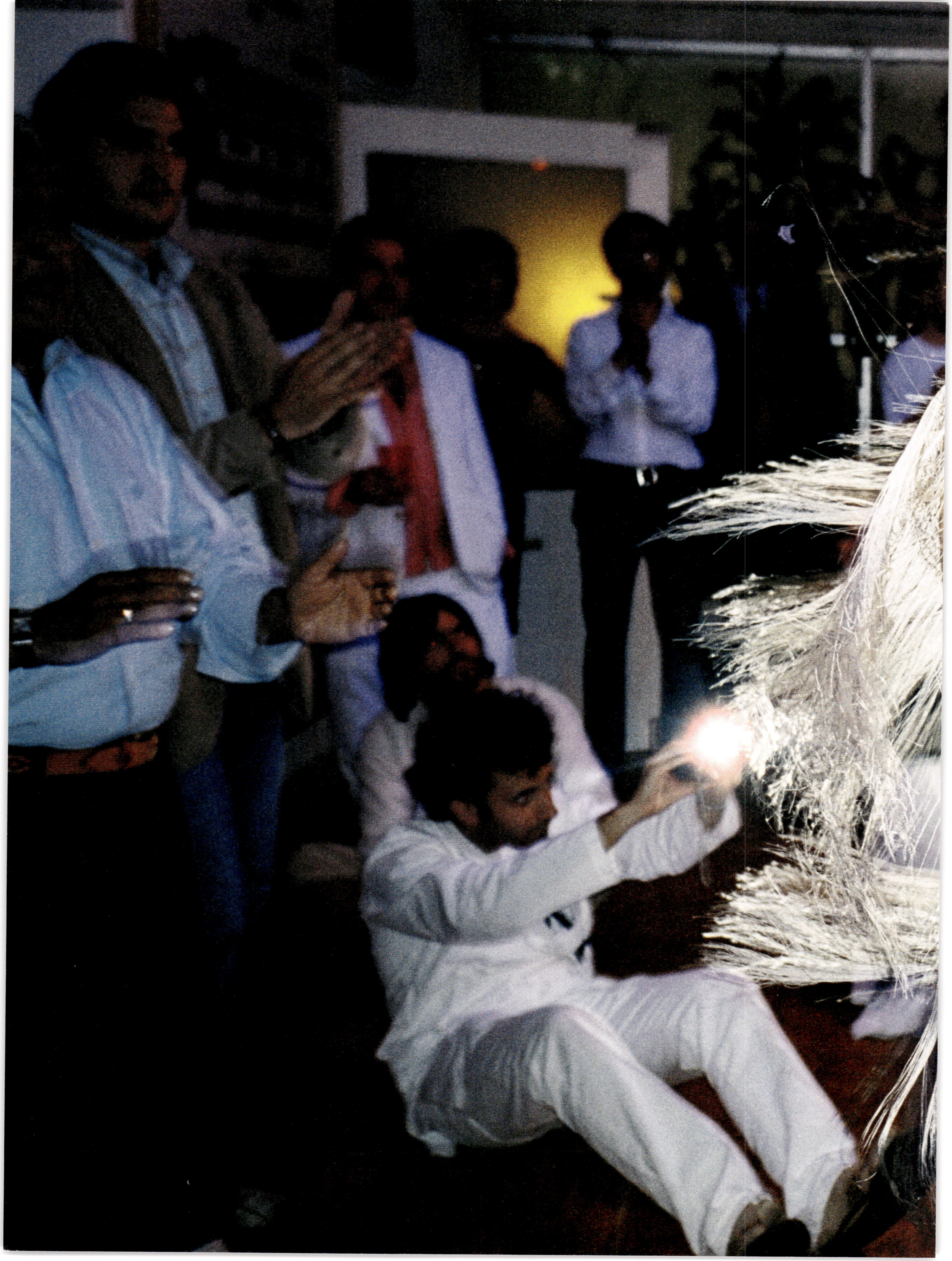

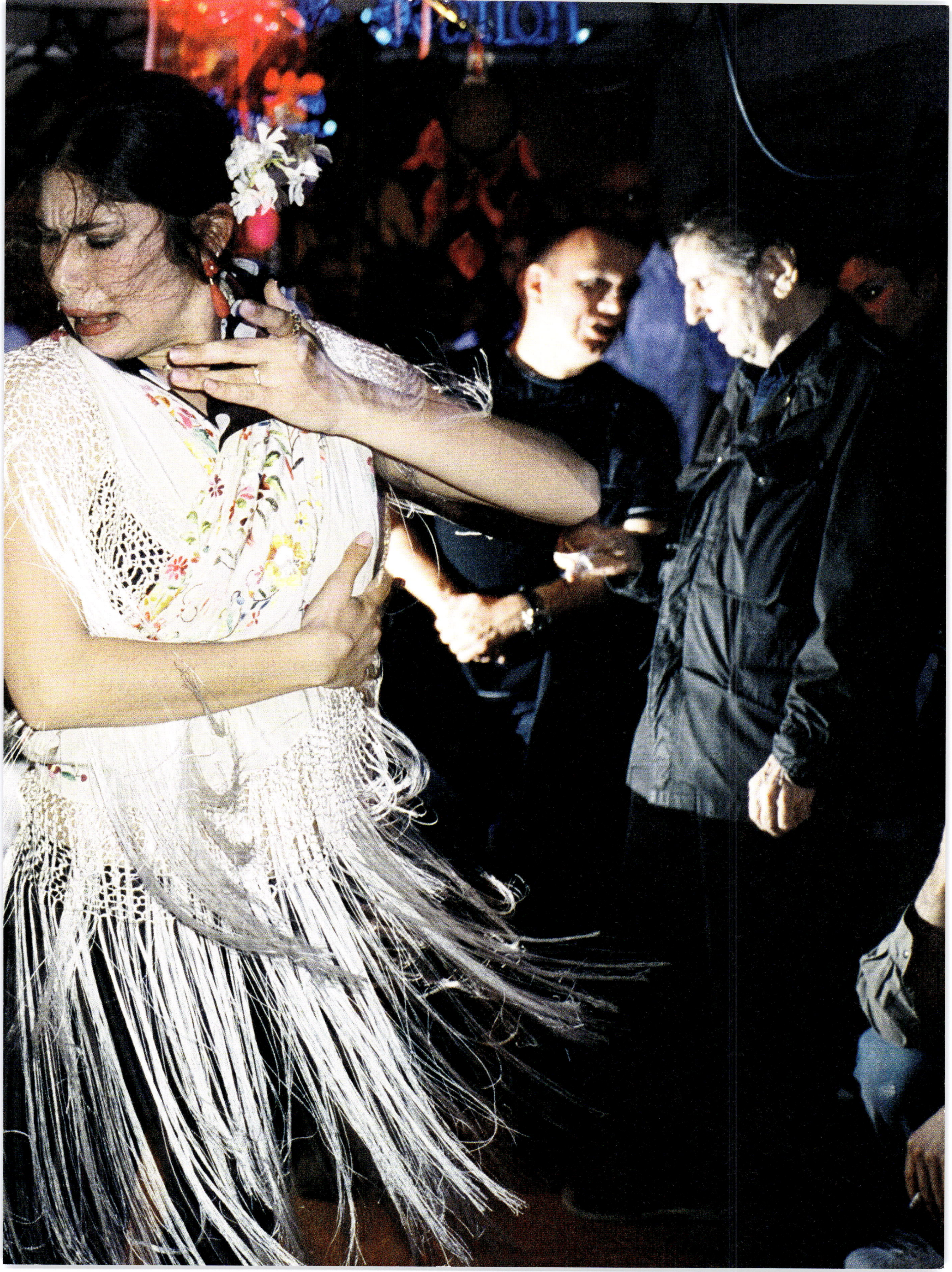

Foreword by Kevin West

If "pussy" is a vulgar word, then it is usually made more so by an adjective. Take the word pairings "fresh pussy" and "smelly pussy." Each is somehow worse than the unadorned noun, and both are equally bad — both are dirty.

But the word pairing "black pussy" inhabits its own linguistic niche, one that is oddly affirmative, thanks to its associations with such related words and concepts as Black Pride, Black Power, Black History, Black Culture, Black Hair, Black Music and so on. Black Pussy is strong. A Black woman (or her drag-queen imitator) might snap her finger and say "you better get out of my face, or I will get all Black on your ass." When Oprah Winfrey blasted "A Million Little Pieces" author James Frye on her television show, that's what she did: she got all Black on his ass. (Another prime artifact of black-pussy fury: Nina Simone's come-to-Jesus testimonial "Mississippi Goddamn.") Black Pussy can smite those who provoke its wrath, just as it can seduce those it desires — a duality of power/allure that pop culture icons such as Hip-Hop diva Missy Elliot and chanteuse Beyoncé have made the pivot of their public personae. Young gay guys boast on the Internet about their Boi Pussies, but that's really wishful thinking — men don't have Pussy Power.

Black Pussy is nonetheless vulnerable as well. It brings to mind acts of violence and postures of servitude: slavery, rape, pornography, "exotic" dances. It creates an atmosphere of fear and loathing. In the spring of 2006, members of Duke University's all-white lacrosse squad were accused of rape by an African-American dancer hired to perform at a student party. The charges were eventually dropped for lack of evidence, but only after the lacrosse team was suspended for the remainder of its season and several of its members were alleged to be rapists in national news reports. Black Pussy is explosive, and liable to erupt at any moment.

So when Jason Rhoades' studio emailed invitations to something called the *Black Pussy Soirée Cabaret Macramé*, one couldn't help but be alarmed and excited. With its grand title, the *Black Pussy Soirée Cabaret Macramé* had the air of event about it, but what sort of event? Would it be pretentious? Smutty? Political? Maudlin? Puerile? Didactic? Incomprehensible? Uplifting? The letter of invitation said it was an evening of charisma-swapping or some such thing, and also noted that guests would be given dinner. The rest was left to the imagination, and my imagination ran wild. Would we get to look at naked women? Would we be asked to take off our clothes? Was this a sex party? When I talked to another person who received an invitation, he referred to the happening in code — "the BP." Circumspection of that kind that hinted at illicit activities and of course further piqued my interest. I emailed Alex Israel, Rhoades' co-host and collaborator on the *Black Pussy Soirées*, to say I'd be delighted to attend.

PUSSY TRILOGY

Black Pussy was begun in 2005 as the third installment of a Pussy Trilogy that has occupied Rhoades since 2000. It began with *Meccatuna*, a project to send a live deep-sea tuna fish on the pilgrimage route to Mecca. (The project was only partially realized: Rhoades sent a case of canned tuna to Mecca, where it circled the Ka'bah before returning to New York.) Next came the grand Pussy Mosque, *My Madinah: in pursuit of my ermitage*, which Rhoades built in St. Gallen, Switzerland, and which coincided with the publication of his book *1724: Birth of the Cunt*.

Black Pussy was first introduced to the public in 2005 at London's Hauser and Wirth gallery. The following year, Rhoades created its "Little Sista" in his studio at 3113 Beverly Boulevard in Los Angeles. This, the *Private Black Pussy* — "private" because accessible by invitation only — was a room-sized, site-specific sculpture that was subsequently modified in subtle ways when it served as the setting for ten Happenings, christened the *Black Pussy Soirée Macramé Cabarets*, that were held during the first half of 2006. "*Black Pussy*" is thus a tripartite name that applies equally to Rhoades' sculpture, the venue housing it and the Happenings that occurred there.

Like Rhoades earlier work, *Black Pussy* relates to the history of Islam, specifically the story of Mohammed's return to Mecca in the seventh century to declare that Islam had but one god, Allah, and that god had no material form. To save his followers from idolatry, Mohammed destroyed 360 pagan idols housed at the Ka'Bah shrine. Mohammed's act of iconoclasm has a loose parallel in the Old Testament Bible story of Moses and Golden Calf, in that both were milestones in the sweep of world history, events that mark the transformation of a primitive animist, polytheistic belief systems into monotheistic religions organized around deistic worship.

But Rhoades' principal interest is the back-story of how and why the Ka'bah had become a center of spiritual pilgrimage. The 360 idols had been gathered at the Ka'bah by wandering nomadic tribes who wished to create a spiritual center in Arabia, but who equally figured to profit from it, since a large and lively market developed around the mosque to sell food and other necessary provisions to faithful visitors. Rhoades views this savvy conflation of piety and commerce as a prime early example of the cynical marketing of religion for reasons of profit.

Rhoades decided the history of the Ka'bah resonated with our contemporary culture's version of idol-worship: the adoration of celebrities. The West has never entirely escaped its pagan past, and even the Catholic Church canonized a crowded pantheon of saints as an outlet for its followers' latent pantheistic impulse. Modern media culture has largely replaced the holy saints with a pantheon of venerated stars such as Paris Hilton and Lindsay Lohan, whom Rhoades refers to as "White Virgins." (Hilton and Lohan are unruly "virgins," to be sure, but one of their sisterhood, Britney Spears, at the beginning of her career famously told interviewers that she was literally still a virgin. For years to follow, radio "shock-jock" deejays joked about who would "deflower" her. Likewise, when Mary-Kate and Ashley Olsen, the pop phenomenon known as the Olsen Twins, turned 18, young men's magazines leeringly announced that they were now "legal." Clearly America is deeply ambivalent about the chastity of its White Virgins.)

For *Black Pussy*, Rhoades recreated the 360 idols of the Ka'bah as neon black-light signs. Half were sent to London, while the other half remained in his L.A. studio, where the signs, which spell out synonyms for Pussy, cast a pale violet glow over the entire installation.

ULTIMATE PUSSY WORD

Upon entering Rhoades's studio, a former retail space between a tattoo parlor and a New York-themed donut shop, one first passes through an antiseptically white room, the Johnny Cash Gallery, where artworks on display can be bought with cash. This antechamber to the *Black Pussy* can be conceptualized as its outer labia — the furthest perimeter of the sacred center. It nonetheless also suggests the *Black Pussy's* dialectic opposite: the White Cock of gravel-voiced country music singer Johnny Cash. As a place of commerce (cash changes hands) the Johnny Cash Gallery is analogous to the marketplace outside the Ka'bah. It is a way-station on the journey to the *Black Pussy*, where visitors have the chance to take a preparatory pause — to buy art or drink from two well-stocked bars — before they leave the profane outer realm of cash/cock for the holy destination inside the *Black Pussy*.

Before they leave the Johnny Cash Gallery, though, guests might flip through a pristine copy of *1724: Birth of the Cunt*. Its bi-lingual introduction begins:

Au commencement était le Verbe. Apres, les hommes trouverent les synonymes

In the beginning was the word. Then men found synonyms.

There follow 1724 synonyms for the female pudendum, printed in Braille-like bumps on paper the pale pink of feminine hygiene products and sex toys. Some of the words are:

Launch Pad
Lawrence of a Labia
Lincoln Tunnel
Lobster Pot
Long-Eye
Lotus Blossom

This is the first indication of the fecundity of Pussy, and of its ineffability. *1724: Birth of the Cunt* demonstrates that language proliferates around Pussy precisely because words fail to adequately describe it. Man cannot subjugate Pussy with words. This may strike some as a lamentable truth and others as a joyous one, but it is a truth not yet acknowledged by the vox populi. The storehouse of language records an ongoing urgent if unsatisfactory search for an appropriate Pussy vocabulary. Like Adam walking through the Garden and naming the Creation into existence, men (and women, too) continue to throw names at the Pussy, as they cling to the inchoate belief that there must be a word equal to the thing itself — the Ultimate Pussy Word.

Since the first Pussy Word Harvest in 2005 in Bogotá, Colombia, Rhoades has gathered some 7,000 Pussy words. The *Black Pussy Soirée Macramé Cabaret* is, on one level, simply a mechanism to continue the Harvest — words are also gathered via the Internet at *Pussy.is* — and presumably the Harvest would end if the Ultimate Pussy Word were discovered, as the Black Pussy would then be complete. But who is to say which language would generate the Ultimate Pussy Word? Or even if the Ultimate Pussy Word, should it ever emerge, could be said aloud? Might it not be unspeakable, as Yahweh, the Tetragrammaton, is the proper name of the God of Israel but cannot be voiced?

Some of the words (in various language) Rhoades has harvested so far include:

Almeja
Baby ATM
Circulus Vitiosus
Dédale
Erva (Hebrew)
Ffanni
Ganha-Pão
He Xhitombo...et cetera...

The list demonstrates the Pussy's unique linguistic profligacy. The number of Pussy words in English, French or Spanish alone far surpasses the several dozen Inuit words for snow — the classic example of a culturally important phenomenon that generate superabundant vocabulary words. Pussy is inexhaustible, a veritable springhead of language. It is *L'Origine du Monde*, as Gustave Courbet named his — scandalous 1866 painting of his lover's naked genitals — a landmark in the history of Pussy art. And yet the Pussy is also a *vagina dentata* that devours all words in its path. It is the womb and tomb of language, to use the familiar Shakespearean rhyme.

Indeed, one might observe Rhoades' ceaseless search for Pussy Words and conclude that there is, in fact, no one Ultimate Pussy Word. Instead, the Pussy Word List might be imagined as a global archive that strives to contain *every* Pussy word. In this case, the list would reach a state of static (and ecstatic) perfection when it assembles all the Pussy words ever uttered in every language, living and dead. The mind boggles at the Borgesian scope of such a volume: the Word List would have to become as large as the universe it attempts to describe, and so it would itself become infinite. The 7,000-word Pussy Word List that Rhoades has thus far compiled hints at the magnitude of such a Universal Archive, but it has barely begun to complete it. Neither has Rhoades yet attempted a taxonomy of Pussy Words. His list is simply an alphabetical registry, beginning with "A Bit of Mutton" and running in a single unbroken column to "Zulo."

A final thought: just as sex offers only temporary relief from the procreative urge, speaking aloud a Pussy word only briefly satisfies the desire to say more Pussy words.

INSIDE THE BLACK PUSSY

After drinks in the Johnny Cash Gallery, Rhoades beckons guests into the inner sanctum of his studio. Here is the Ali Baba's cave or self-storage unit of his imagination, a self-contained space of creative abundance, a treasure chest, a secret garden. It is the chicken and the egg of Rhoades' artistic production. Seen from certain angles, it could be mistaken for a dorm room, or the Merry Pranksters' garage, or a riotous medina or a country-western store disheveled by a tornado.

This is the actual sculpture entitled *Black Pussy*. It fills a large, high-ceilinged room with various materials, some of which are obviously meaningful (a homemade aluminum knock-off of Jeff Koons' stainless steel *Rabbit* [1986]), even if others have a more obscure significance, such as:

Cowboy hats in various colors, Indian Dream Catchers hung with false fox tails and real feathers, a vintage *How the Grinch Stole Christmas* t-shirt, camel saddles, loose bundles of long coarse fiber the color of Rapunzel's hair, photographs from previous *Soirée Macramé Cabarets* including amateur beaver shots, bales of cheap woven blankets used as low stools, a Chinese scholar's stone with the price tag ($350 +tax) still attached, hundreds of hookah pipes from a seized cargo shipping container, a corn cob stuck in a terra cotta candlestick, a pair of cast-resin bull testicles, rubber stamps (Sweet Potato Lips, Beanie Bootie, African Palace), deer antlers, rolls of ribbon (marked: 15 cents/yard), an empty bottle of 1965 Charles Krug Napa Valley Cabernet Sauvignon, a vase with dried branches, a frozen yogurt machine, Black Pussy self-adhesive stickers, a Casio digital camera (non-functioning), Mexican donkey cart flower pots used as candles, several photo albums, a big bed with a white duvet, a water pipe (bong), Venetian glass bananas and eggplants, a low stage made of plywood and mesh fabric for gym shorts, a small Hammond organ with sheet music, small brass pyramids engraved with scenes of ancient Egyptian life, a dried palm tree trunk, a network of black or orange extension cords attached to 250 neon "black light" signs that spell out Pussy words.

As the eye begins to seize on specific objects, there's a natural impulse to assign them significance.

Some suggest Pussy puns:

Cowboy hats (genuine beaver)
Camel saddles (camel toe)
Dried branches (pussy willow)

Still other items seem to pair up, as if to show how the *Black Pussy* encompasses contradiction within its abundance:

Beaver shots / bull's testicles — female / male
Palm tree / glass bananas — nature / artifice
Hookah pipes / wine bottle — Eastern/Western hallucinogen
Scholar stones / cowboy hats — Eastern virtue / Western virtue or contemplation / action or enlightenment / violence

And then, upon further observation, some of these pairs of items seem to align themselves as if to suggest loose thematic patterns:

Felt hats / Dreamcatchers — Cowboys / Indians
Dreamcatchers / Donkey Pots — Handicraft / consumer good
Donkey Pots / Koons Rabbit — Mass produced / unique or global commerce / local market or cheap / valuable or even kitsch / art
Koons Rabbit / Scholar's stone — Western/Eastern abstraction

Of course with the example of Koons' work we realize that such categories as mass produced/unique and kitsch/art are already in play. Still, the real *Rabbit* is inarguably an iconic artwork worth millions of dollars, while the Donkey Carts are faux folkloric trinkets sold as inexpensive souvenirs in tourist markets (The *Black Pussy* also contains bits of paintings by Jean-Michel Basquiat, another icon of the Eighties art world in New York.) Even so, the *Black Pussy* proves to be grandly indifferent to such distinctions as kitsch/art or cheap/valuable; it posits the Donkey Carts and the Koons Rabbit as equivalents. Both are reproductions and both represent, on some level, the base world of commerce at the Ka'bah market, rather than the elevated realm of the idols inside.

The Donkey Cart and Koons Rabbit are equivalent in another sense that isn't as readily apparent: both are hand-made readymades. The Rabbit reveals its status as a knock-off, since it is crudely fashioned in aluminum — a spoof of Koons' shiny surfaces and industrial fabrications. The origin of the Donkey Carts is more complex. After Japan surrendered to Allied Forces on August 14, 1945, an Allied military force occupied the country until April 28, 1952, when the San Francisco Peace Treaty went into effect. During that time, the war-torn nation reactivated its traditional porcelain factories to produce inexpensive ceramics for export to Western markets. Donkey Cart pots, styled after the popular souvenirs originally made in small Mexican workshops, were among those items mass-produced for export. The pieces often bore a "Made in Occupied Japan" stamp of origin. For *Black Pussy*, Rhoades bought a group of vintage Occupied Japan Donkey Carts on eBay and, reversing the process by which such souvenirs had left Mexico decades earlier, sent them to be knocked off by small factories in Guadalajara.

While certain free-market idealists may take pleasure from this example of capital's efficient flow around the globe towards favorable labor markets, pessimists will note that international trade has darker repercussions, as well. Since the terrorist attacks in New York on September 11, 2001, America has felt vulnerable to attack from outside, and nowhere more so than in its ports, which are largely unguarded openings or passages into the body of the nation. Policing the ports has proven to be an impossible challenge due to the vast volume of trade they handle. Rhoades evokes this looming threat of terrorist attack with the many hookah pipes in *Black Pussy*, which were among the contents of a seized cargo container. They may initially suggest, innocently enough, that the *Black Pussy* will take us on a hallucinogenic dream journey to Arabia. But they also remind us that Saudi Arabia is a source of the fundamentalist Islamic threat — a homeland of terrorists' bombs as well as exotic tales.

Be that as it may, the Donkey Carts play a vital function at *Black Pussy*. During the *Soirée Macramé Cabaret*, Rhoades demonstrates a device called the Spukaki Machine, first developed for *My Madinah*, The apparatus comprises a nozzle hung from a step-in waist harness, and it droops between the legs like a meaty phallus. For *My Madinah* it was used to shoot a stream of hot glue, but for the *Black Pussy* Rhoades modified it to squirt a hot wax that has been perfumed with one of two subtle fragrances, Black Pussy or White Virgin. (Developed by Ezra Woods, the Nose of the Black Pussy, the scents are derived from such vital essences as Paris by Paris Hilton perfume.) Rhoades fills Donkey Carts with Spukaki to make Donkey Cart Candles, and he also allows guests to strap on the Spukaki Machine to make their own candles, and thus indulge their fantasies of sexual prowess, as they take charge of a giant penis that spews in perpetual orgasm. They may not realize they are also mimicking the labors of assembly-line laborers in Japan or Mexico who earlier produced the Donkey Cart souvenirs

Of course *Black Pussy* guests, unlike their counterparts on minimum-wage assembly lines, get to enjoy the result of their labor immediately, when Rhoades invites them to share a final treat: a delicious Shoegurt dessert, which is frozen yogurt served in a Donkey Cart fitted into the guest's left shoe. Is Shoegurt an edible Spukaki simulacrum, just as Spukaki's correlative is semen? A potentially unsettling thought for those who are squeamish or for anyone who would normally rather "spit" than "swallow." Rhoades describes both Spukaki and Shoegurt as "vegan," which may be an ironic tribute to the hypersensitivity or even hypocrisy of guests, and it raises the odd question of whether semen is vegan.

THE VOICE OF THE BLACK PUSSY

Modern-day *saloniste* and libertine, Rhoades always wants guests to be comfortable at the *Black Pussy*, and he resists imposing rules on their visit. Early in the *Soirée*, he says by way of introduction:

The most important thing tonight is that you enjoy yourself. Please feel free to take off your clothes, touch yourself, or me, or Alex. Let yourself wander, wonder, and maybe weep. Don't be shy, we're all family here in this special place that we call the Black Pussy.

There is, all the same, a program of scheduled activities. Planted guest Bettina Korek, a friend of the Rhoades studio, helps novice guests negotiate the experience of *Black Pussy,* and she encourages them to participate in their first group activity, which binds them into the "family" Rhoades wishes to create. It is literally a binding experience: Macramé.

Weaving fibers is one of the oldest human skills, and indeed basket-making and cloth-making are archeological harbingers of early civilizations. Since prehistory, basketry and textiles have been valuable in the household (food storage, clothing), in ritual (such as burials) and in the marketplace (the Silk Road, a 5,000 mile trade route that stretched between China and Europe, takes its name from the ancient trade in fine textiles.) In many cultures across time, weaving and other related skills have belonged principally to the sphere of women's labor, whereas men have claimed the manufacture of goods using hard, valuable materials including metal and stone. As late as the mid 20th century, women of the Western world continued to make significant contributions to their home economies with needlepoint and knitting, and if such skills are today largely exercised only as leisure activities (hobbies), in many other parts of the world, weaving remains a vital household chore and an economically important job.

Macramé, a technique of tying knots that originated among sailors, blossomed as a national pastime in the 1970s, just at the moment when ERA discredited the retrograde notion of "women's work" and Women's Libbers proclaimed their independence from traditional domestic roles. As a group activity at *Black Pussy*, Macramé reminds participants of the timeless labor of generations of women and encourages them to reflect on late 20th-century gains in women's social and economic status. The *Black Pussy* Macramé wall-hanging is nonetheless an artifact of the here-and-now: Rhoades offers strips of vintage t-shirts as the Macramé material. And while he posts diagrams that illustrate the basic Macramé knots — the square knot, the double half-hitch — he encourages guests to improvise their own personal knotcraft. Thus each addition to the Macramé wall-hanging is personal and unique, like a signature in a guest-book.

Once Rhoades and his guests have "tied the knot," the principal activity of the evening can begin: the Pussy Word Harvest. Rhoades goes through the crowd with a microphone, like a tent revival preacher beseeching the faithful for true testimonials, and his guests make offerings that are perverse, descriptive, hilarious and sometimes demonstrative of a spontaneous poetic flair, as in:

Groove Tube
Mrs. Spincter's Next-Door Neighbor
Spasm Chasm

My contribution was "Succotash Pie," which caused a friend who accompanied me to say disdainfully, "Oh, you are so Southern," as if conflating food and sex were a particularly Southern depravity. Apparently it isn't:

Beef Curtains
Cherry Poptart
Cream Puff
Double Cheeseburger
Escargot dans la Coquille
Fish Taco
Grilled Cheese
Hairy Clam
Pan Dulce
Tuna Tartar

New Pussy words, especially rare or recondite discoveries, get announced from stage with a shout of glory: scat singer Anita, backed by the Black Pussy house band, belts them out like the oracle of Udaihu. Although the words do not come from her, in her song she reveals the guests' words back to them, since she is the authentic voice of the *Black Pussy*.

Other performers follow later. Sometimes there is a local band such as blackblack, unselfconscious high-school anger angels, who wail little pop songs that are as concise and earnest as anything ever recorded on a 78. The False Bono, when he appears, performs an acoustic set of U2's greatest hits. Once there was a very special visit from José Maria Cano, co-founder of Mecano, a seminal Spanish pop band of the 1980s. (Cano also penned the international song hit "Hijo de la Luna," the theme song for the Real Madrid soccer team and the opera "Luna," which was performed by Placido Domingo.) Cano composed a series of new songs for the *Black Pussy*, and painted them on a heroic scale for display in the Johnny Cash Gallery. The anthem "He Is Showing Me at his *Black Pussy*" is written for countertenor — the highest male voice that soars up into female range — and Cano lead *Black Pussy* guests through a rousing sing-along:

I am very happy because,
Because Jason Rhoades
is showing me,
Because Jason Rhoades
is showing,
Is showing me,
He is showing me,
At his Black Pussy.

The beauty of the song is that it works for everyone: Jason Rhoades is showing us all at his *Black Pussy*.

By the end of the night, we come to understand that the evening's activities — Macramé and Cabaret — aren't mere activities to amuse Rhoades' guests. *Black Pussy*, the sculpture, is an incomplete work that is finished by the presence and participation of guests when they contribute their charisma and perhaps leave behind some trace of themselves — a knot in the wall-hanging or a song. Through their participation, *Black Pussy* at 3113 Beverly Boulevard becomes the crucial locus of activity in Rhoades' creative universe. It is the vehicle and the vessel of an artistic process, the yonic portal that funnels his imagination and collect his guest's charisma — a Charismacatcher that functions, like the handicraft Dreamcatchers that are its symbol, to gather the intangible energies of life into concrete existence.

ELECTRIC PUSSYLAND

A neon black-light sign above the Cabaret stage spells out the words "Live in the Black Pussy." One isn't sure whether "Live" rhymes with "jive" or with "give." "Live" like "jive" is probably the intended sense given its placement over a musical stage (as in "live at the Apollo"), but on reflection I prefer "live" like "give" even better. This second sense suggests how the *Black Pussy* is not just a place to visit, but an experience that will permanently affect our perception, much as a pilgrimage to Mecca to circle the Ka'bah is a life-changing moment for the devout, a journey towards enlightenment.

The electric sign "Live in the Black Pussy" and the 250 other neon signs spelling out Pussy words are crucial components of Rhoades' work. Their illumination suggests this "enlightenment" of high spiritual achievement — what the faithful seek at the Ka'bah, and perhaps what Rhoades' guests are seeking in their own lives. But the light of the *Black Pussy* is an oxymoronic "black light," which encompasses both light and its opposite, the White Virgin as well as Black Pussy. (Paparazzi snaps of White Virgin idols like Jessica Simpson adorn some of the Black Pussy signs/idols.)

Like the Ka'bah's Idols, the Idols of the Black Pussy emit a mysterious, even sacred energy. And while each may be called by a different name, all transmit the same uniform light, since there is but a singular Divine Energy, complete and perfect in itself. The various Pussy Words are but so many names for the Godhead they represent, which is the source of light and dark and everything else, truly *L'Origine du Monde*. This Universal Pussy, if you will, may have 7,000 names, but behind each is the same Creator, a Matriarch of the Universe known to initiates by the name Black Pussy. Visitors to the *Black Pussy Soirée Cabaret Macramé* bask in Her black light.

The invitation to the *Soirée Cabaret Macramé* asks guests to dress in white, and Rhoades himself wears a suit tailored by Reto's in Zurich from 560-threadcount Egyptian cotton sheets, so that he moves "like a white glow" as the ancient poets described the guardian of the Ka'bah. The black light of the Idols shows as a pale purple glow against white clothes, and the guests appear as a host of White Virgins as they circulate.

Through the course of the evening, photographers Alexia Pilat and Josh White document the *Black Pussy* and deliver their film to Naked Nathan in his on-site darkroom. The pictures he develops are later added to the sculpture or slipped under Plexiglas panels on the floor to be trampled underfoot like forest leaves.

And yet there is a crucial detail: the pale ultraviolet glow of the Idols — the glow of enlightenment — cannot be captured on film. There is no way to fully document the *Black Pussy*. It remains intact in the memories and oral histories of those who have been "live at the *Black Pussy*," and continue to "live in" it.

At the end of the night, Rhoades lets guests choose a clean Donkey Cart Spukaki Candle to take home as a souvenir. Originally a base object from the world of commerce/cash/cock outside the *Black Pussy*, the Donkey Pot is now sanctified as a vessel for the fragrant Spukaki. When we go home and light the Donkey Pot Candle, we will again be enlightened by the fragrance of its melting wax and be reminded once more of the subtle, mysterious, ineffable experience known as the *Black Pussy*. It is our own private Burning Bush, and it flickers with the spark of enlightenment.

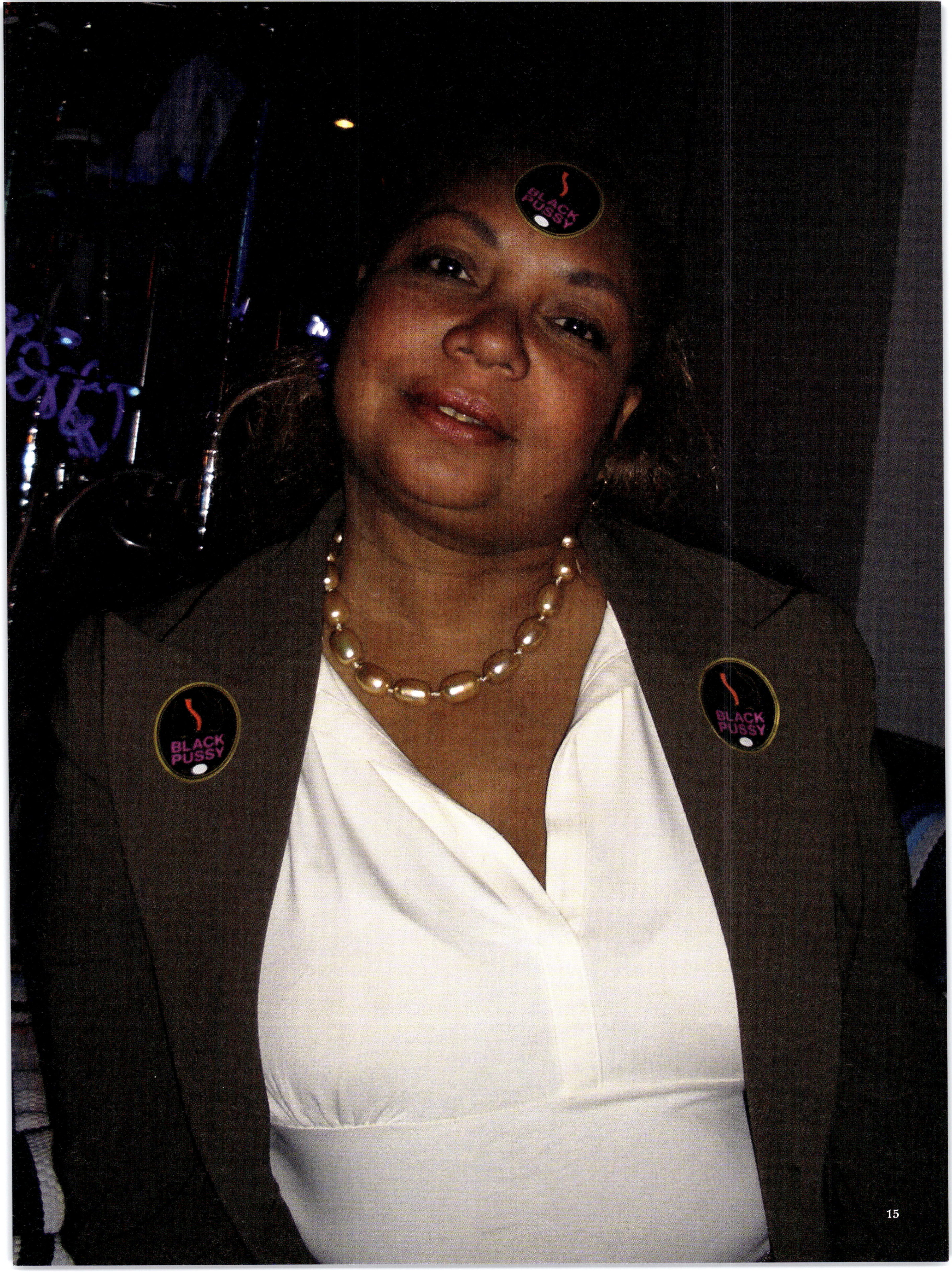
BLACK PUSSY
BLACK PUSSY
BLACK PUSSY

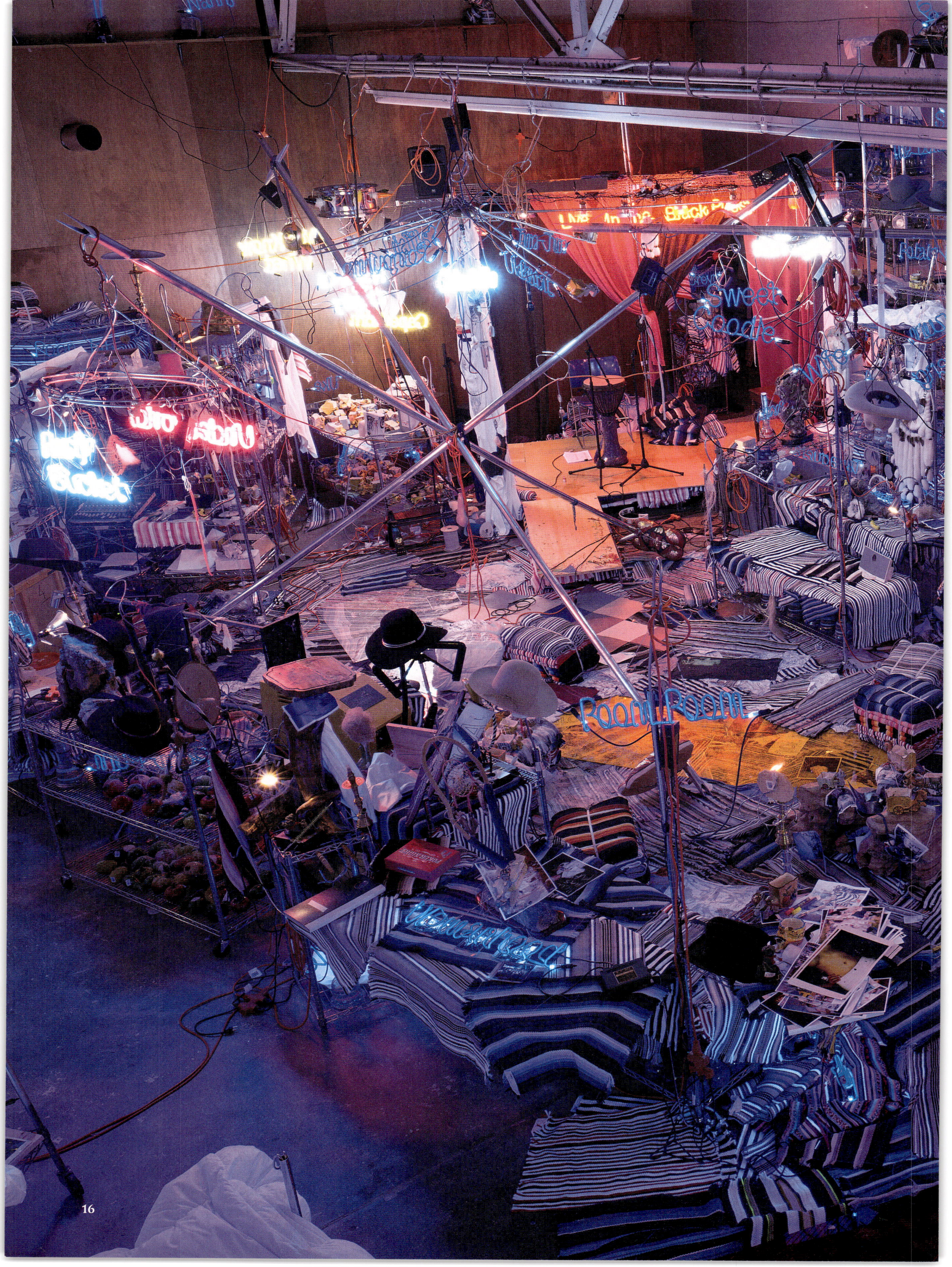
Sweet
Goodie
RoomRoom

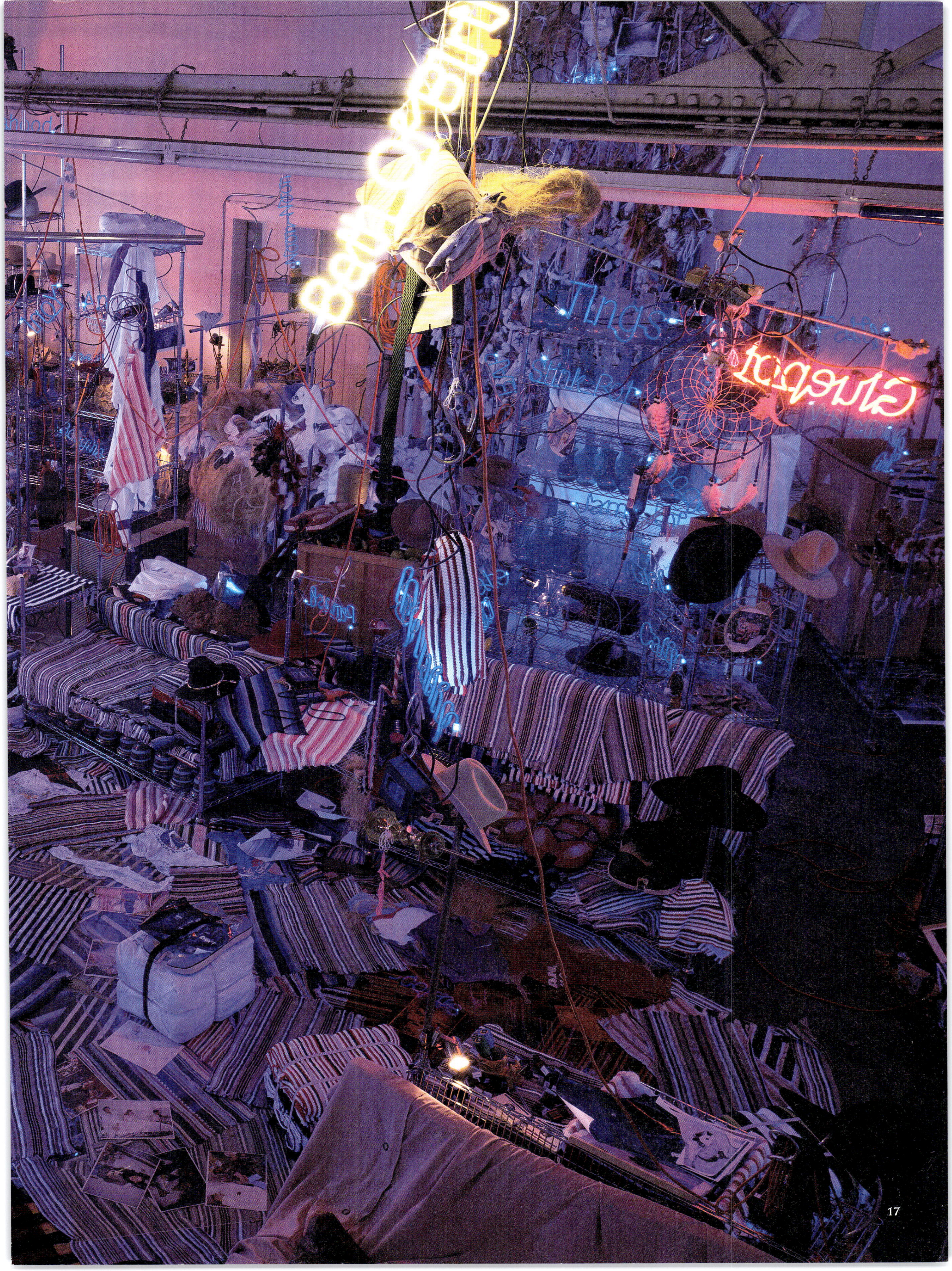

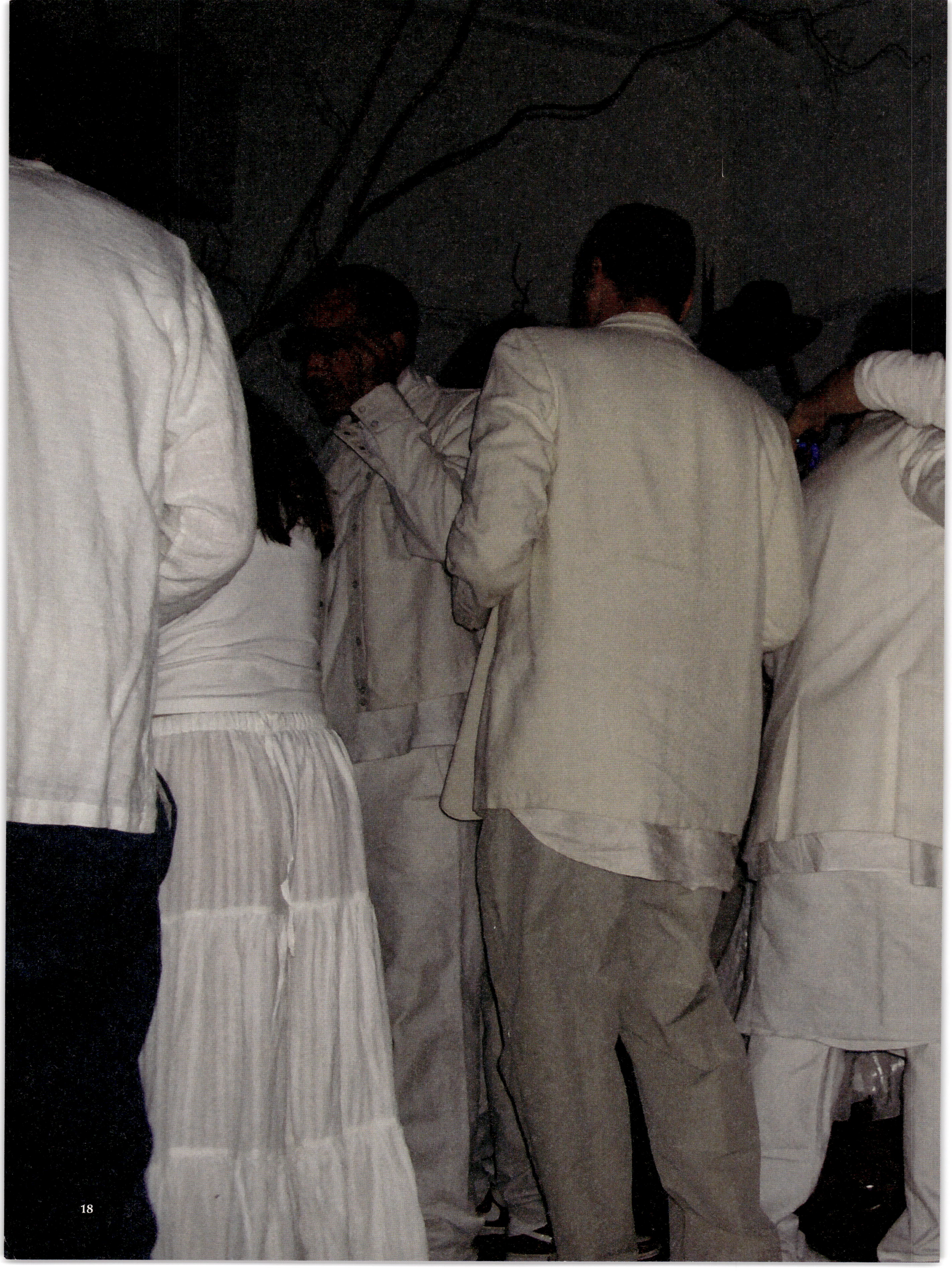

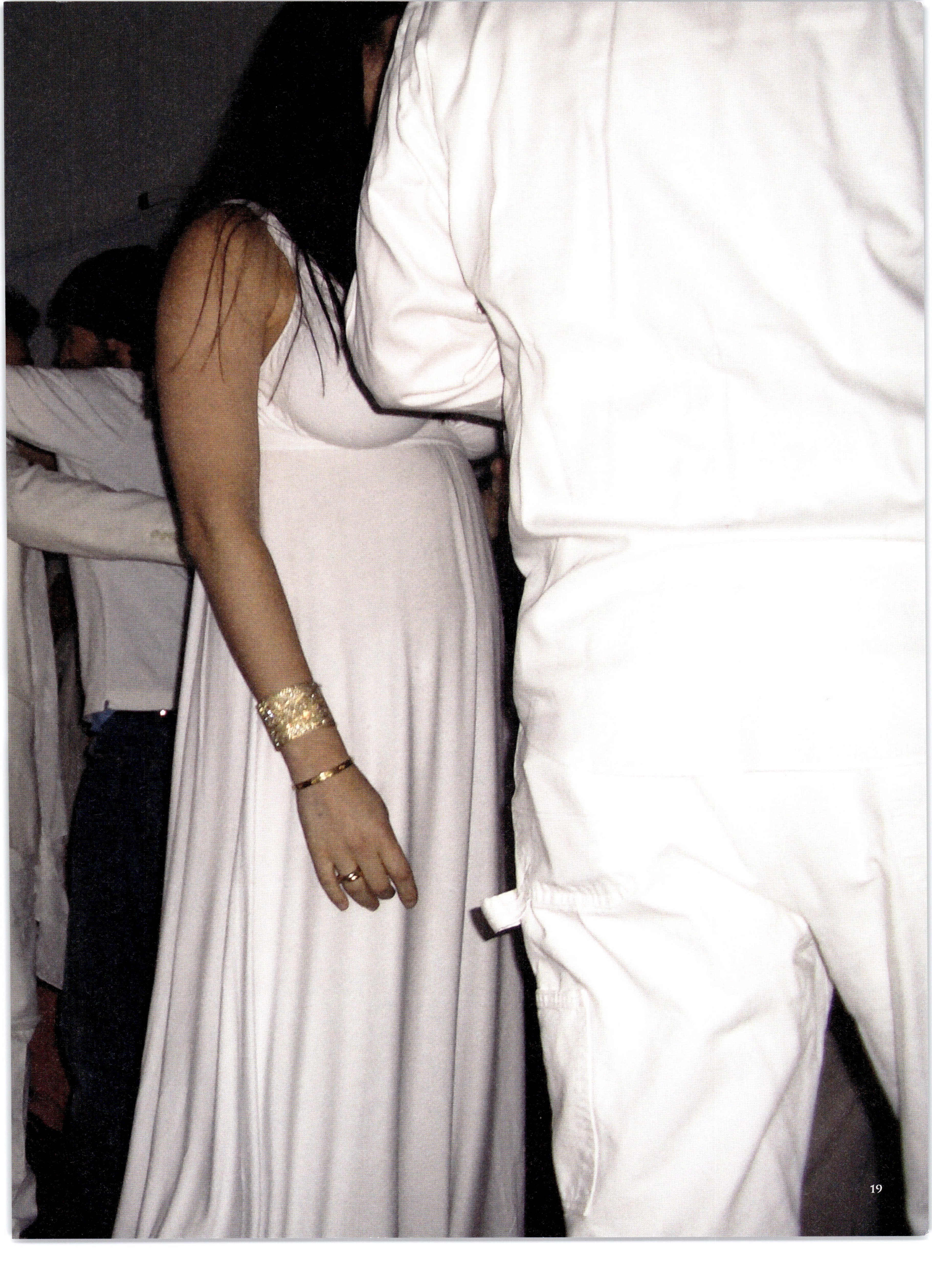

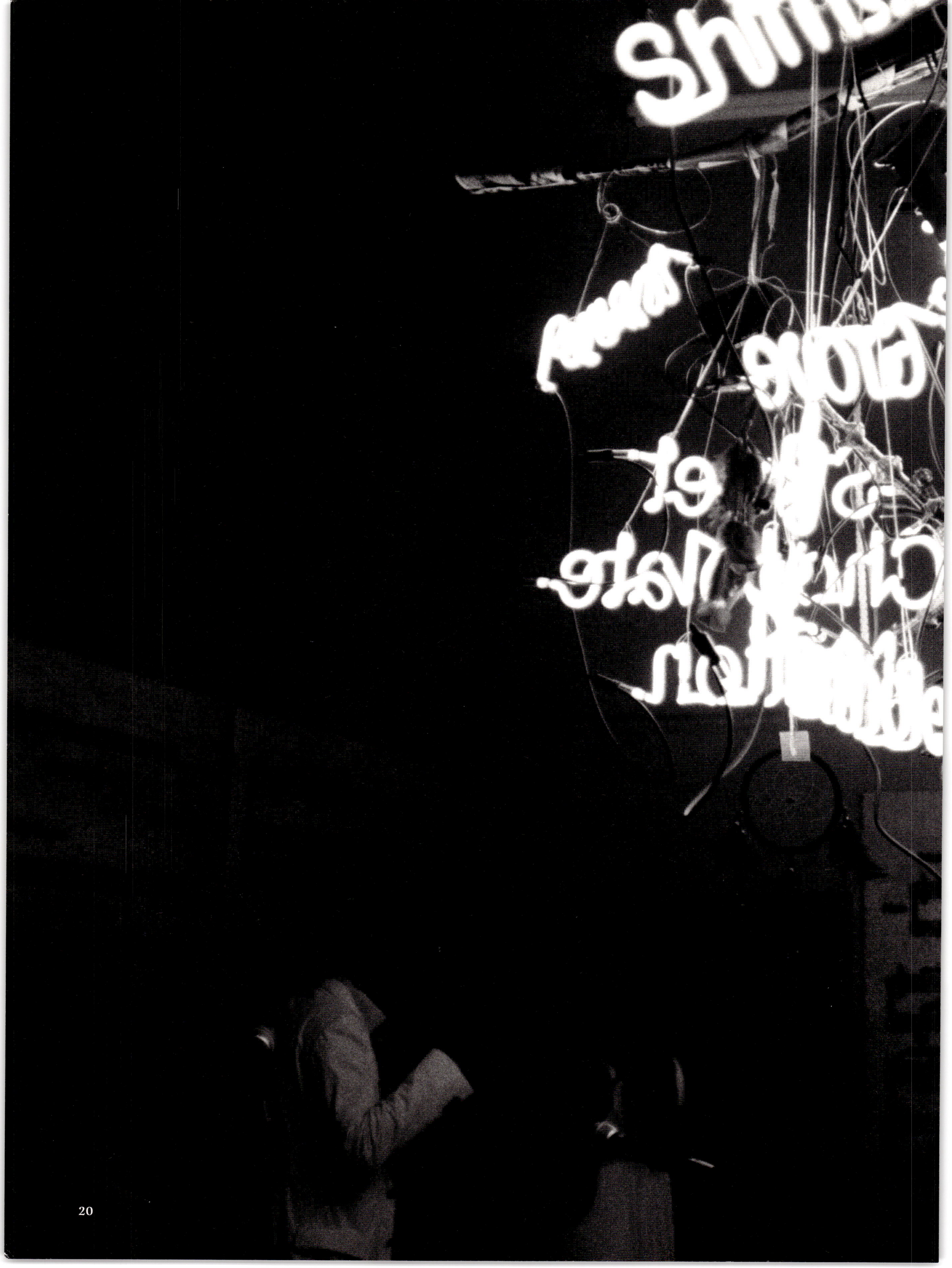

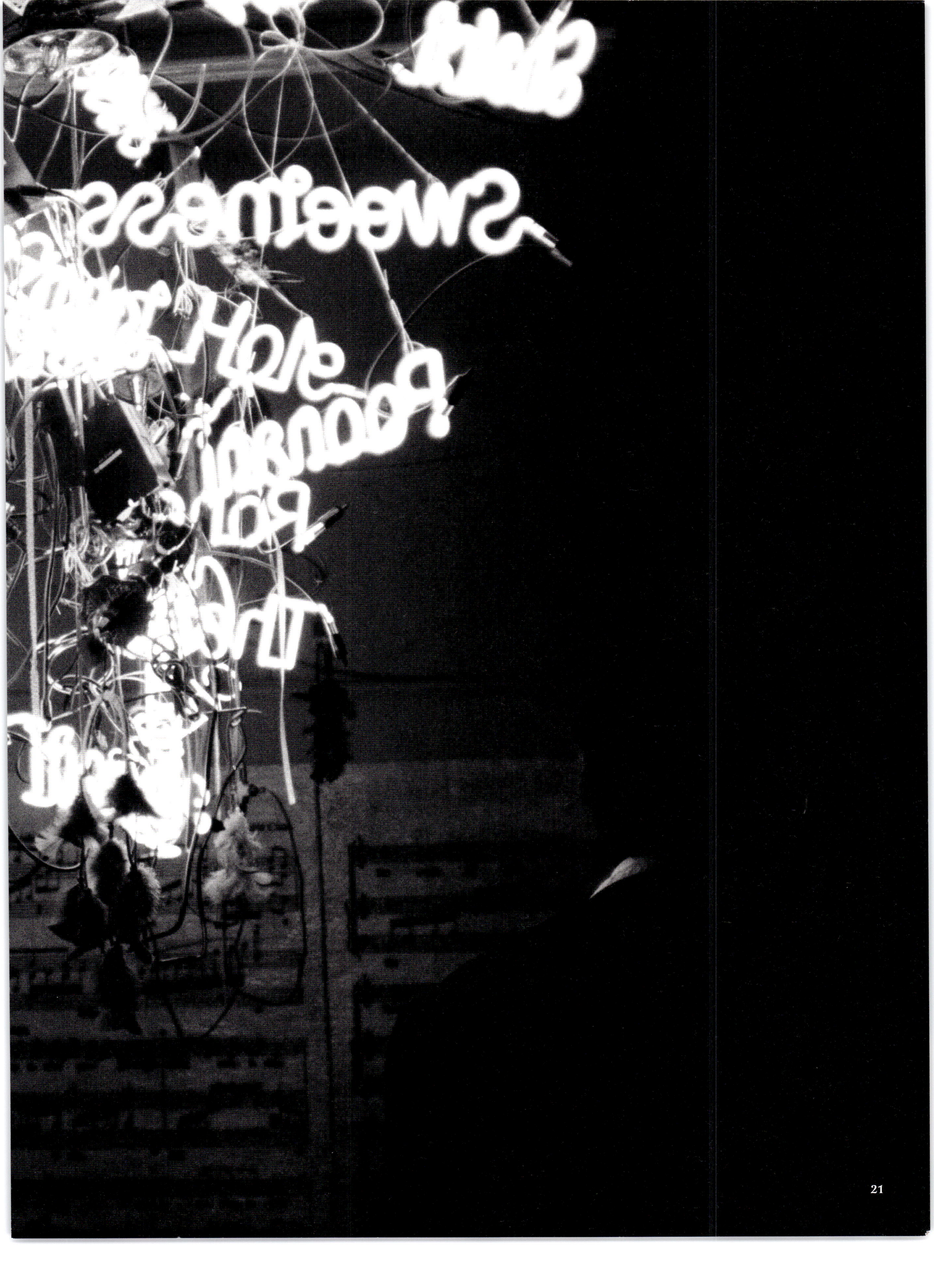

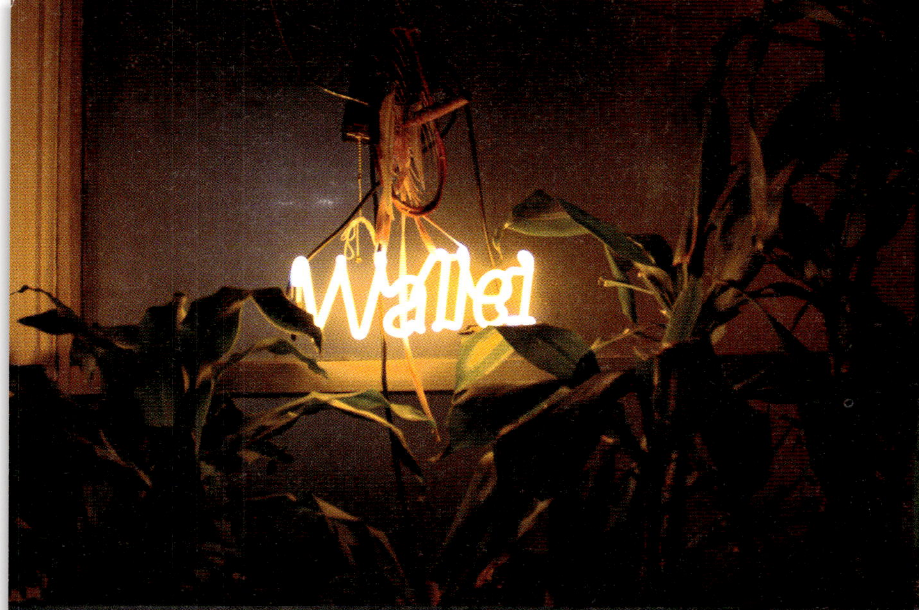

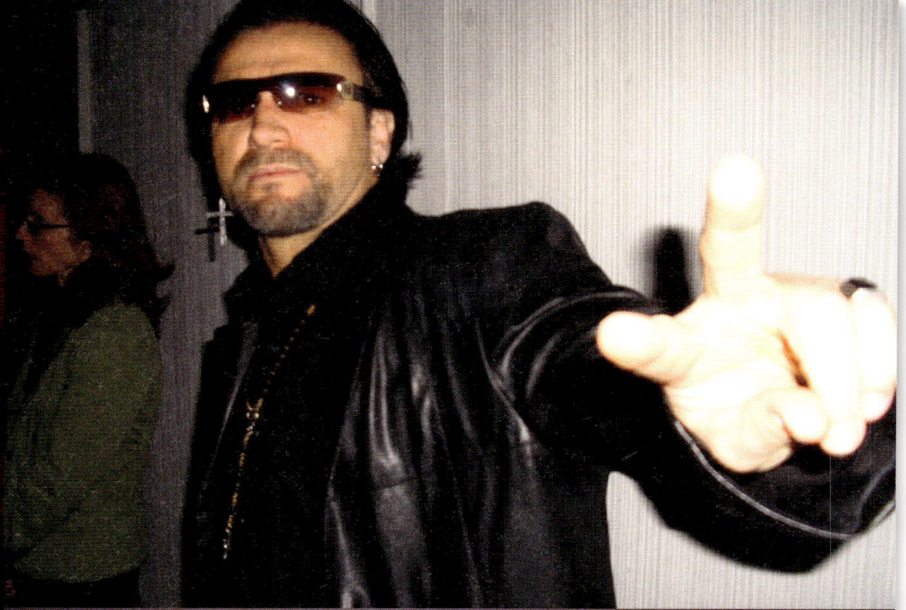

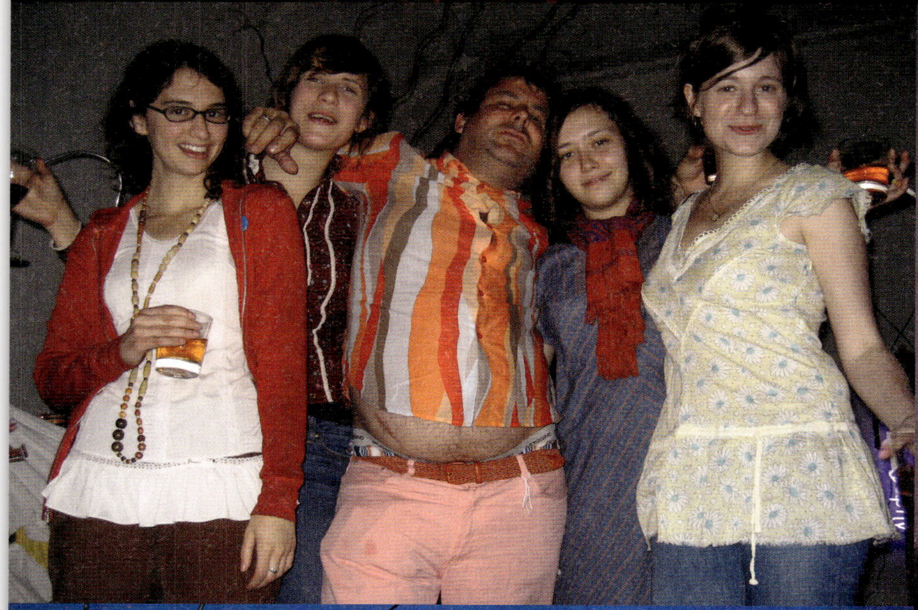

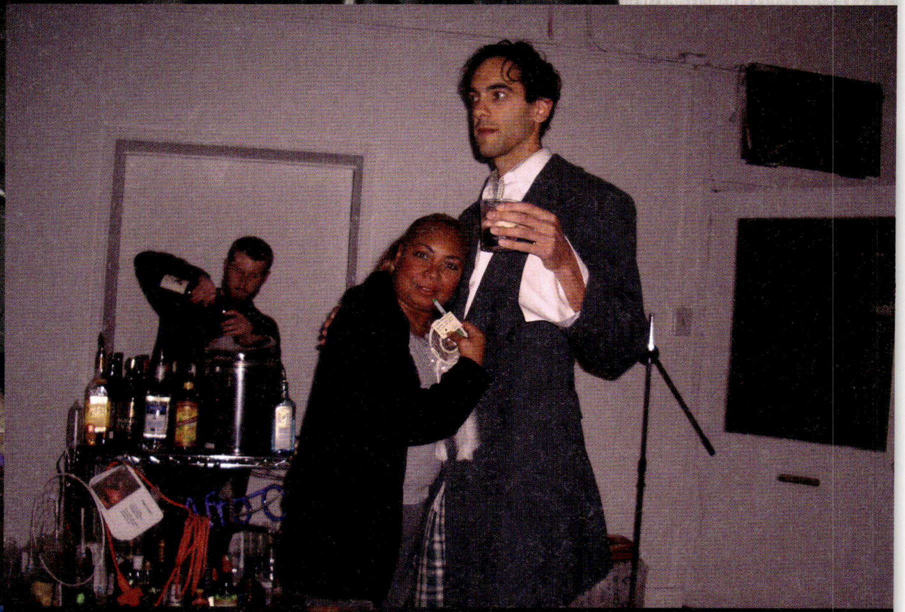

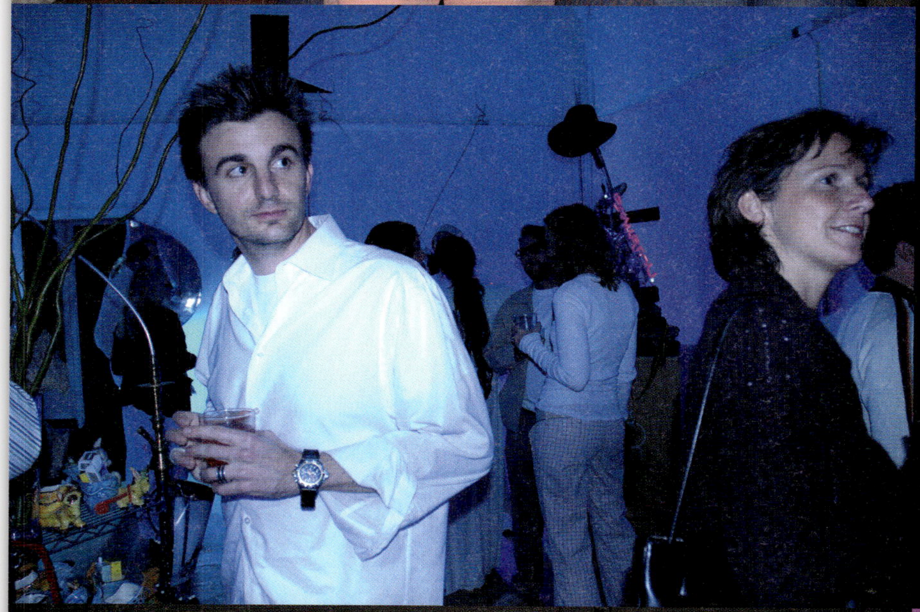

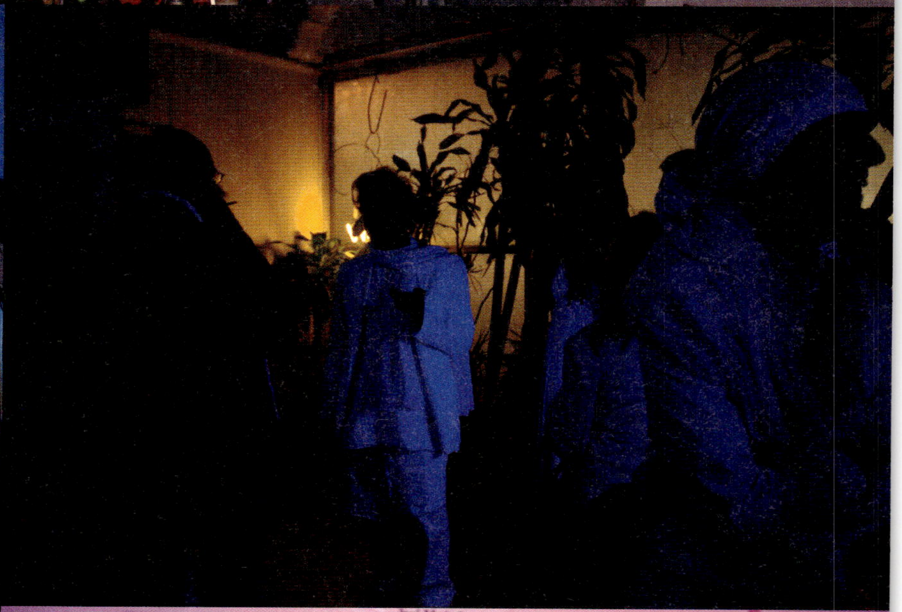

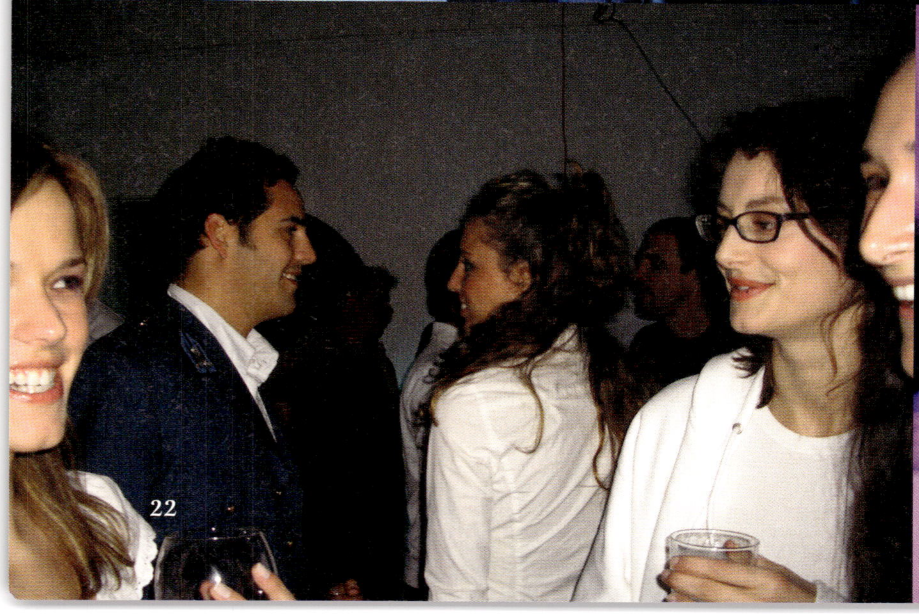

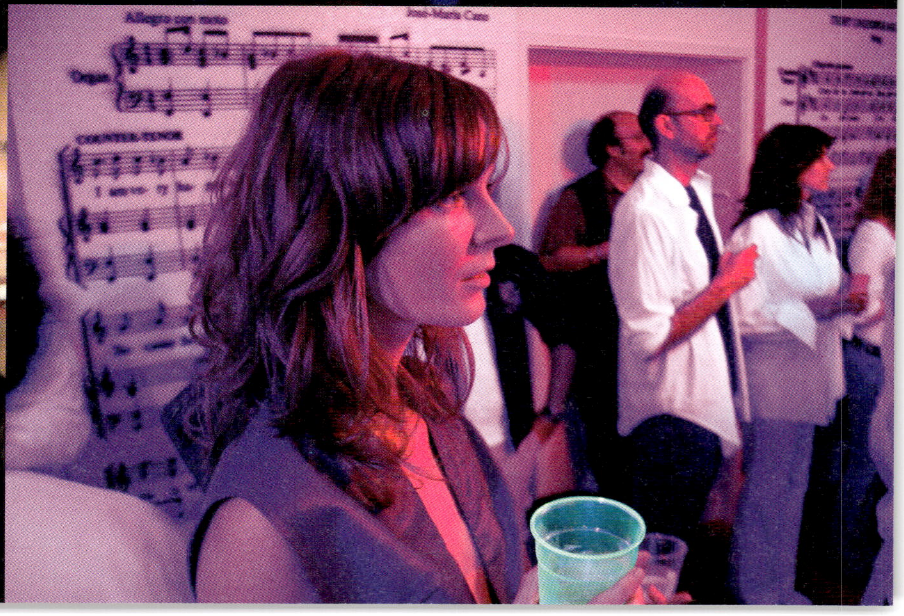
Allegro con moto
Organ
COUNTER-TENOR

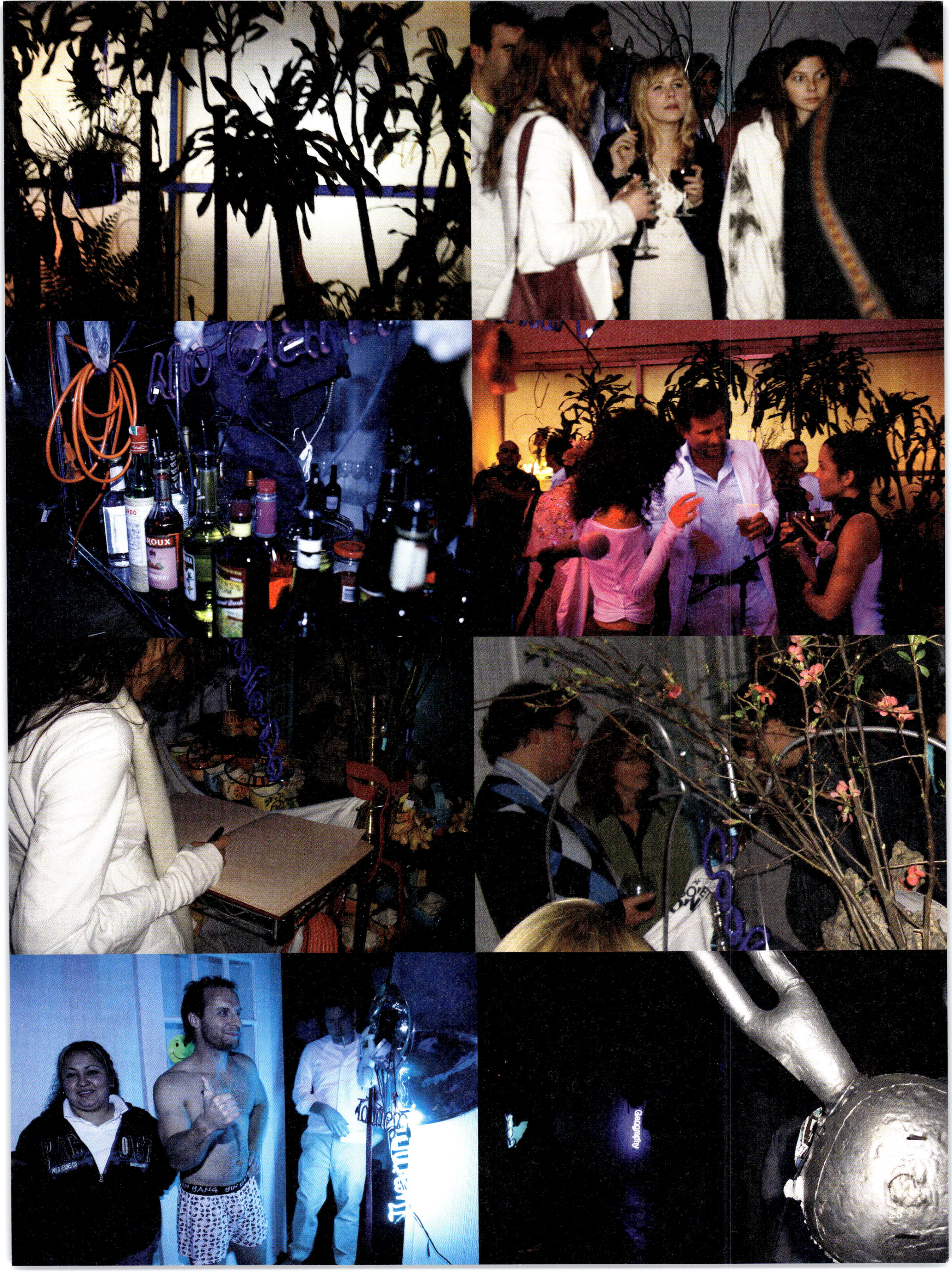
Geography

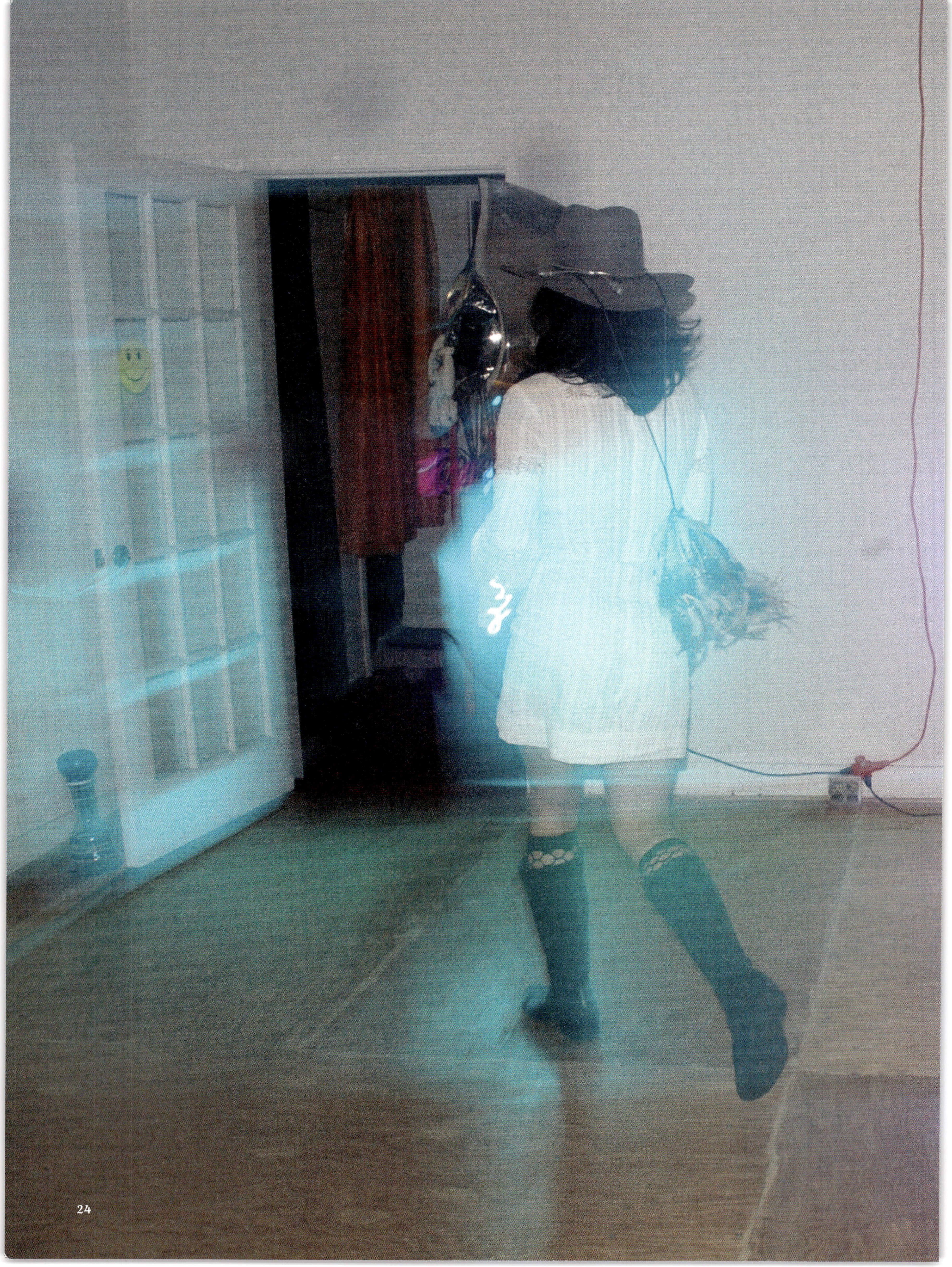

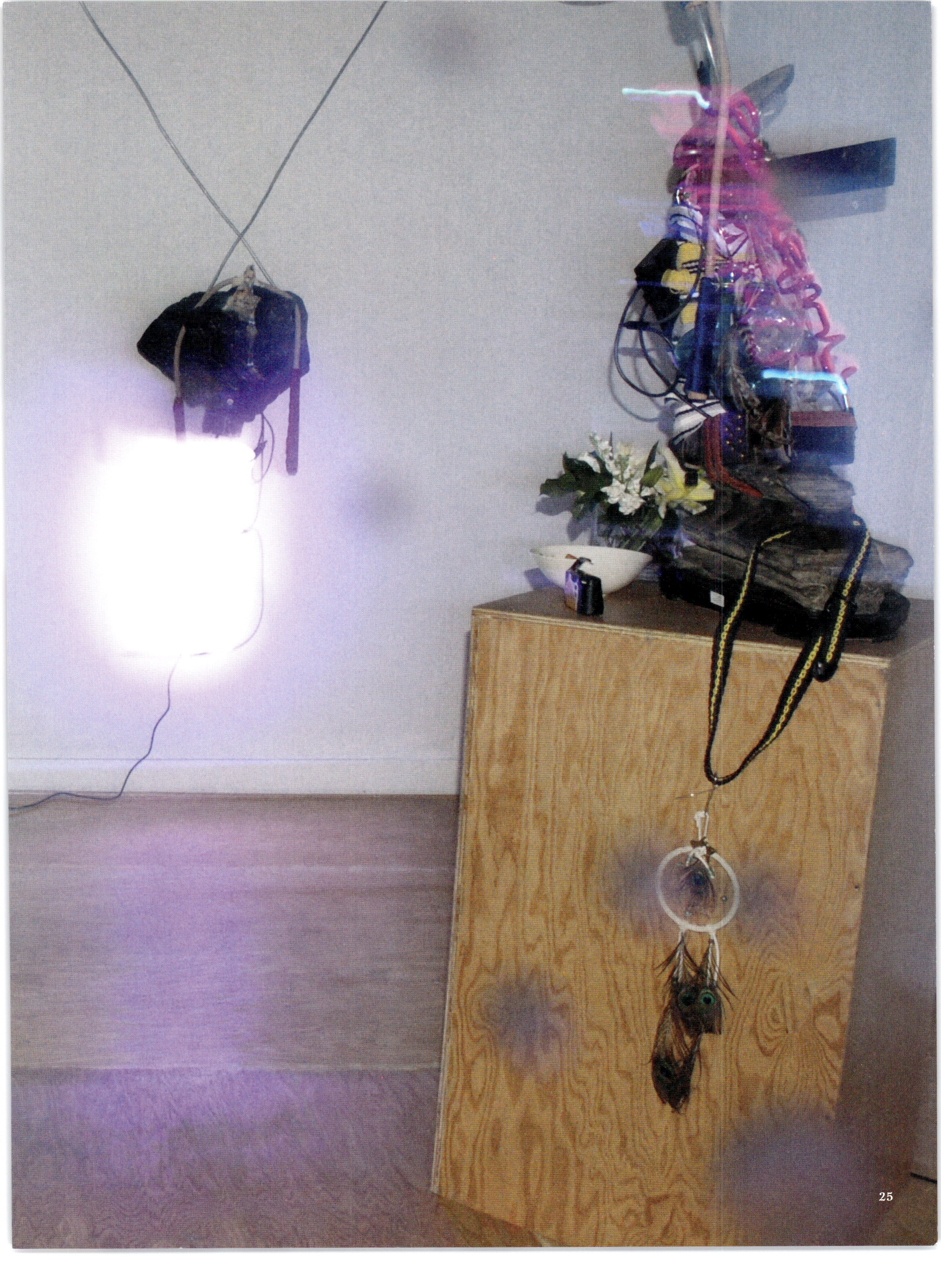

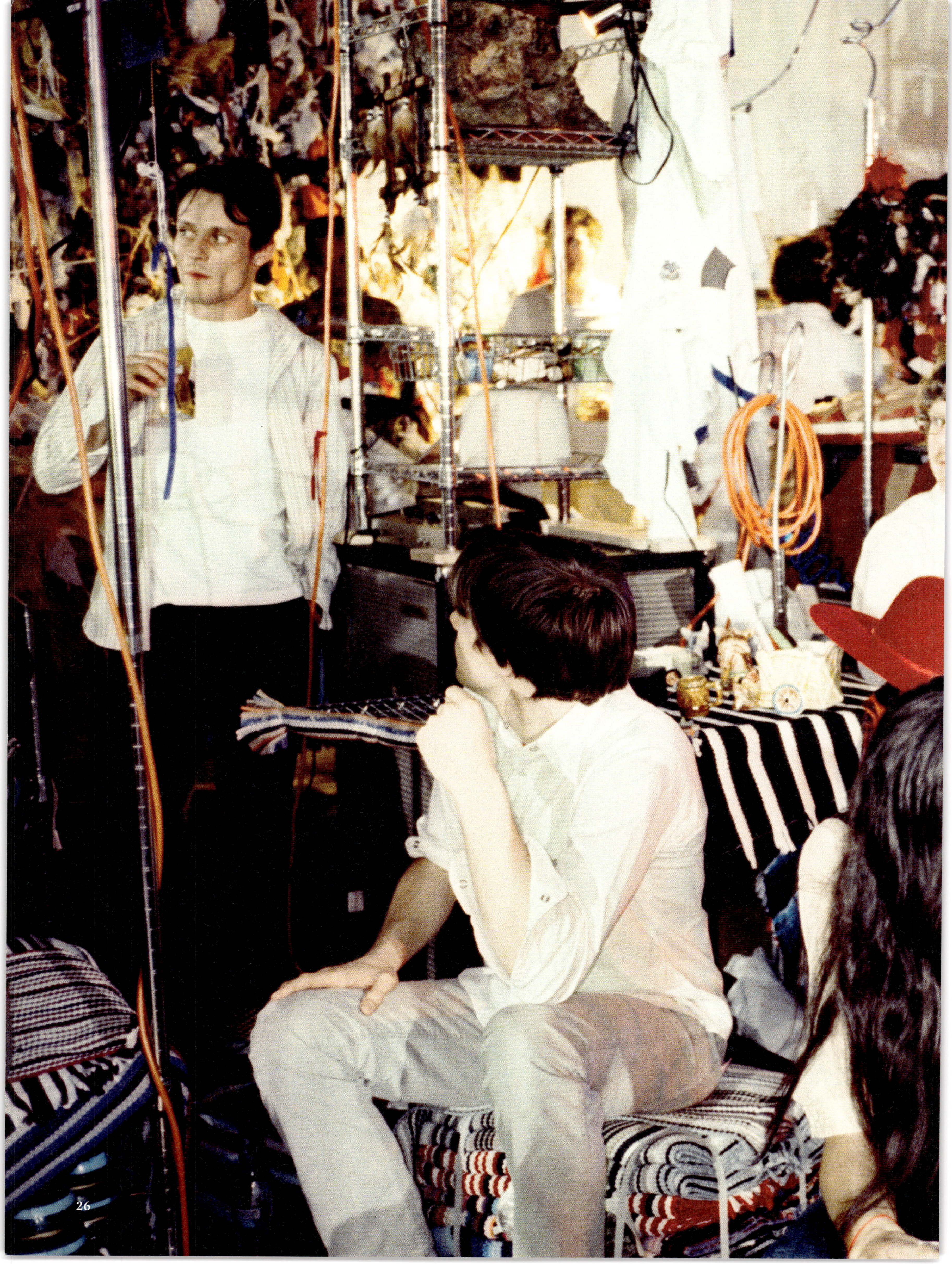

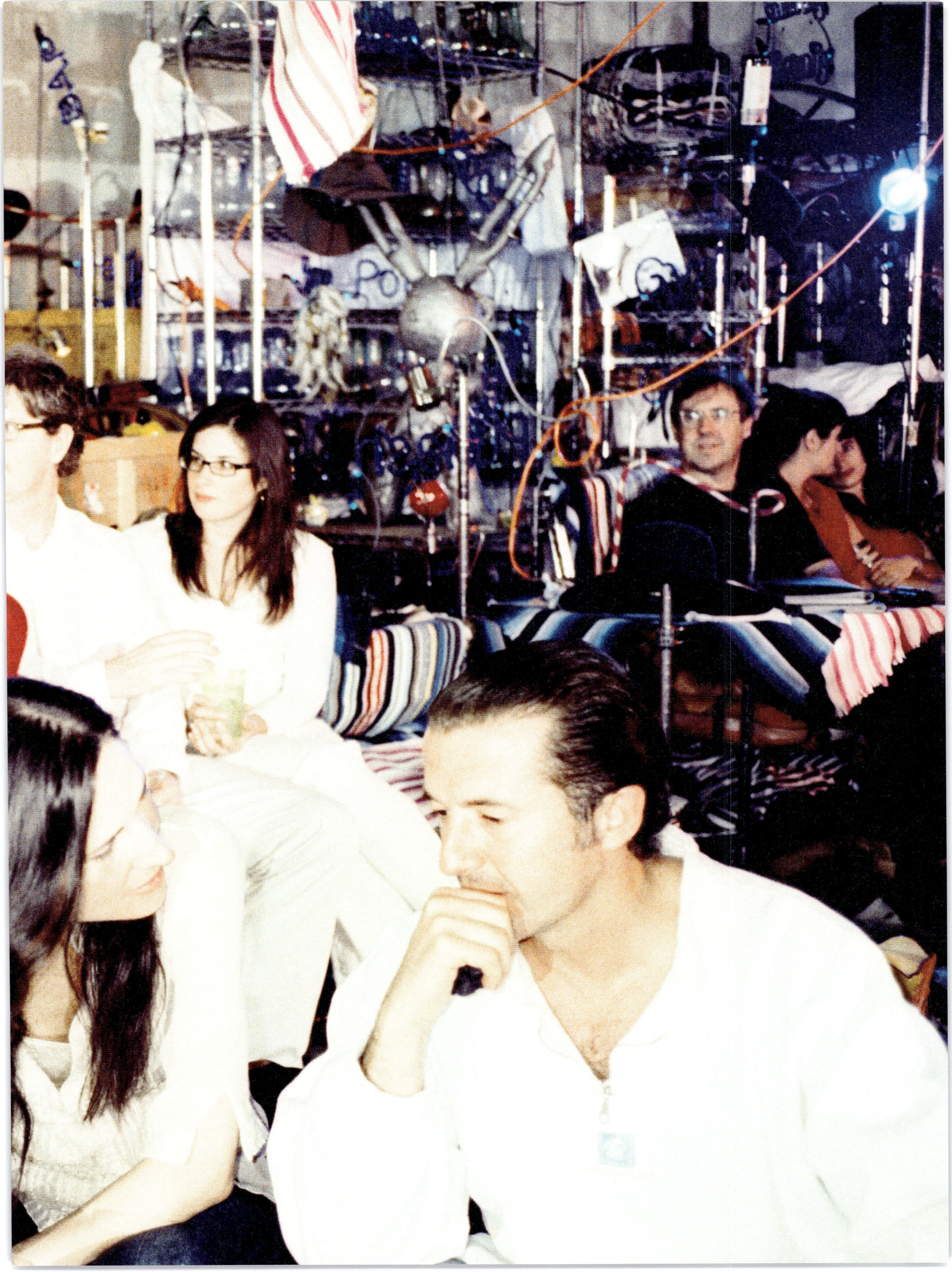

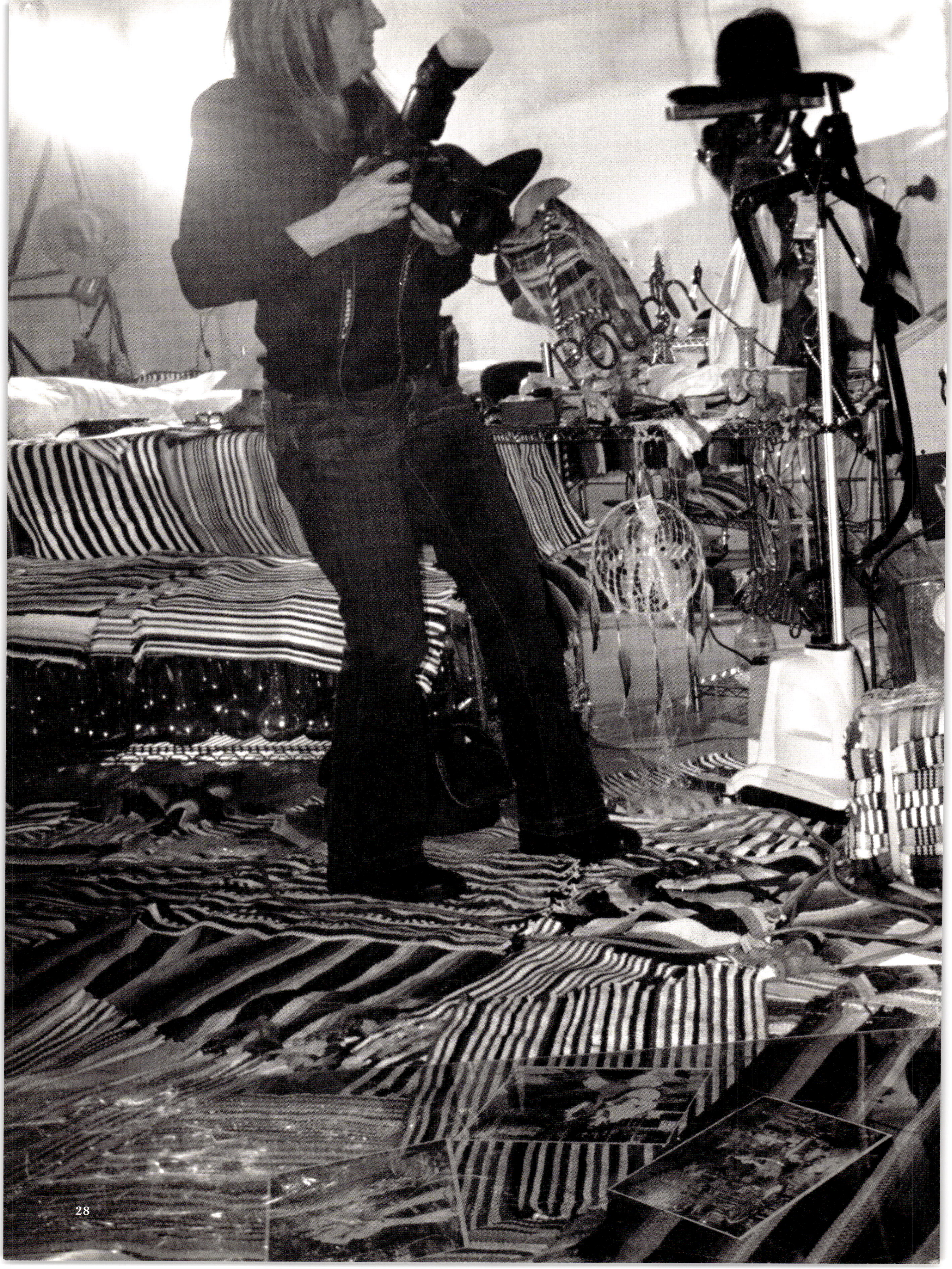

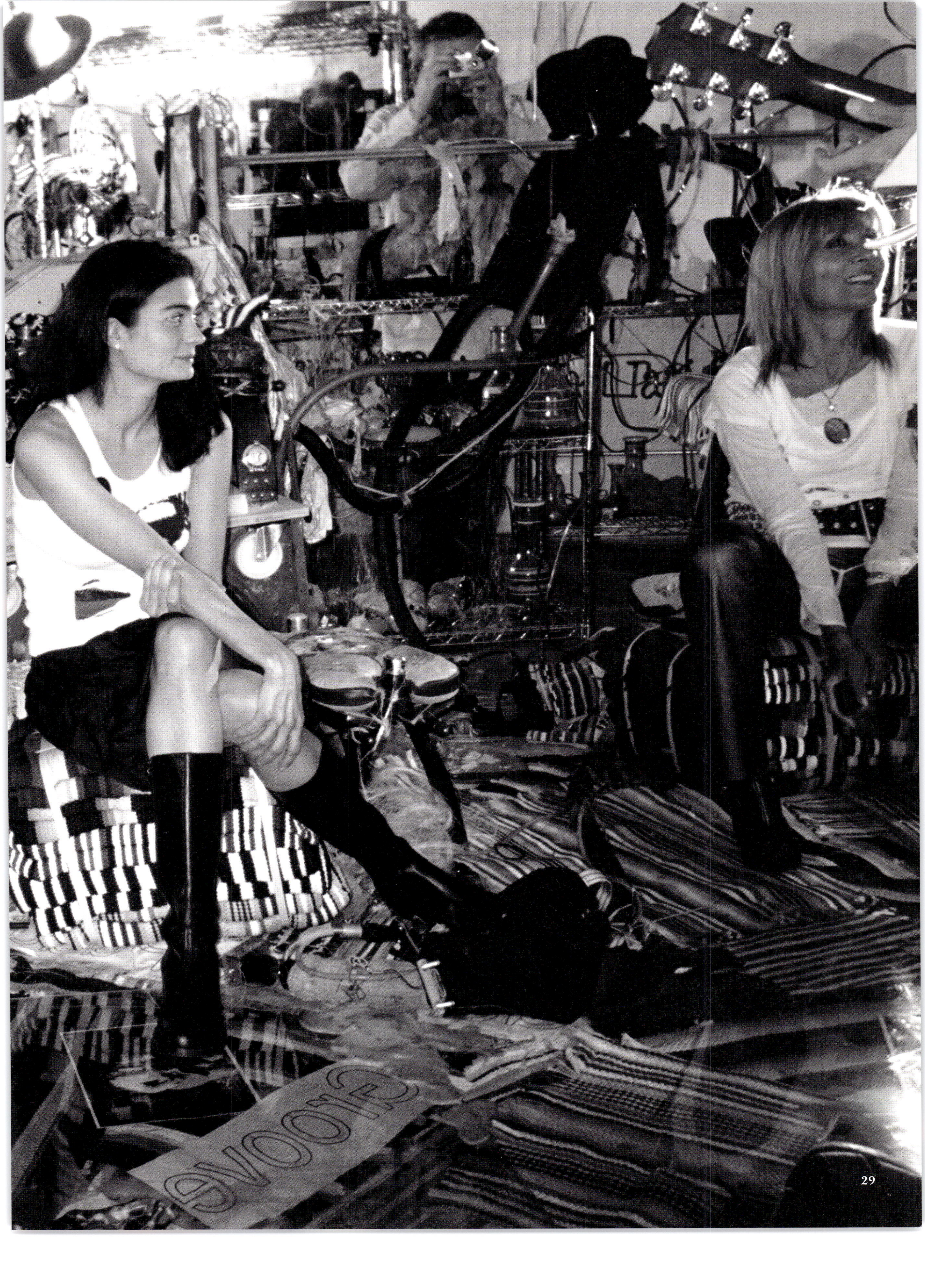

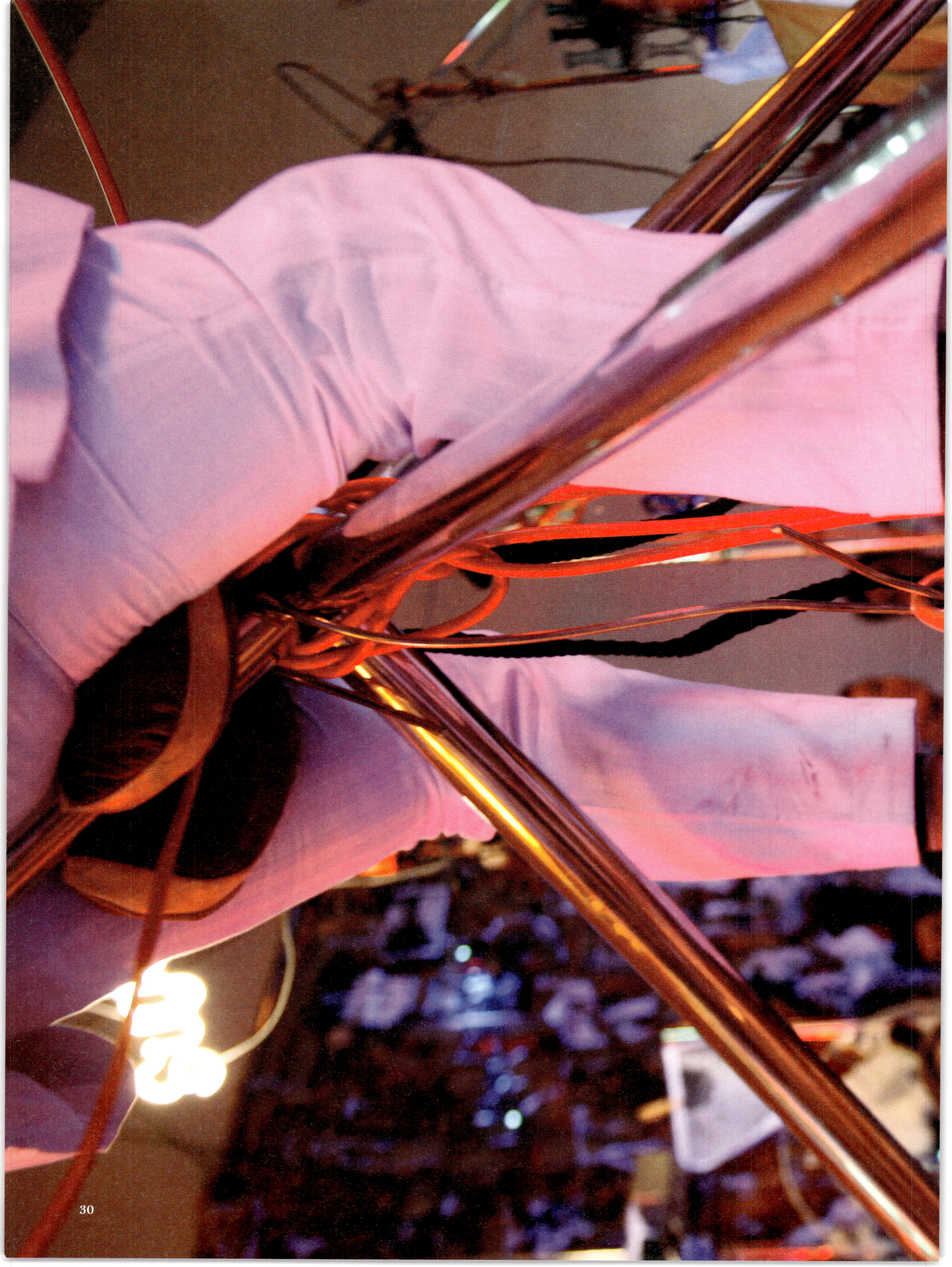

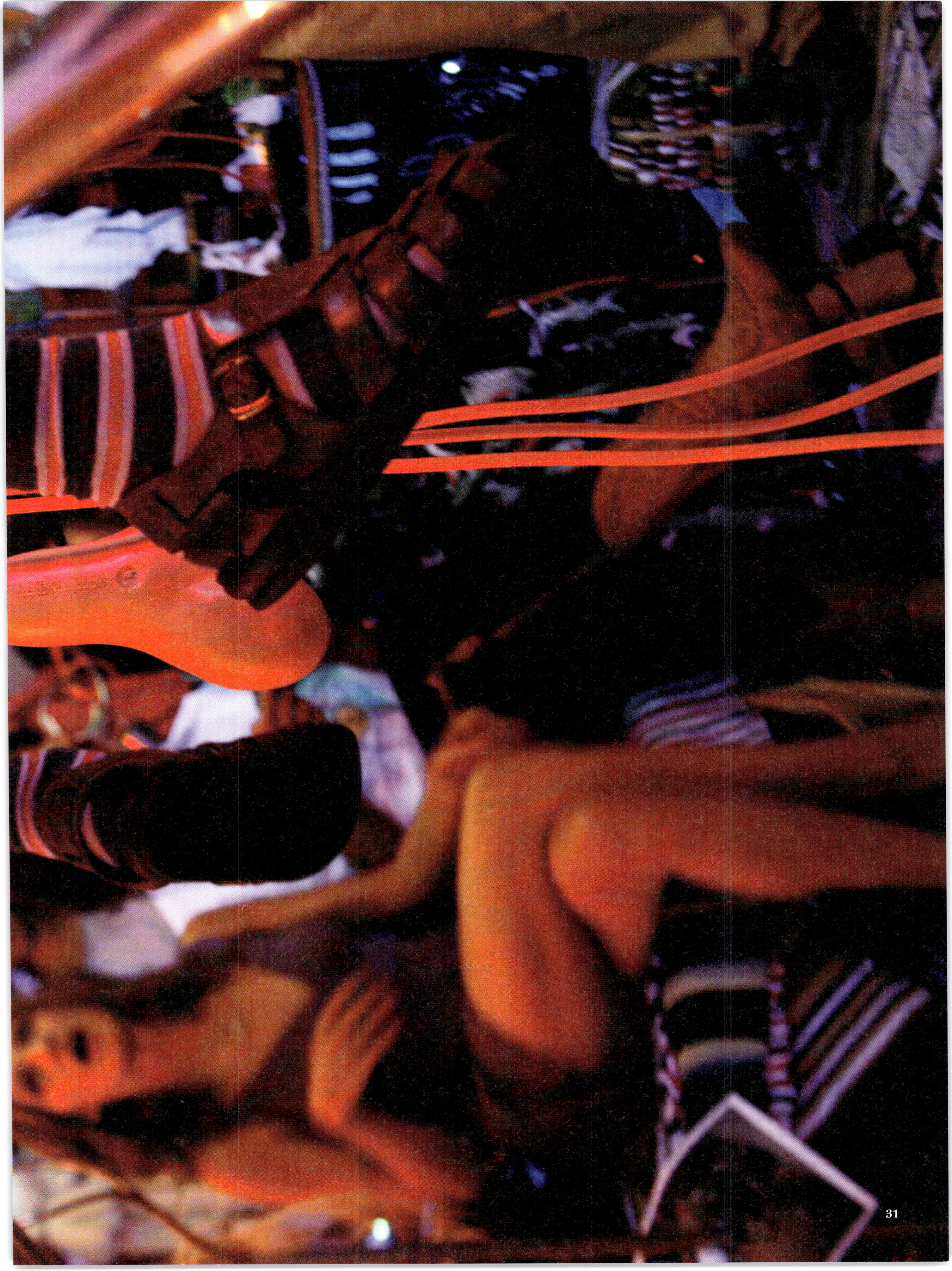

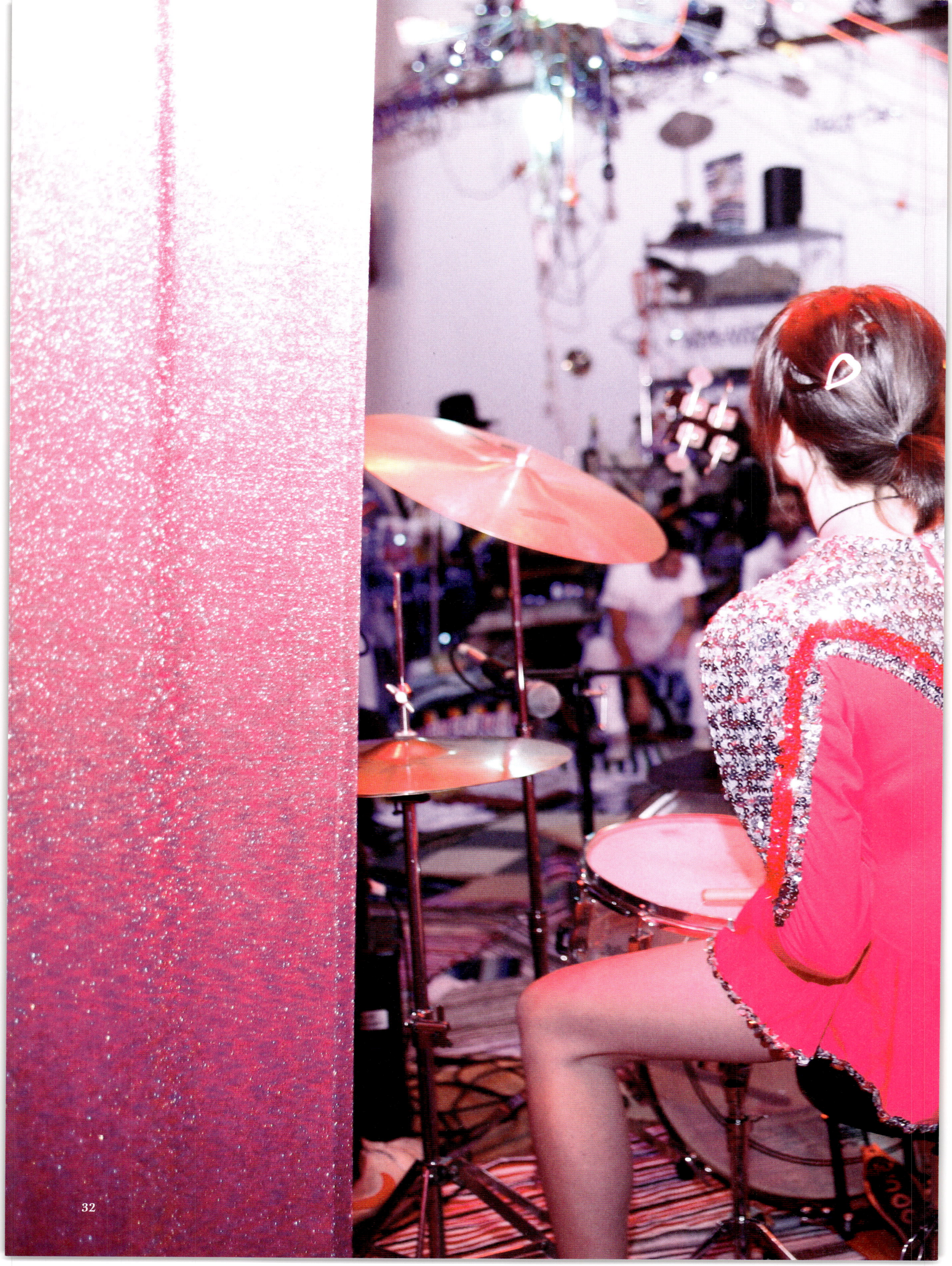

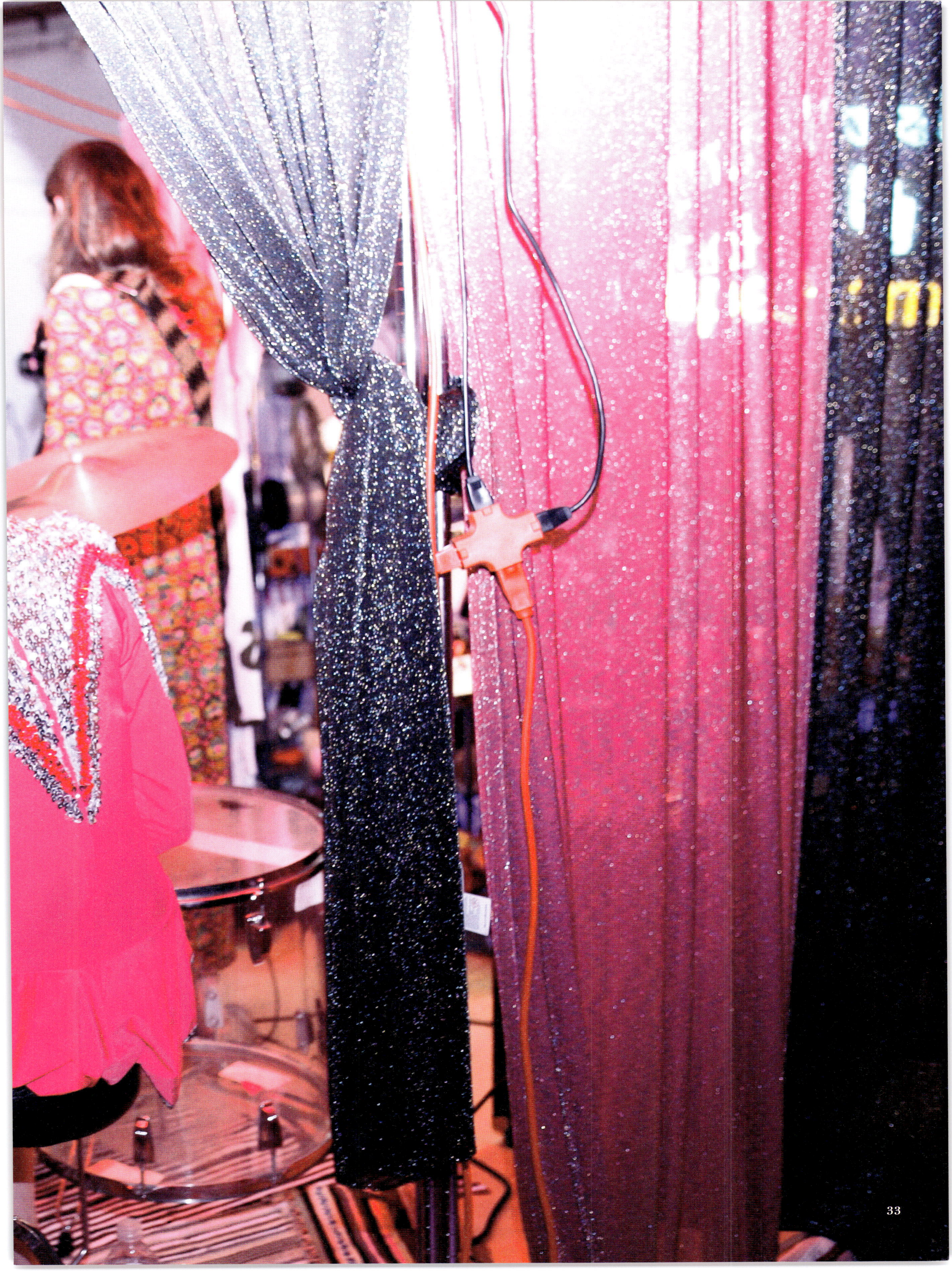

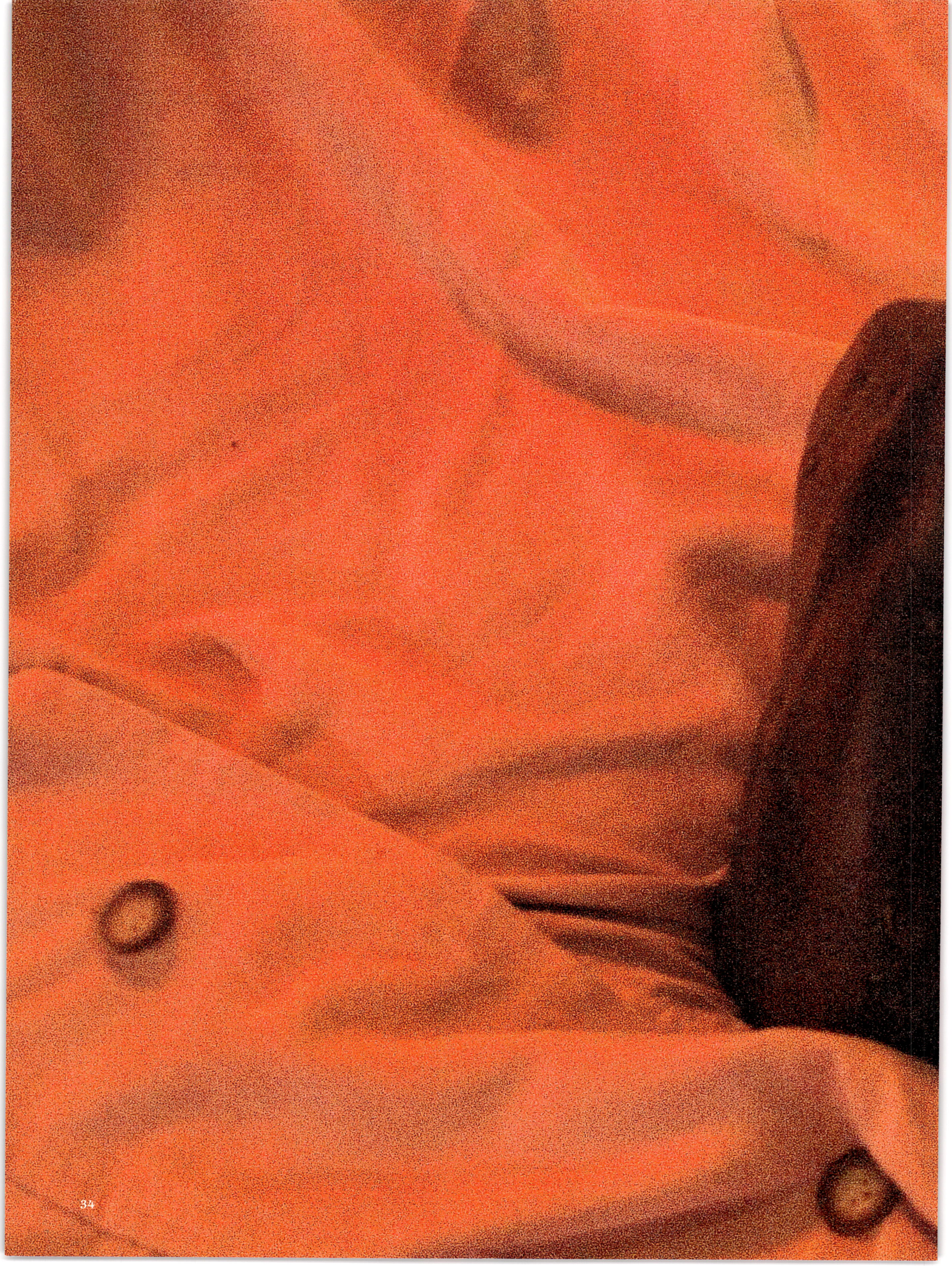

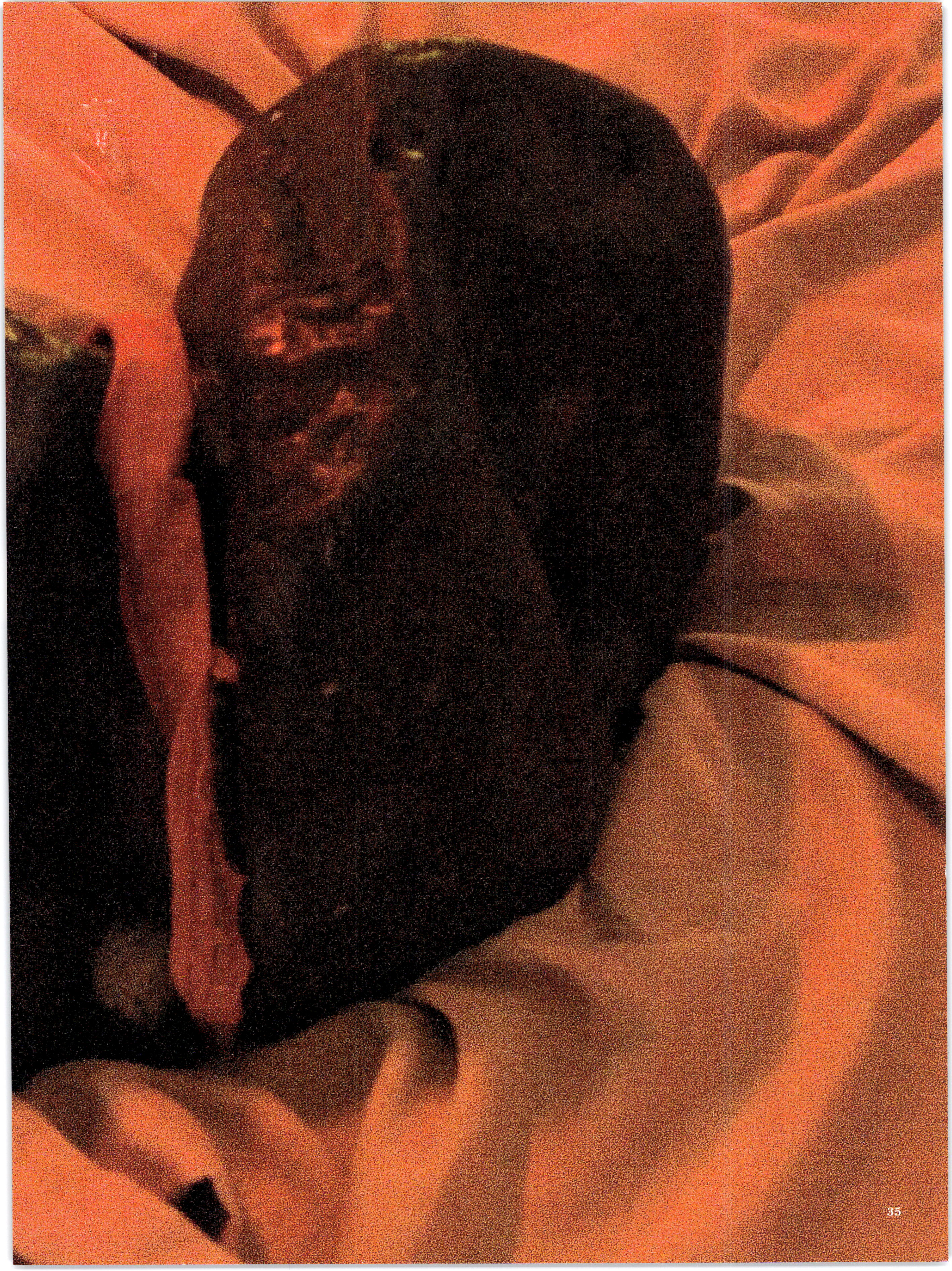

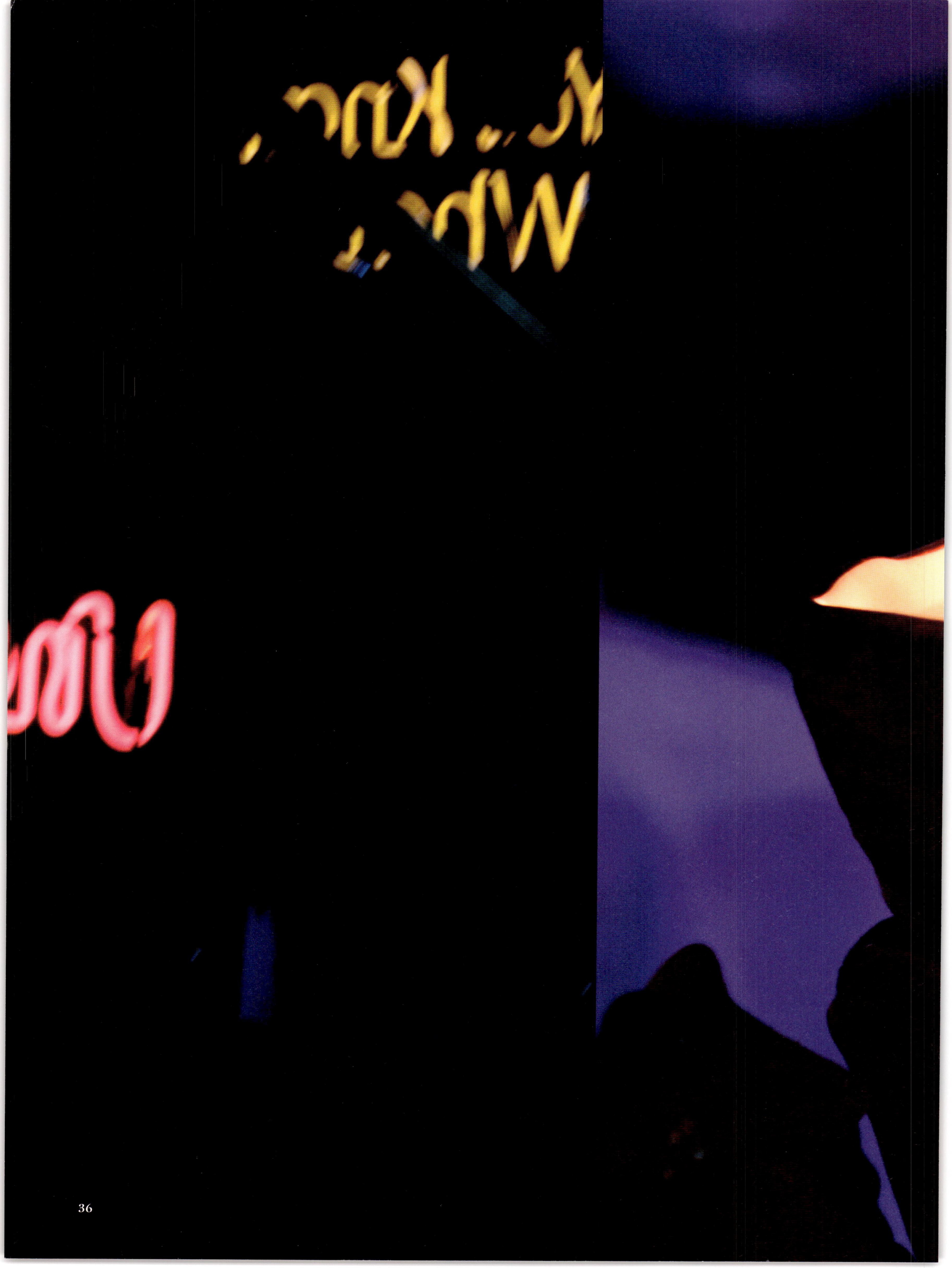

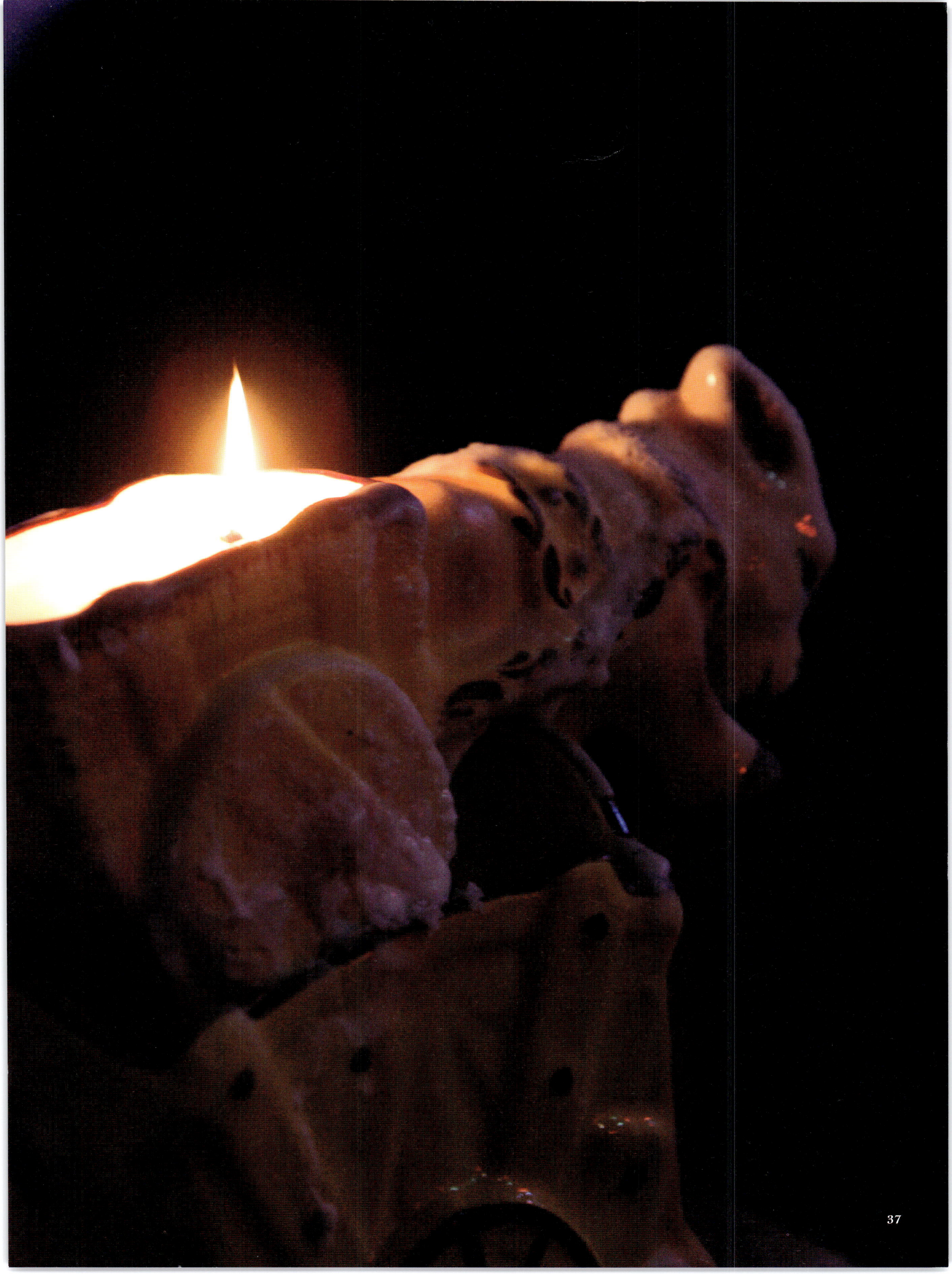

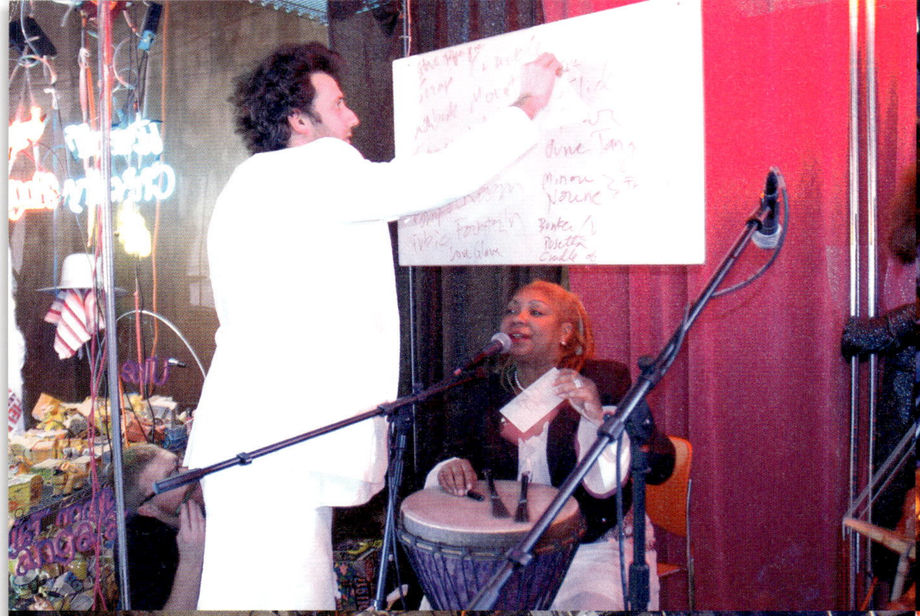

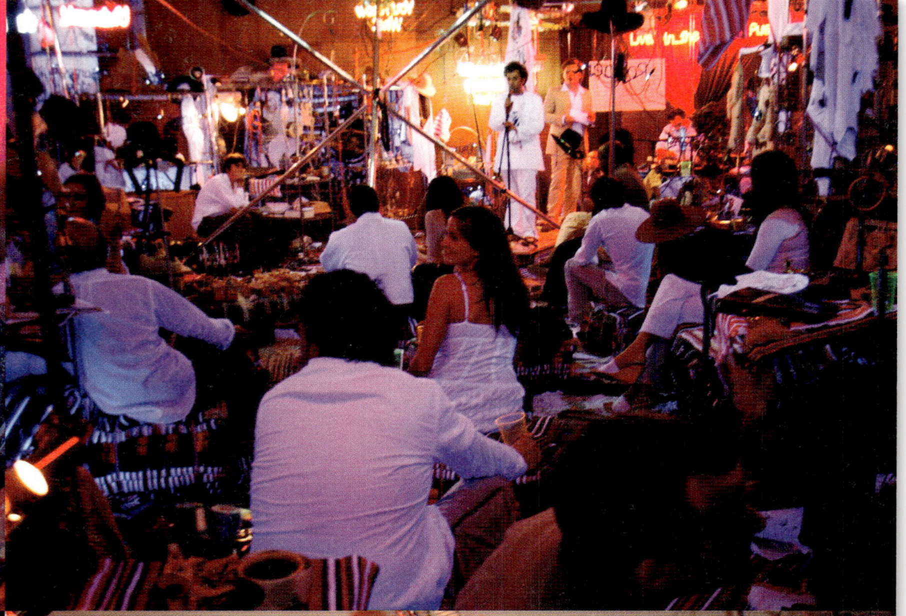

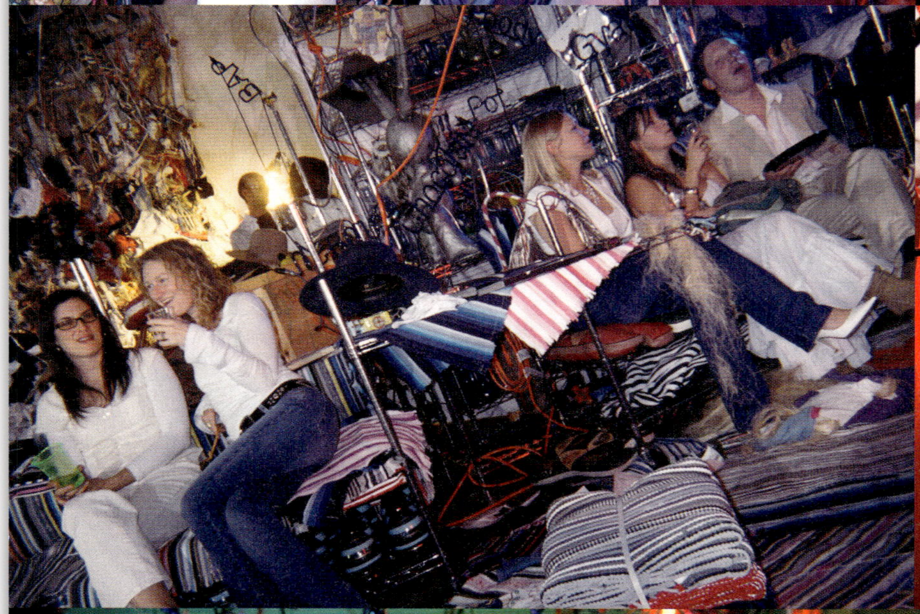

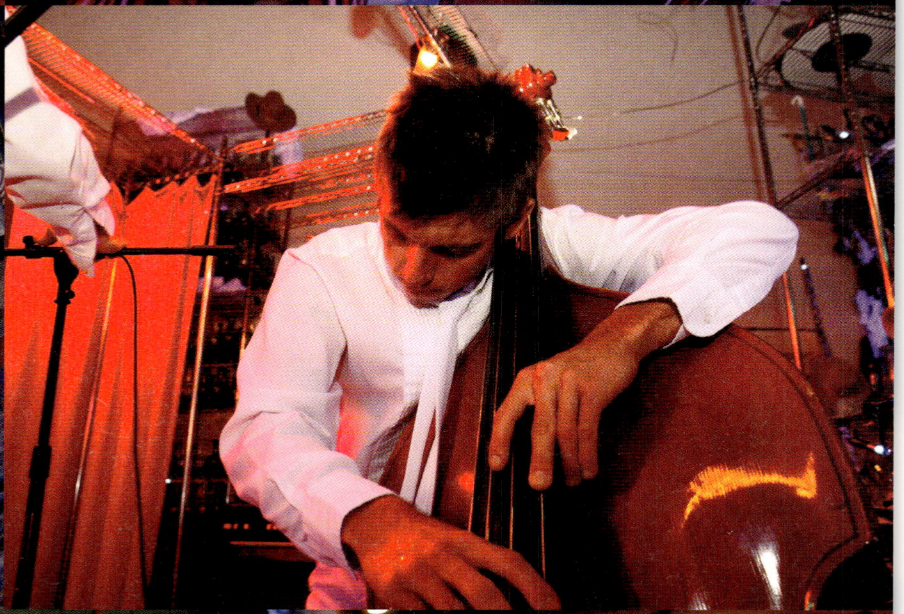

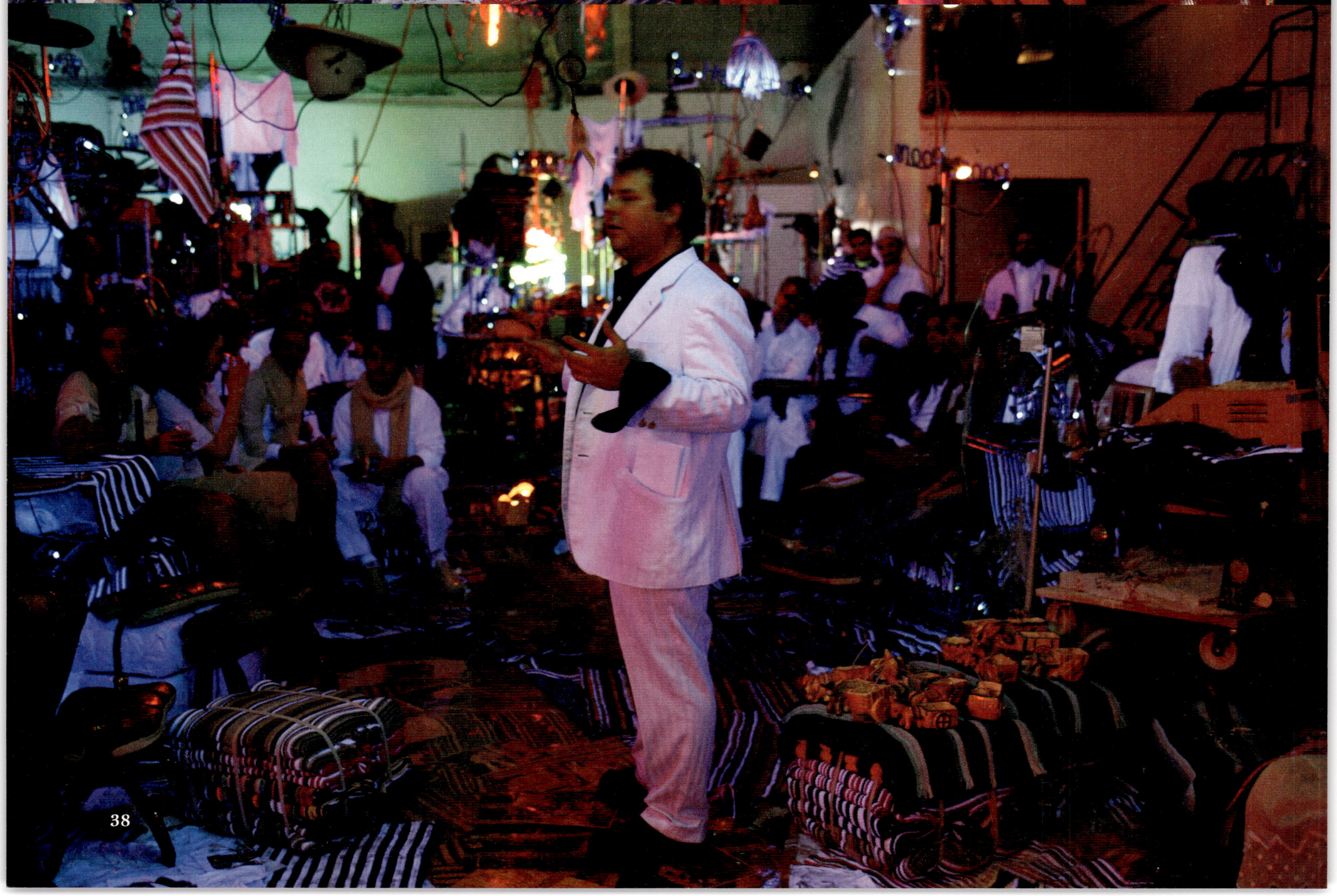

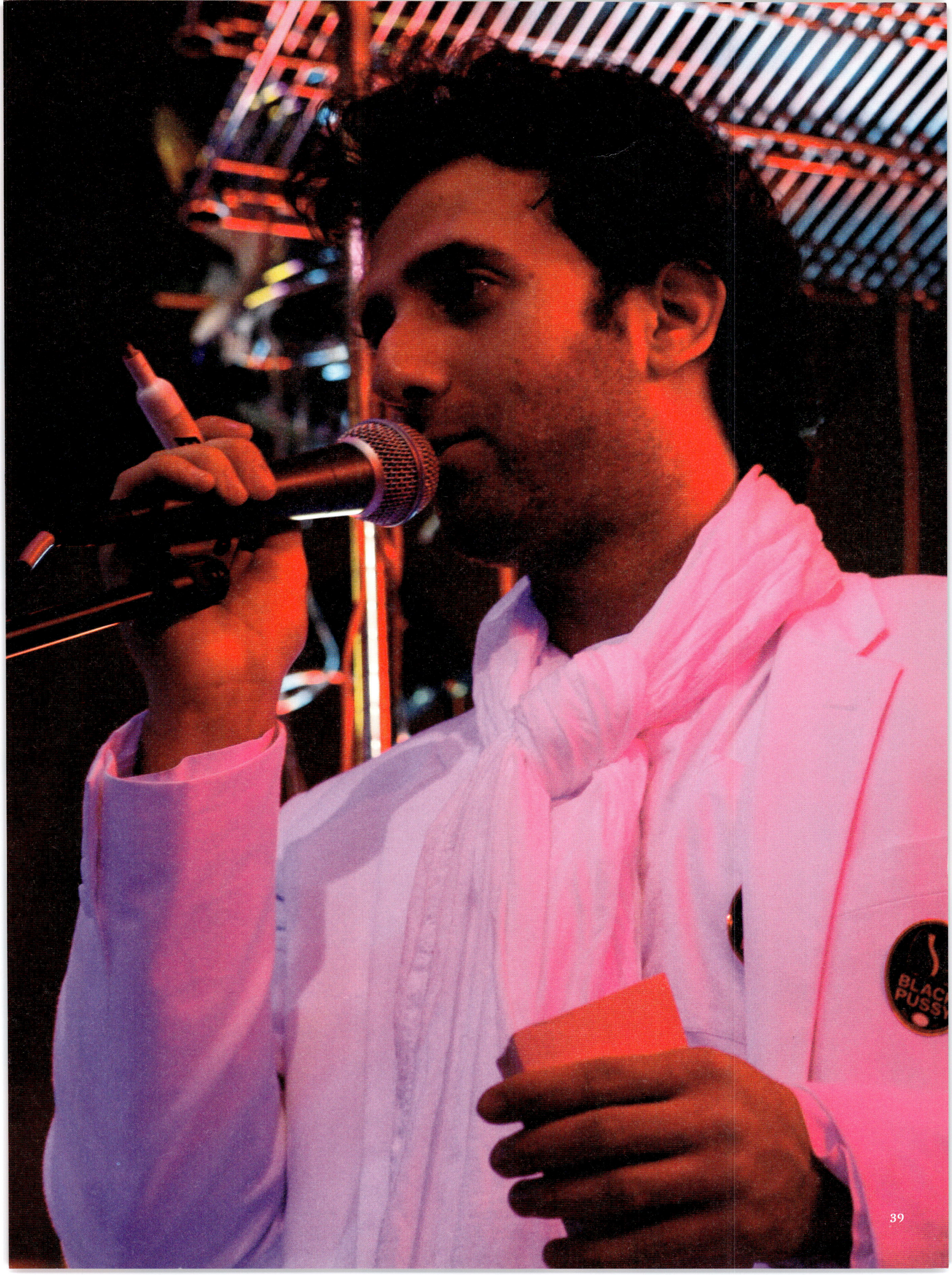
BLAC
PUSS

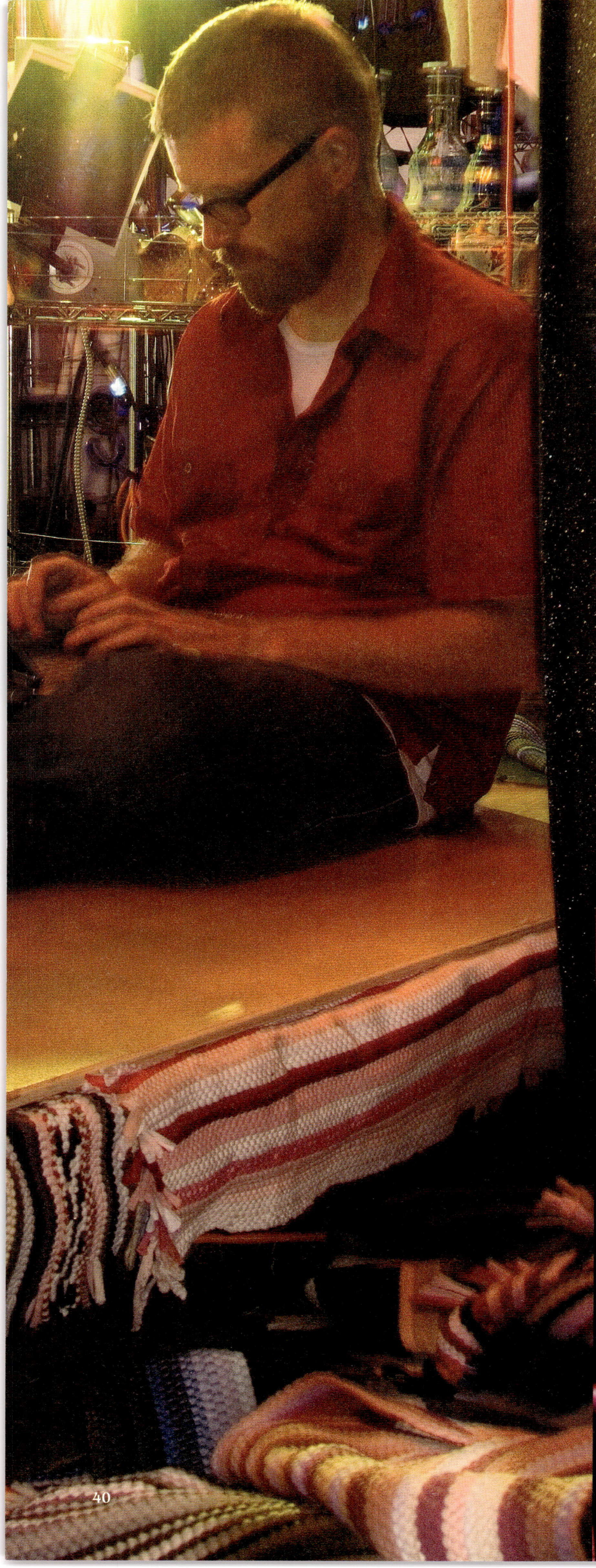
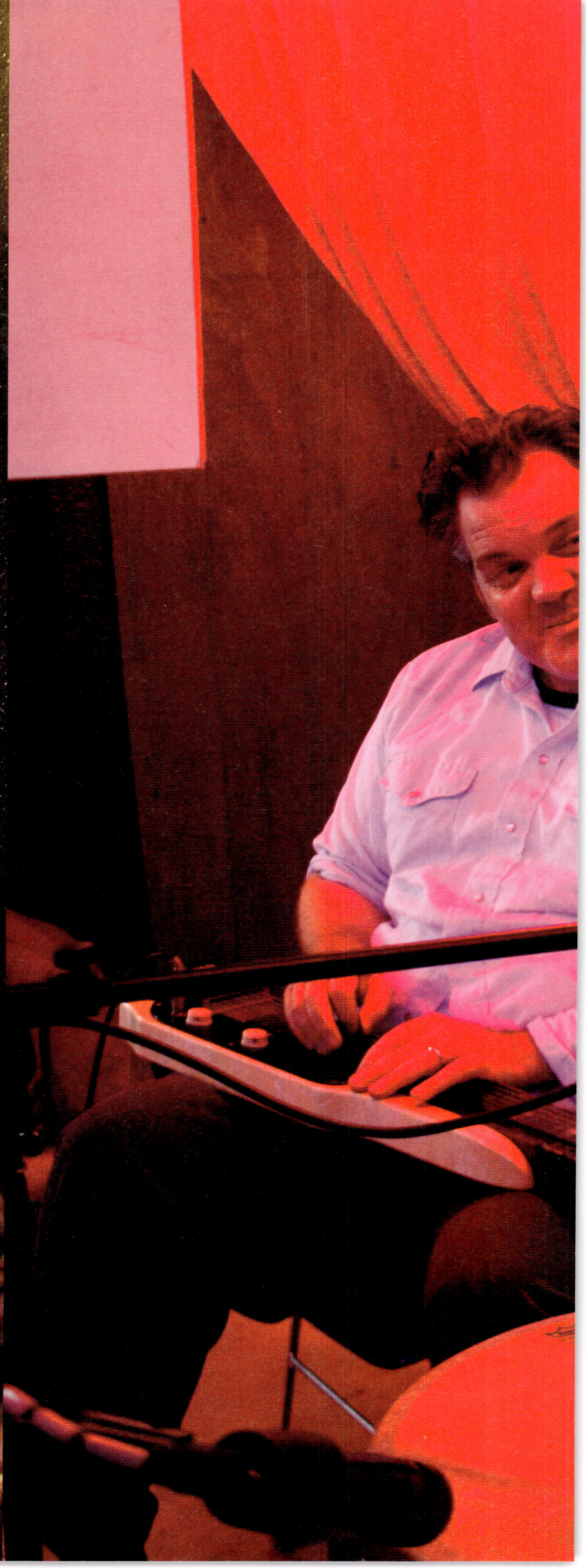

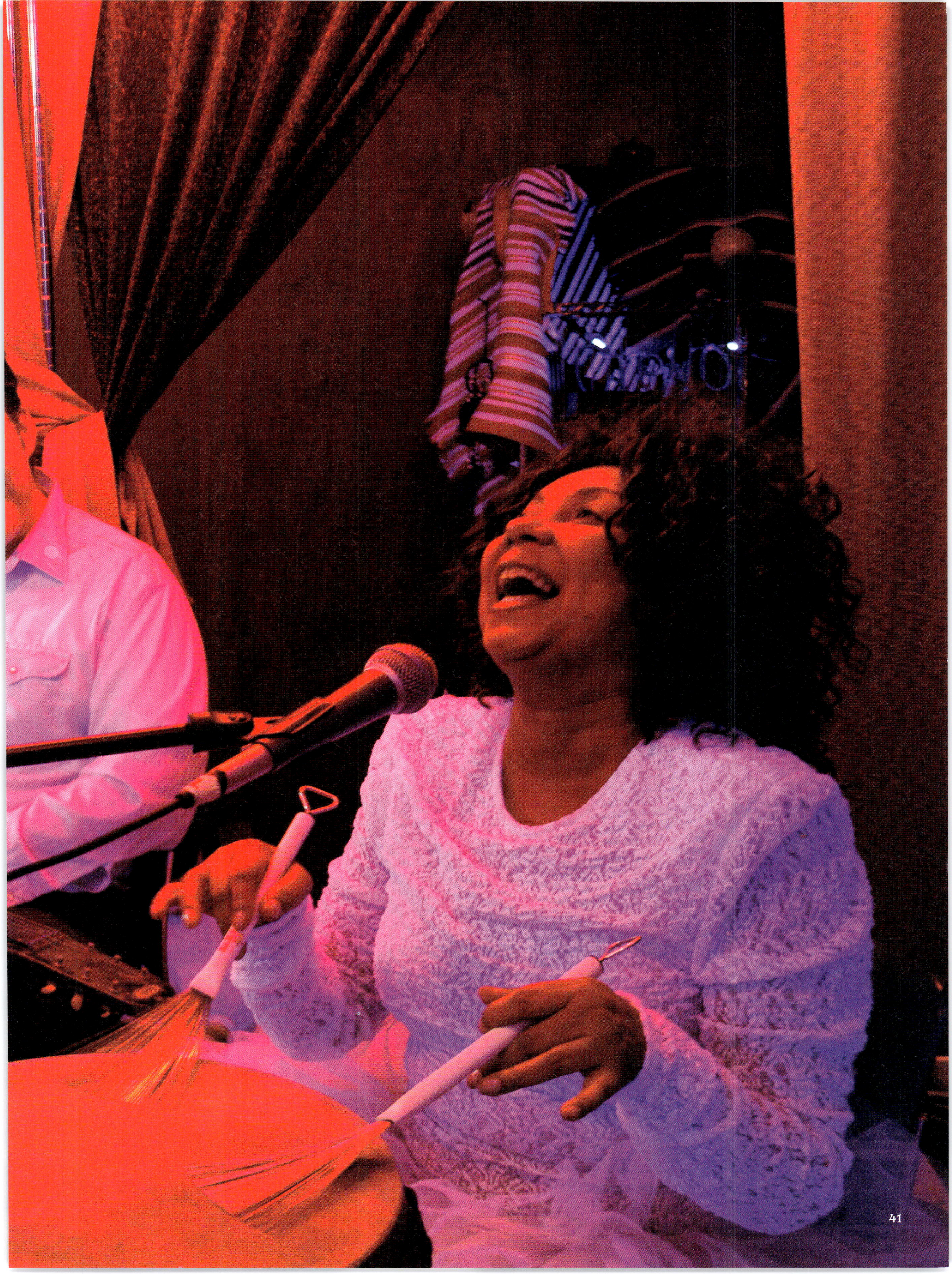

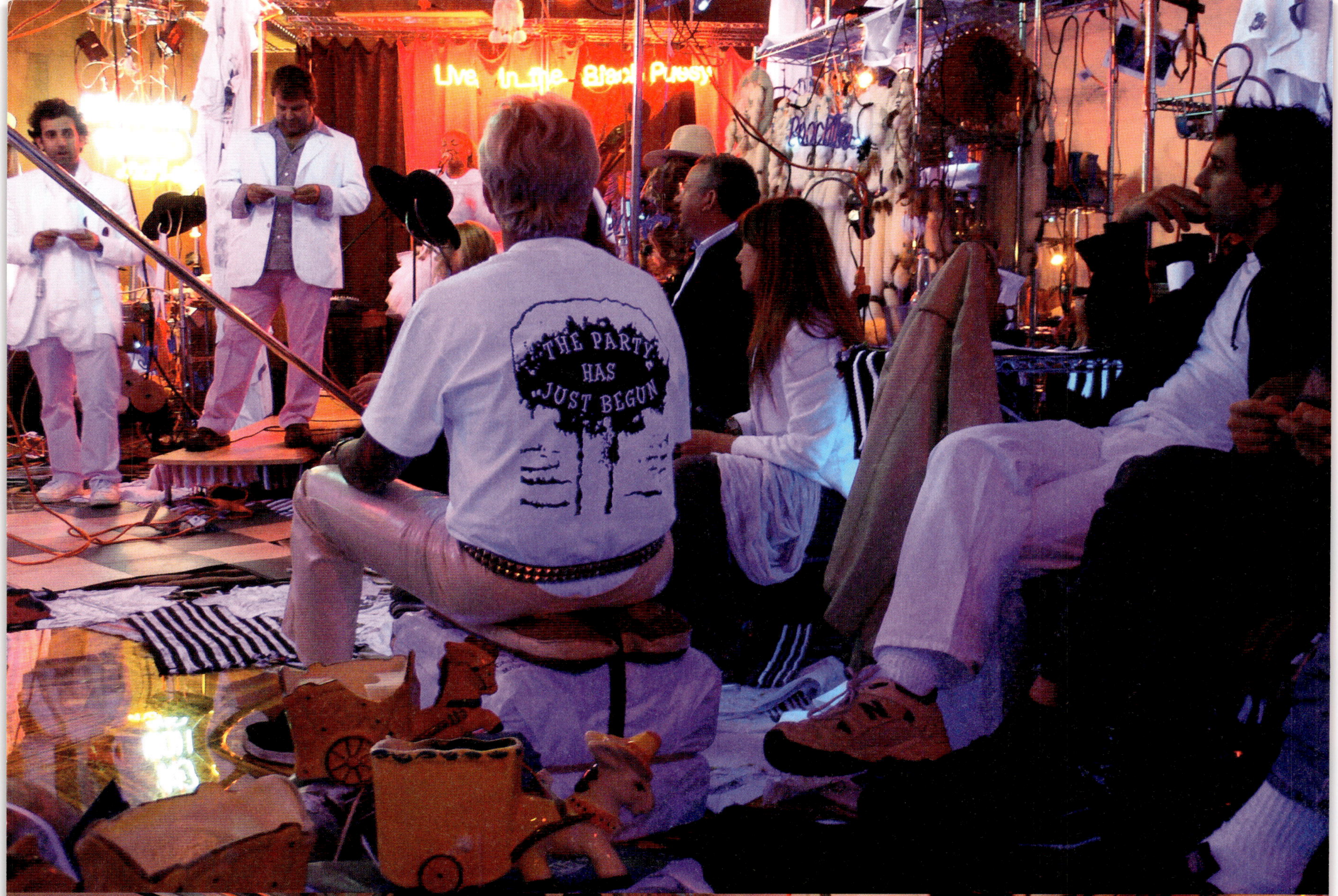
THE PARTY HAS JUST BEGUN

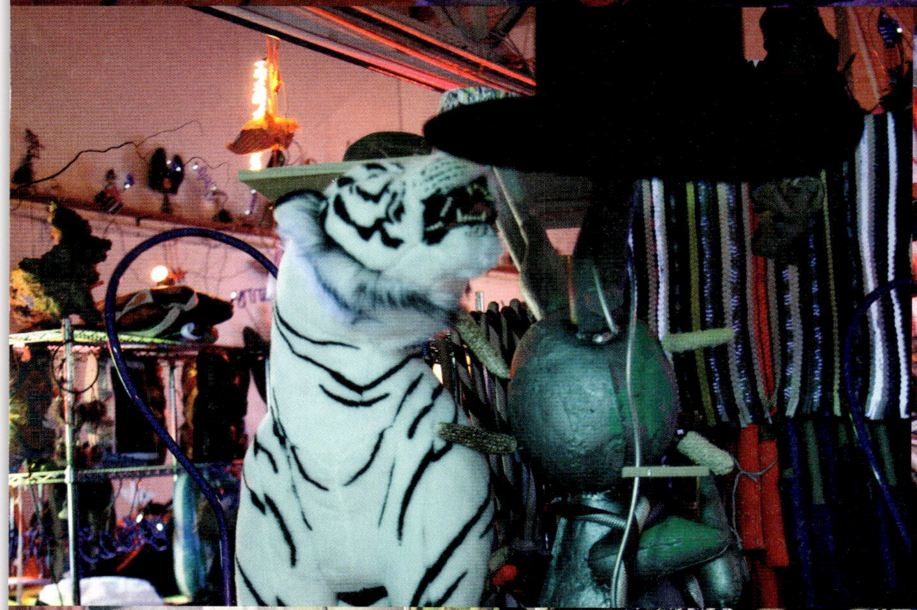

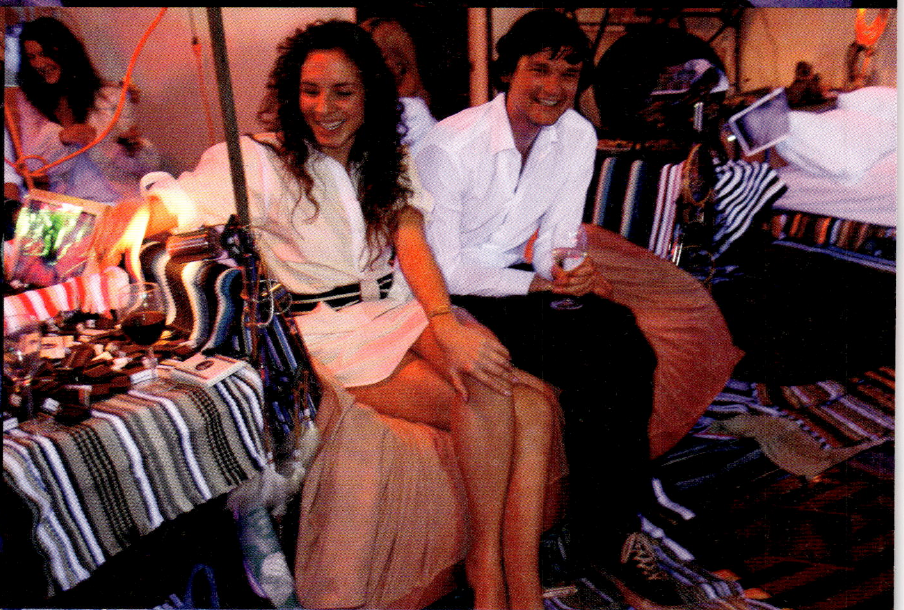

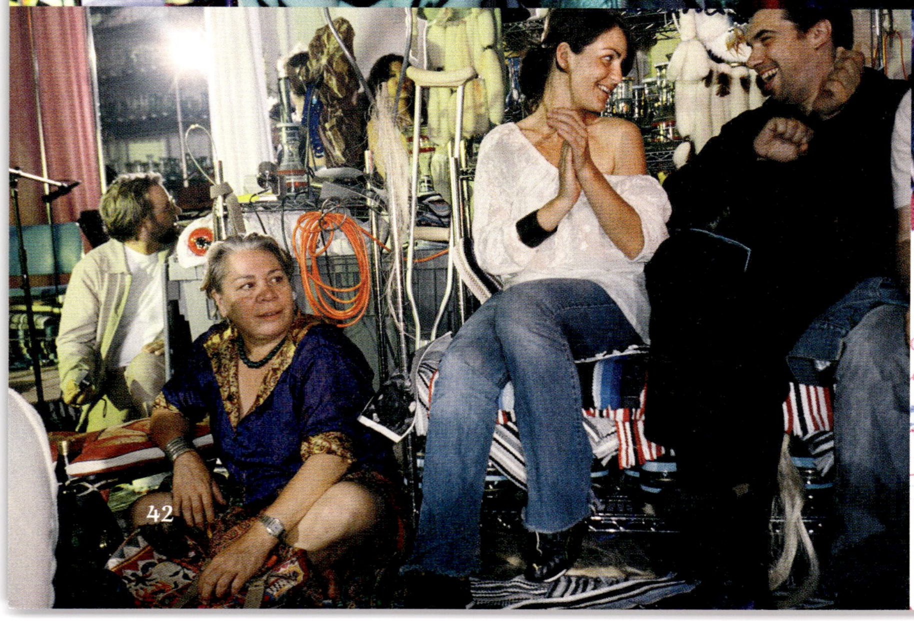

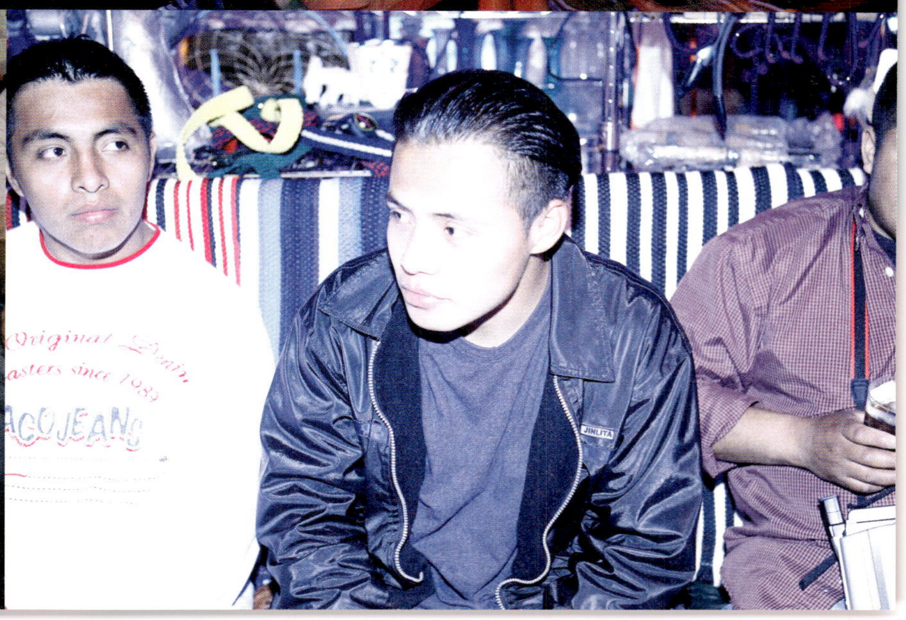

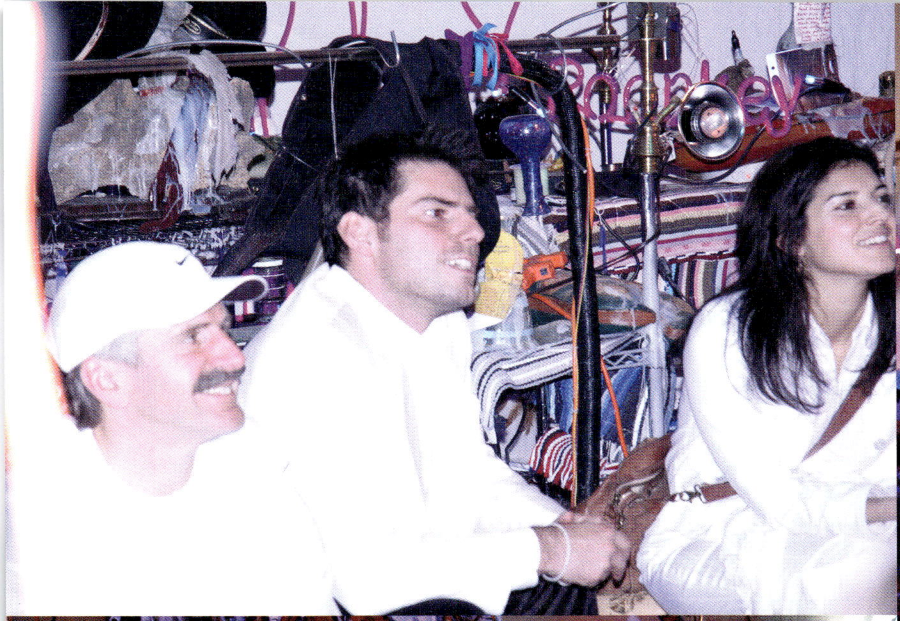
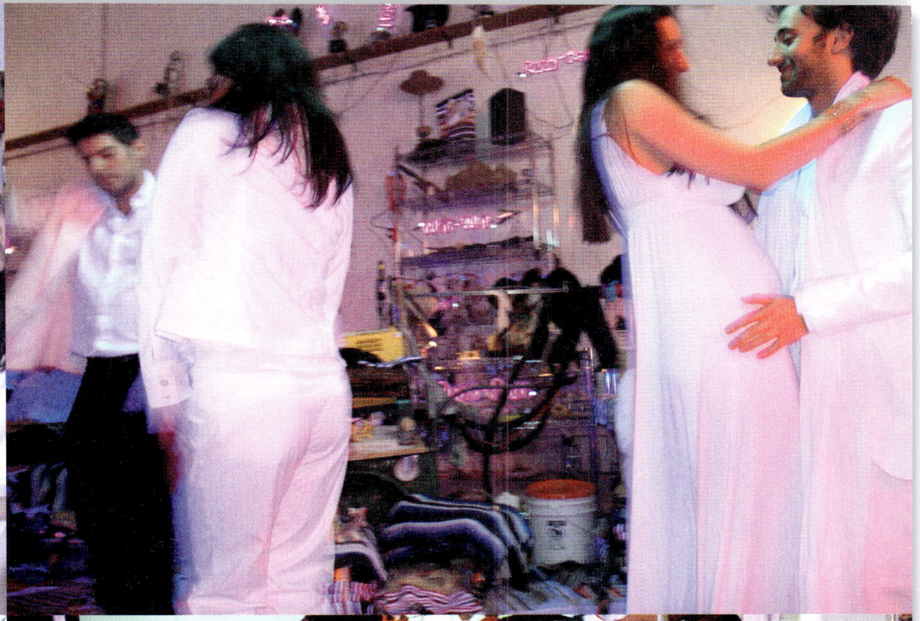
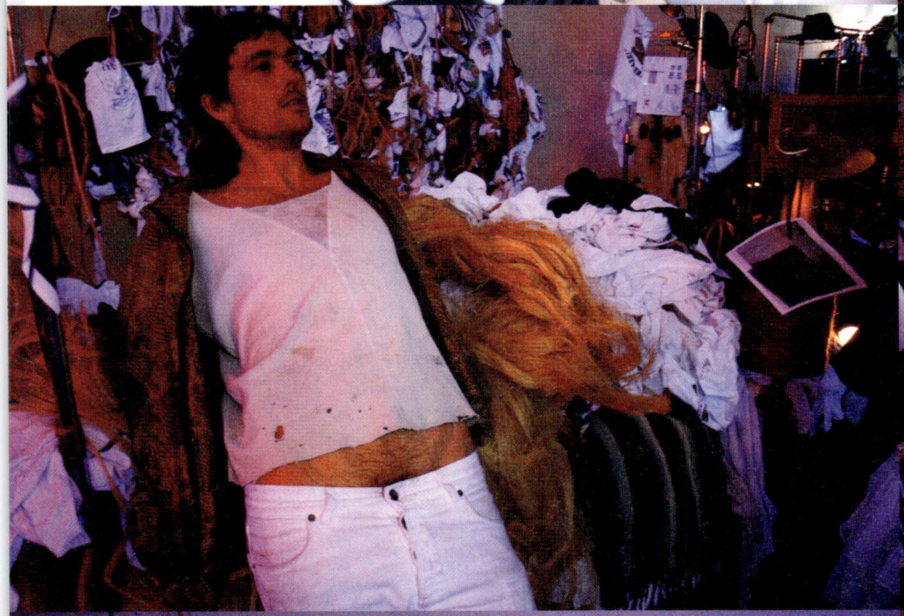
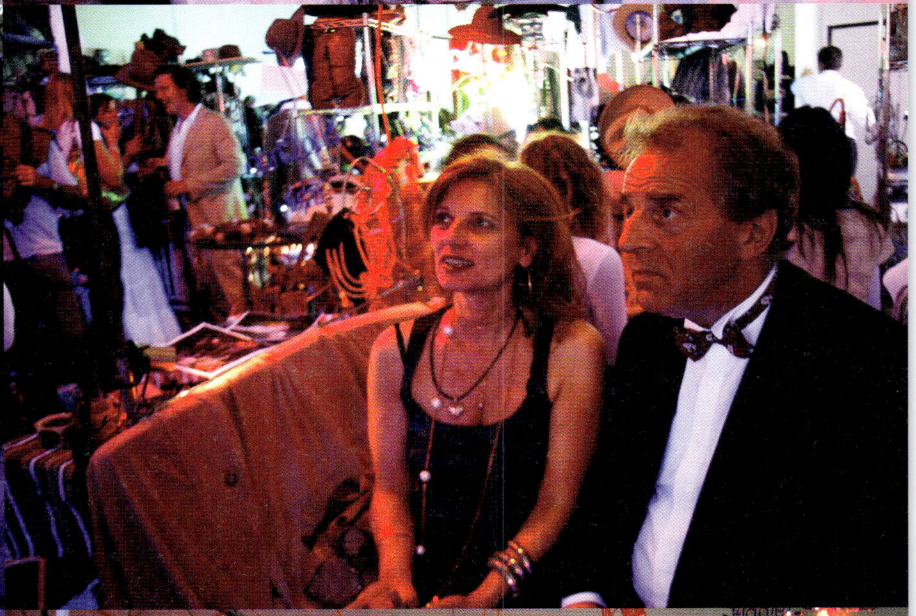
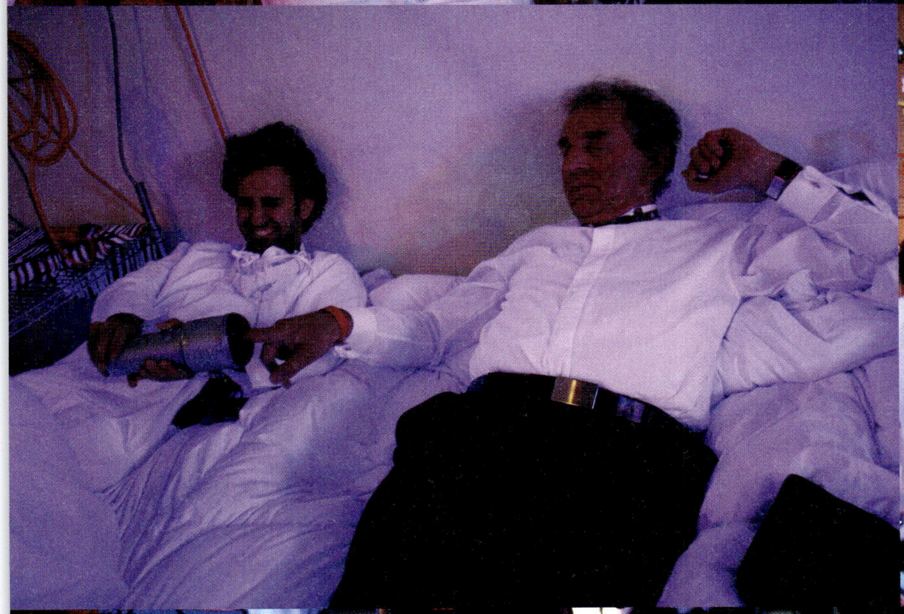
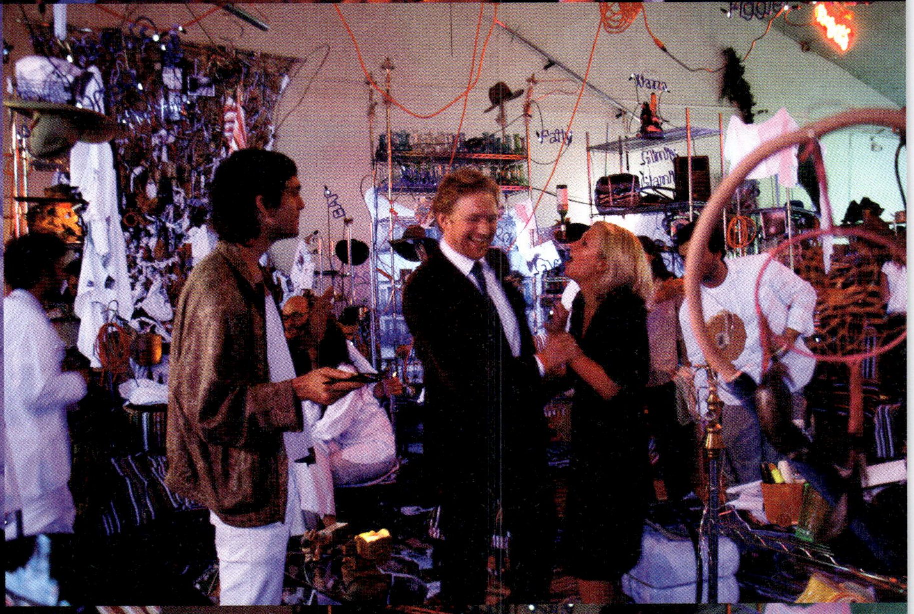
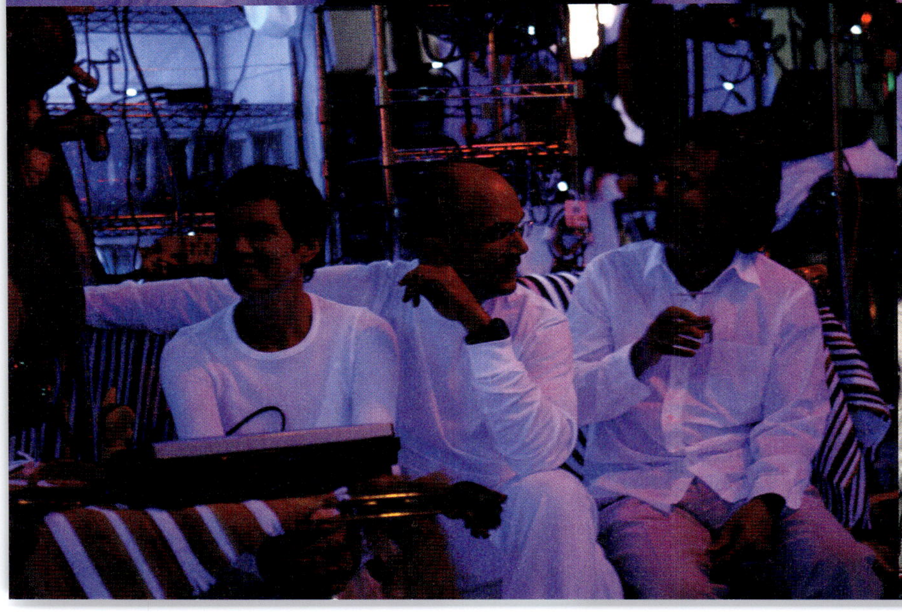
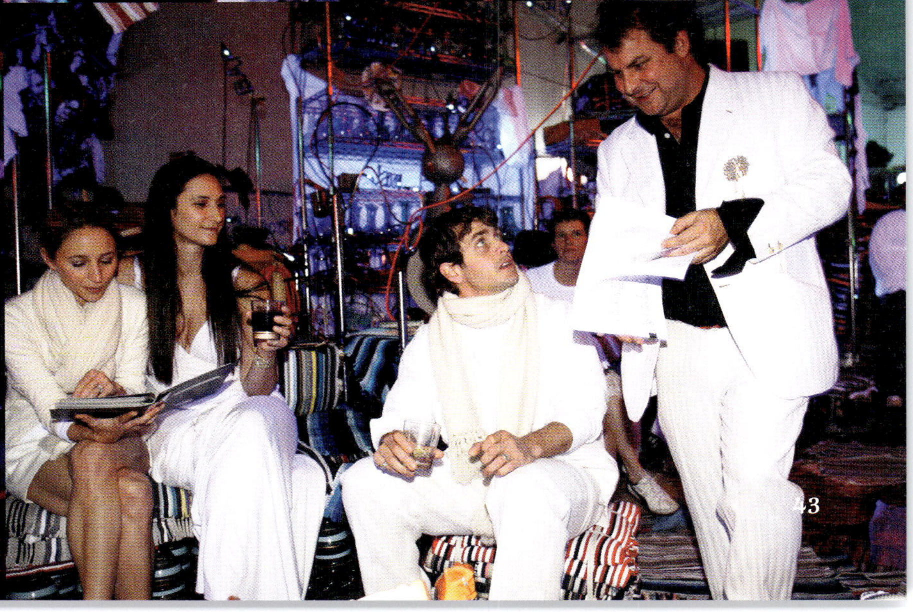

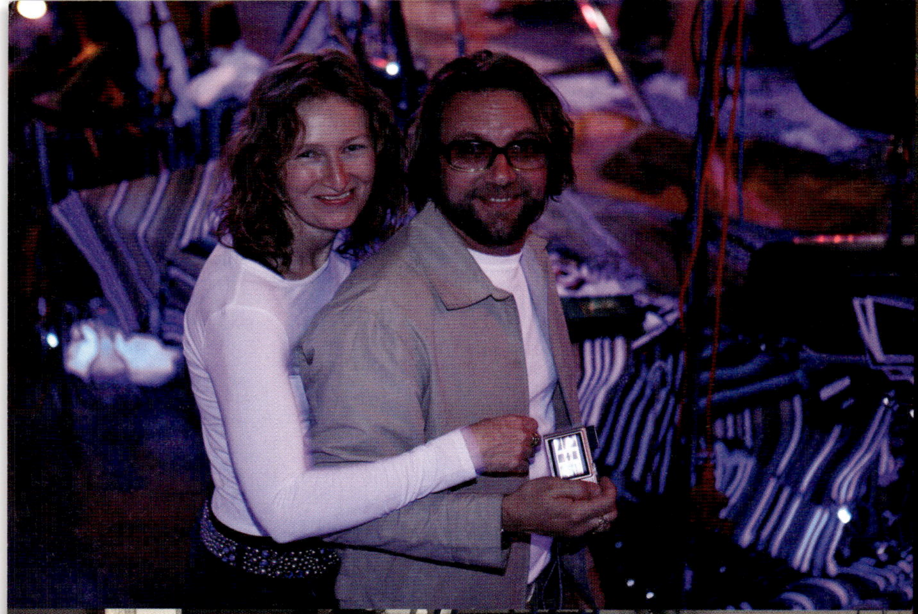
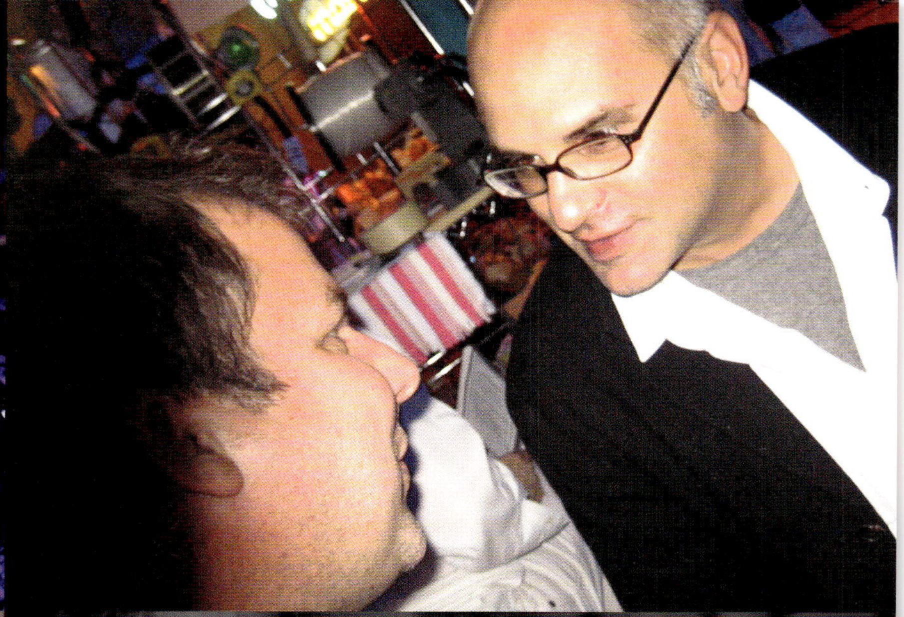
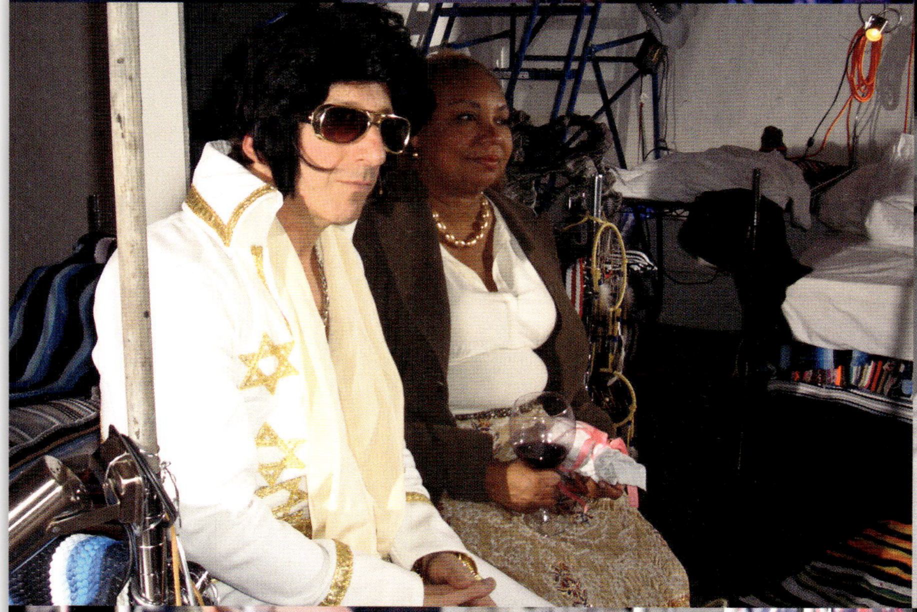
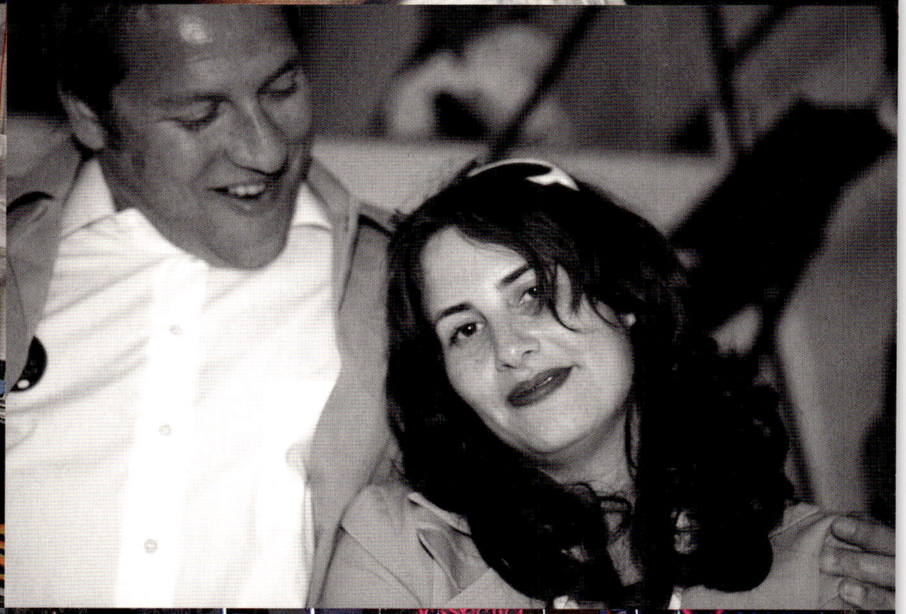
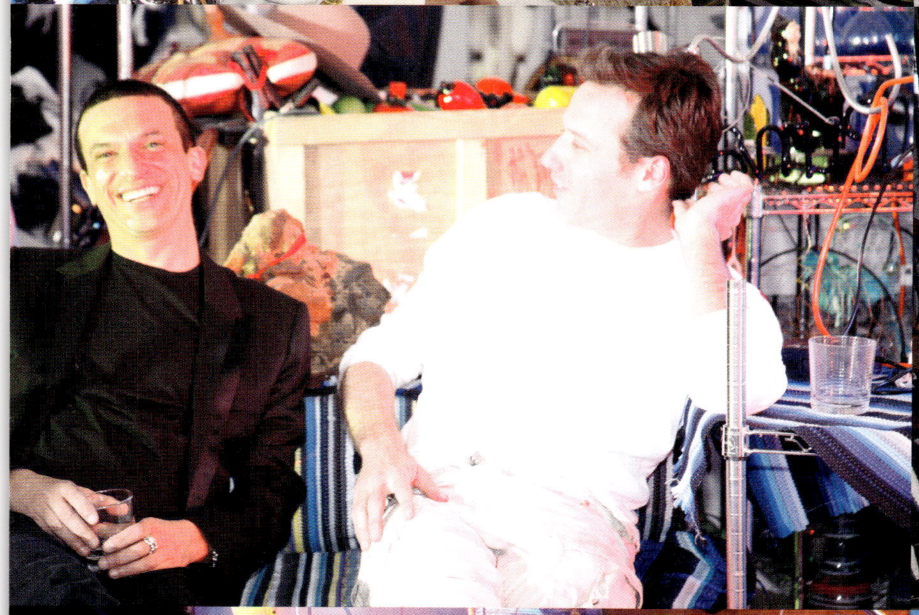
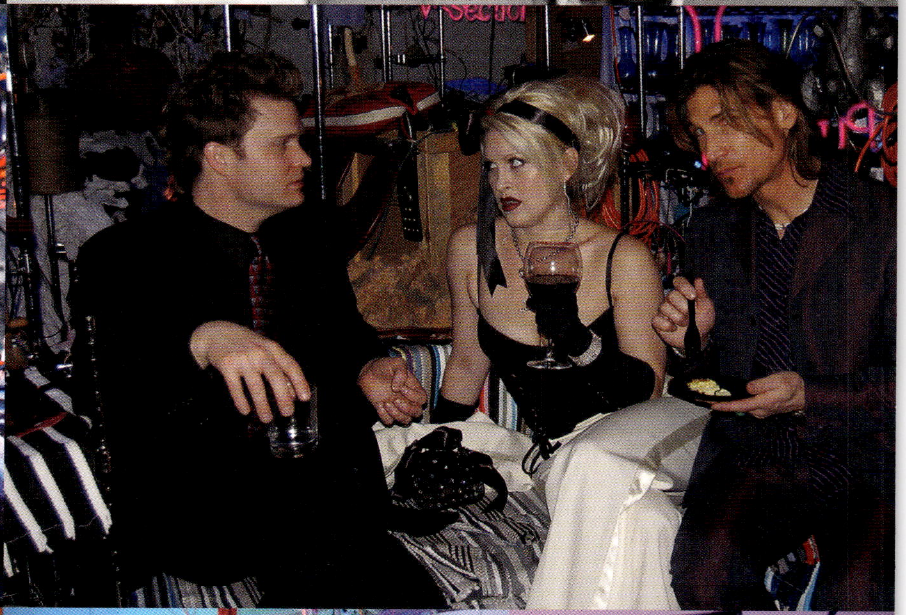
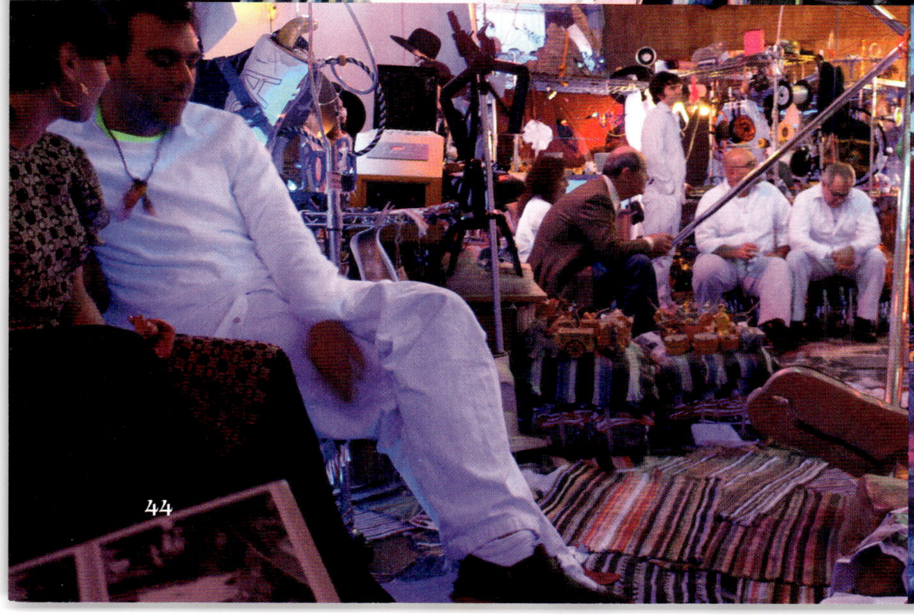
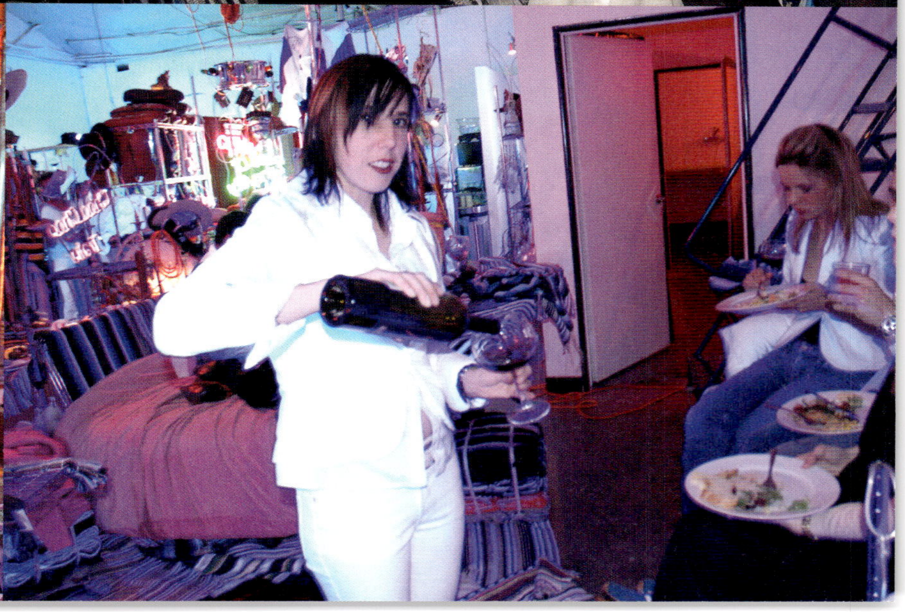

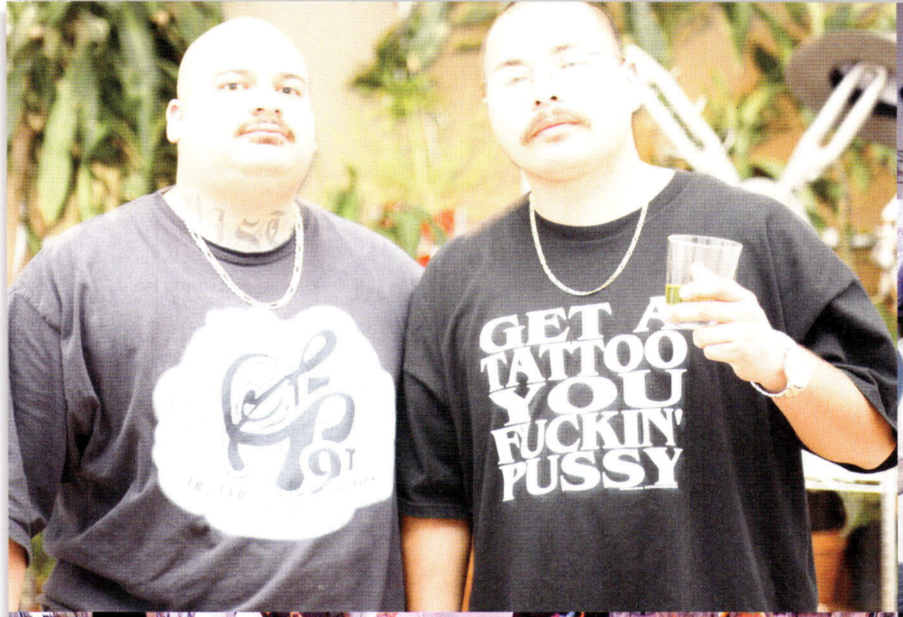
GET A
TATTOO
YOU
FUCKIN'
PUSSY
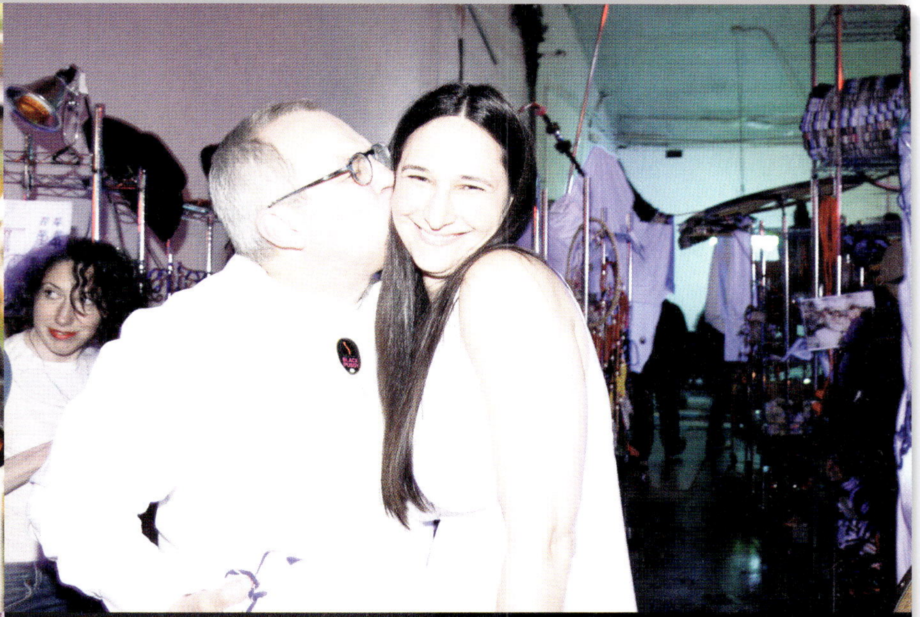
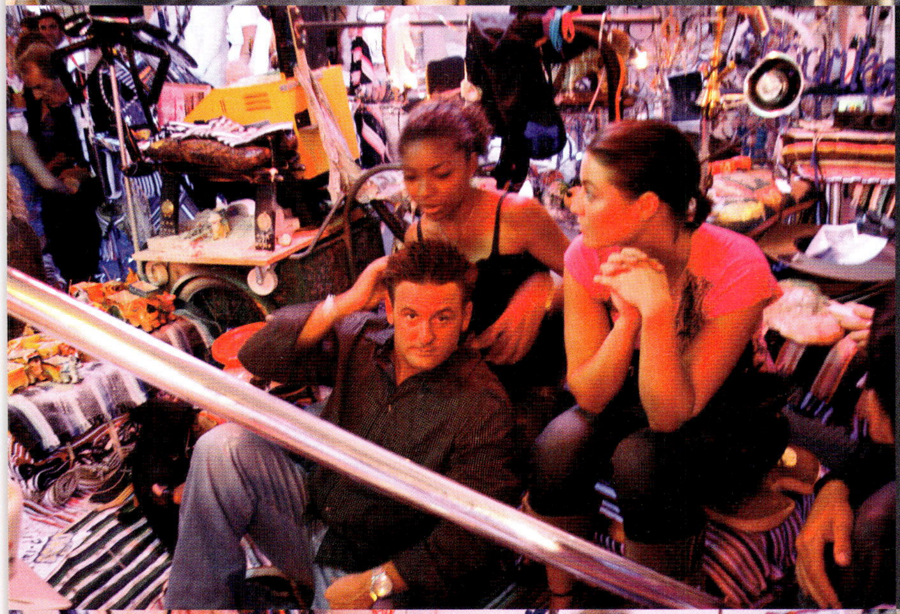
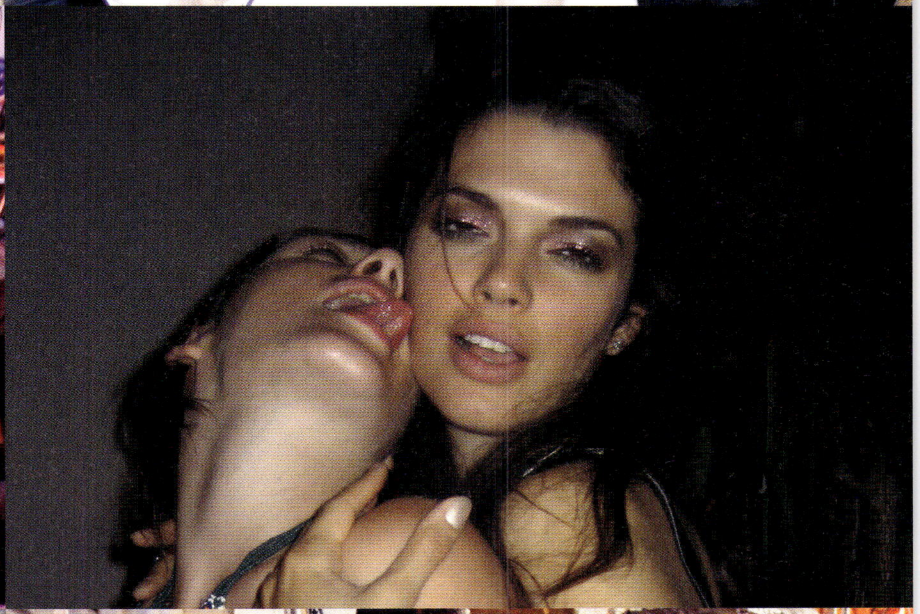
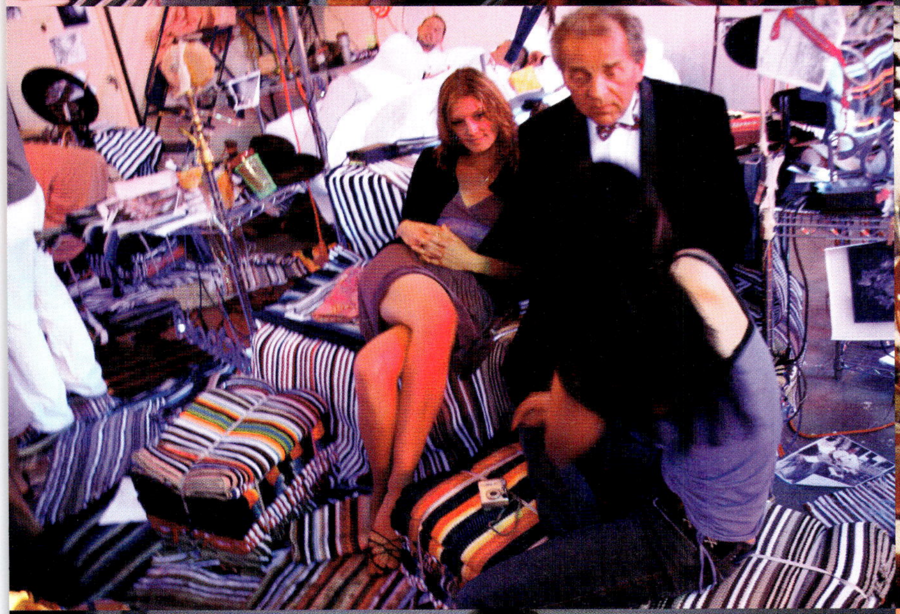
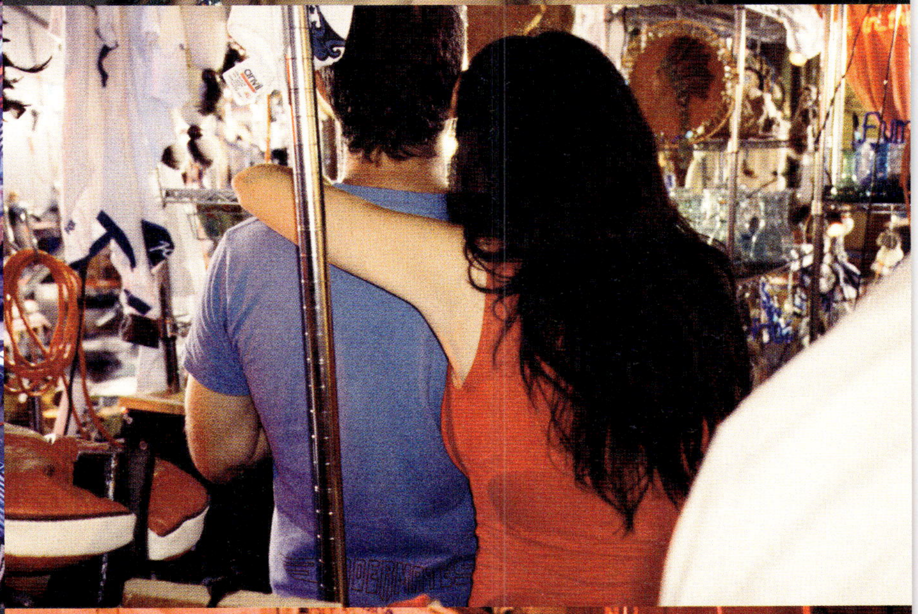
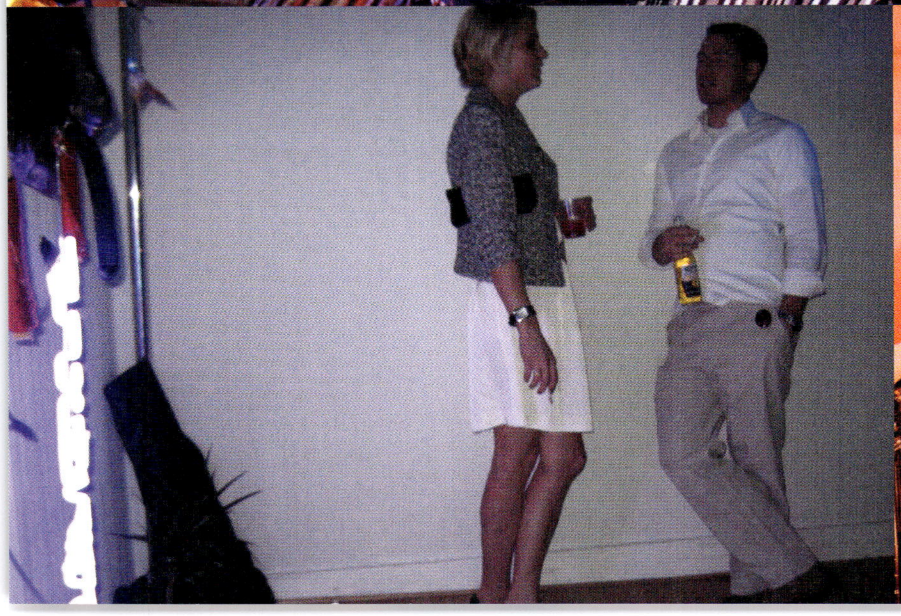
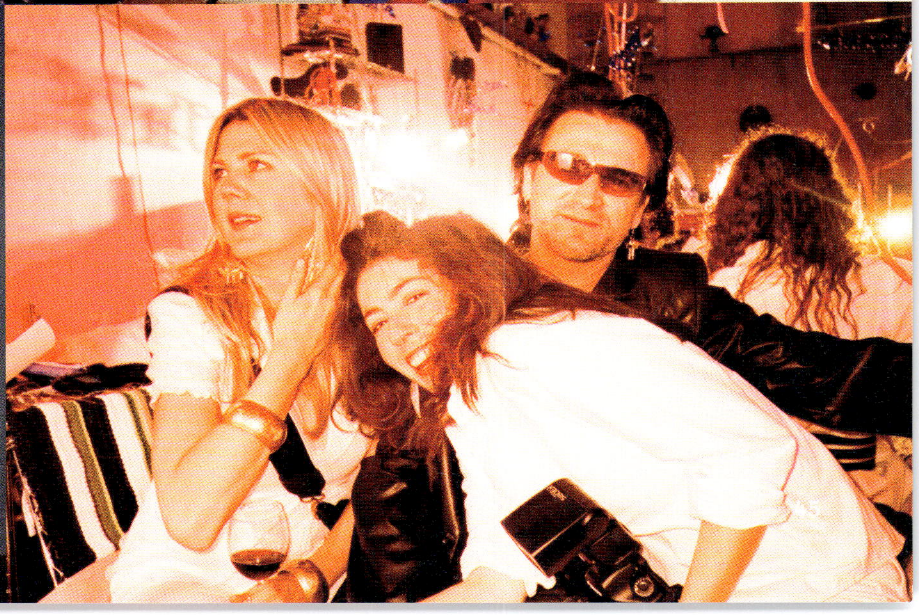

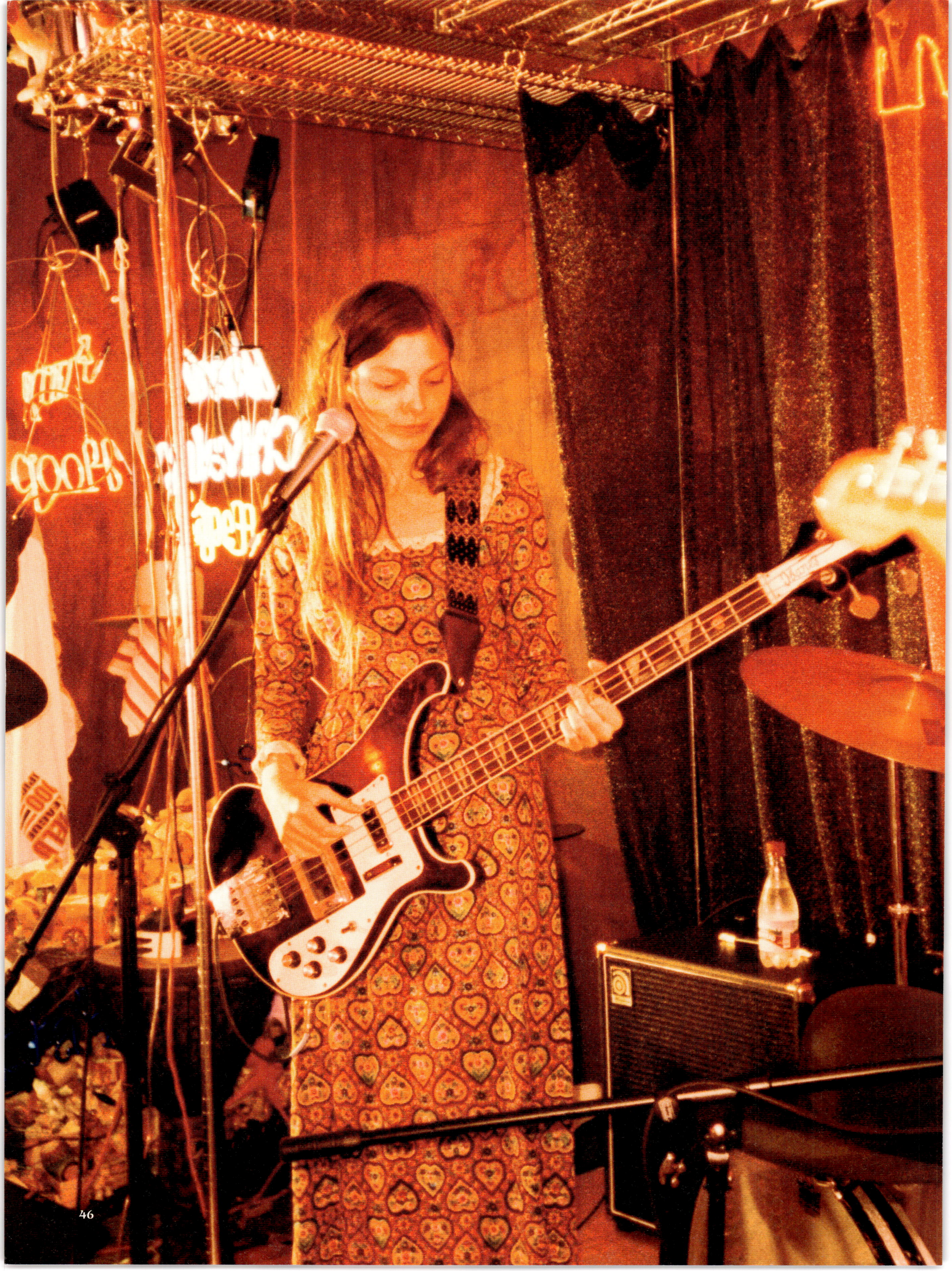

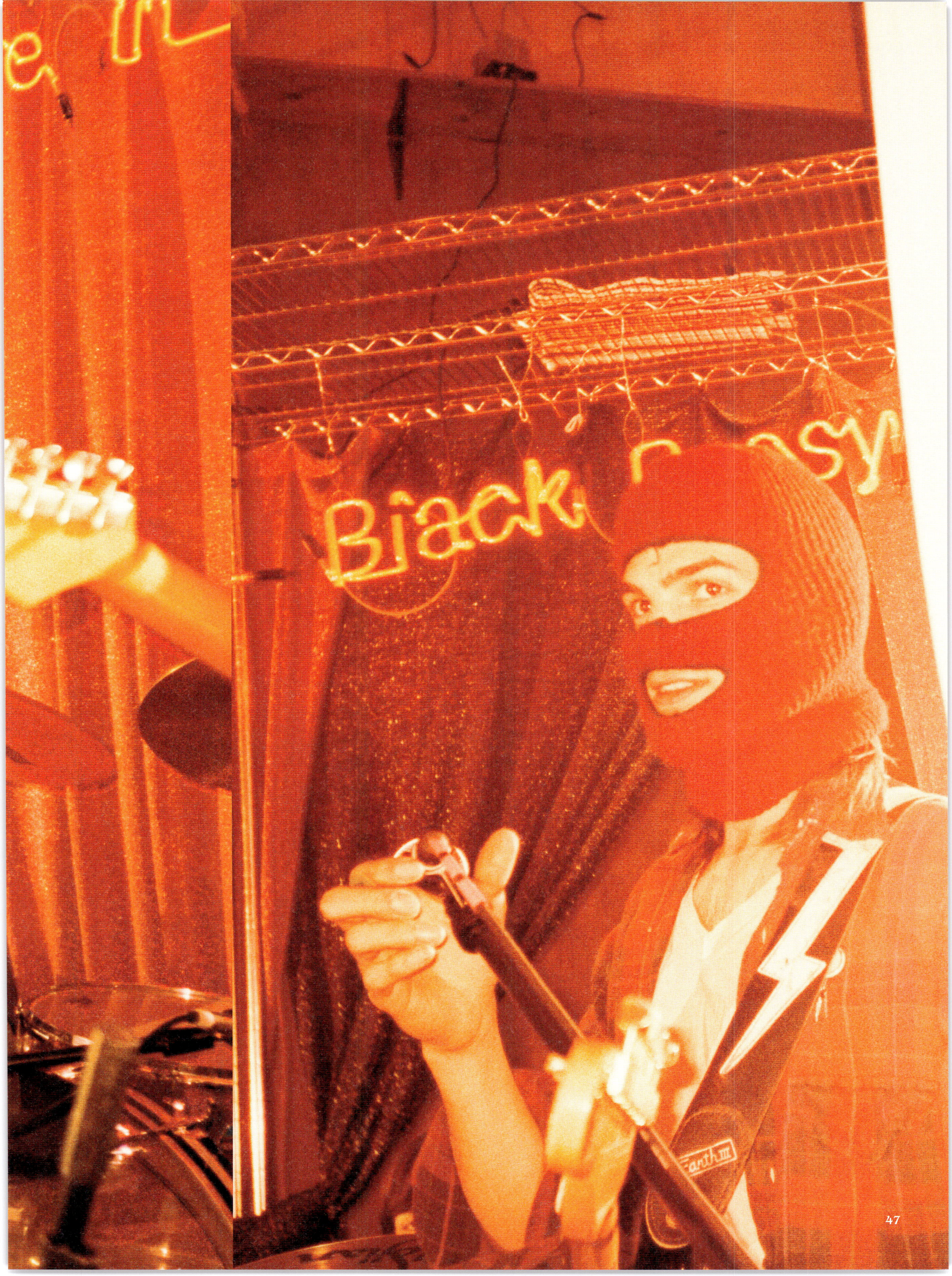
Black

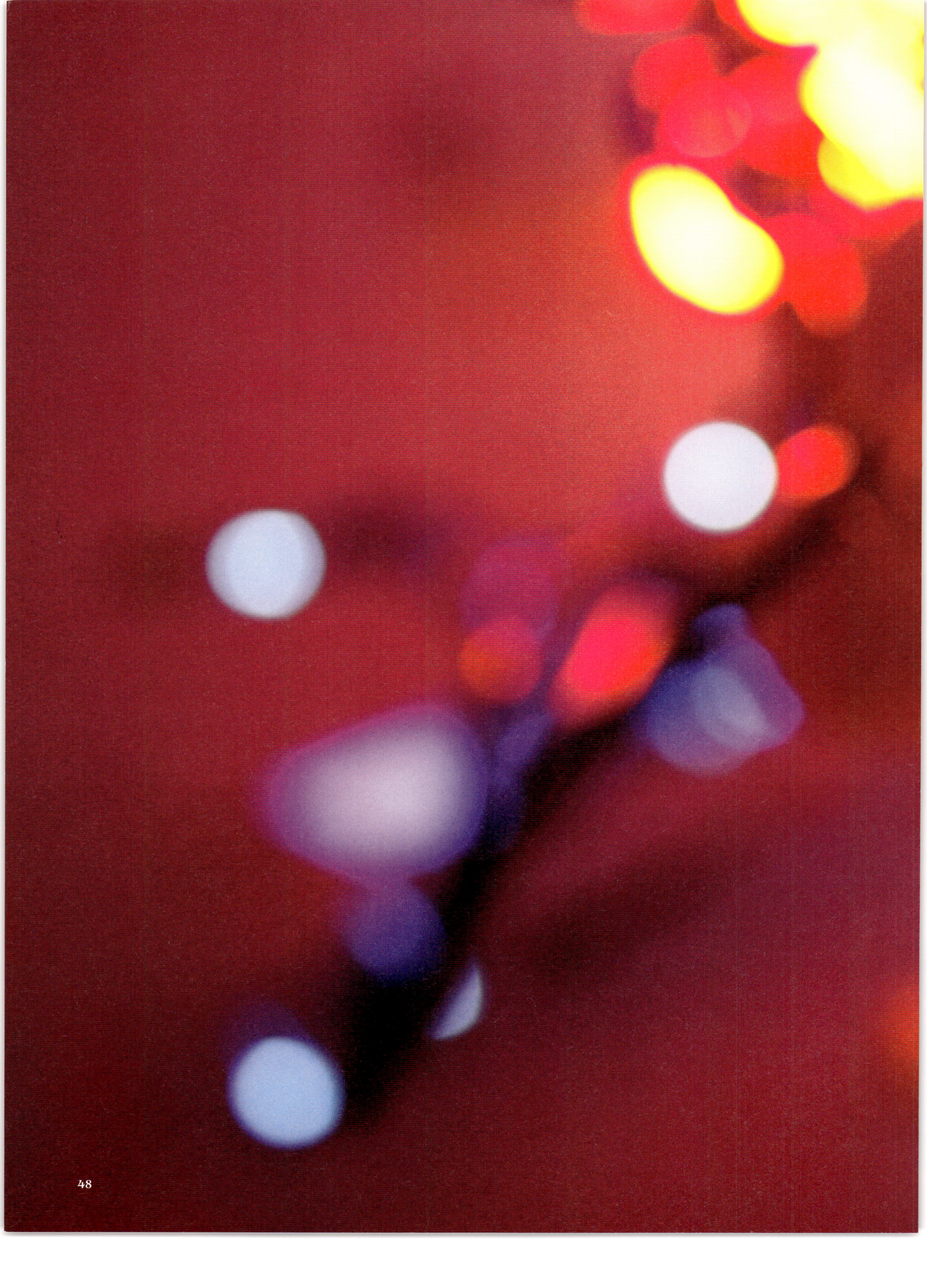

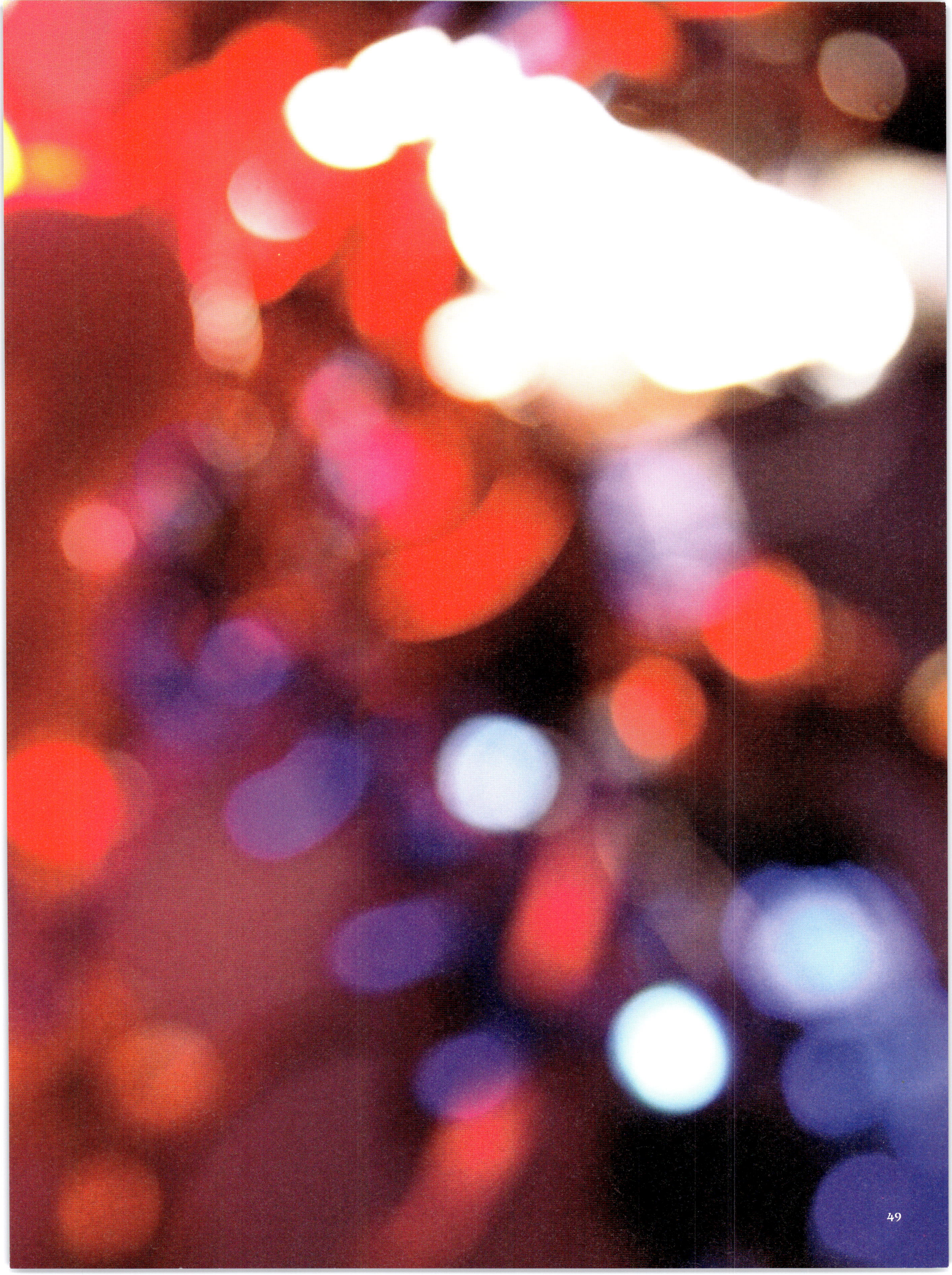

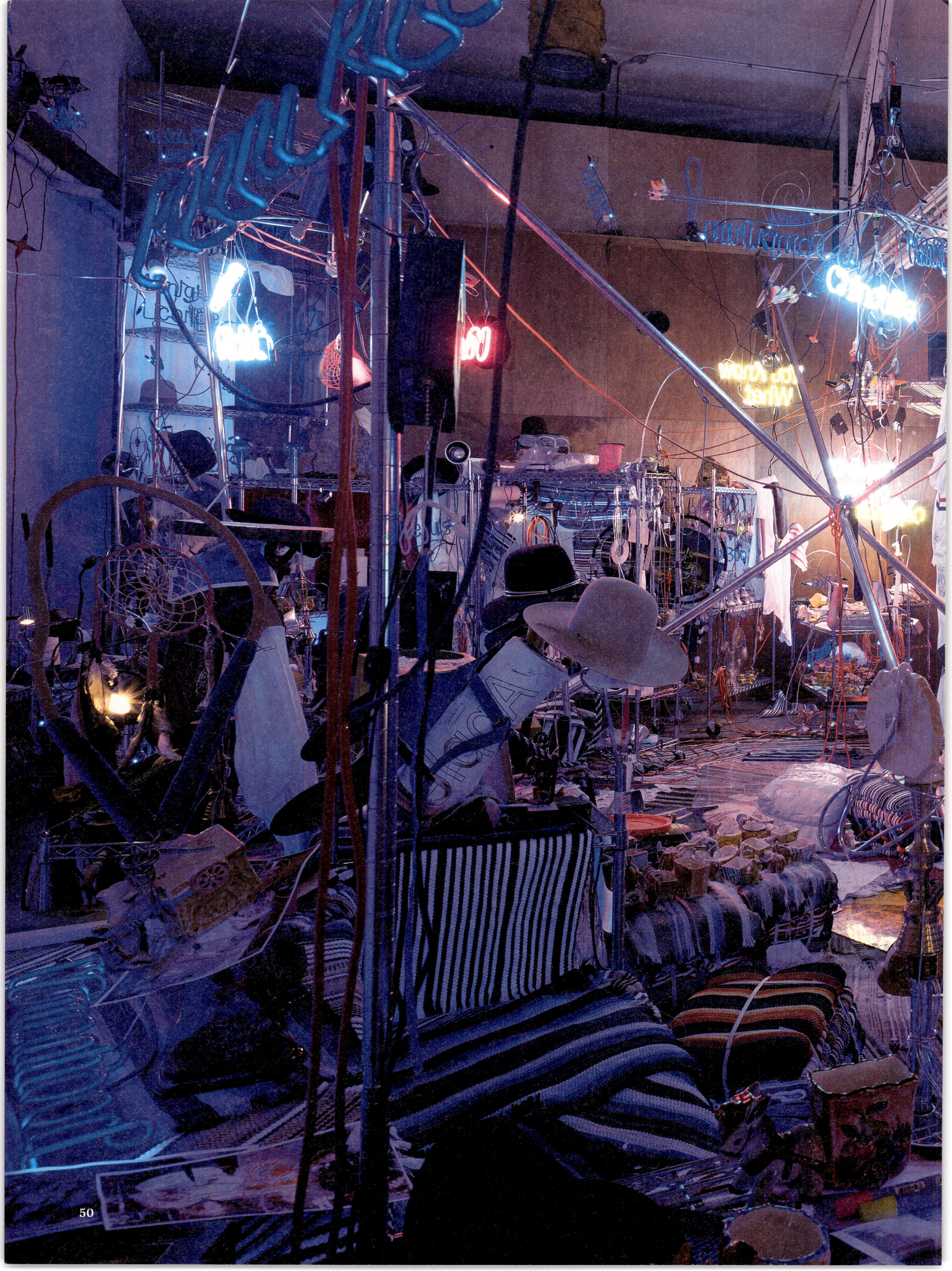

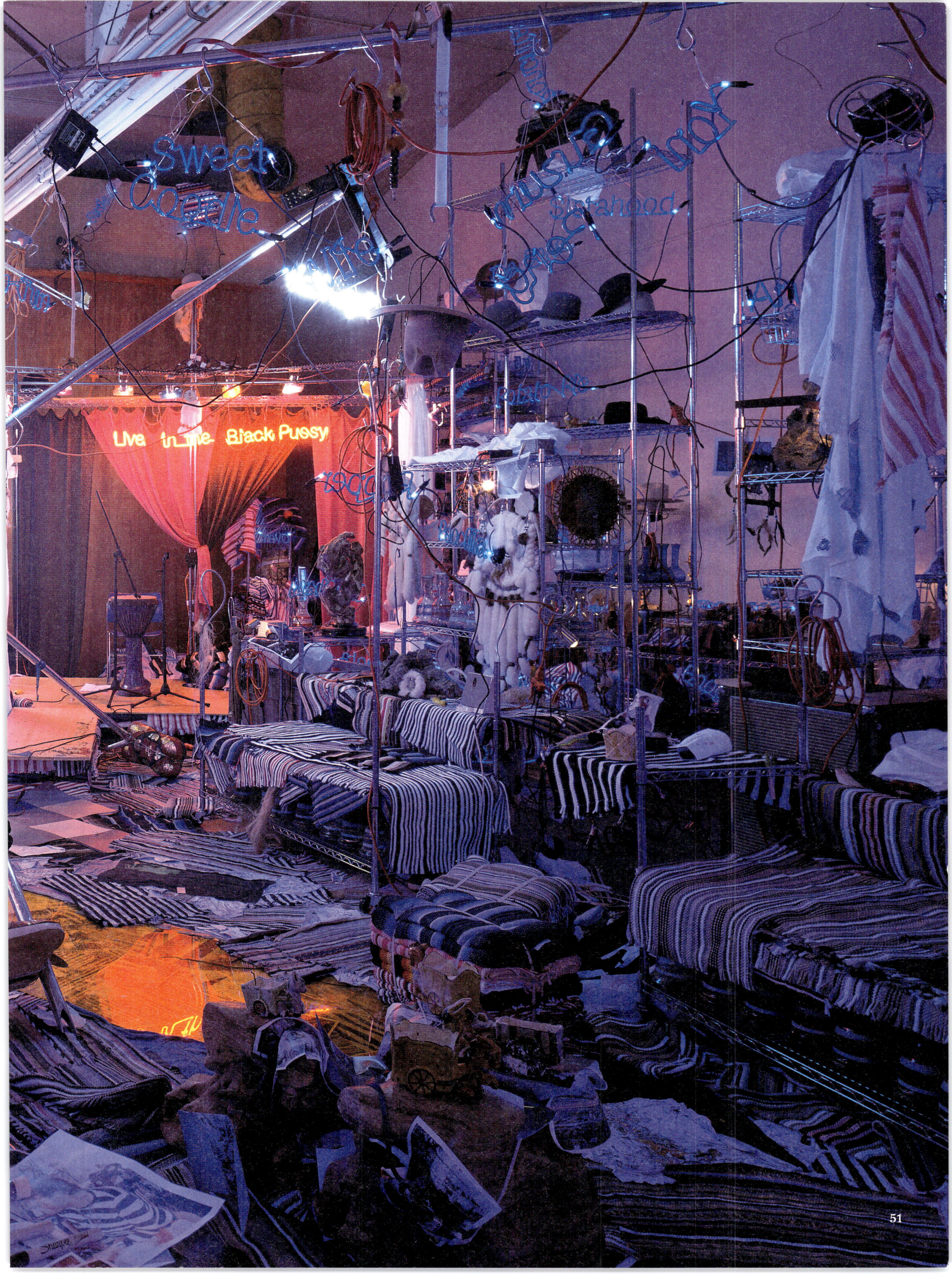
Sweet
Live in the Black Pussy

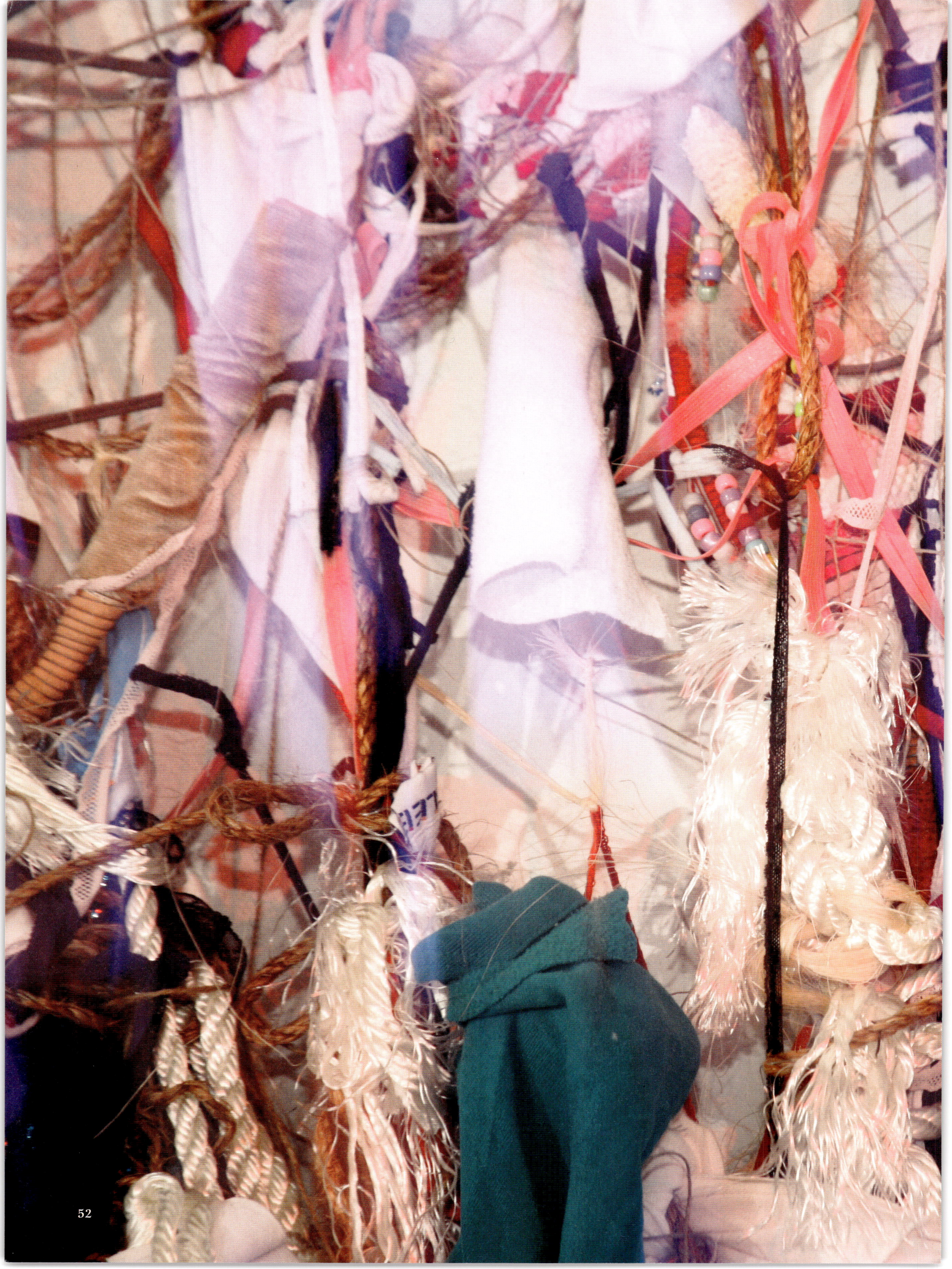

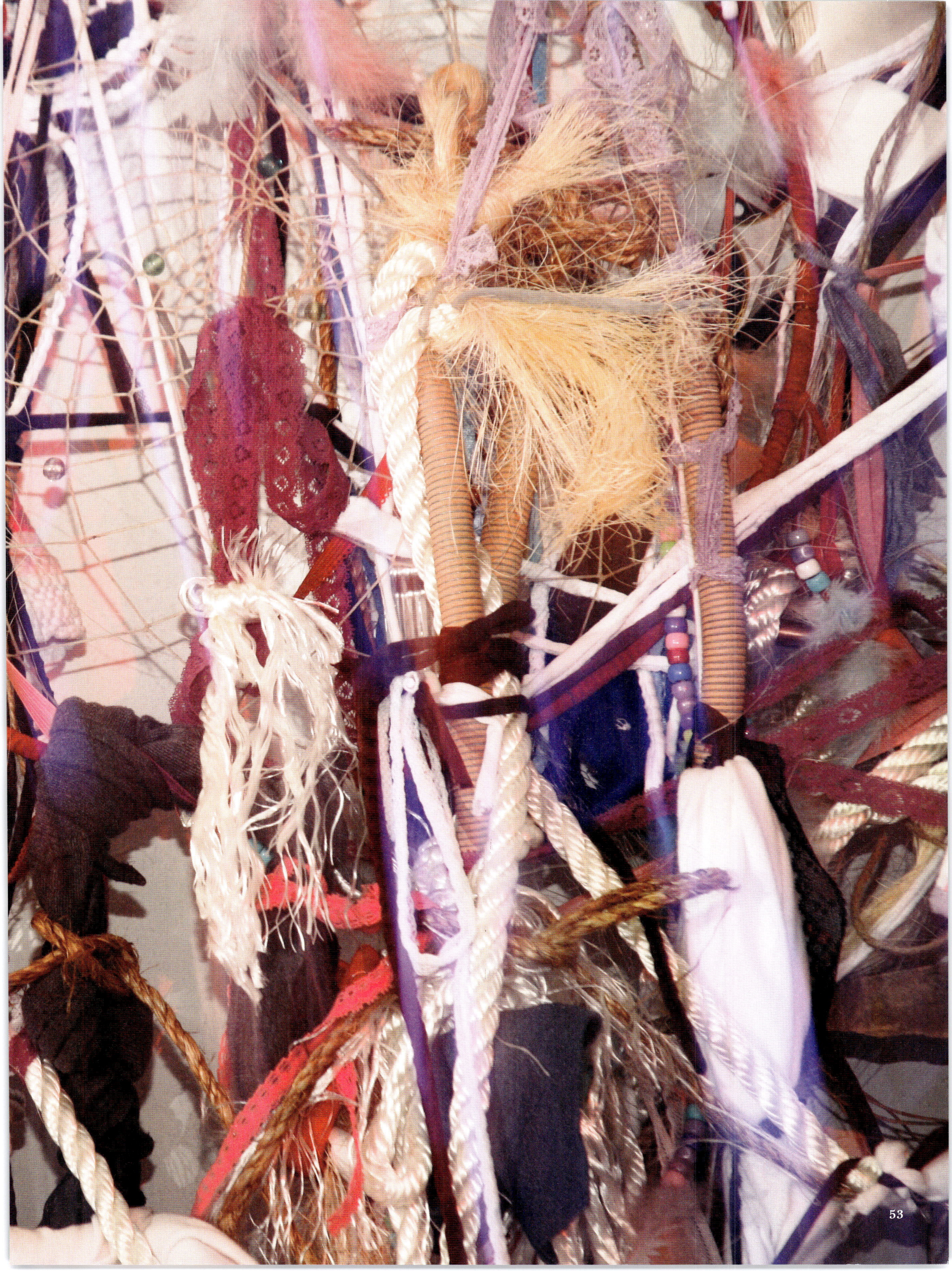

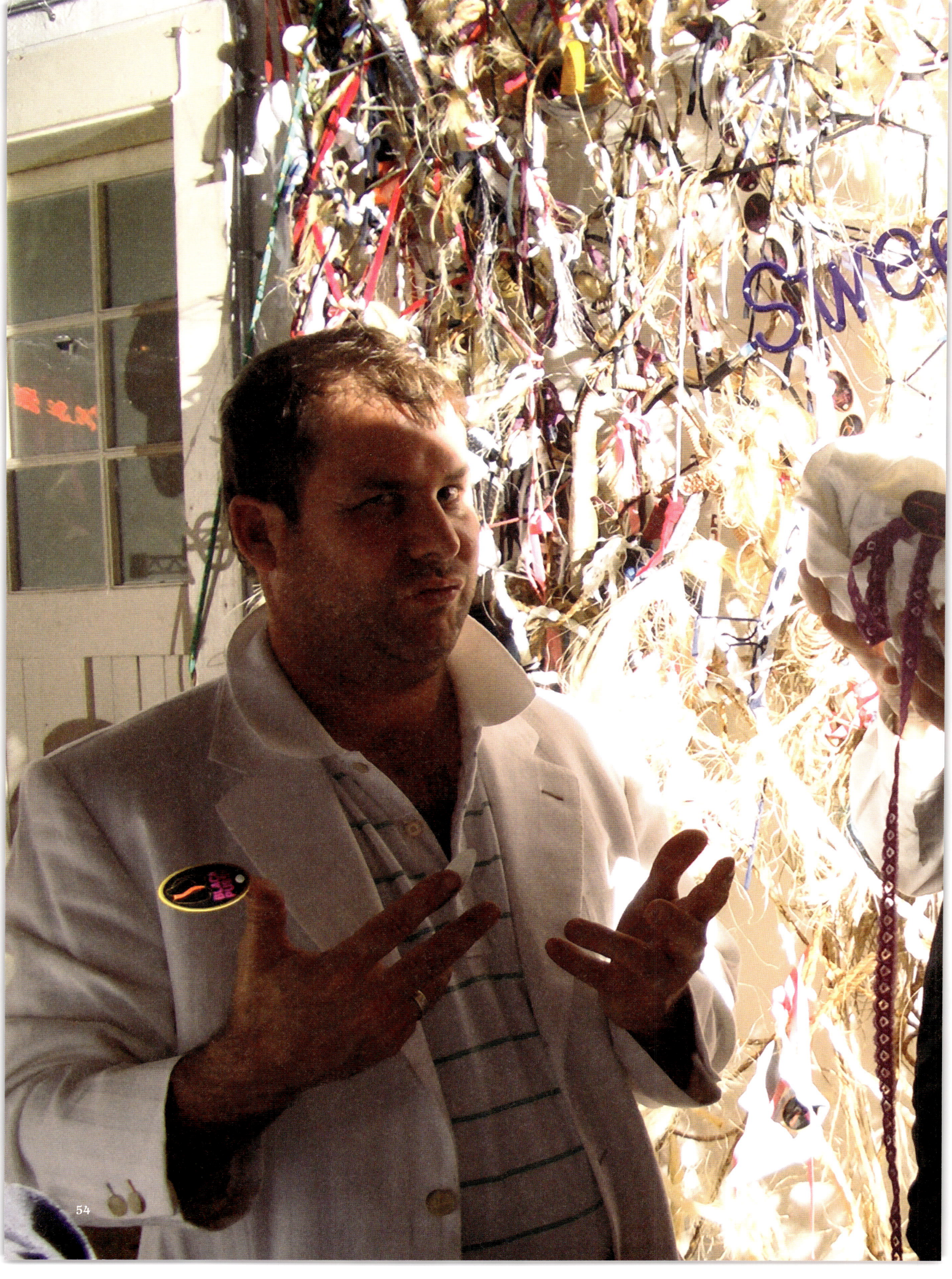

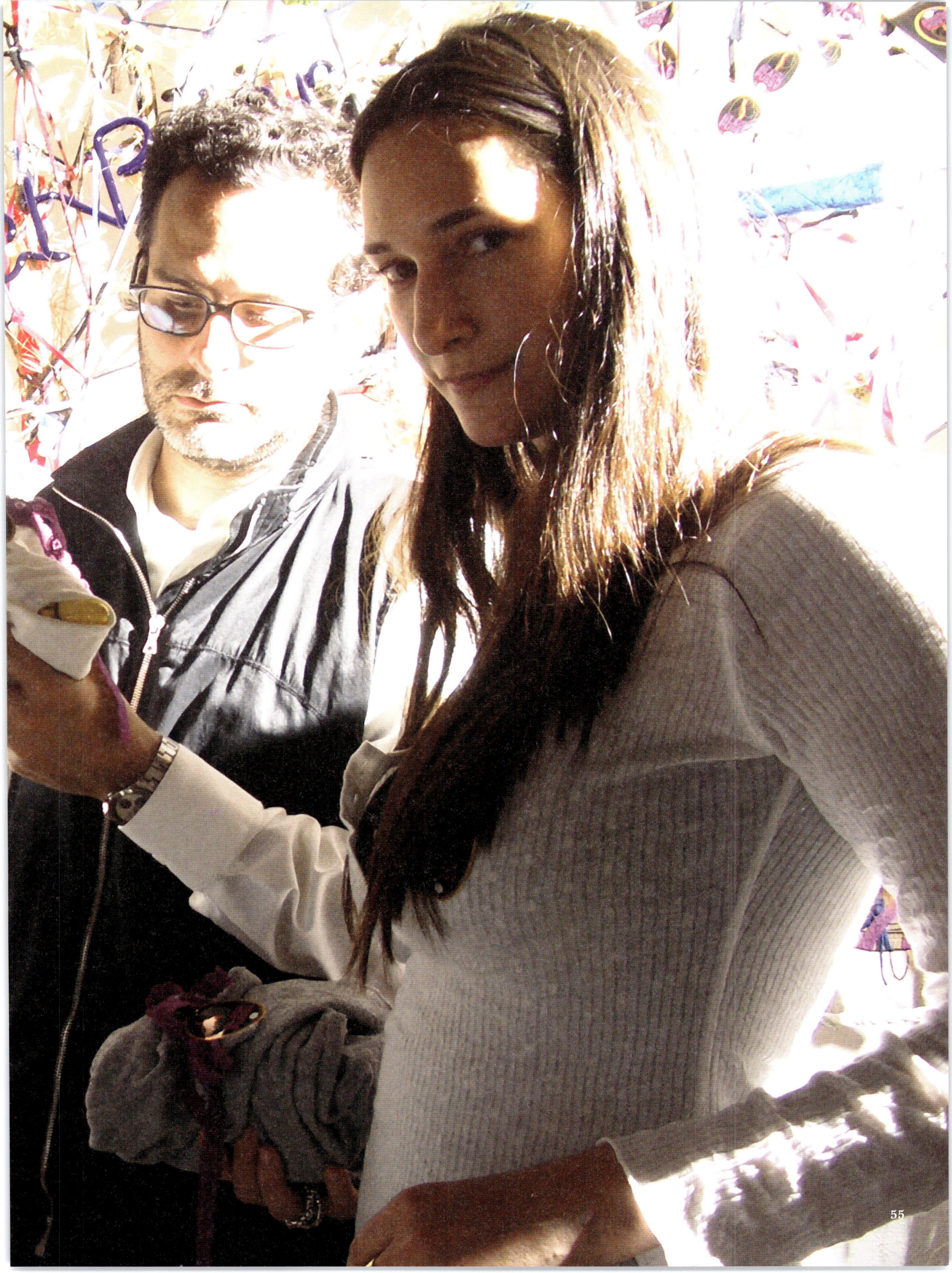

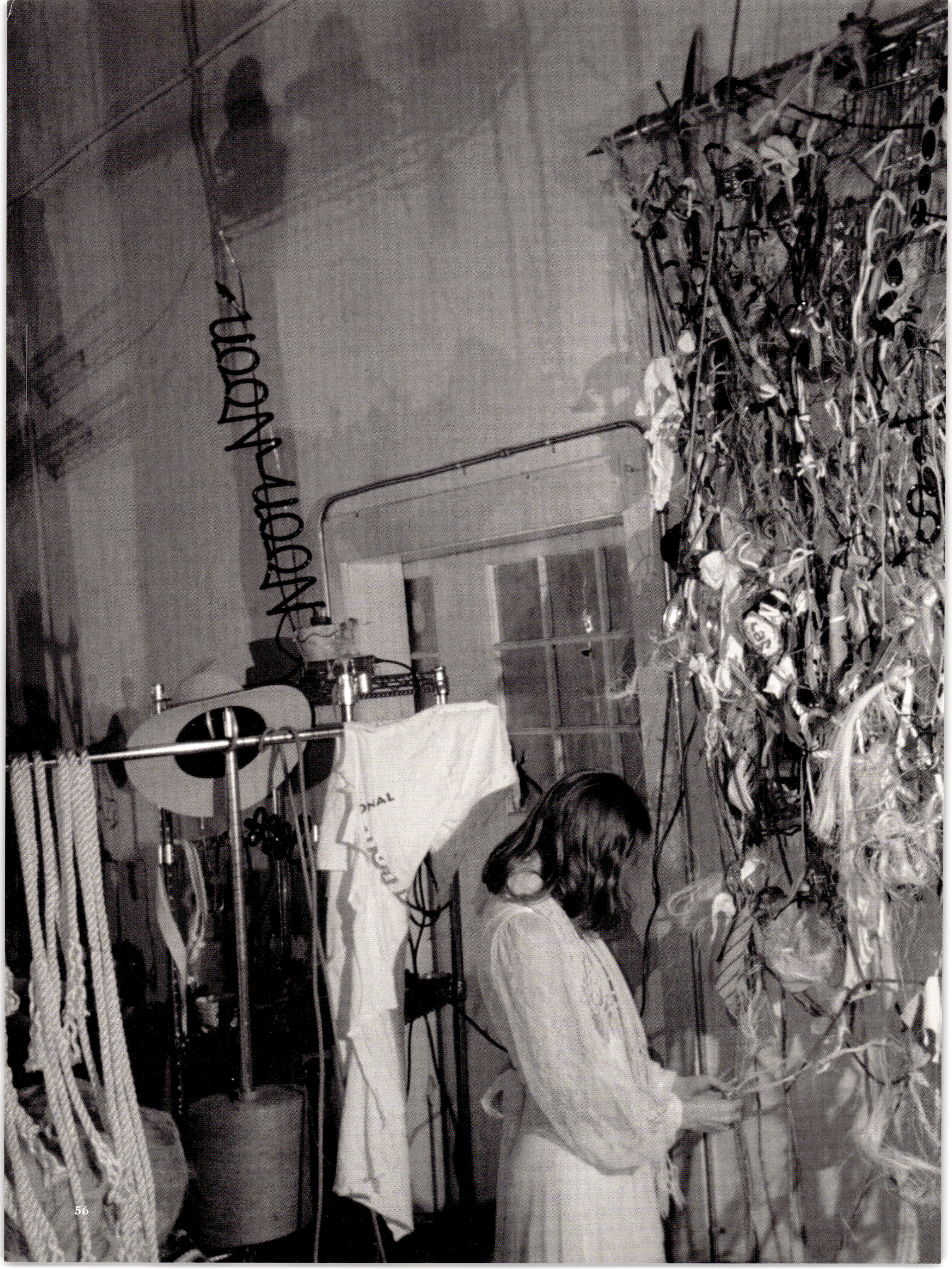

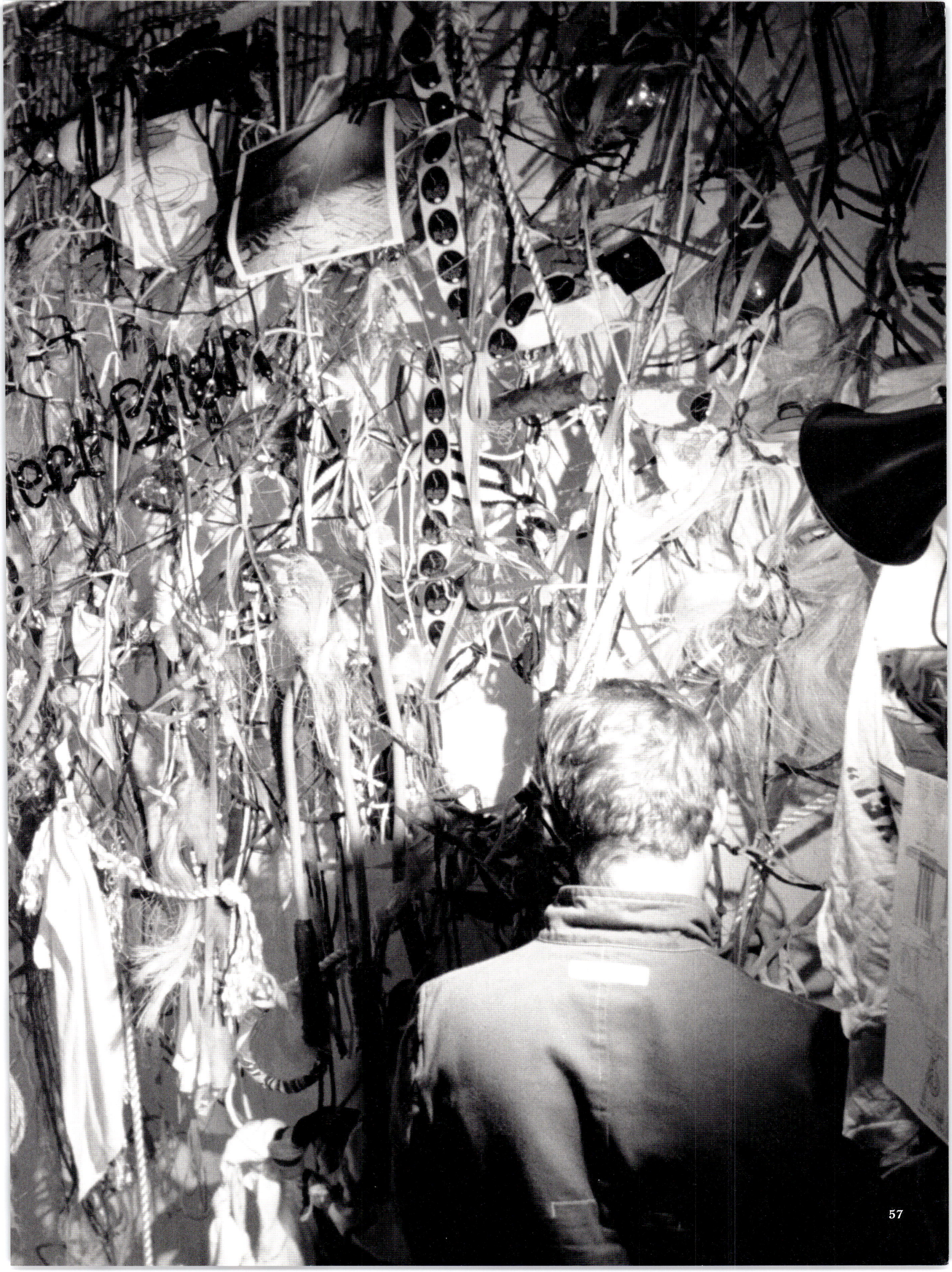

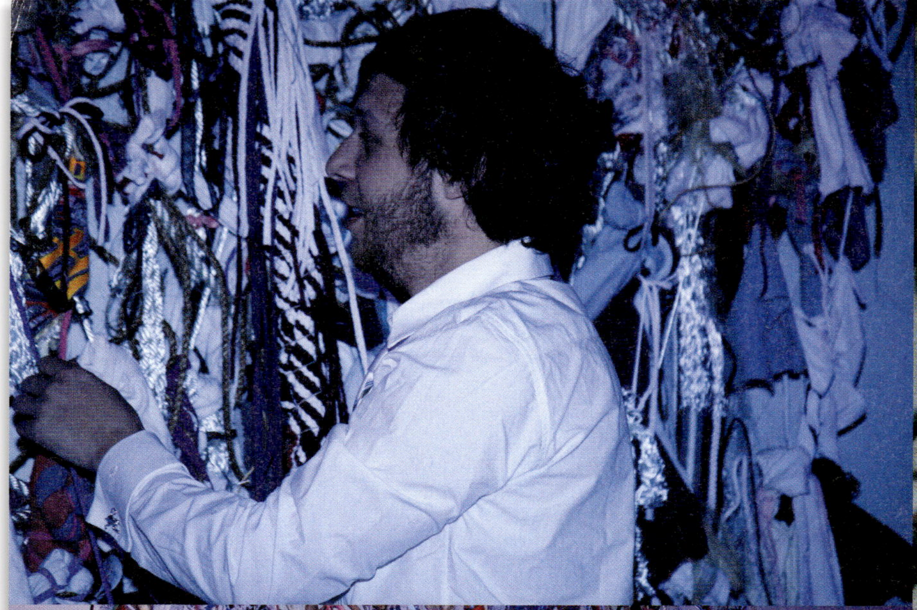
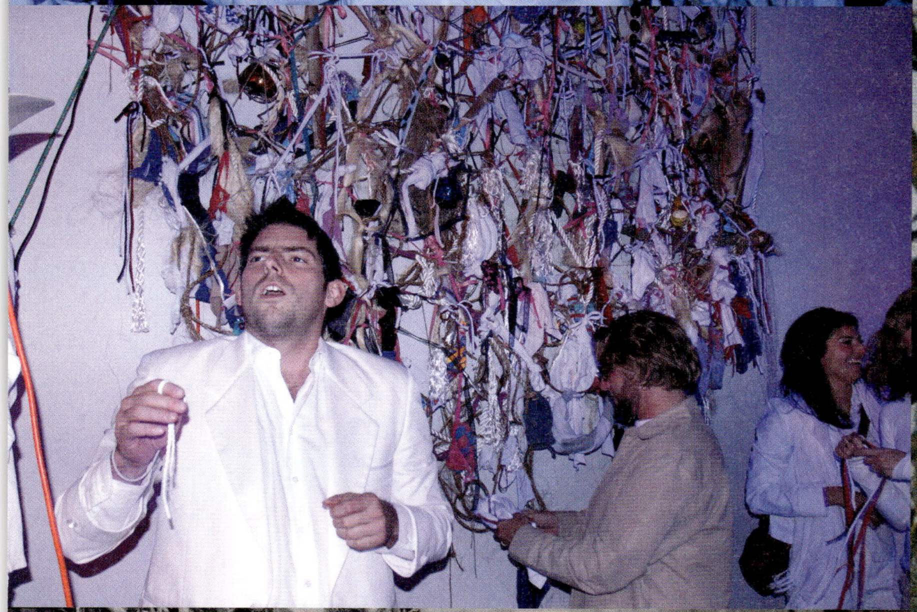
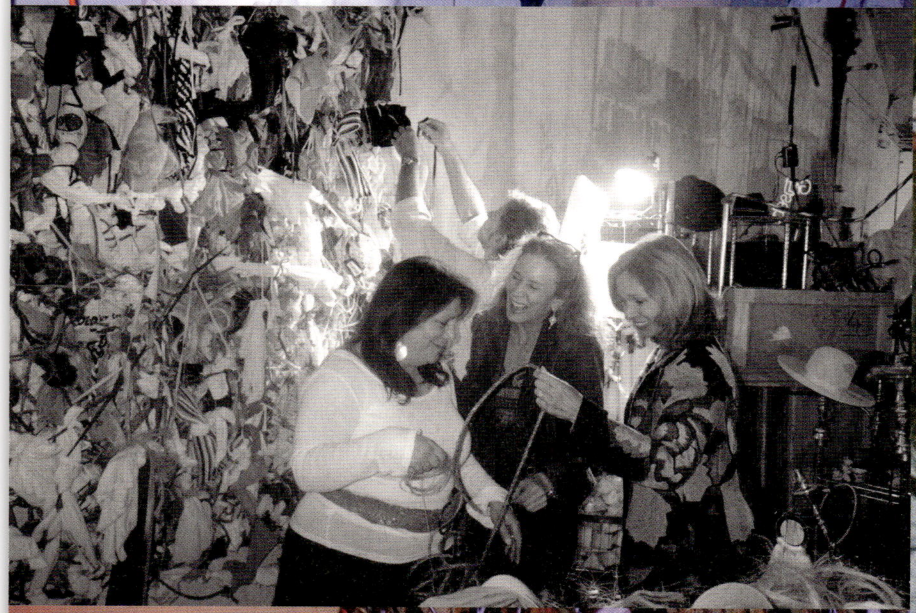
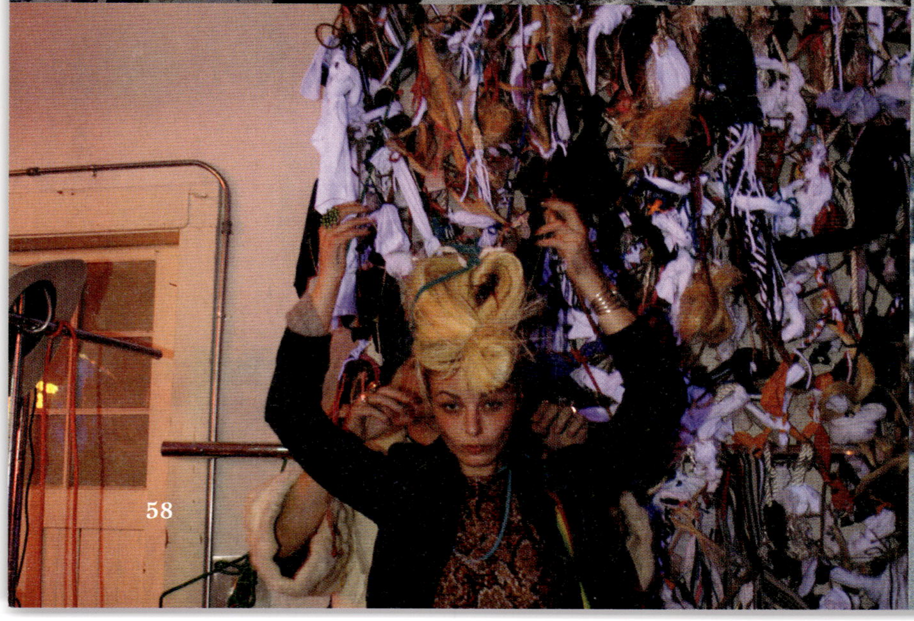
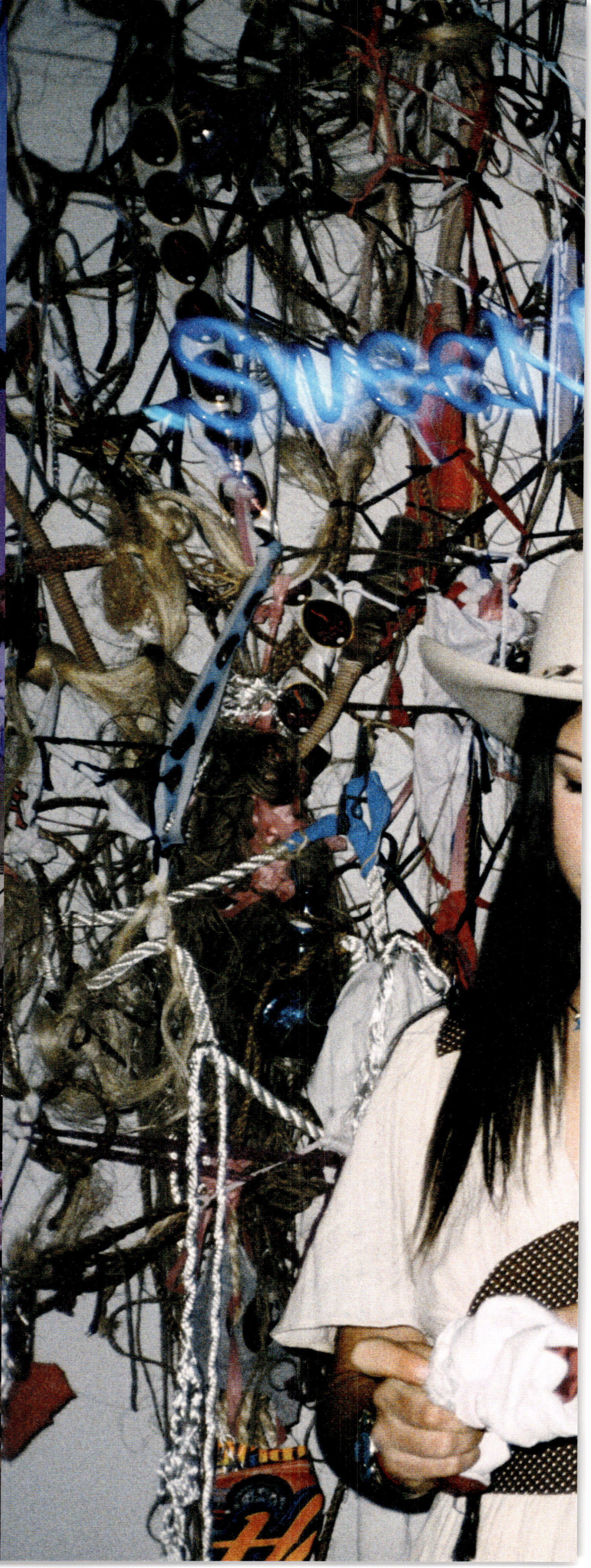

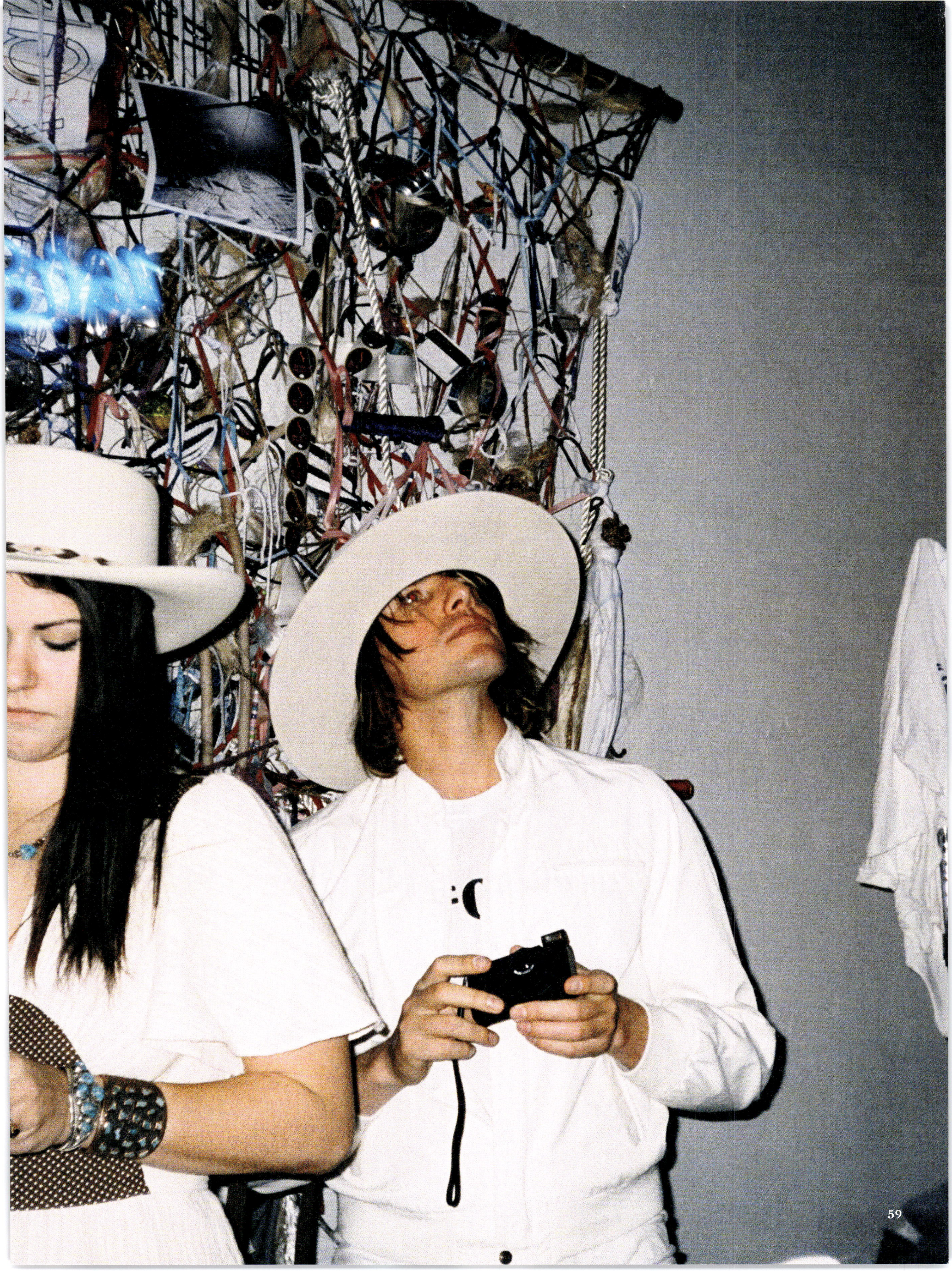

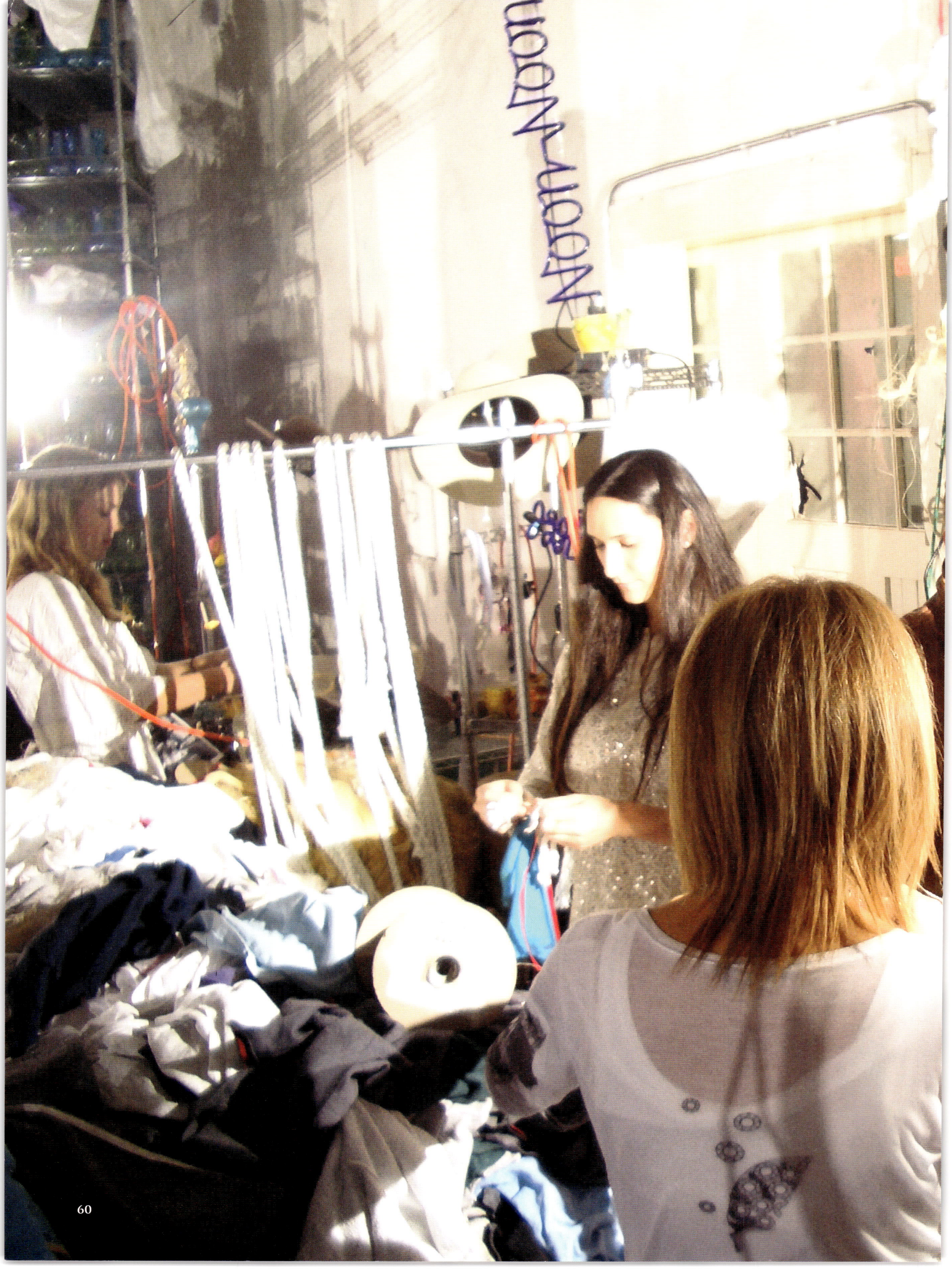

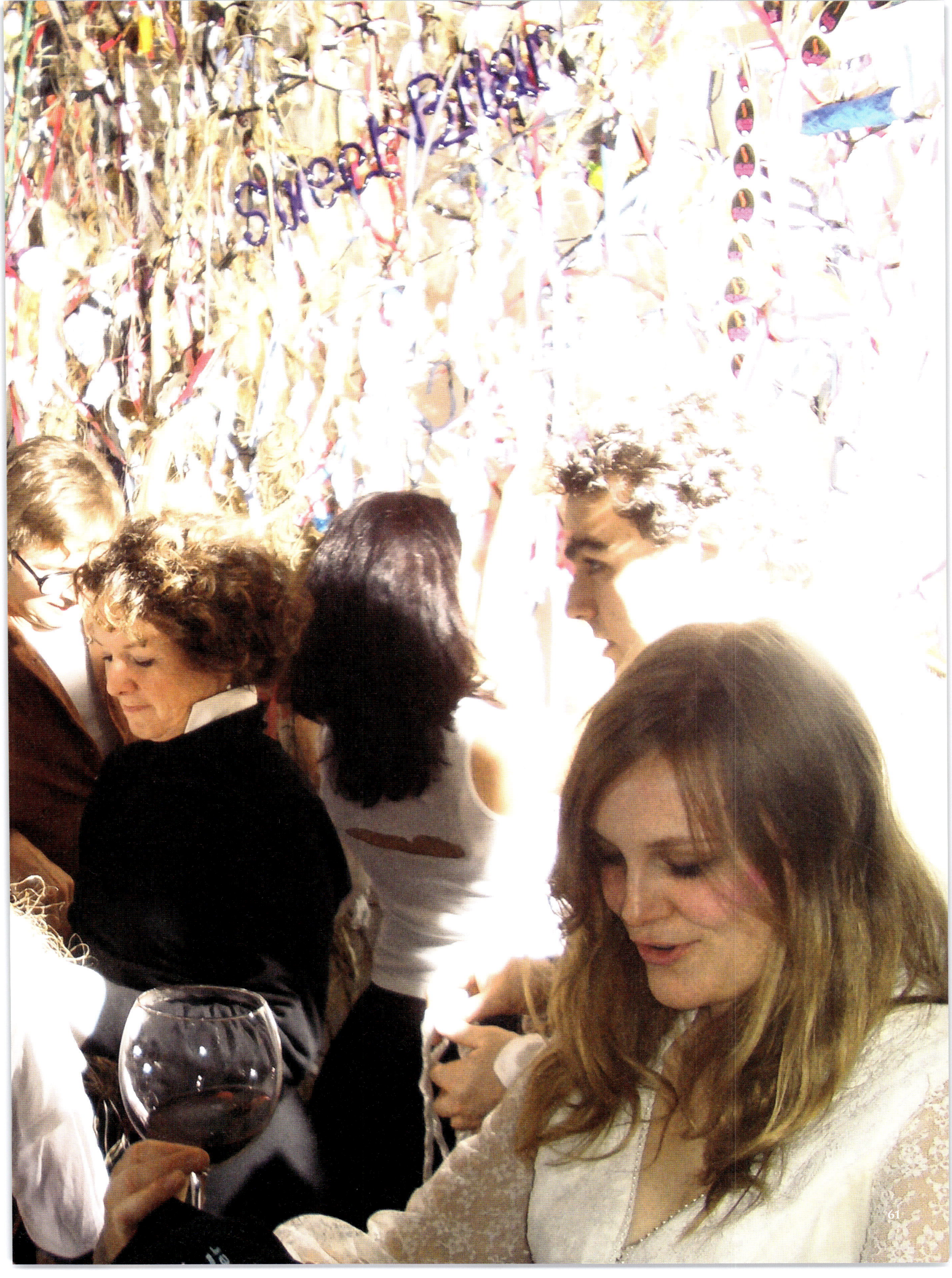

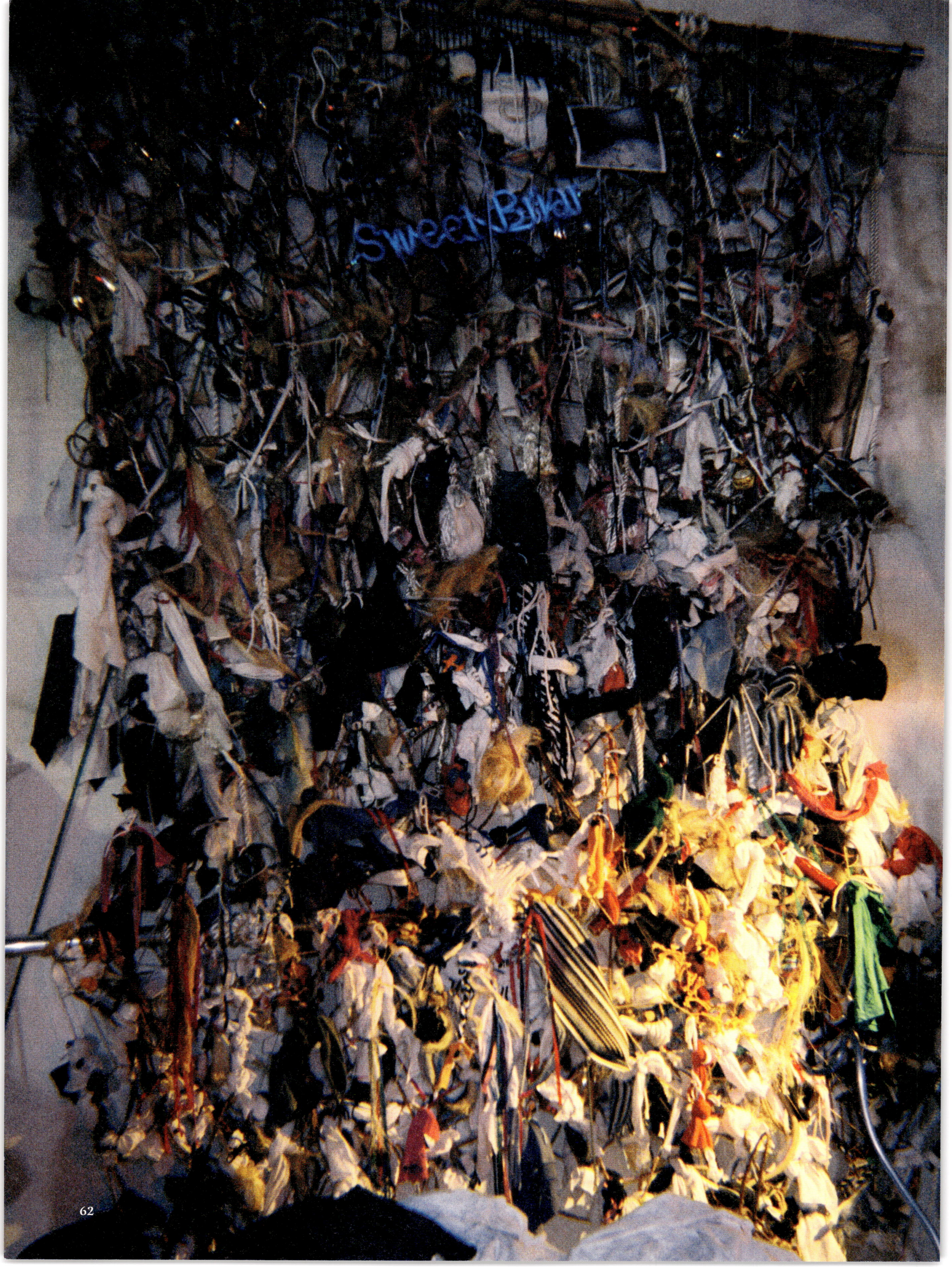

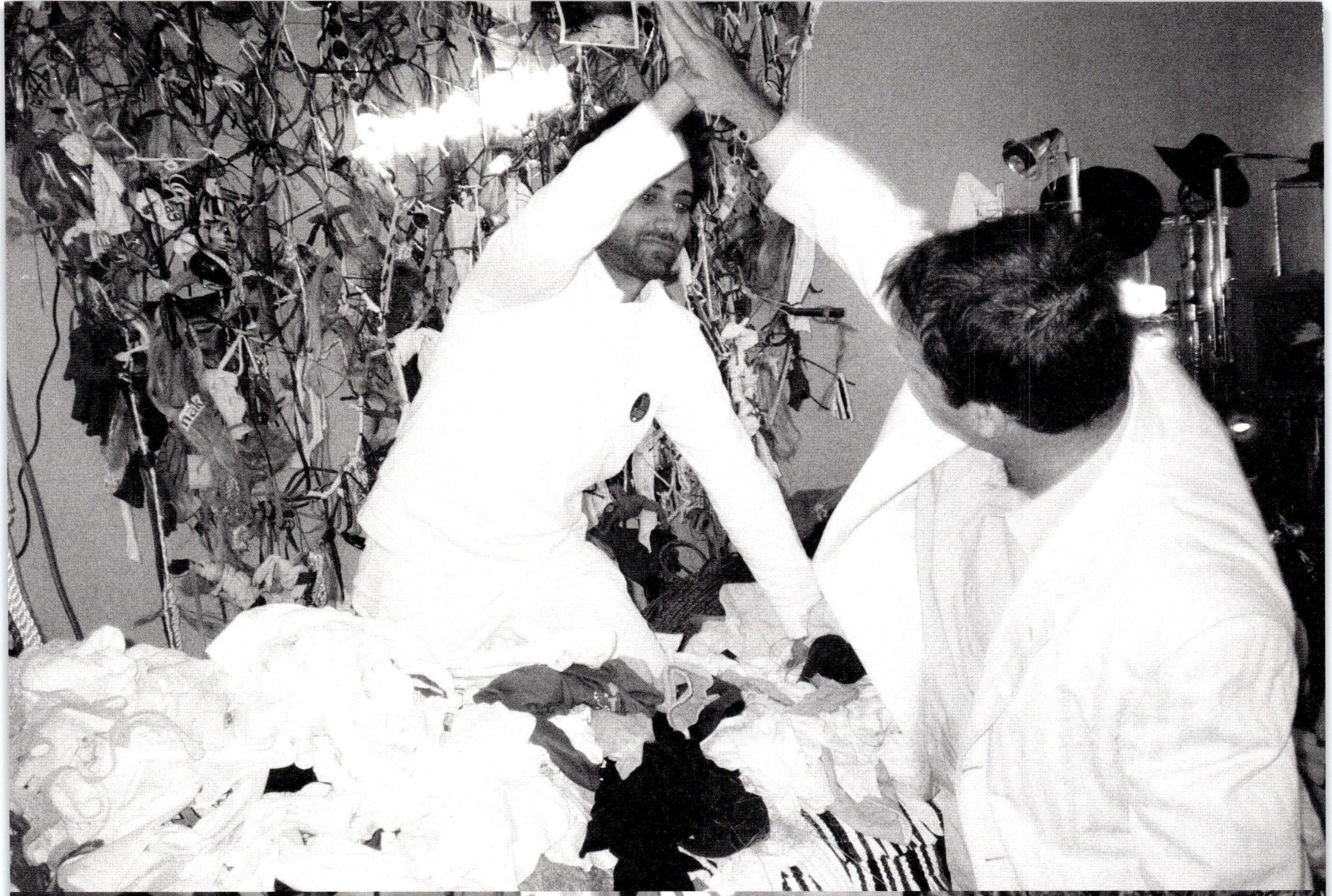

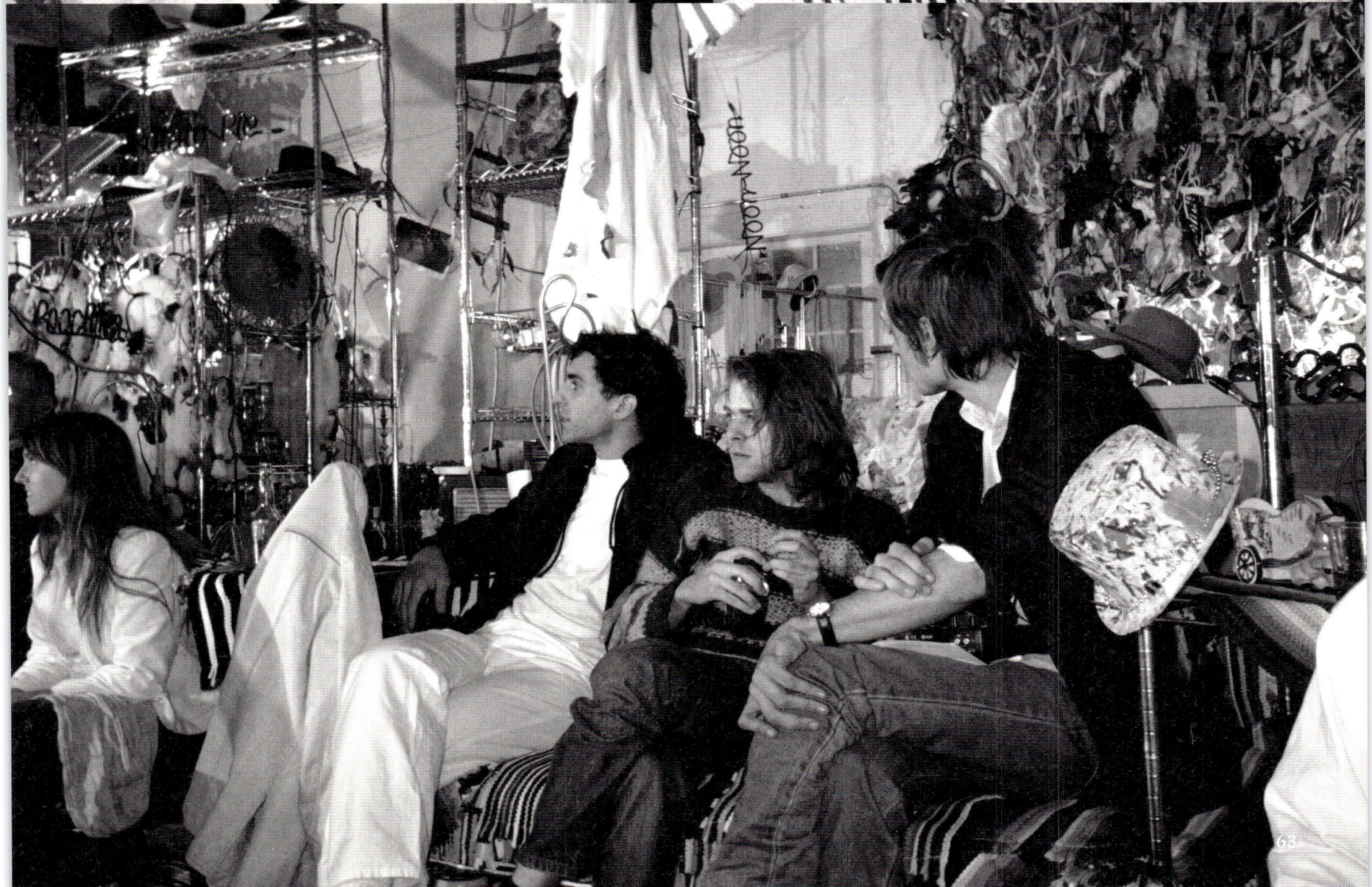

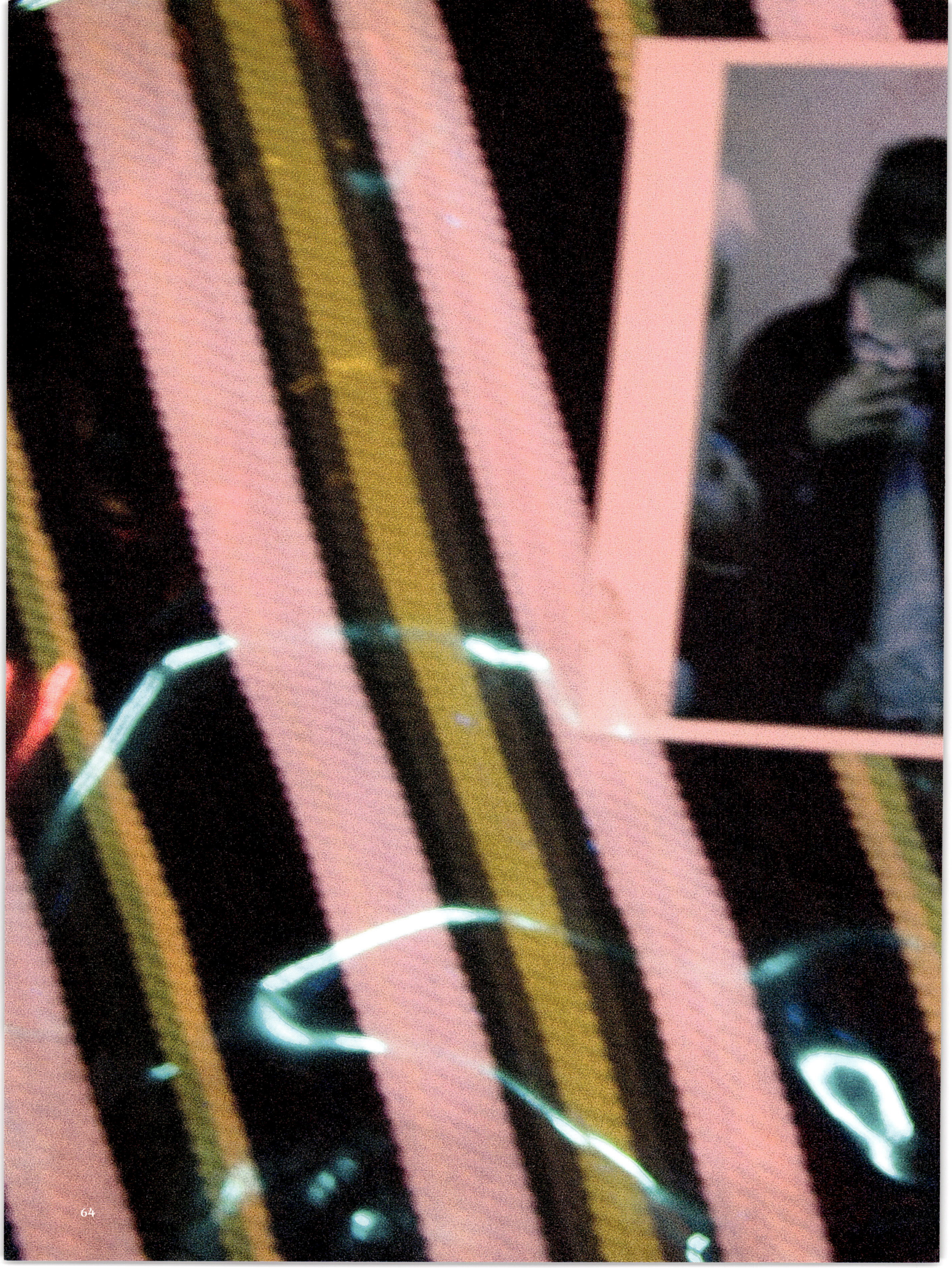

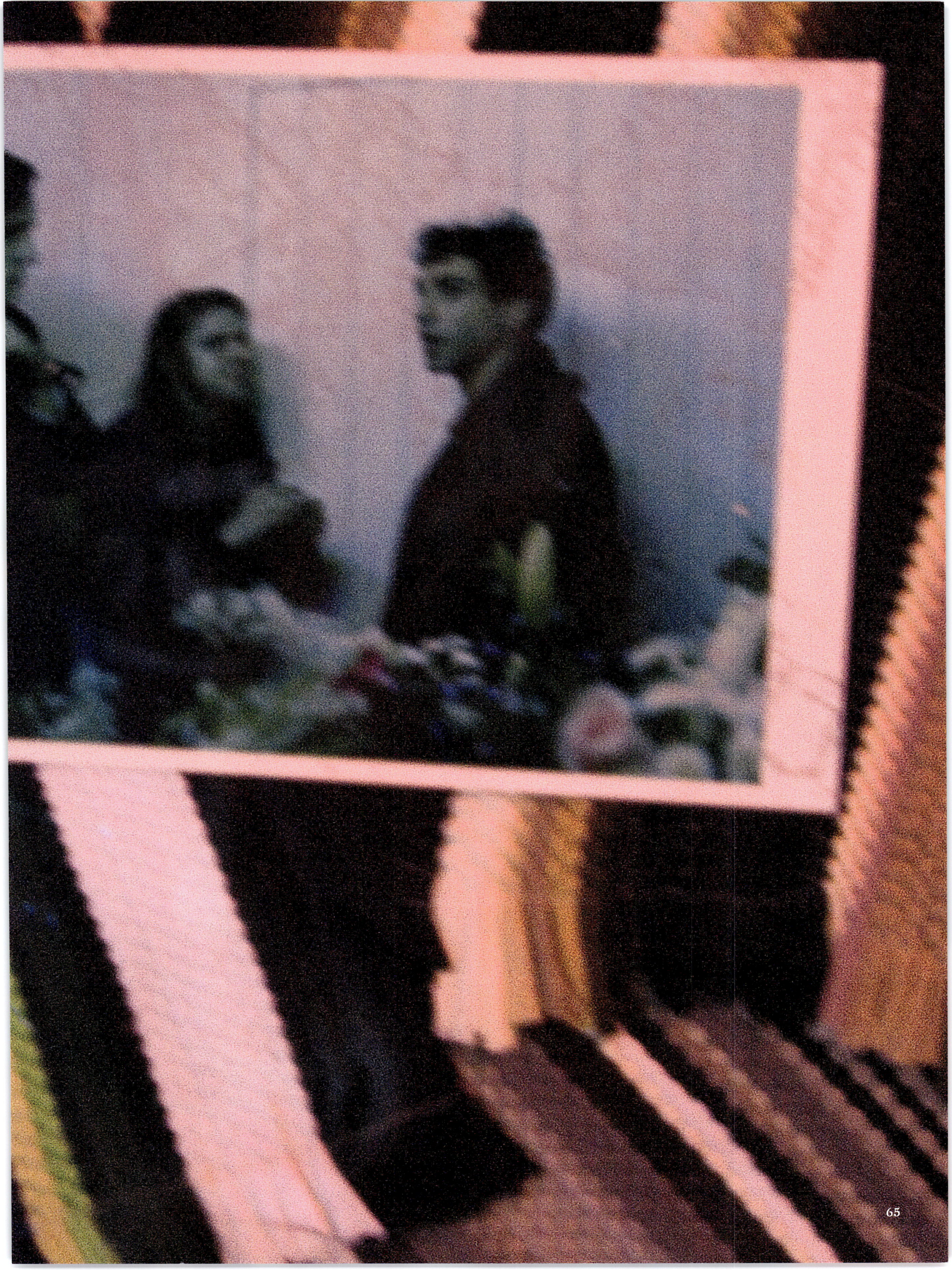

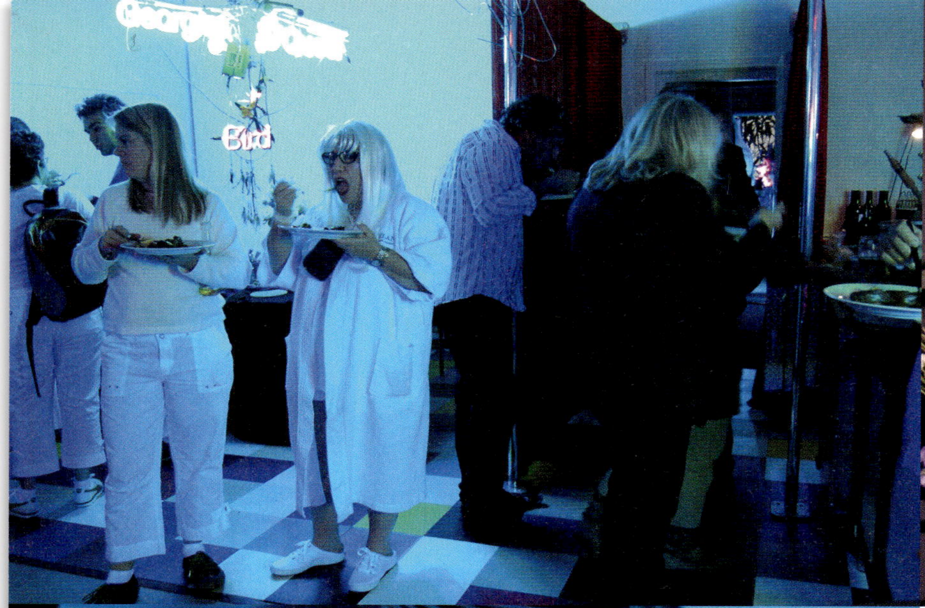
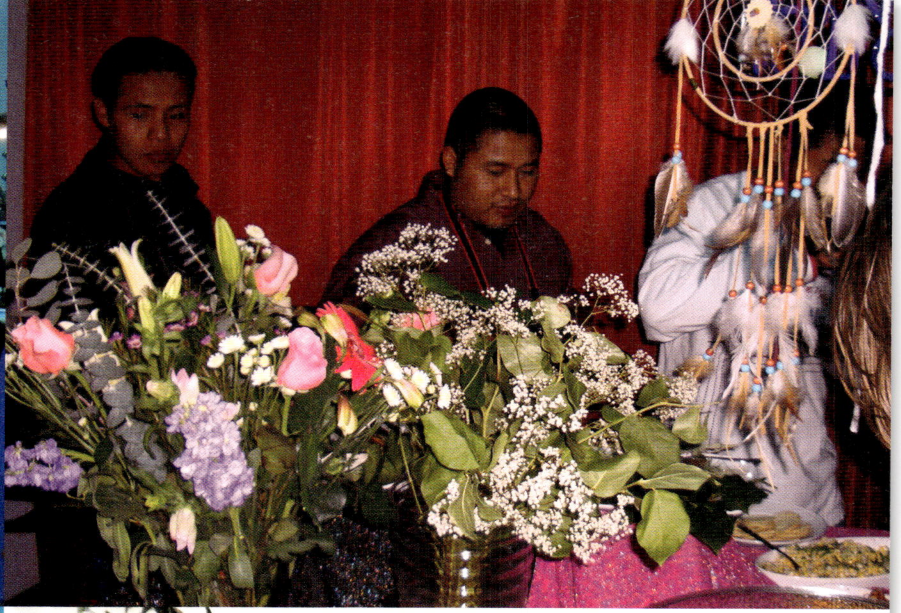
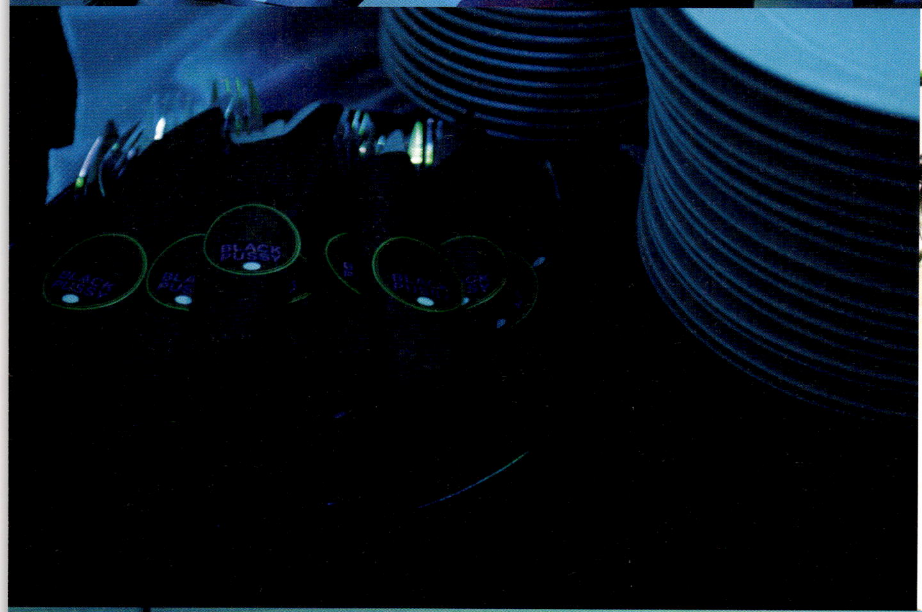
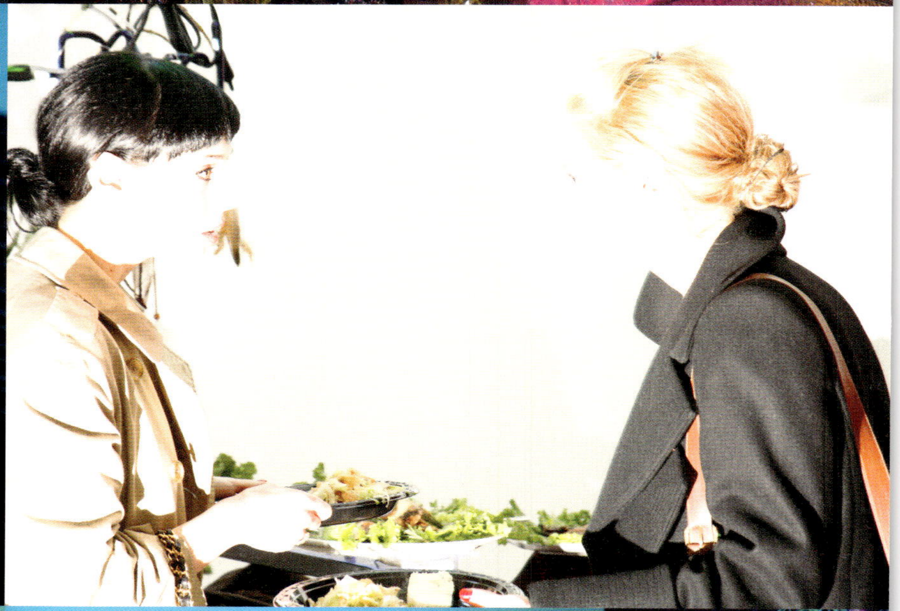
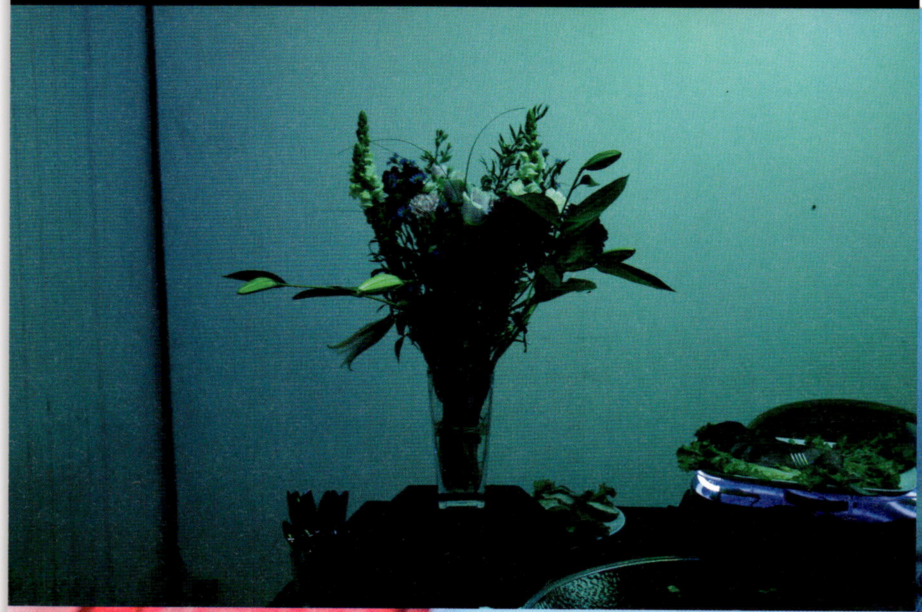
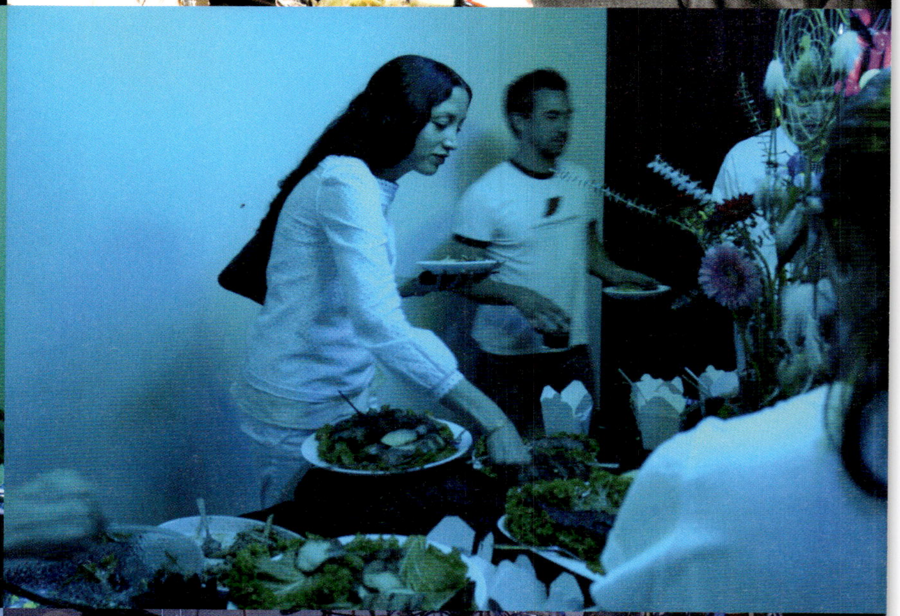
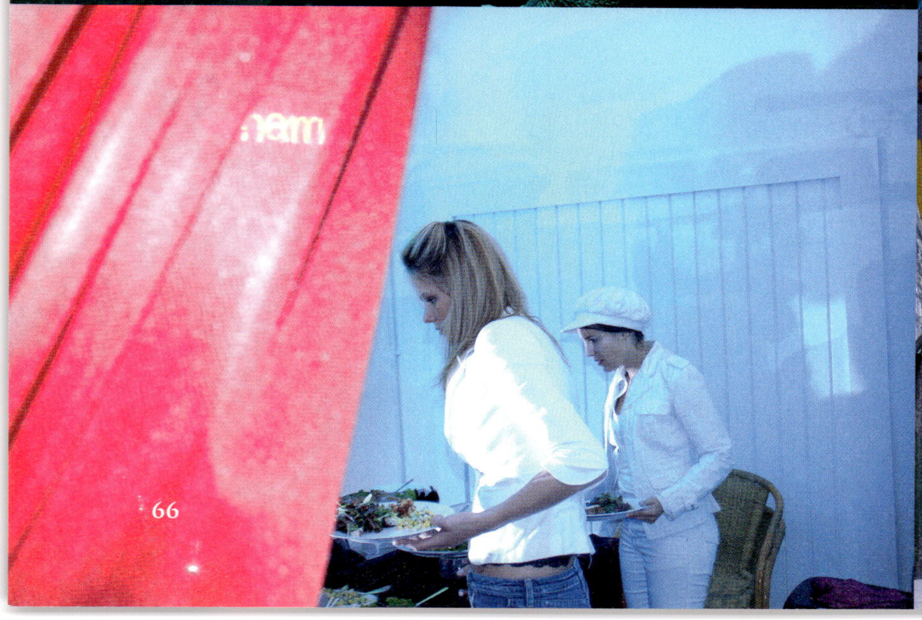
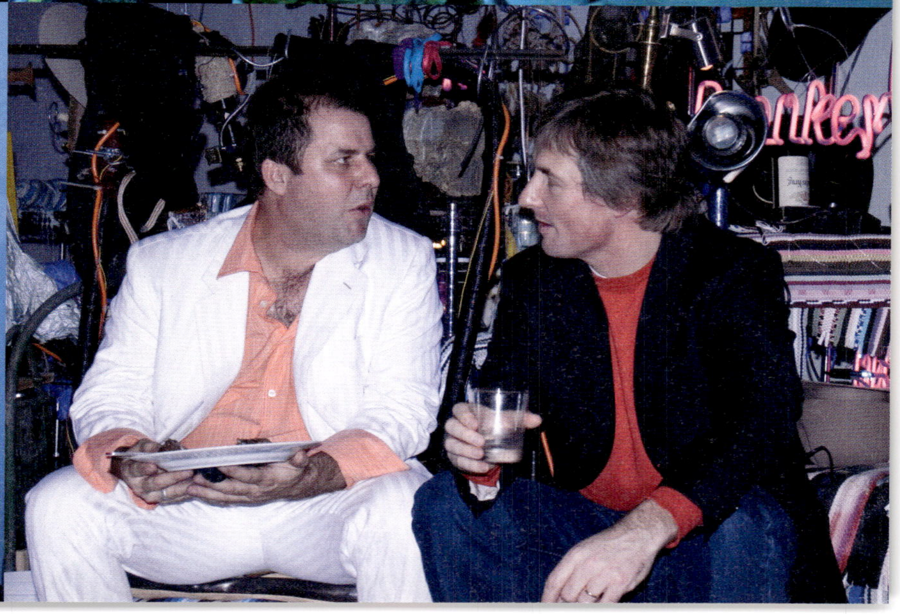

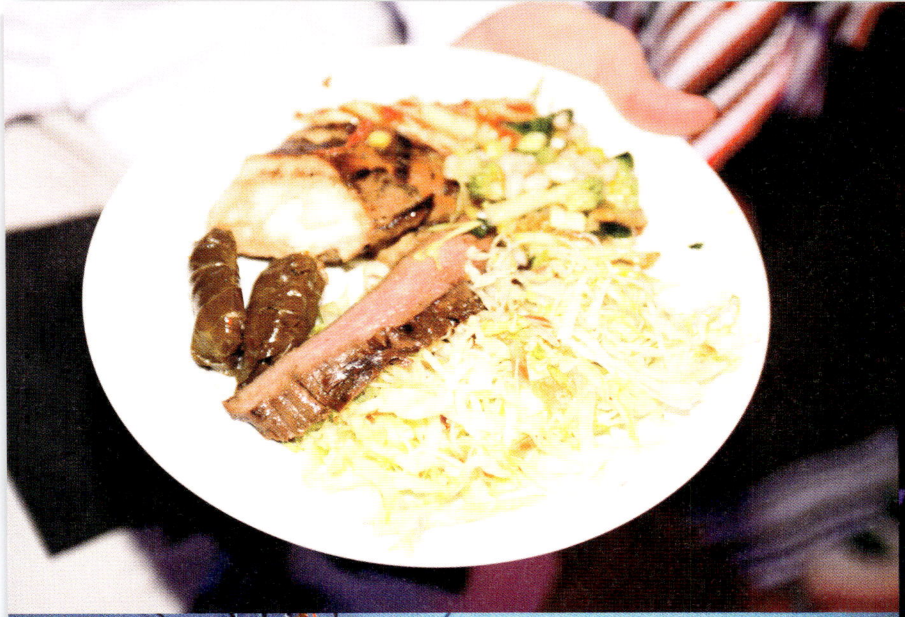

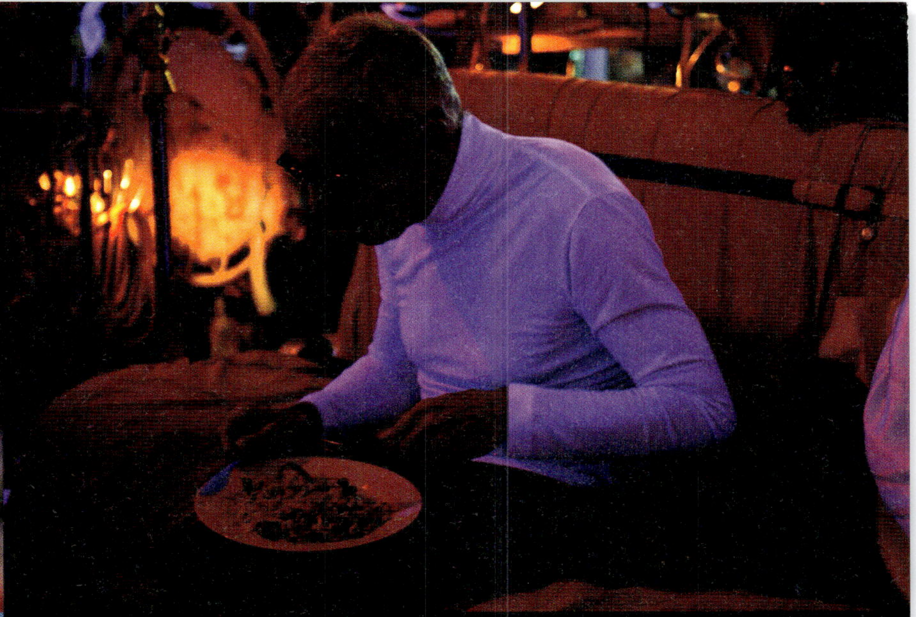

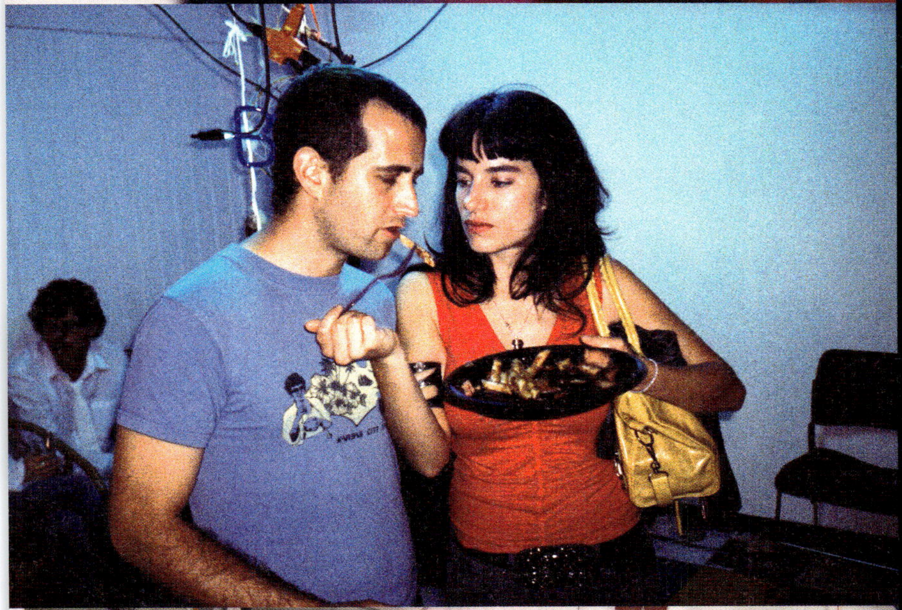

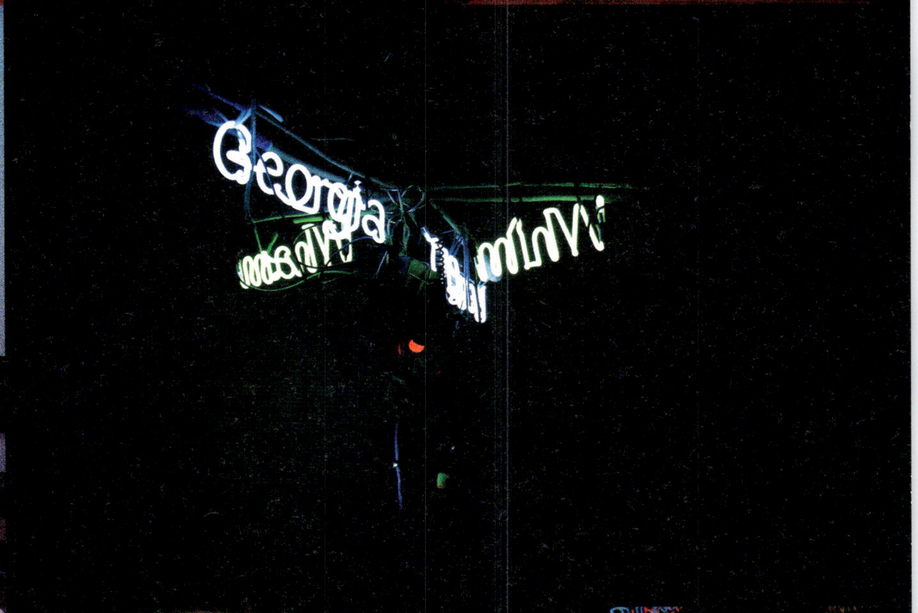
Georgia

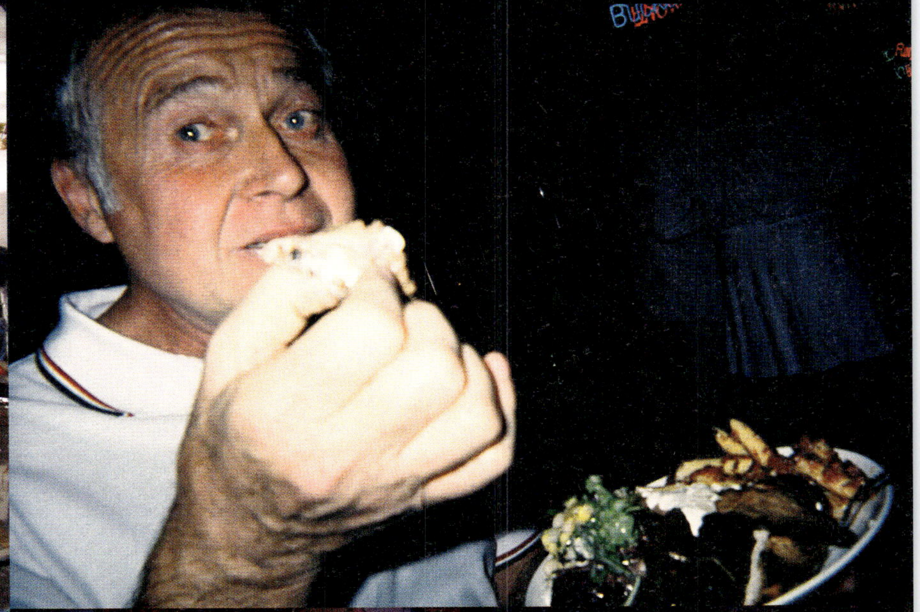

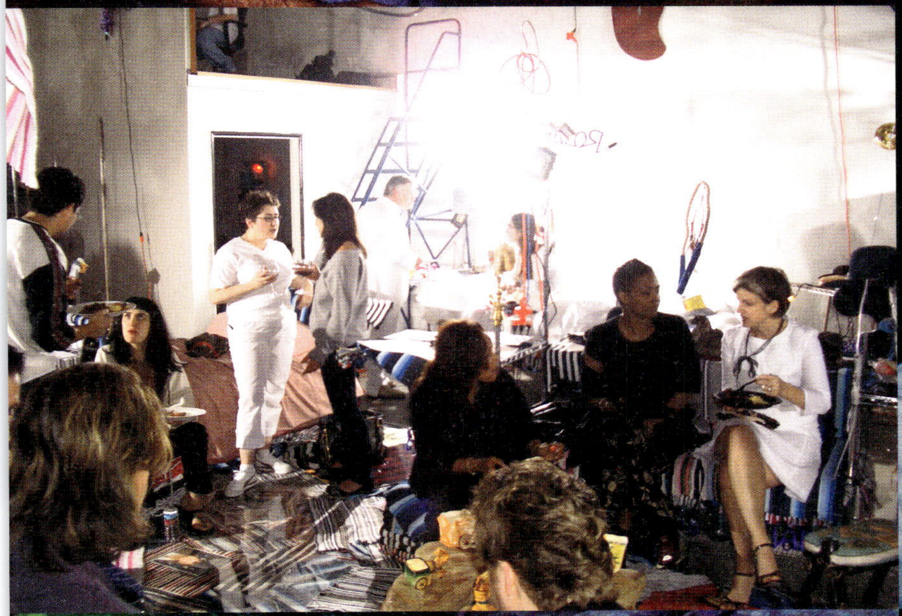

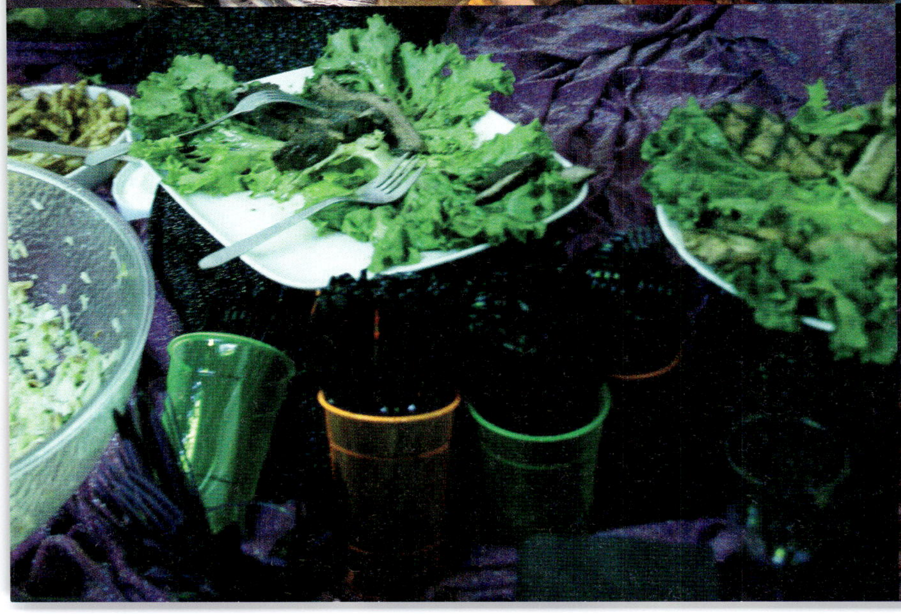

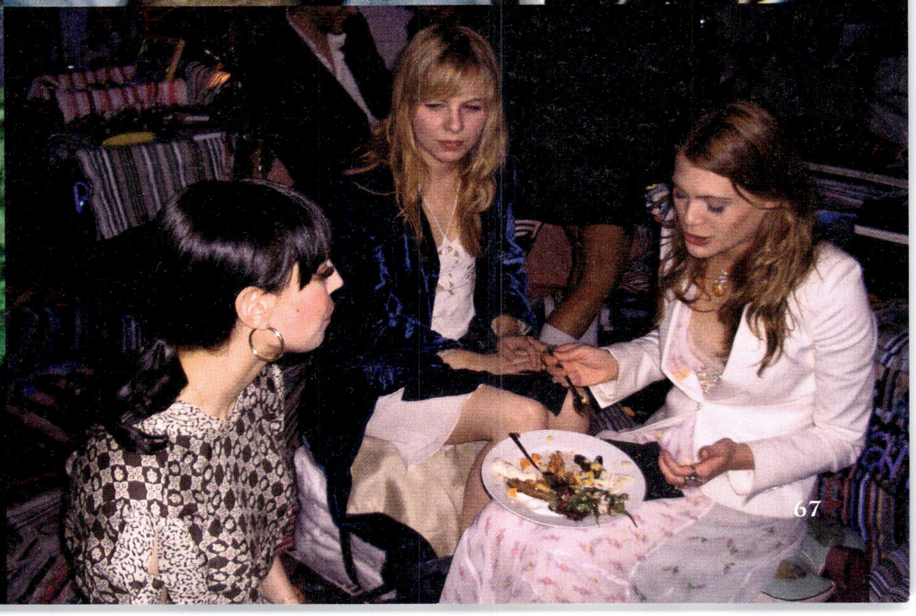

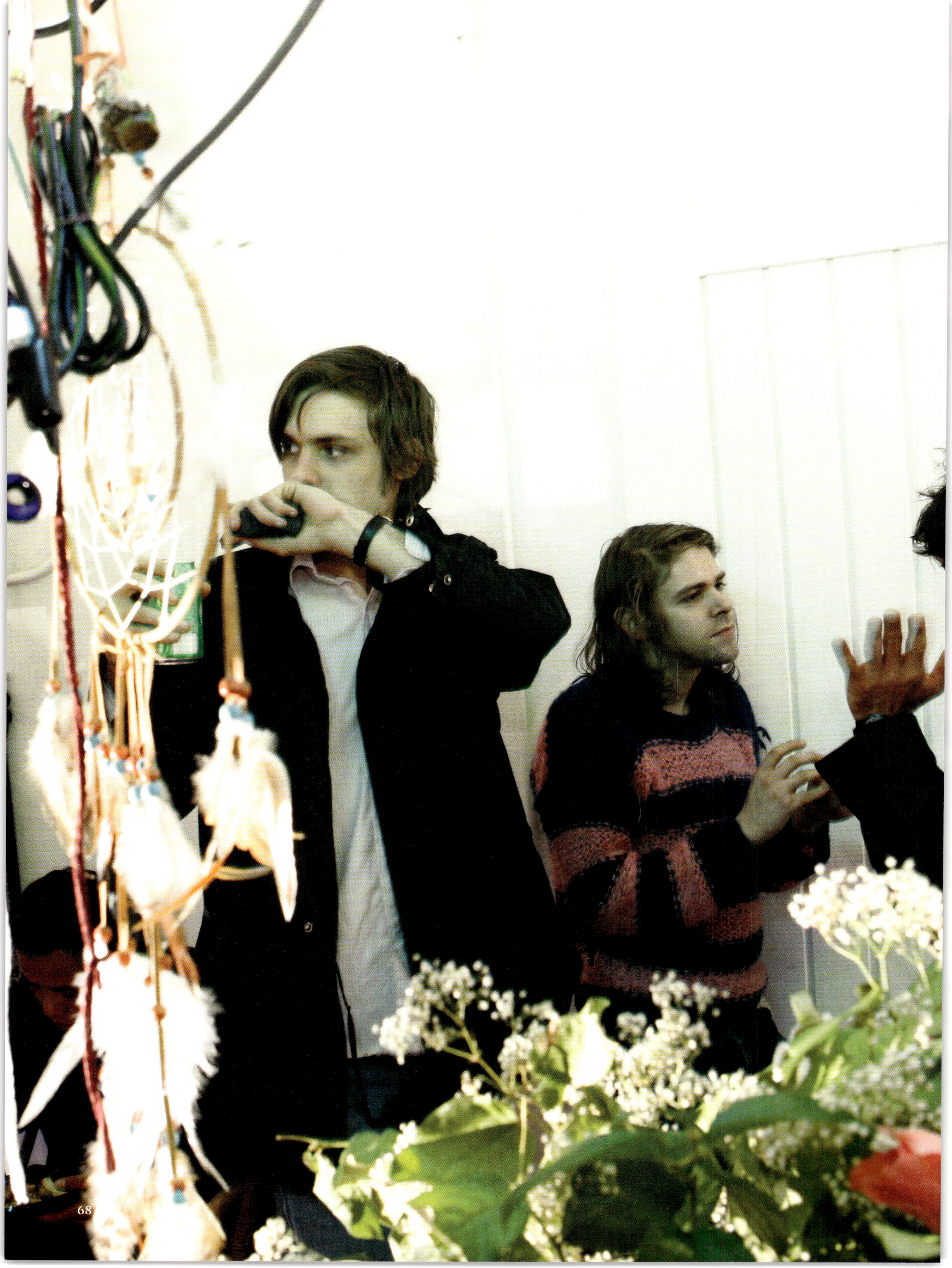

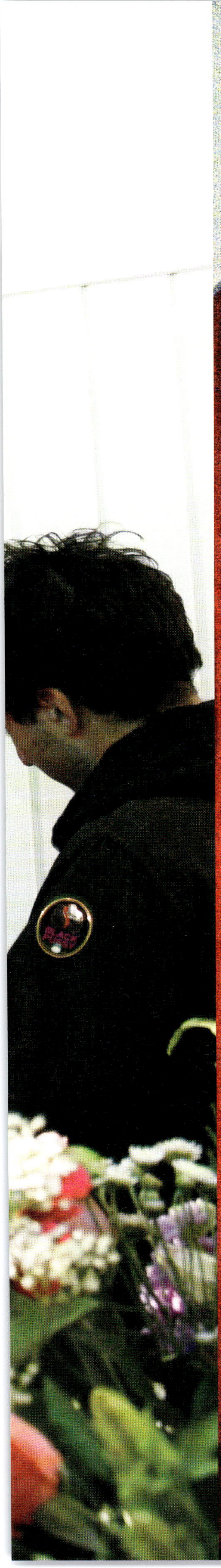
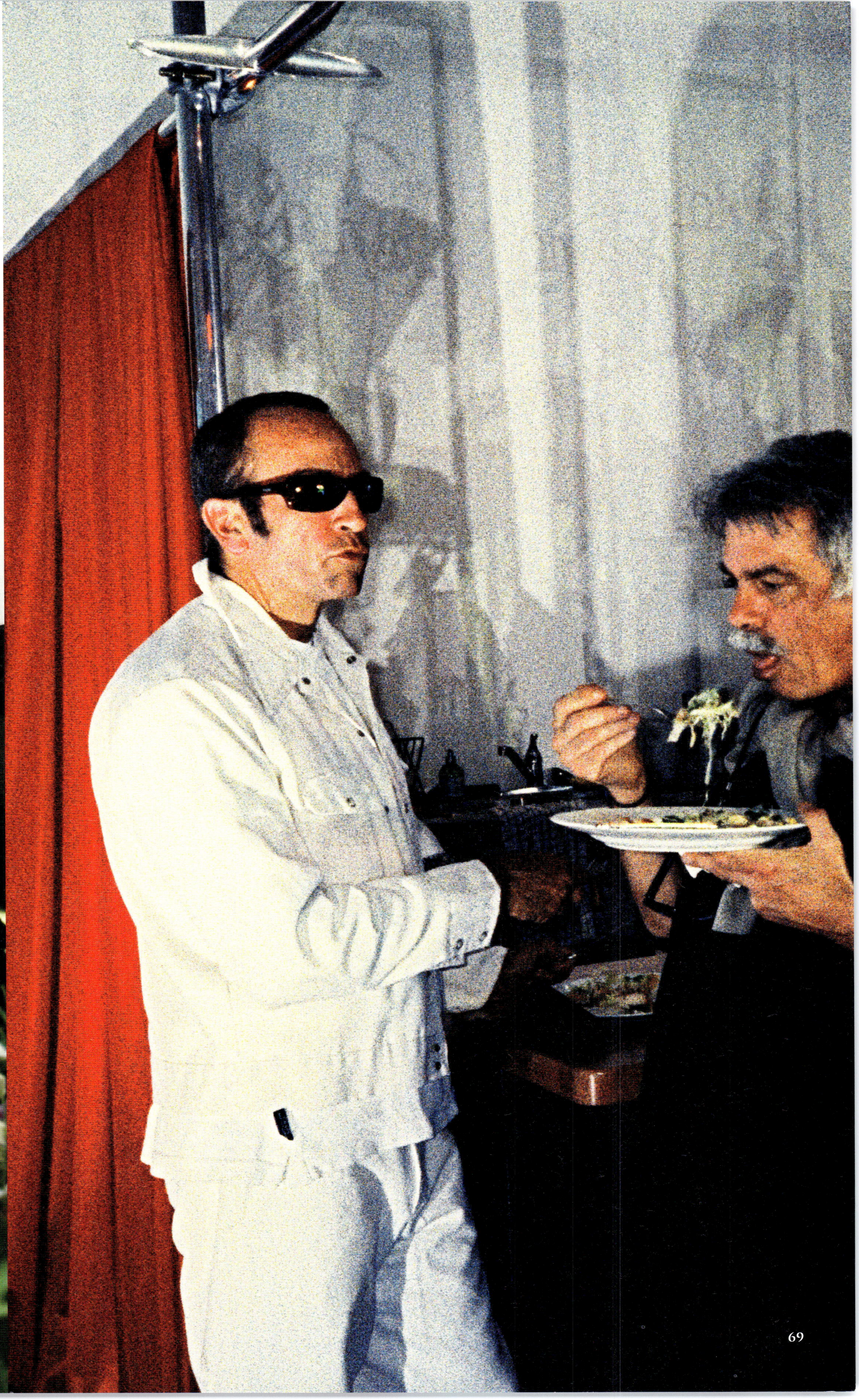

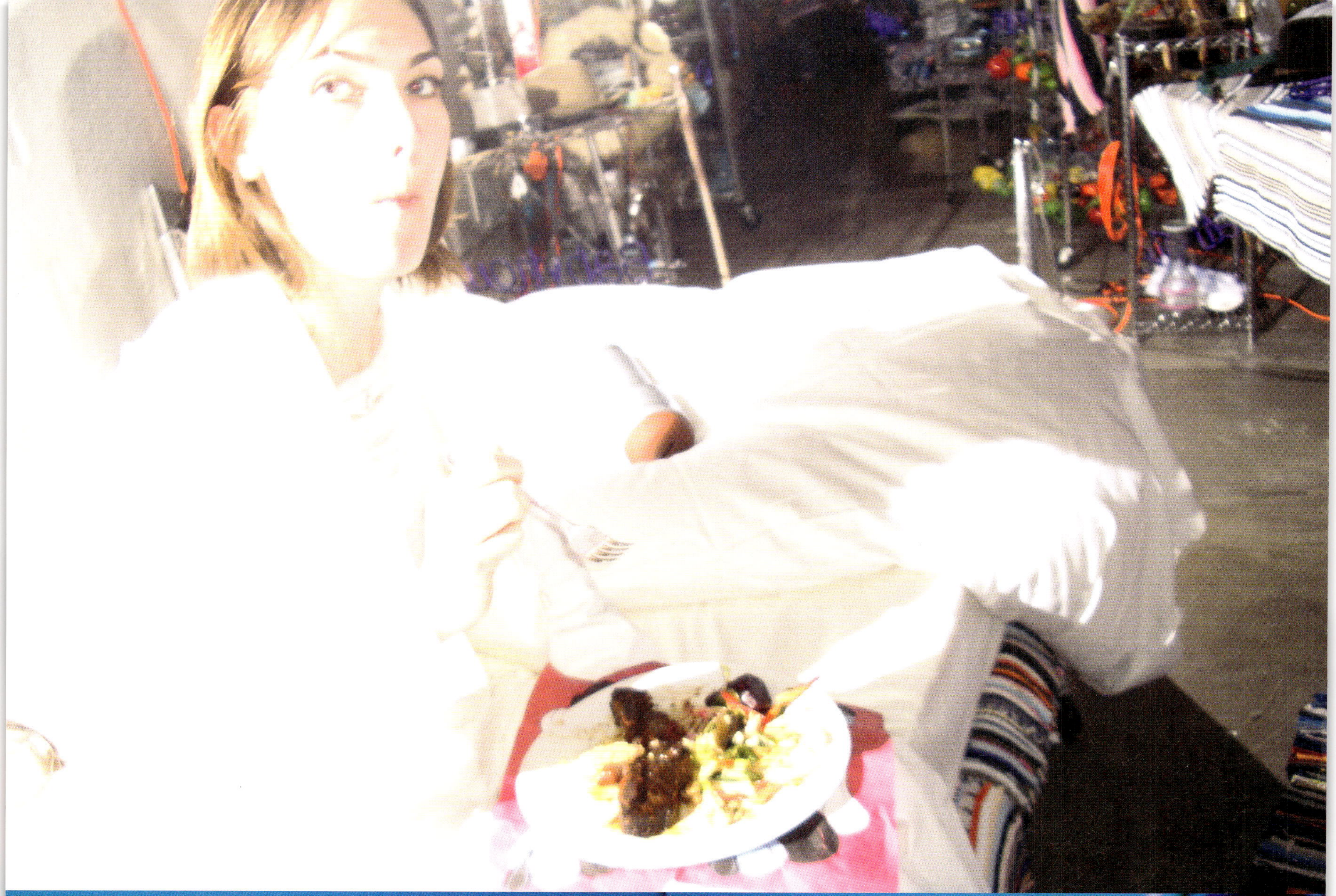

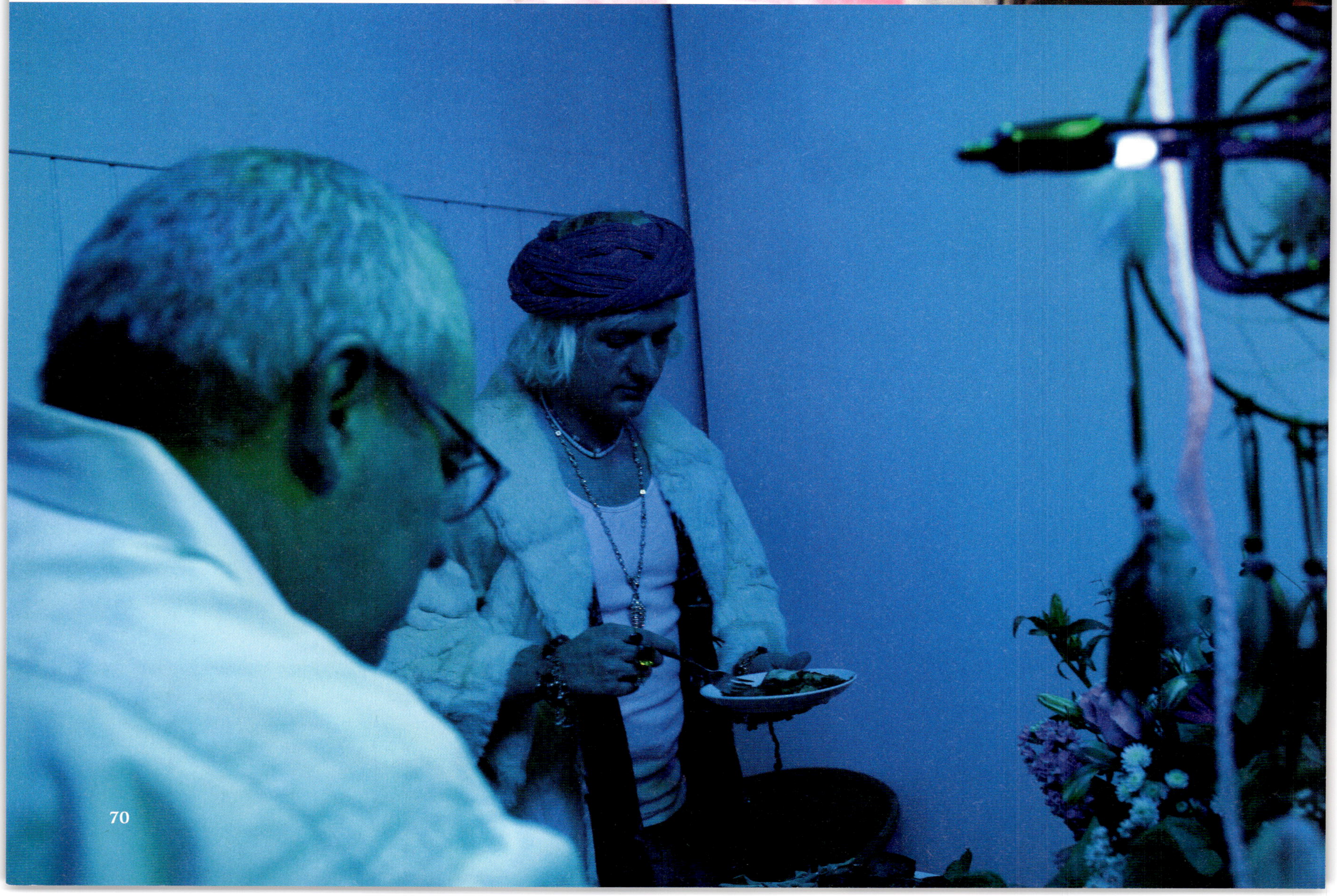

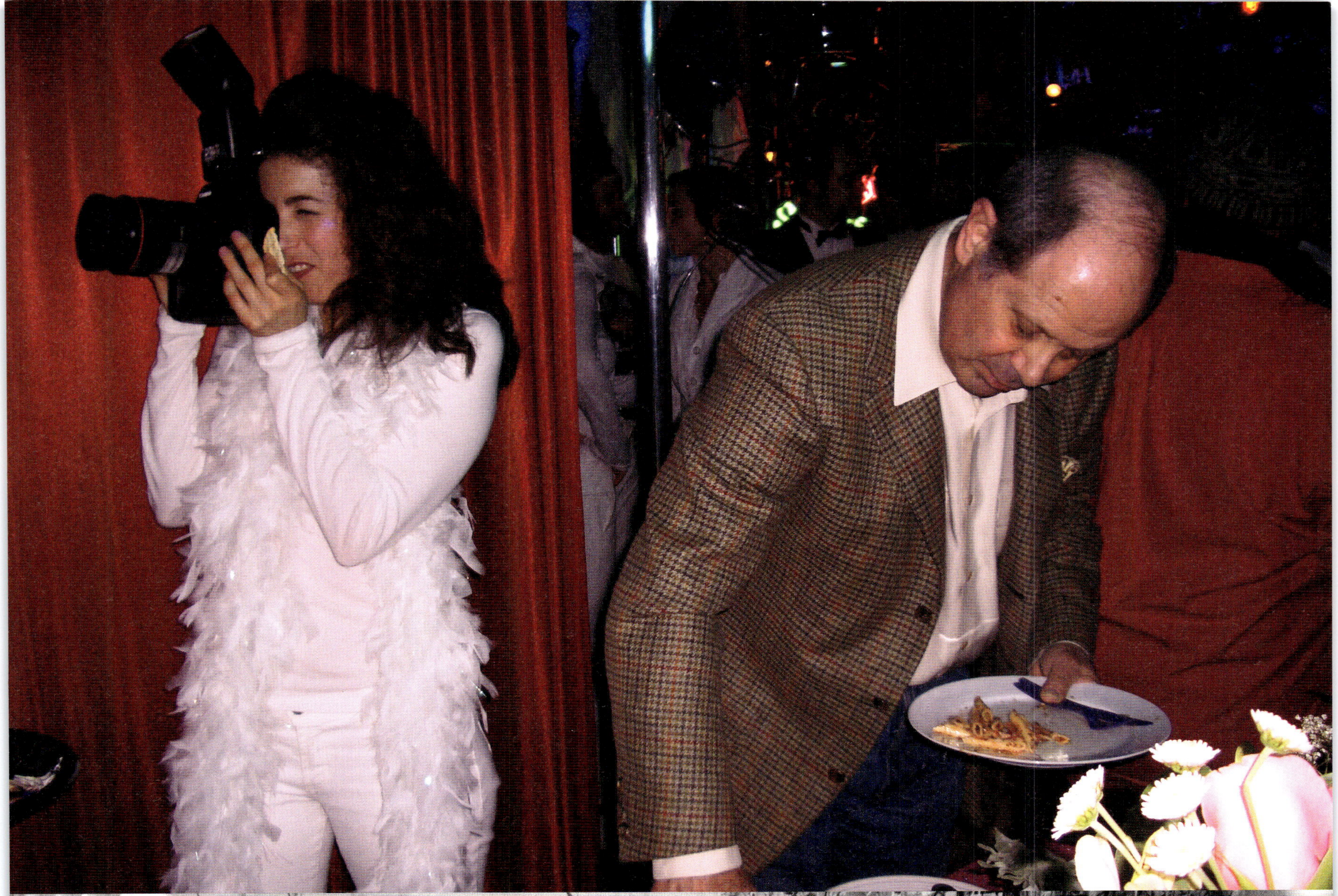

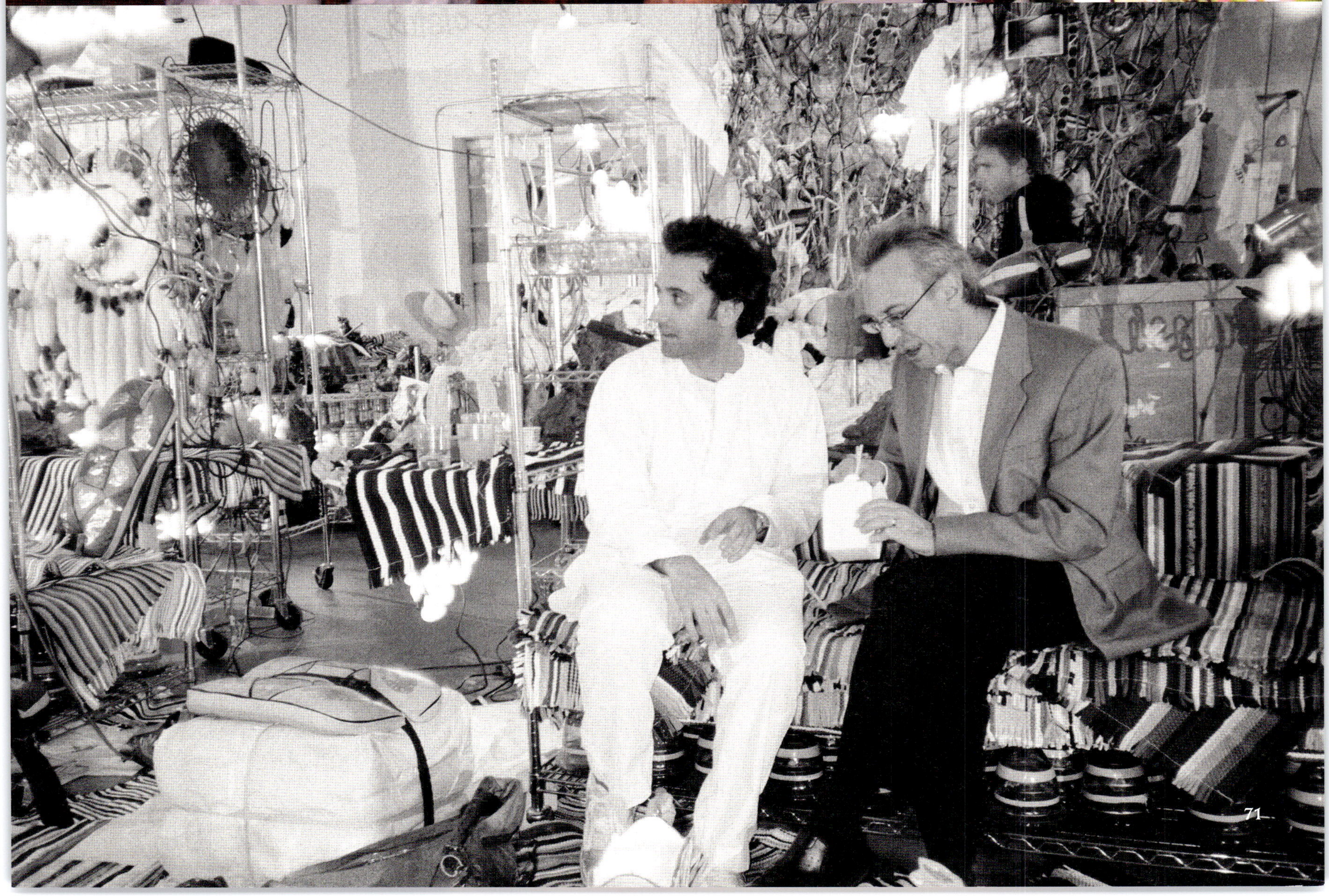

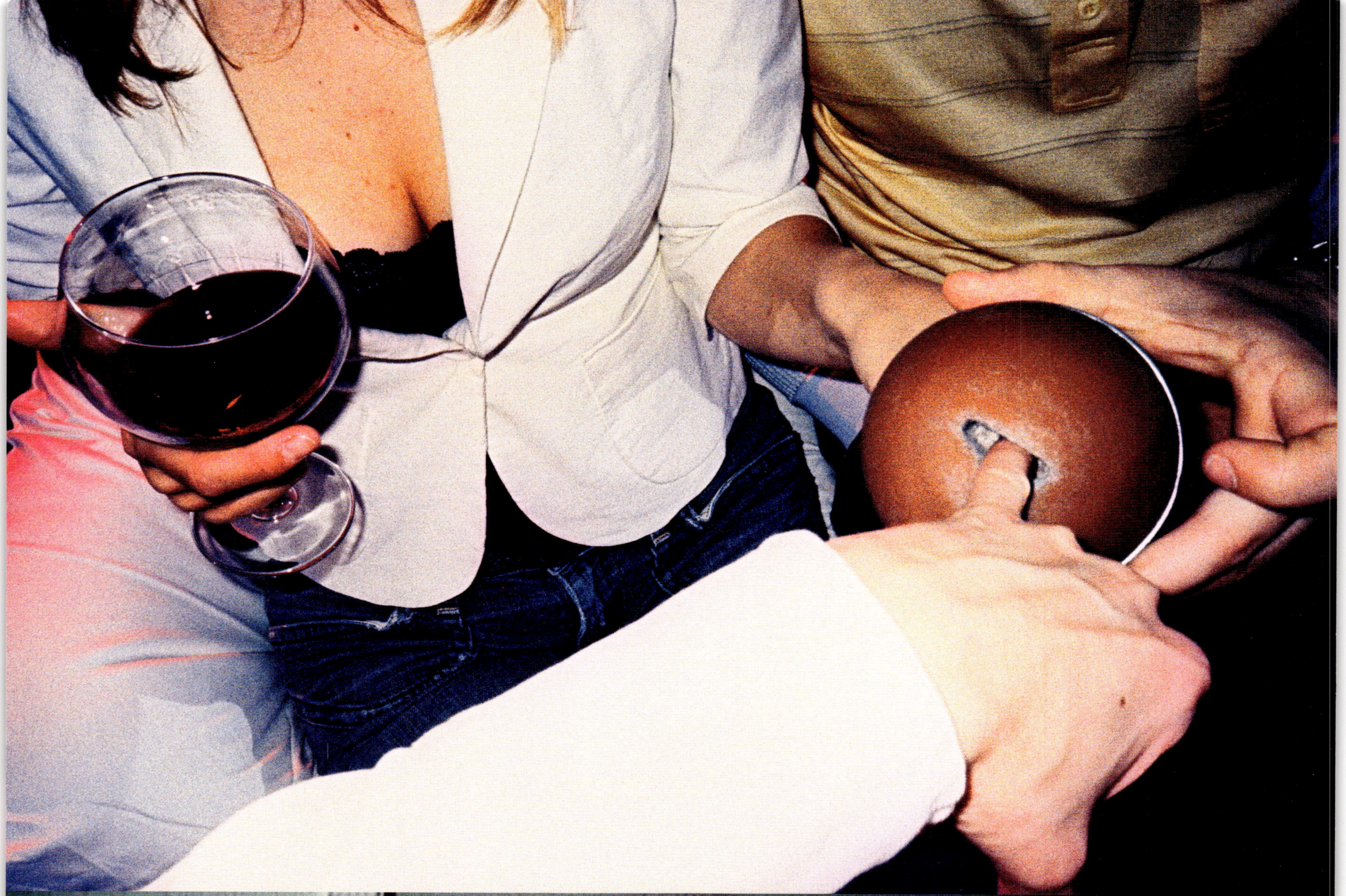

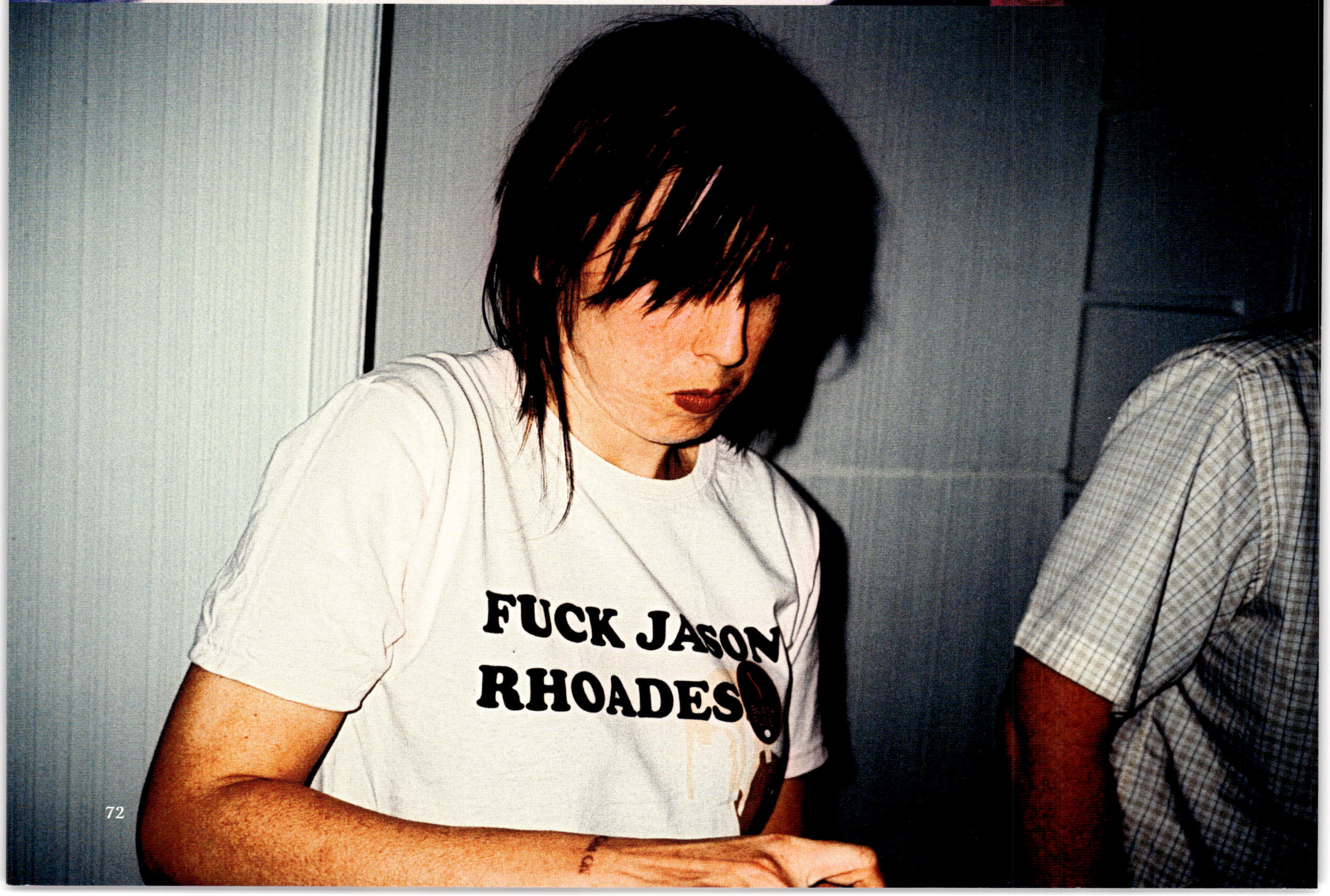
FUCK JASON
RHOADES

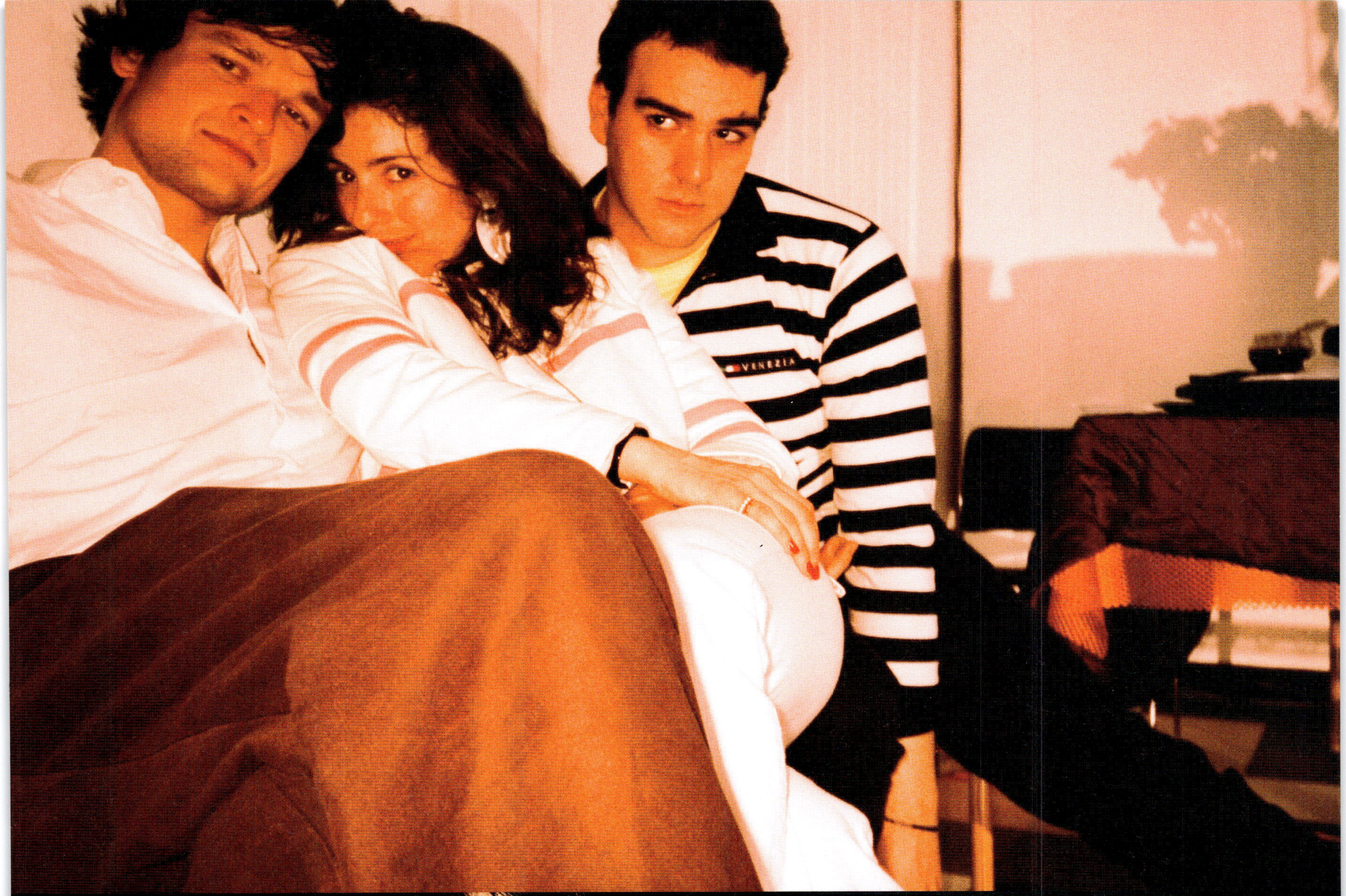
VENEZIA

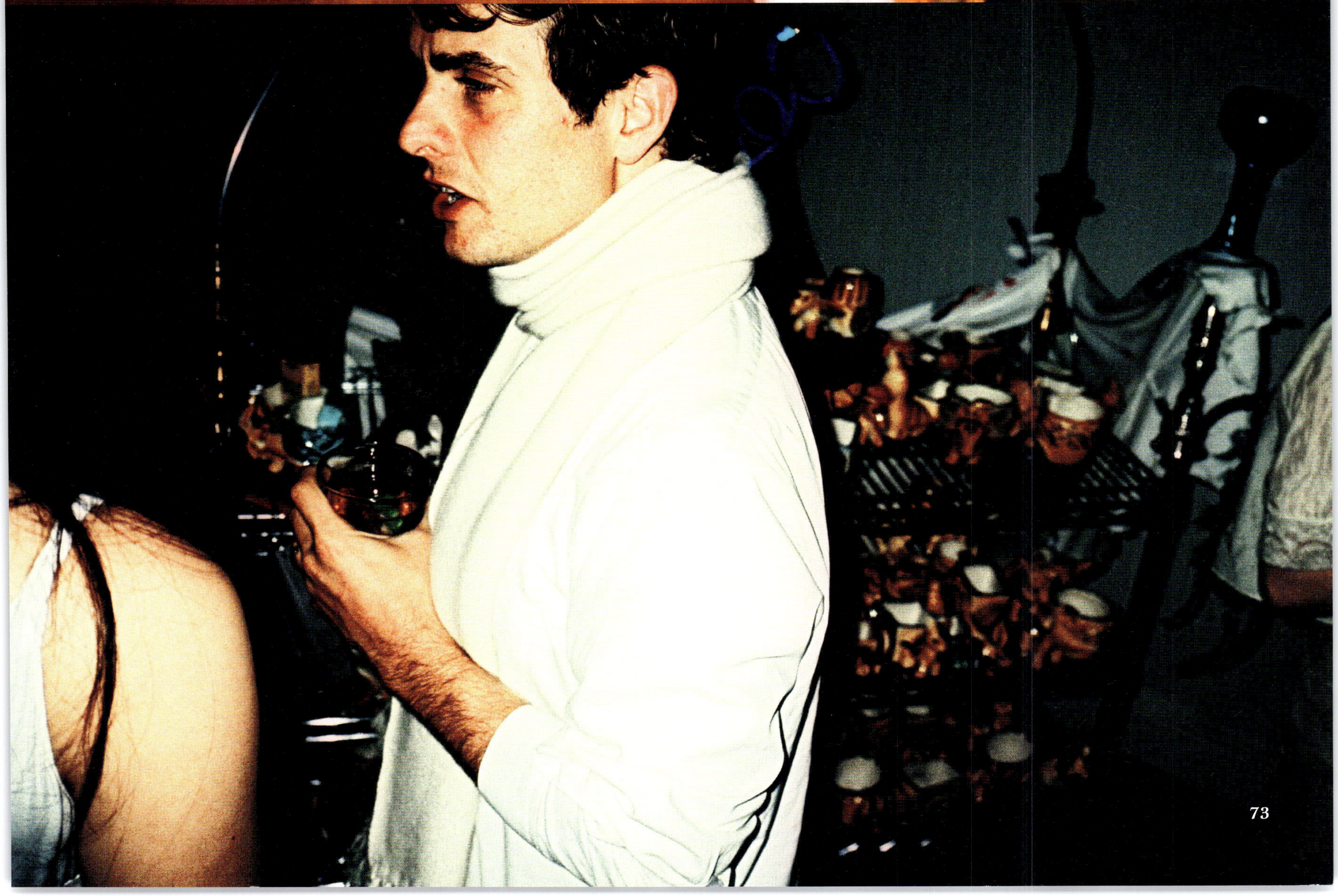

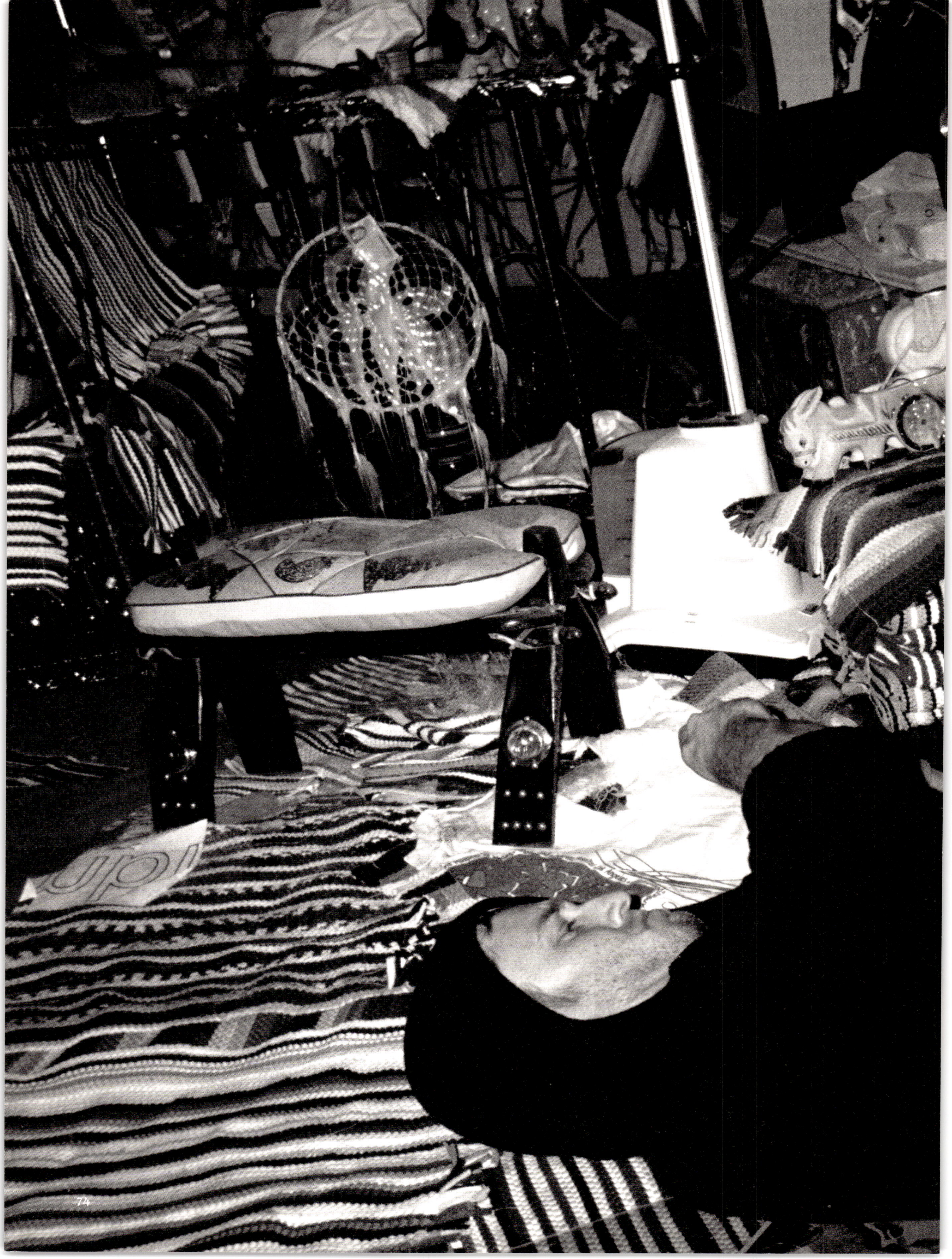

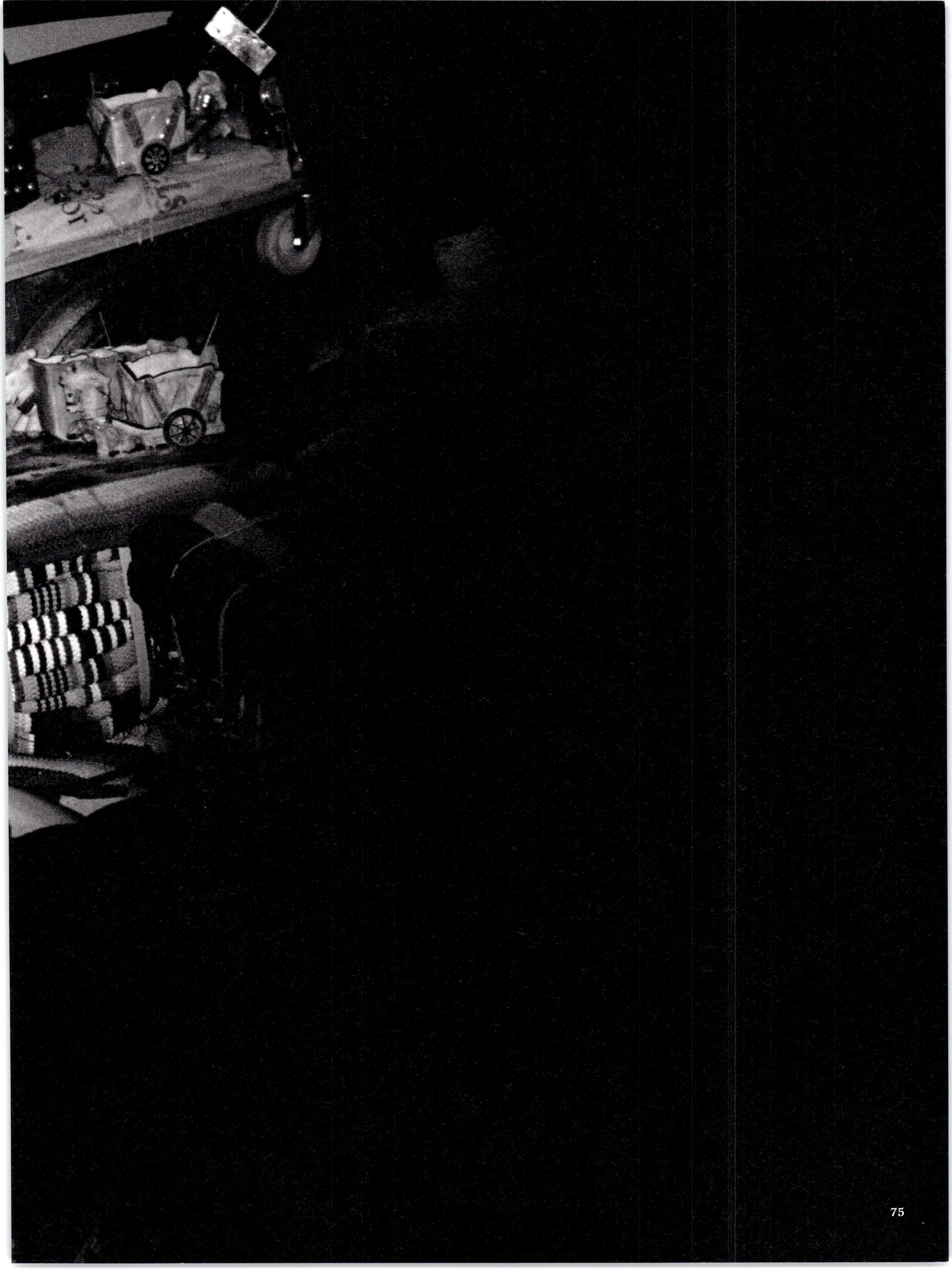

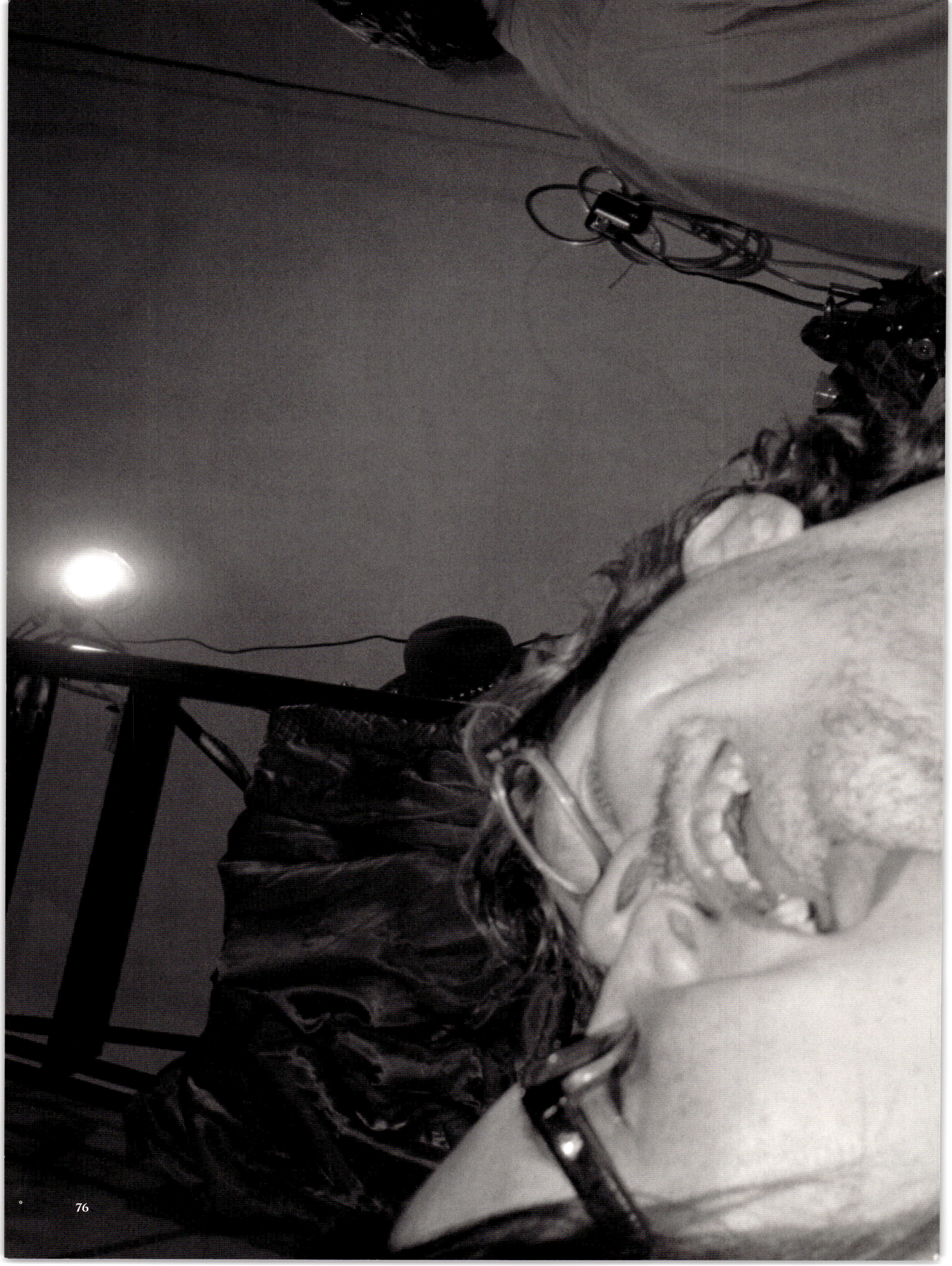

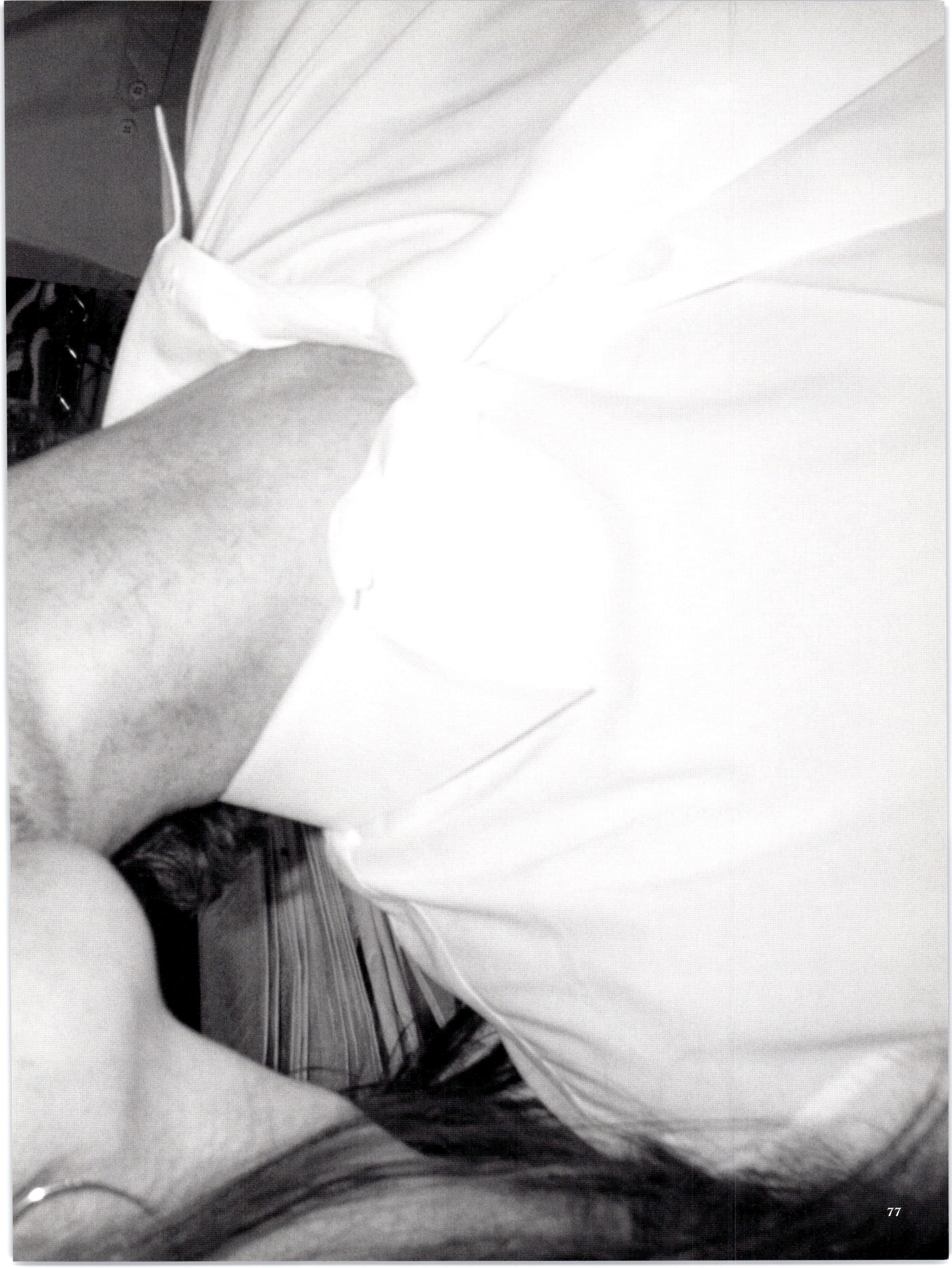

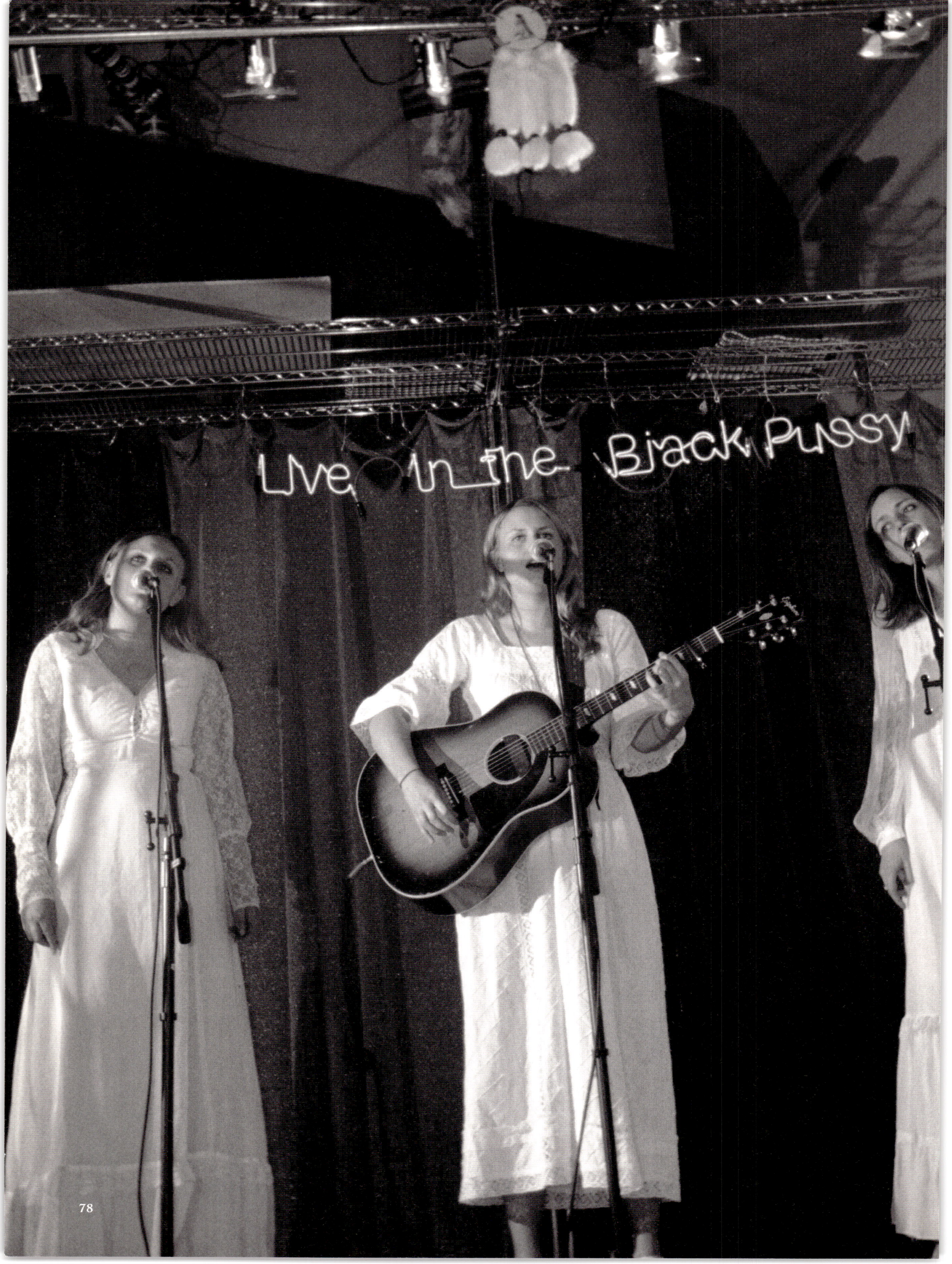
Live in the Black Pussy

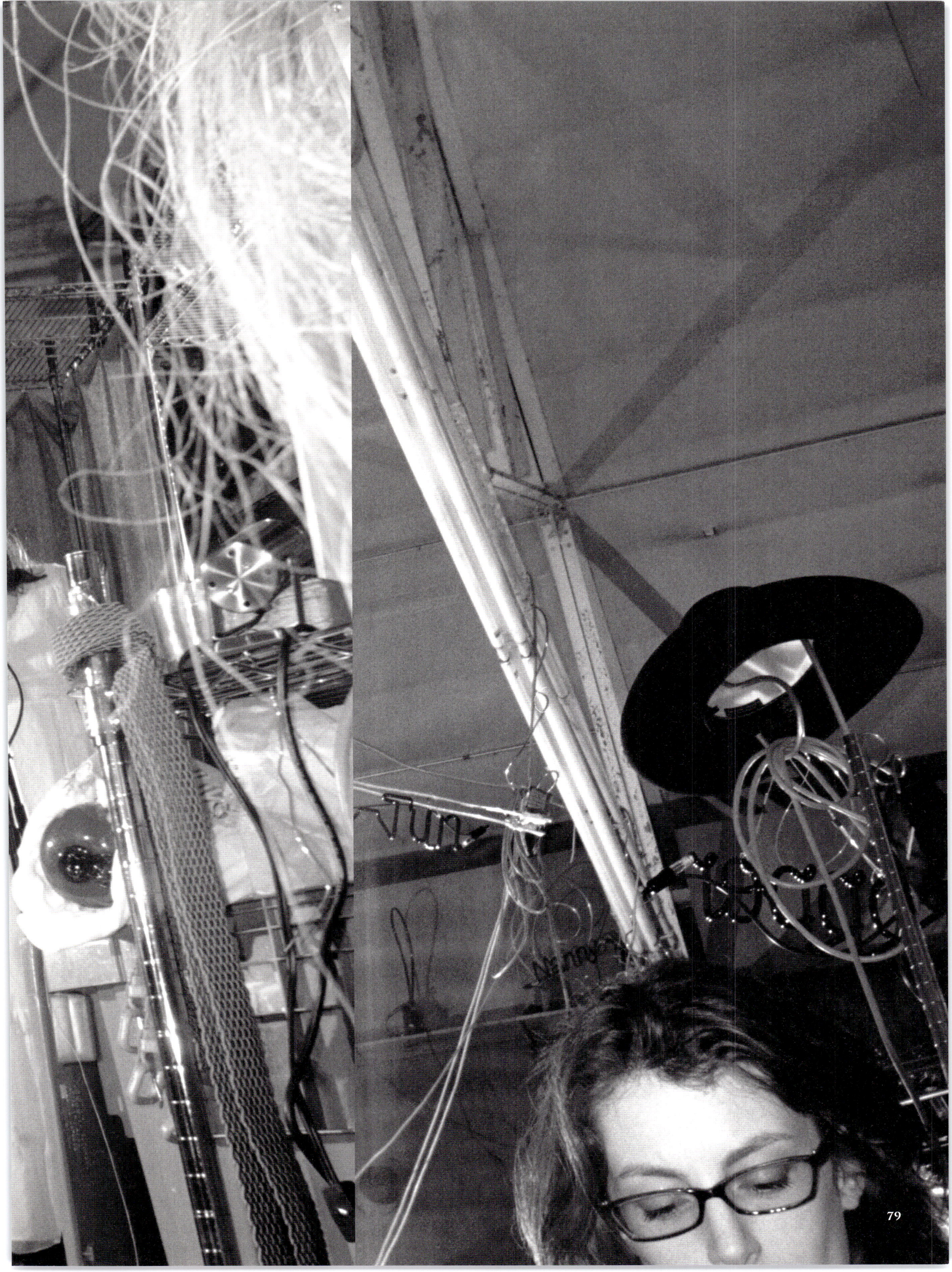

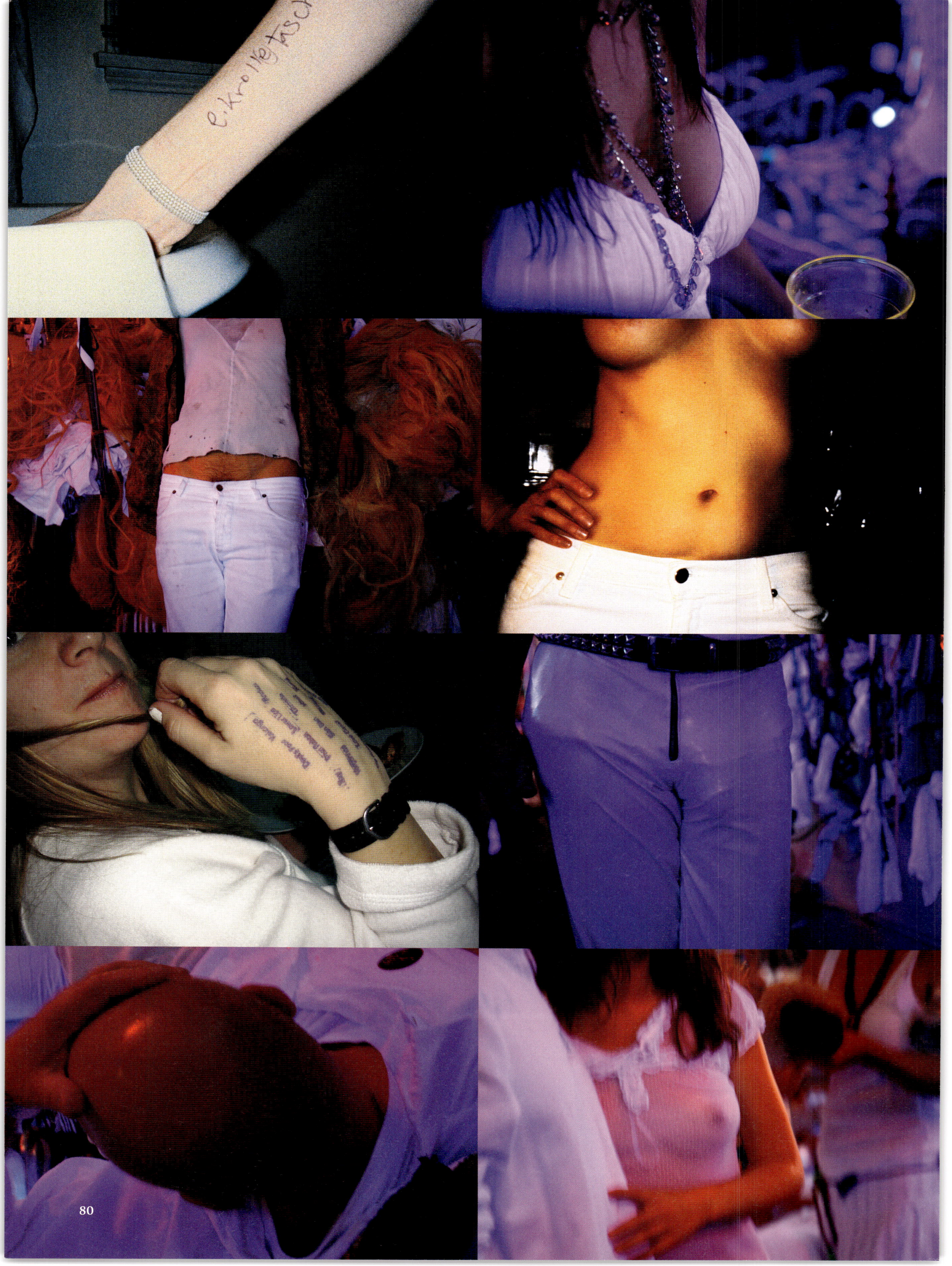

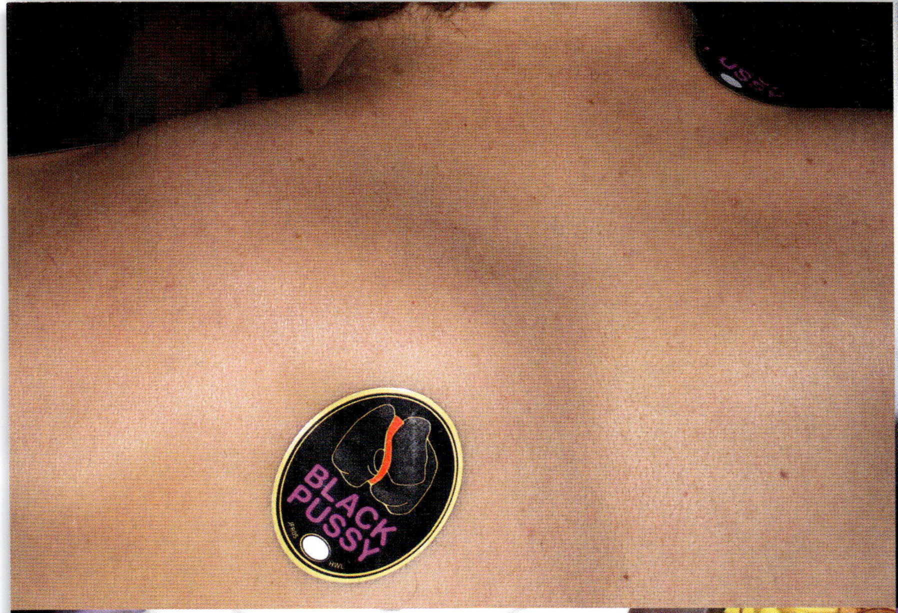
BLACK PUSSY
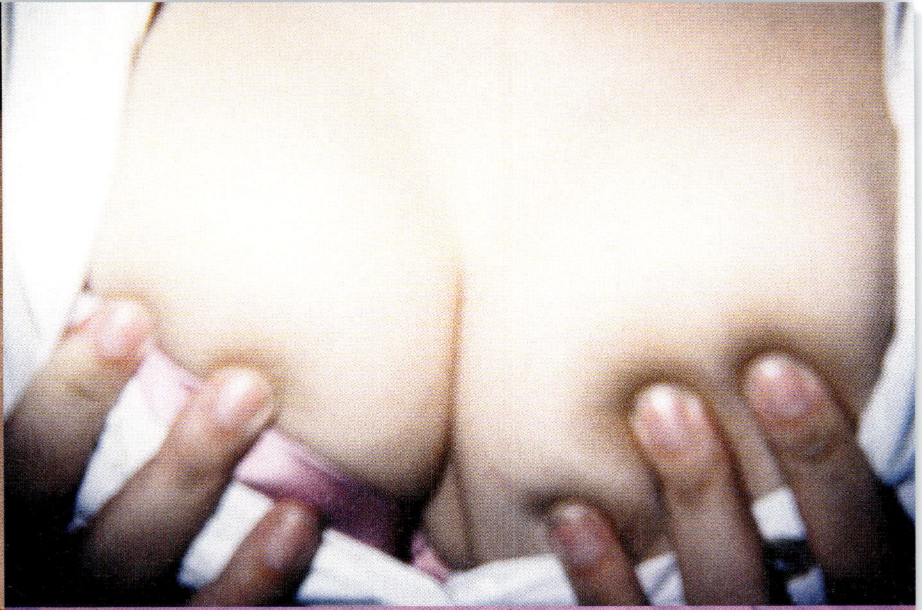
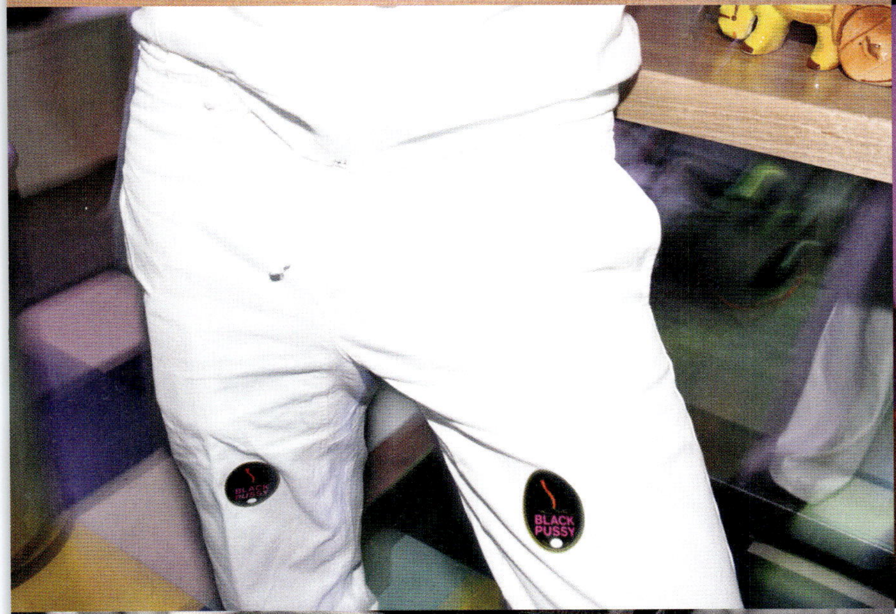
BLACK PUSSY
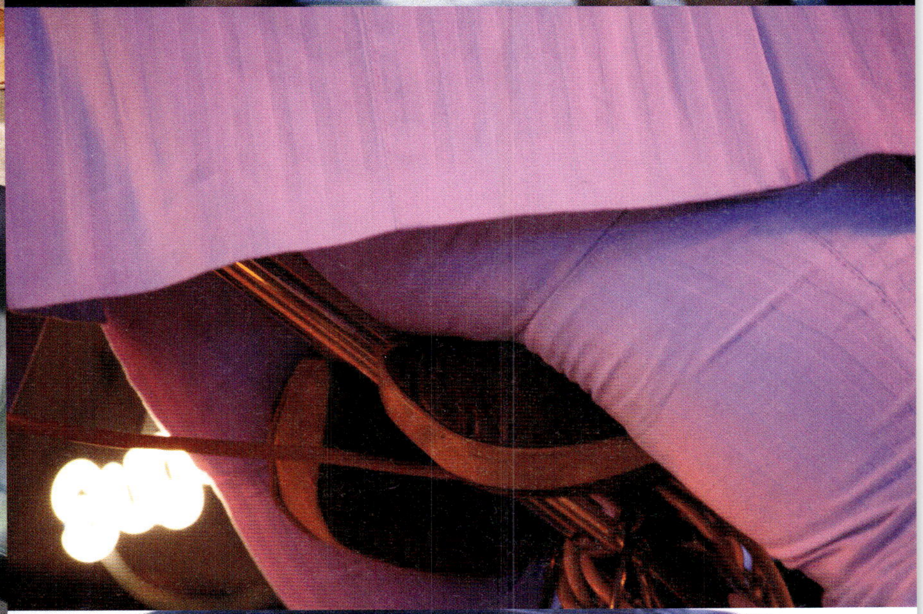
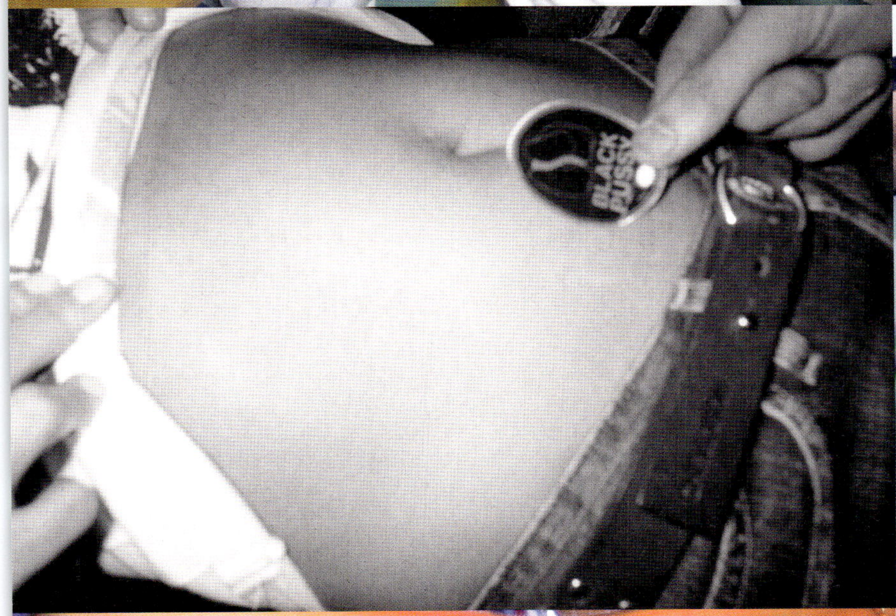
BLACK PUSSY
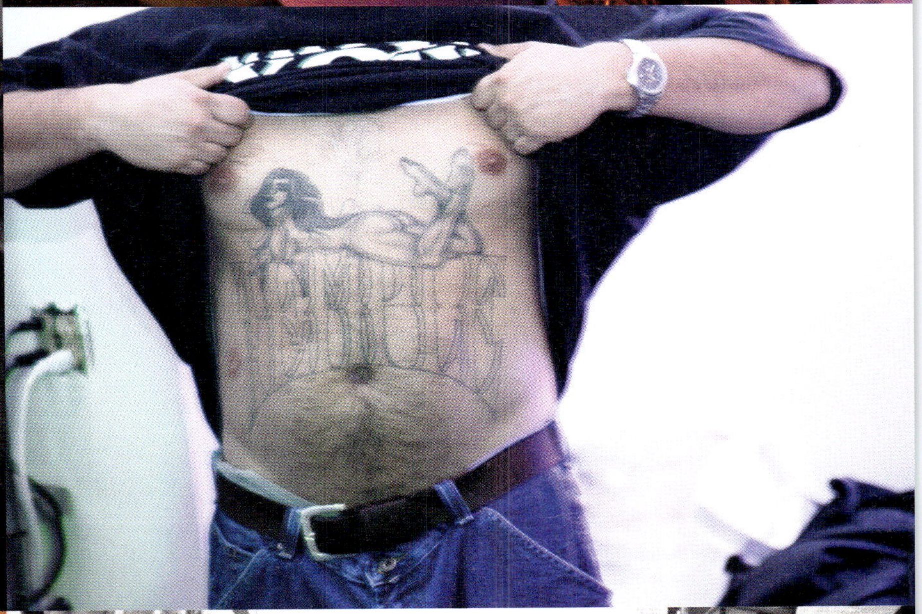
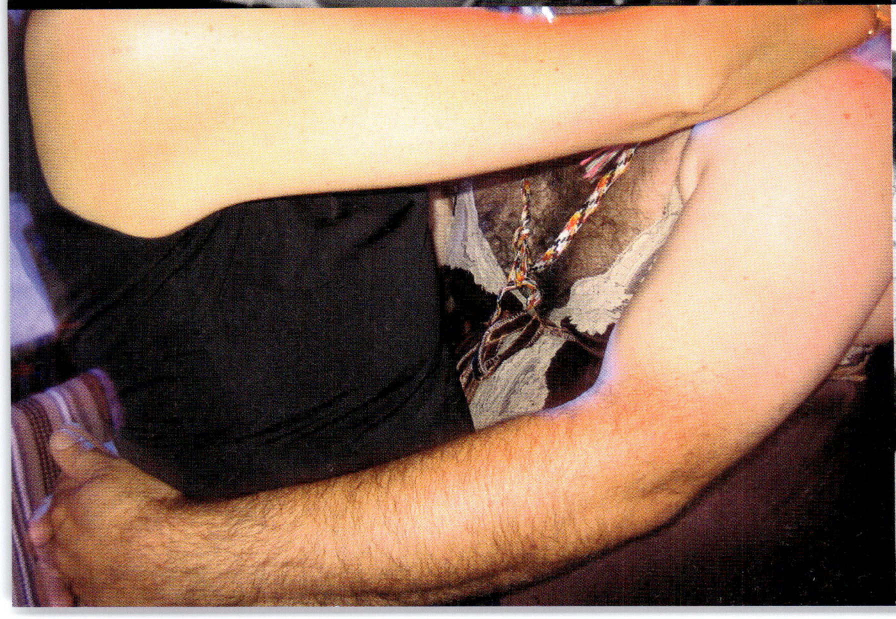
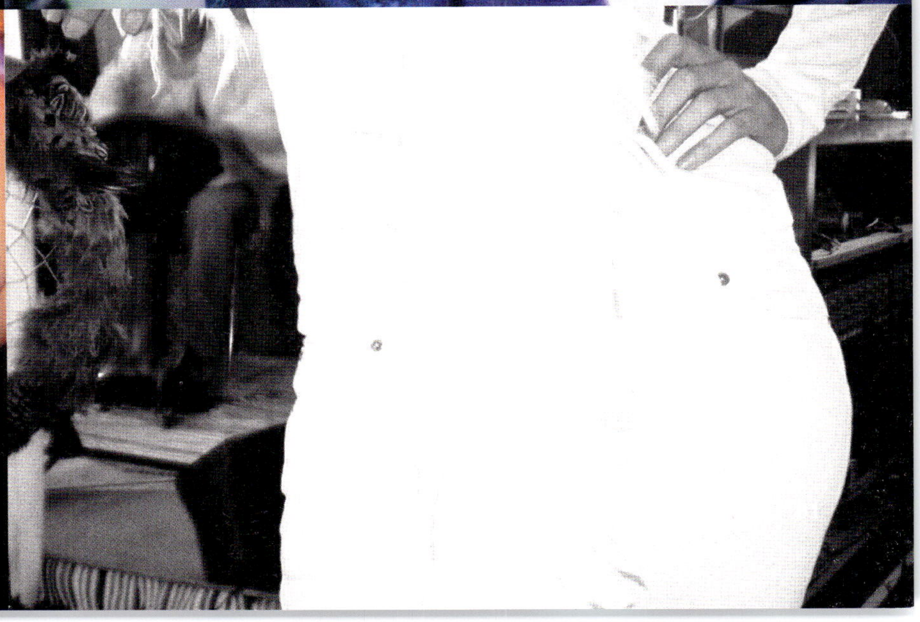

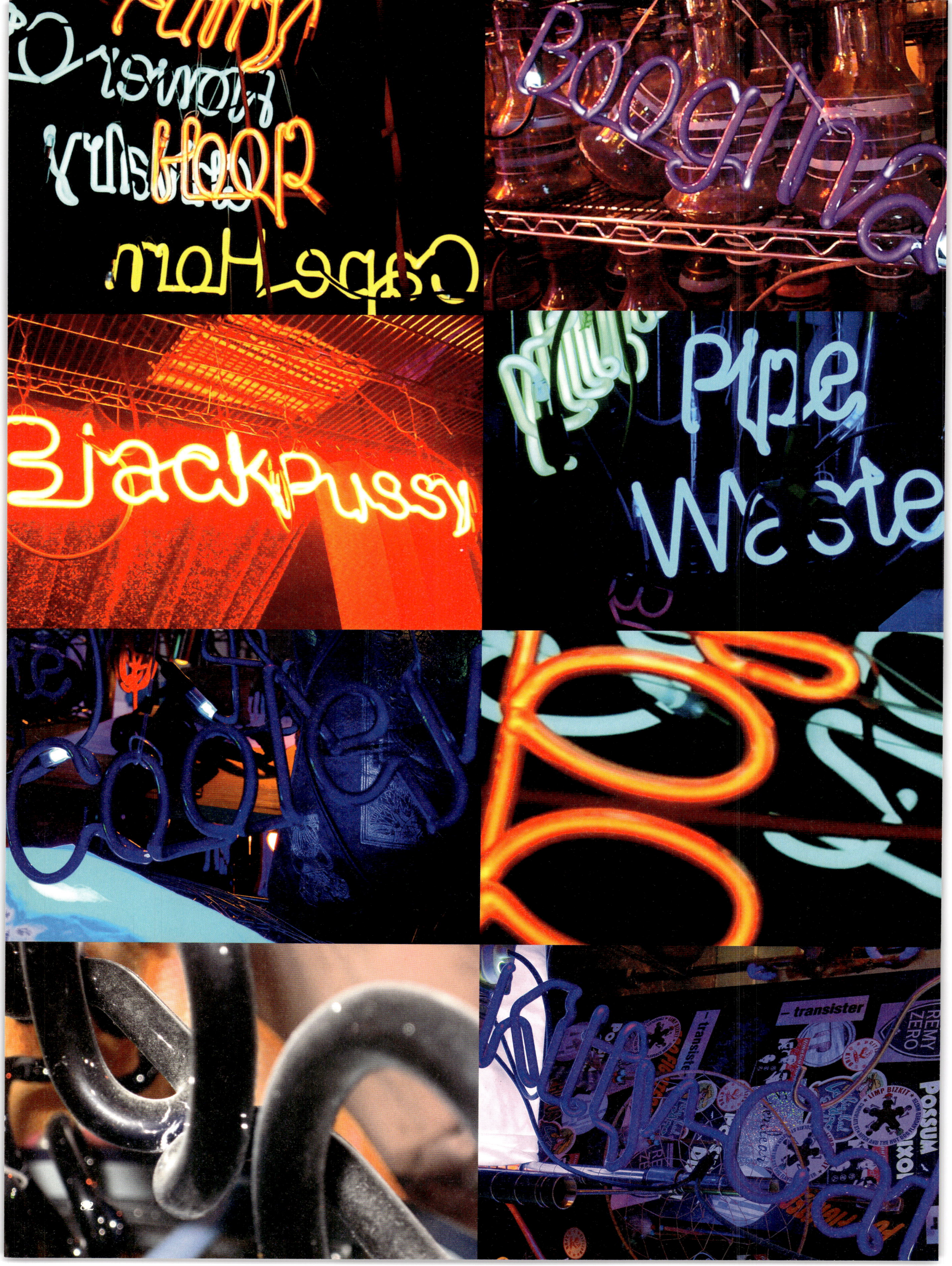
Black Pussy
Pipe
Waste
— transister
REMY ZERO
POSSUM DIXON
LIMP BIZKIT

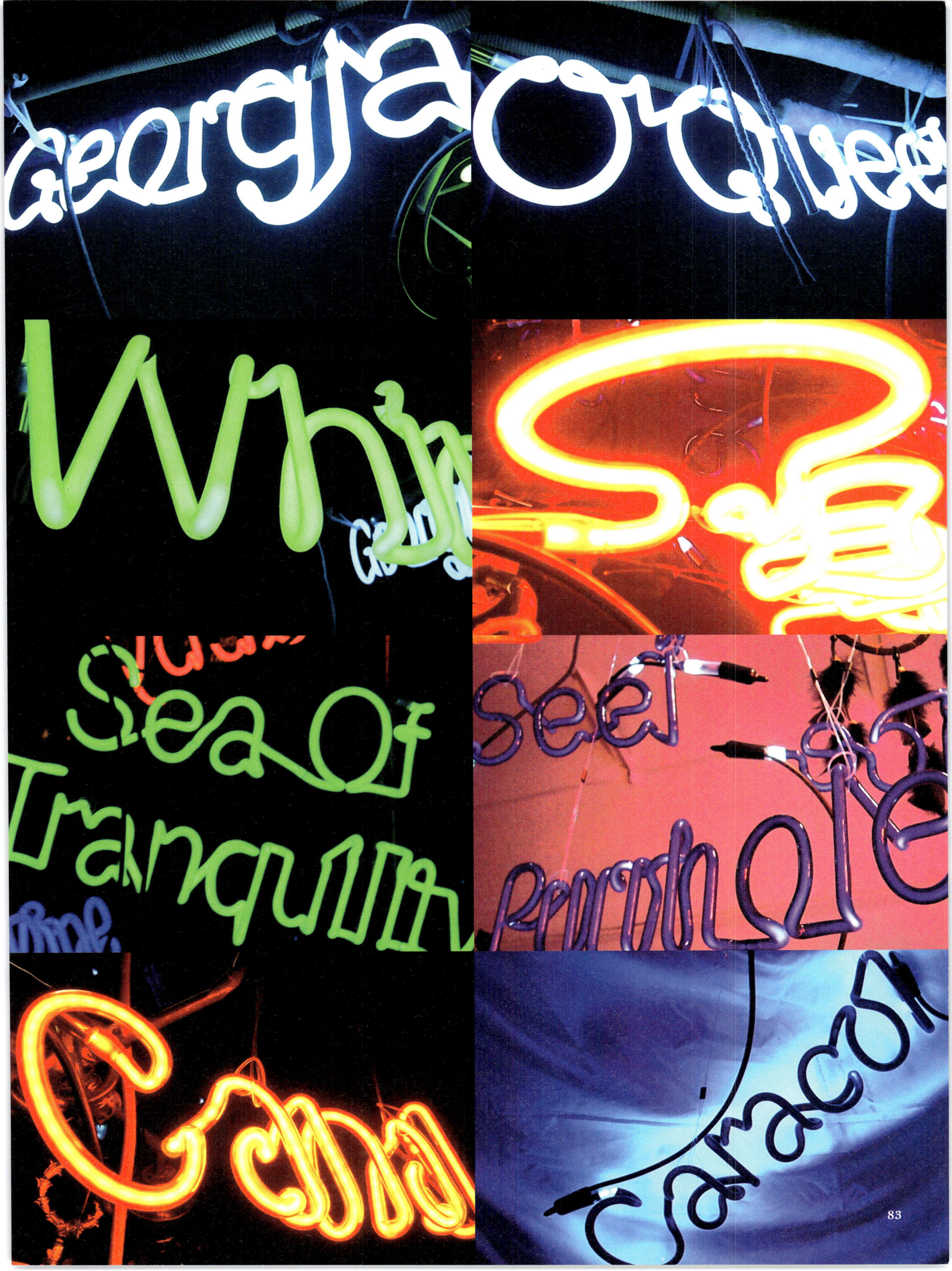
Georgia
Sea Of

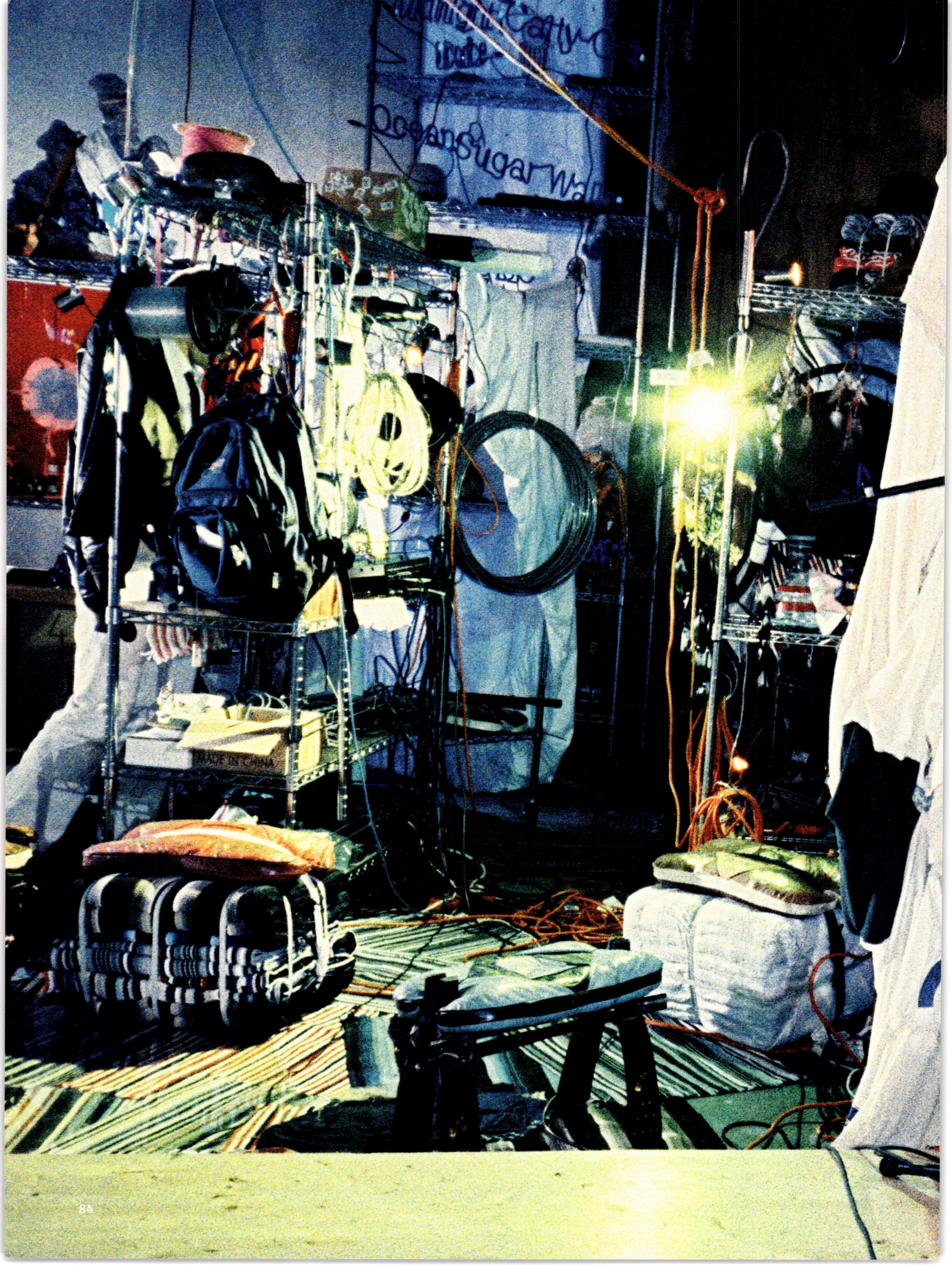
MADE IN CHINA

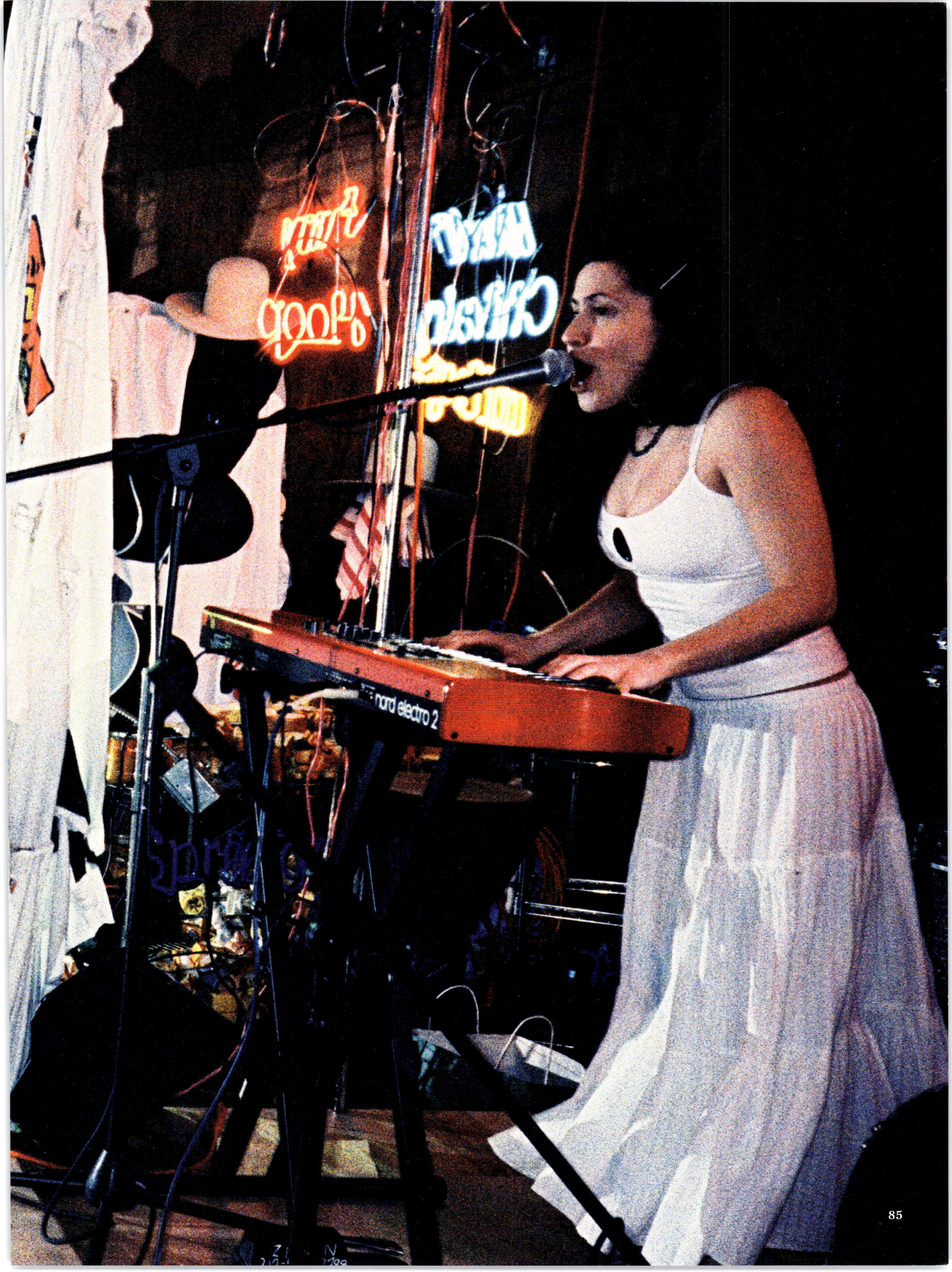
nord electro 2

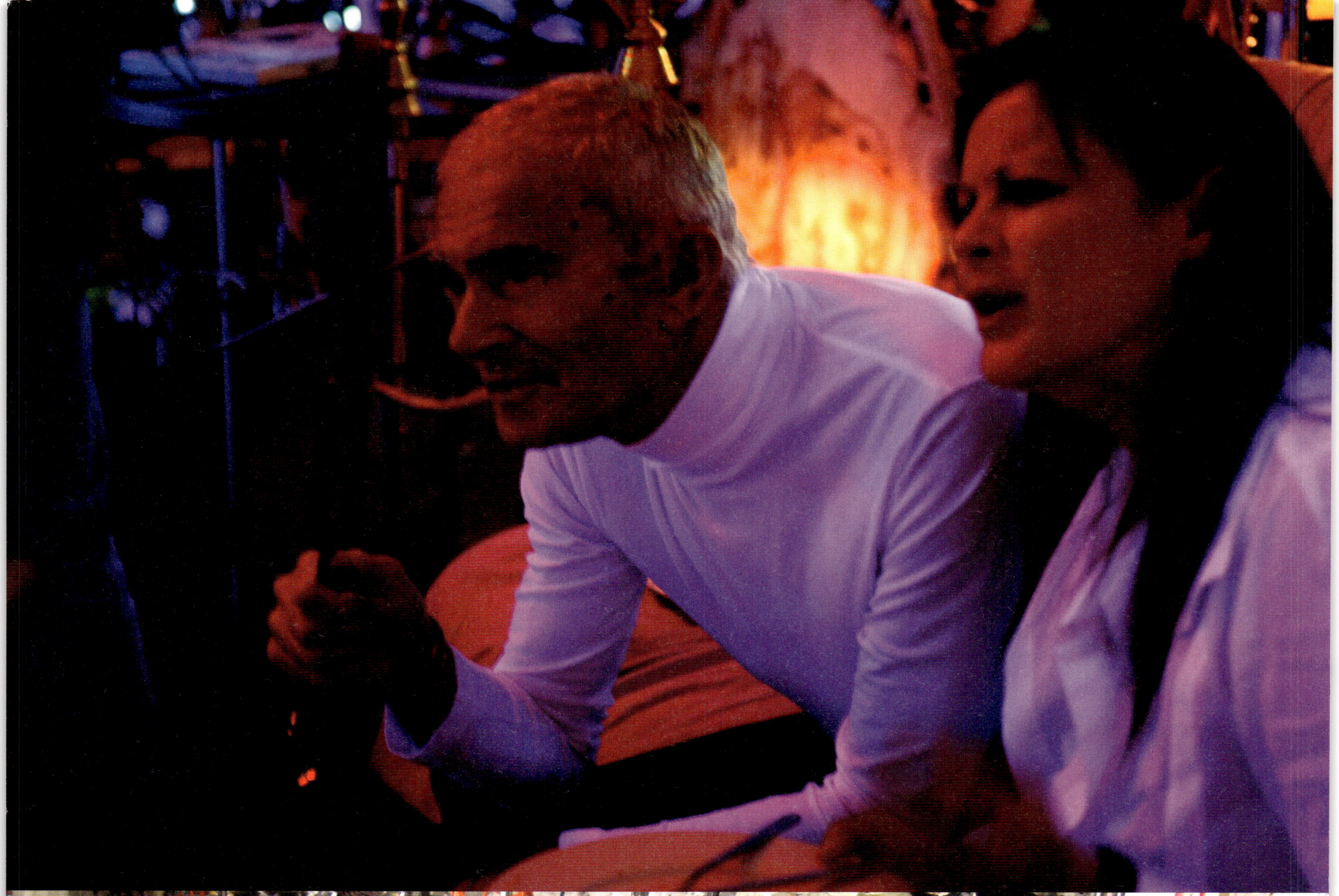

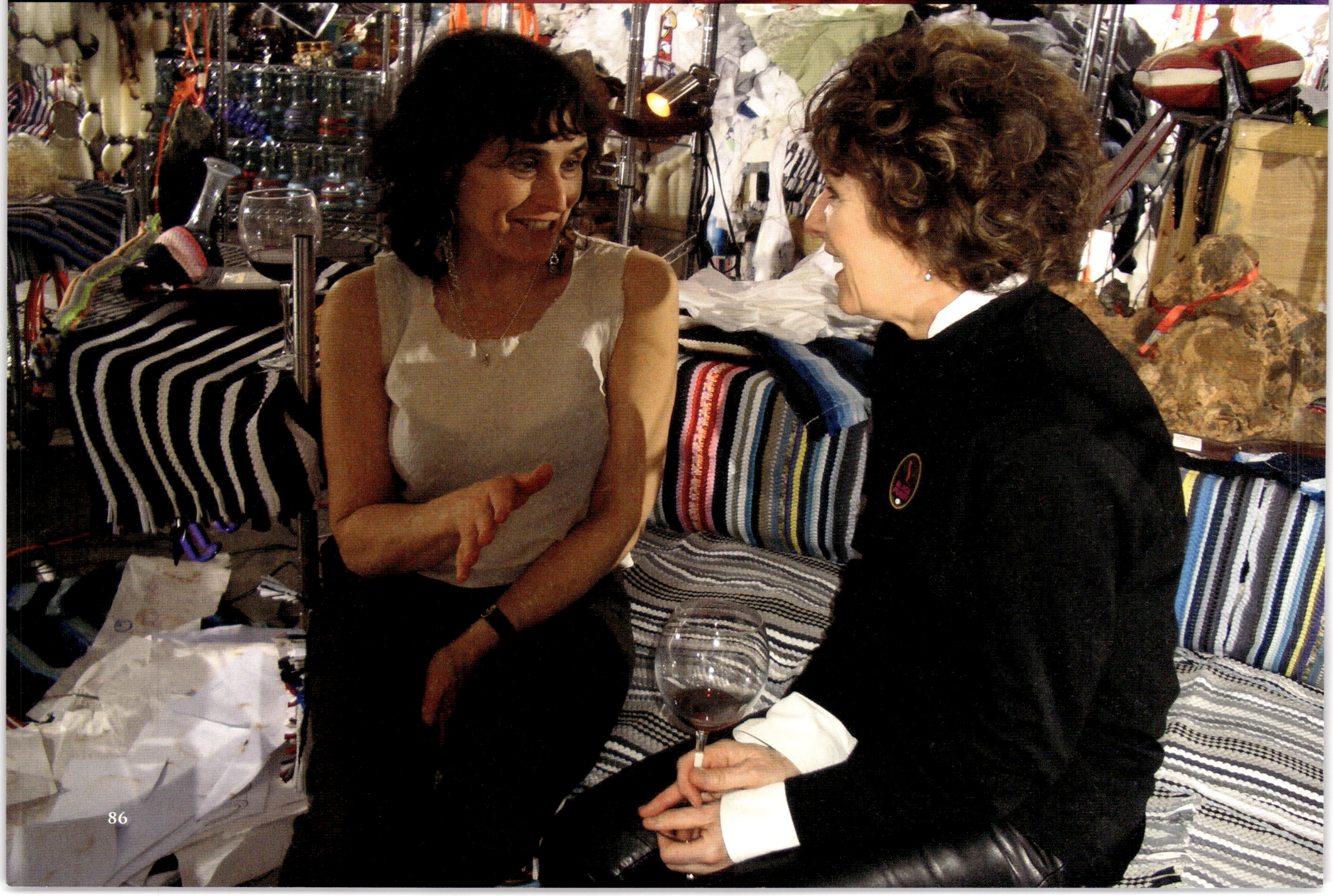

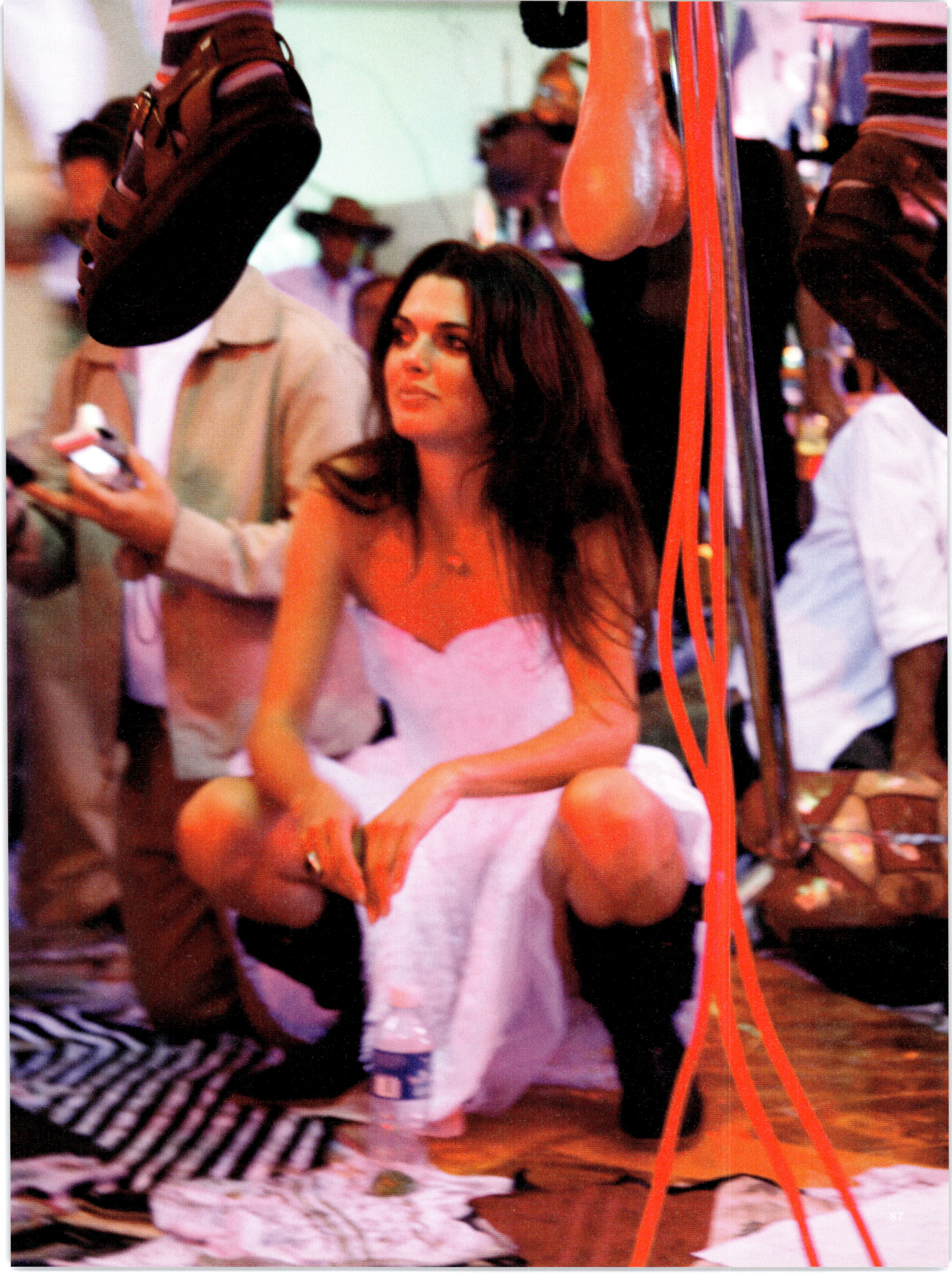

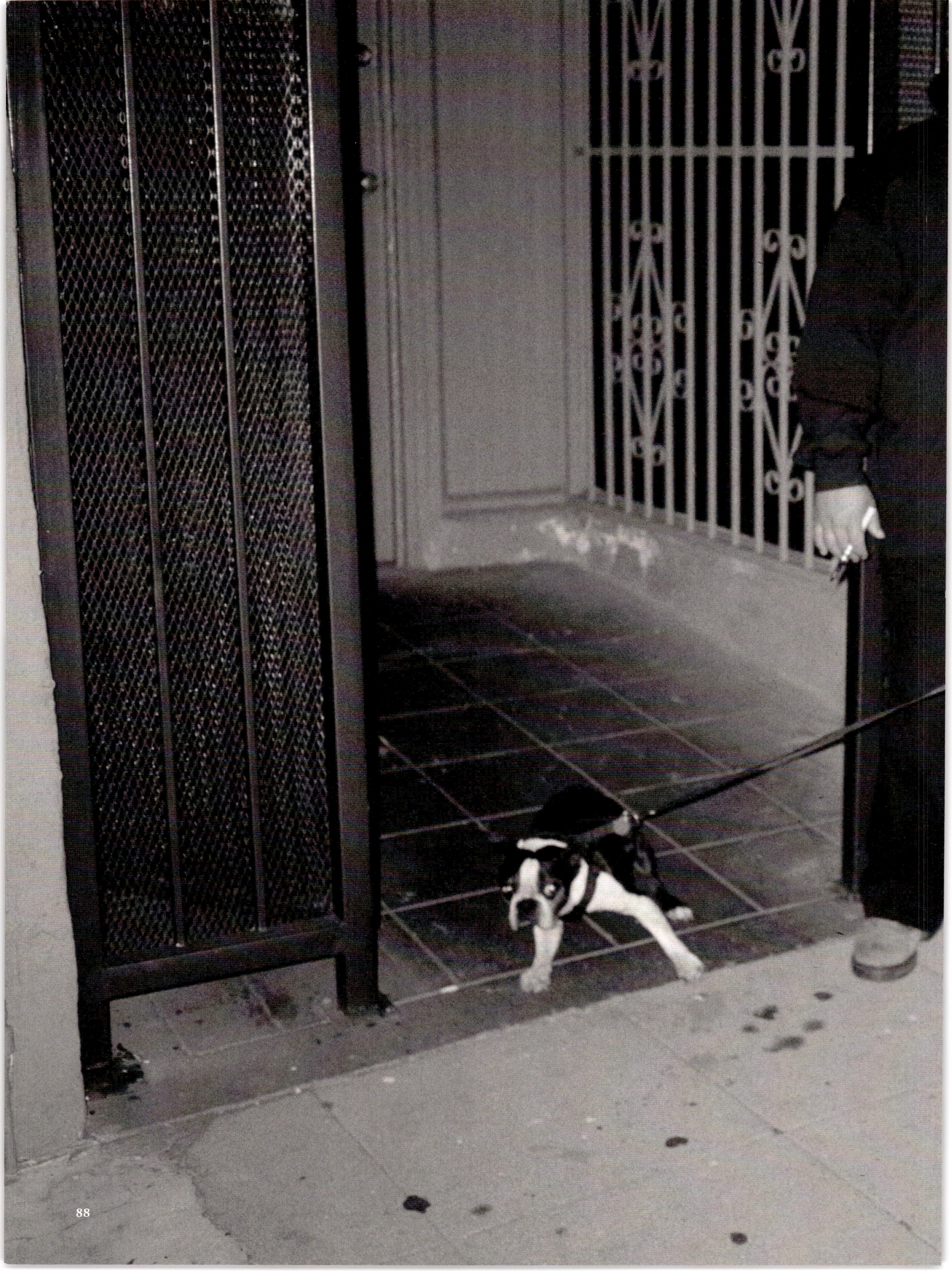

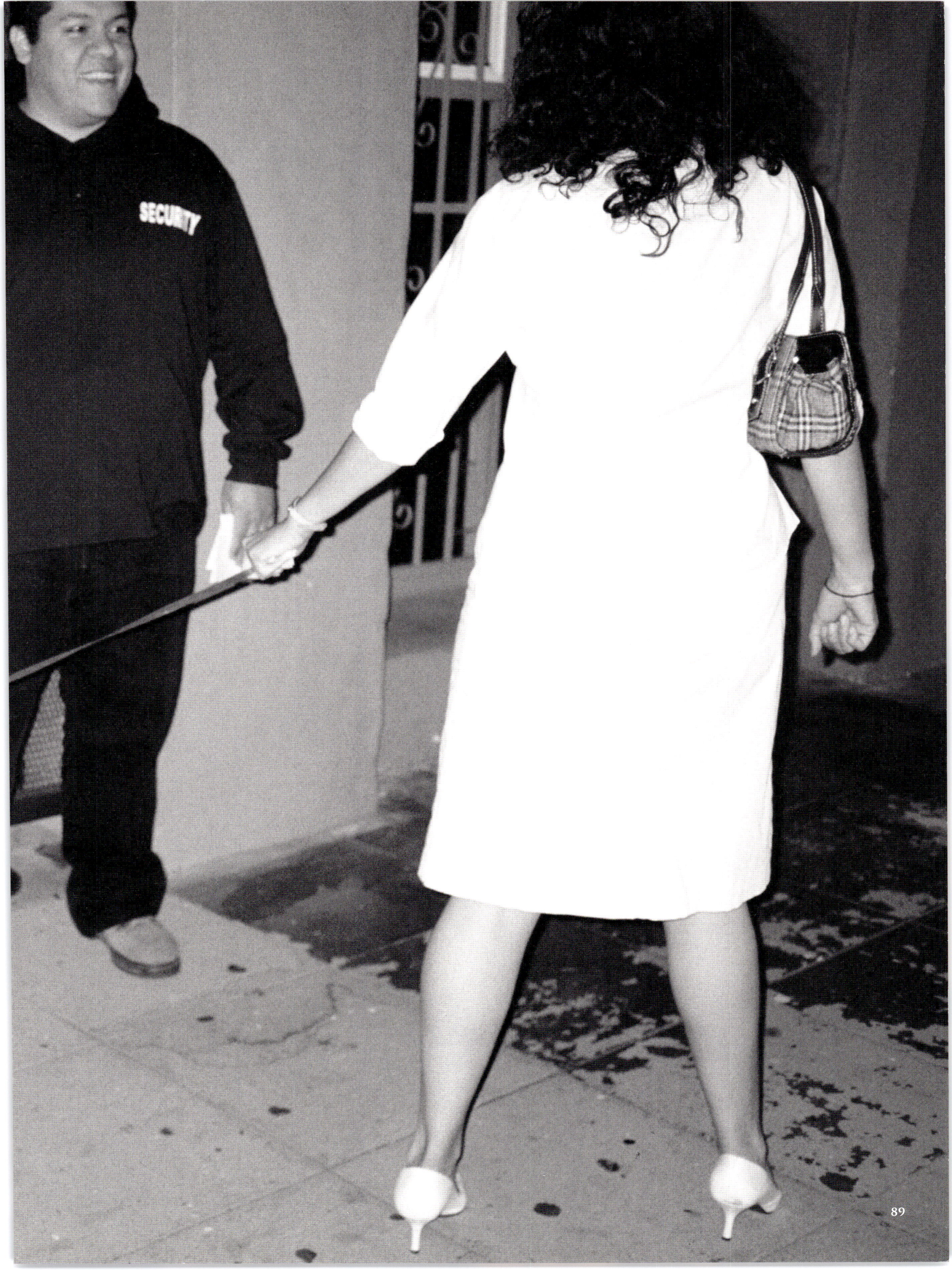
SECURITY

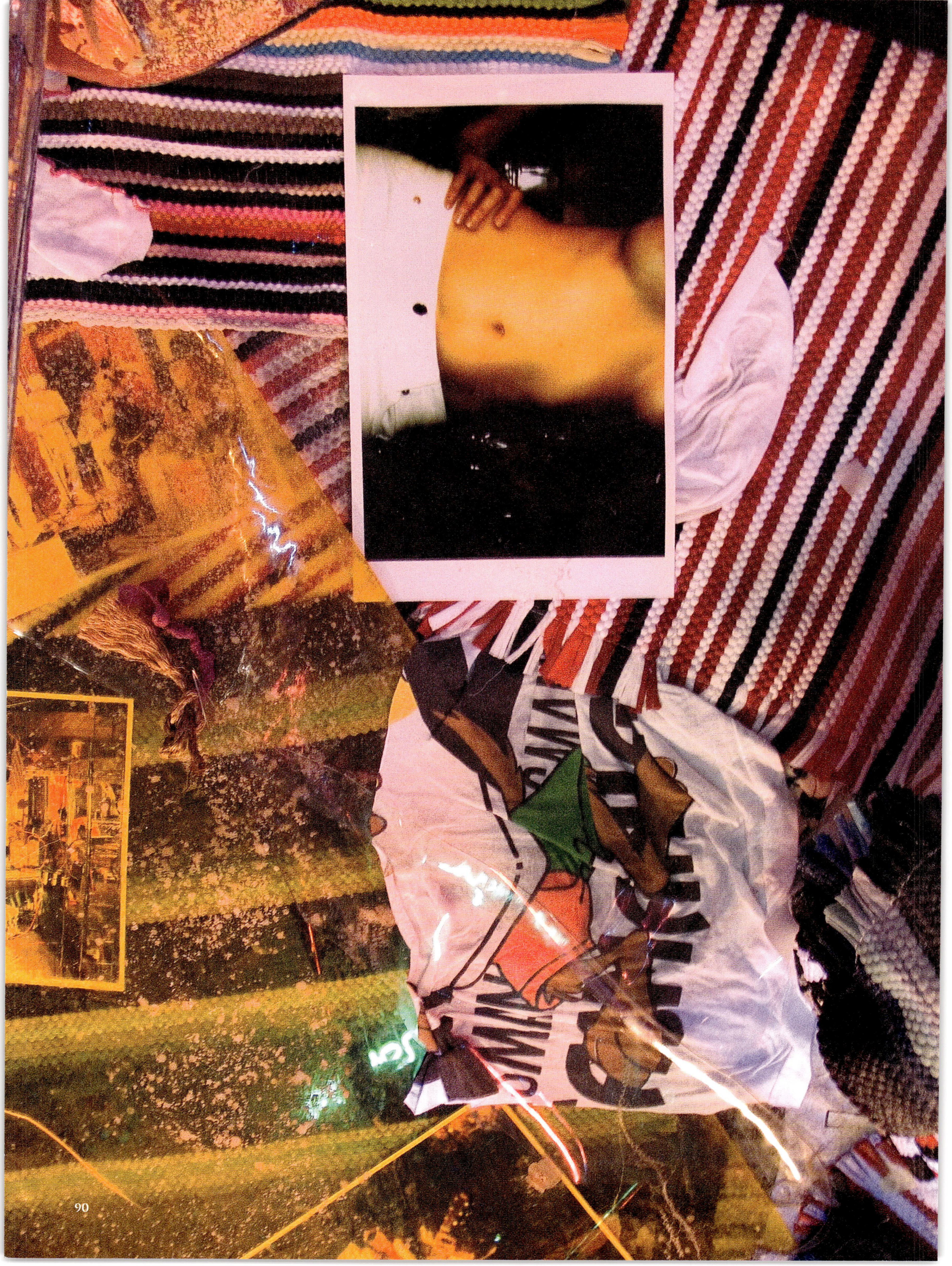

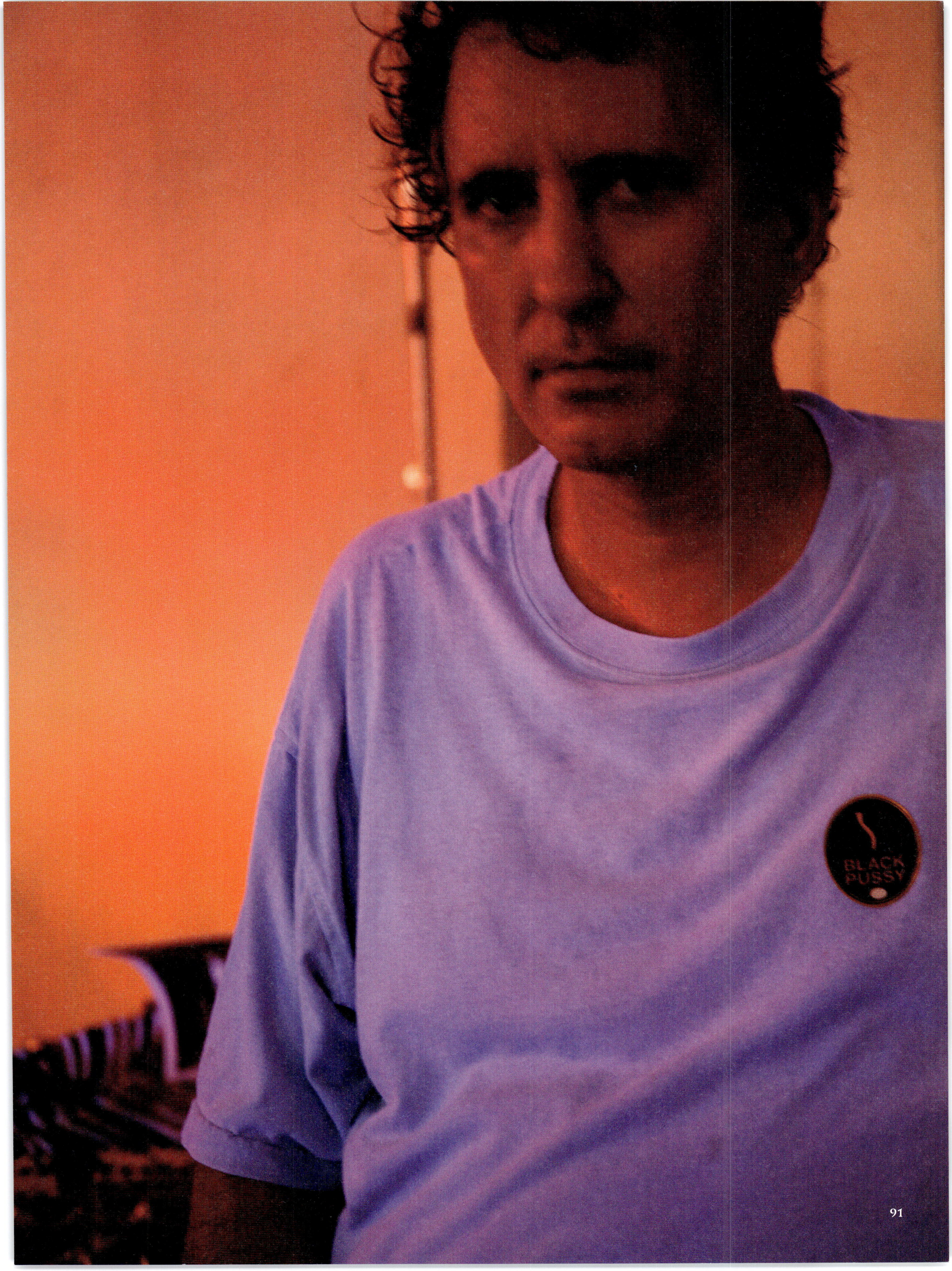
BLACK
PUSSY

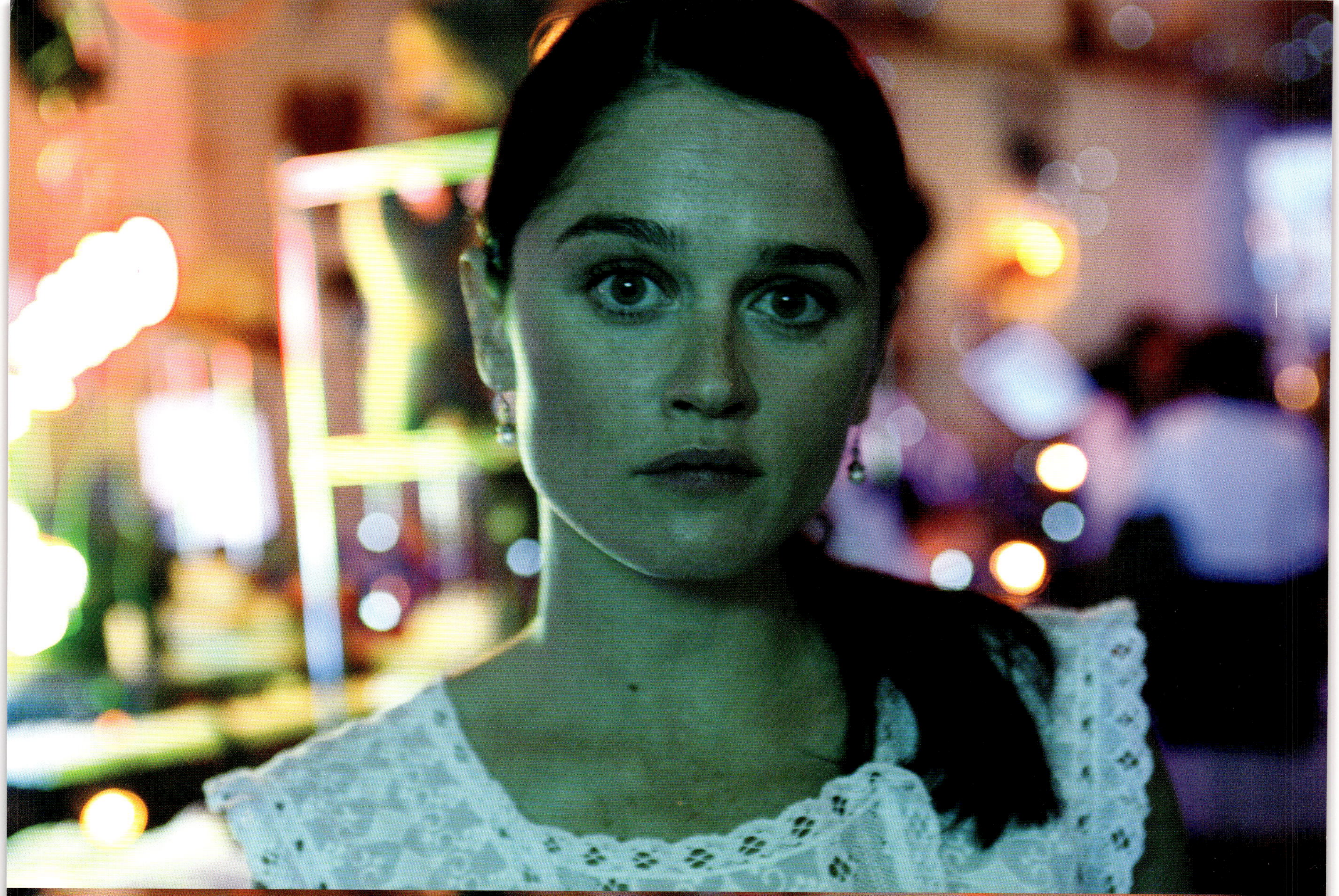

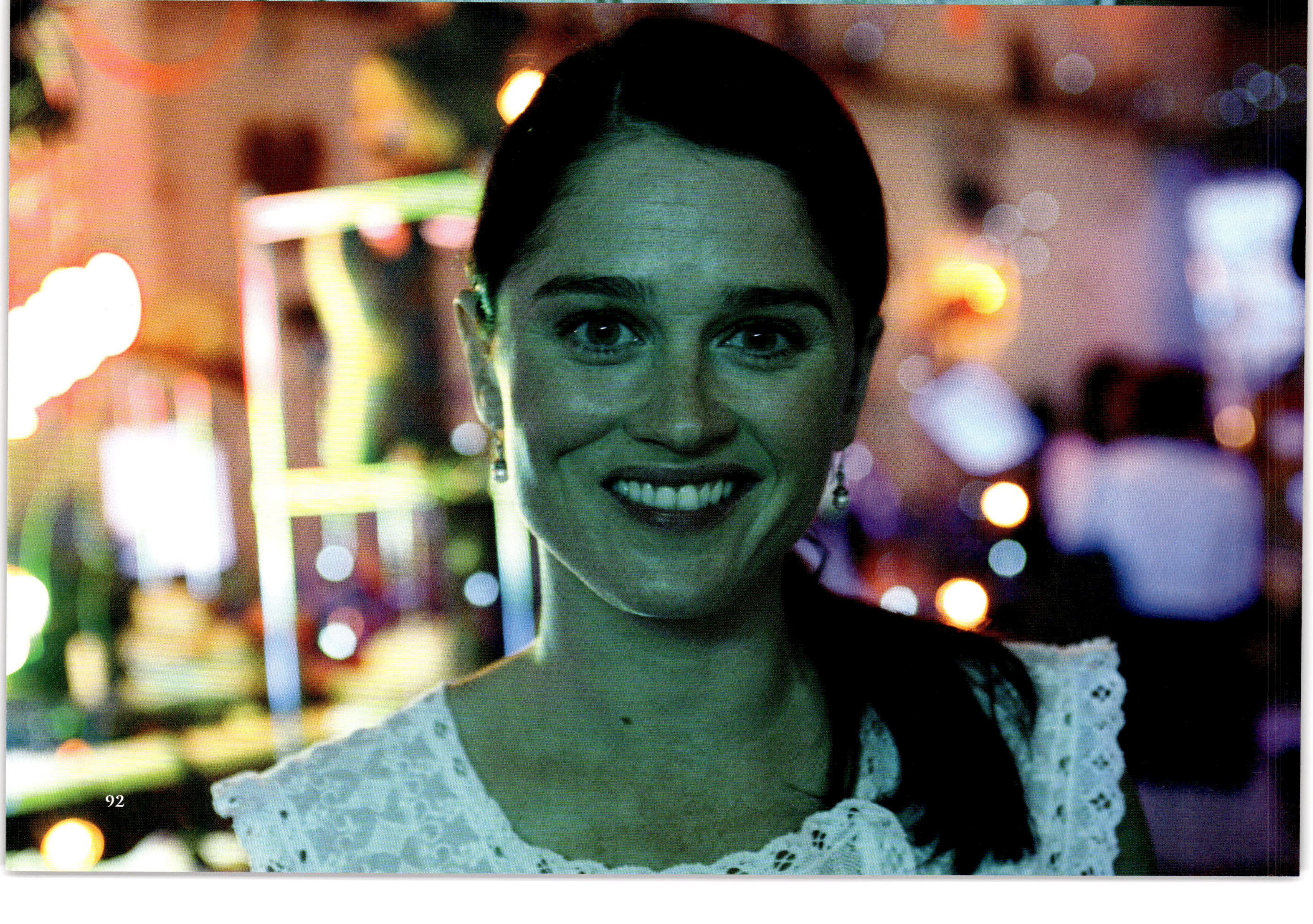

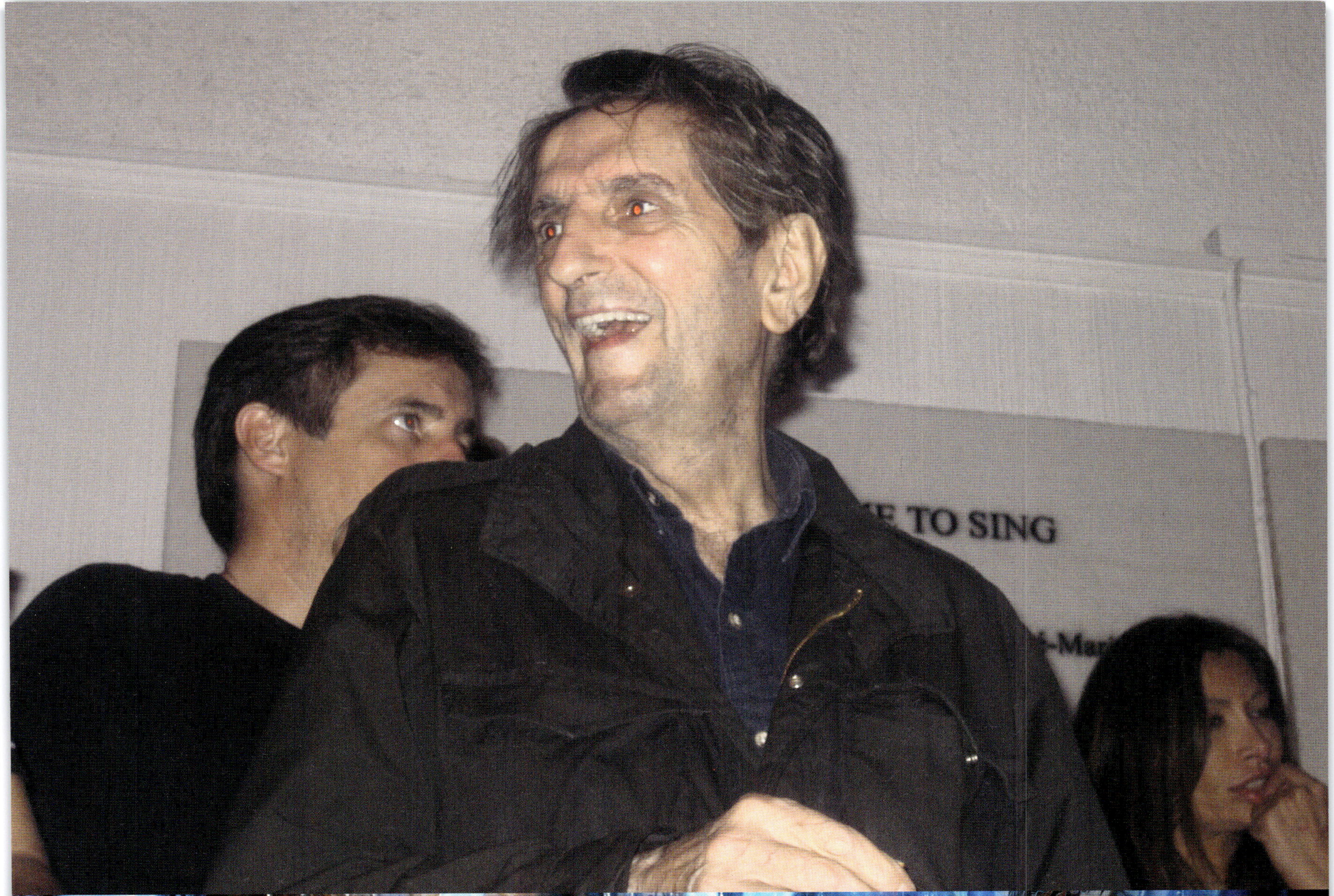
TO SING

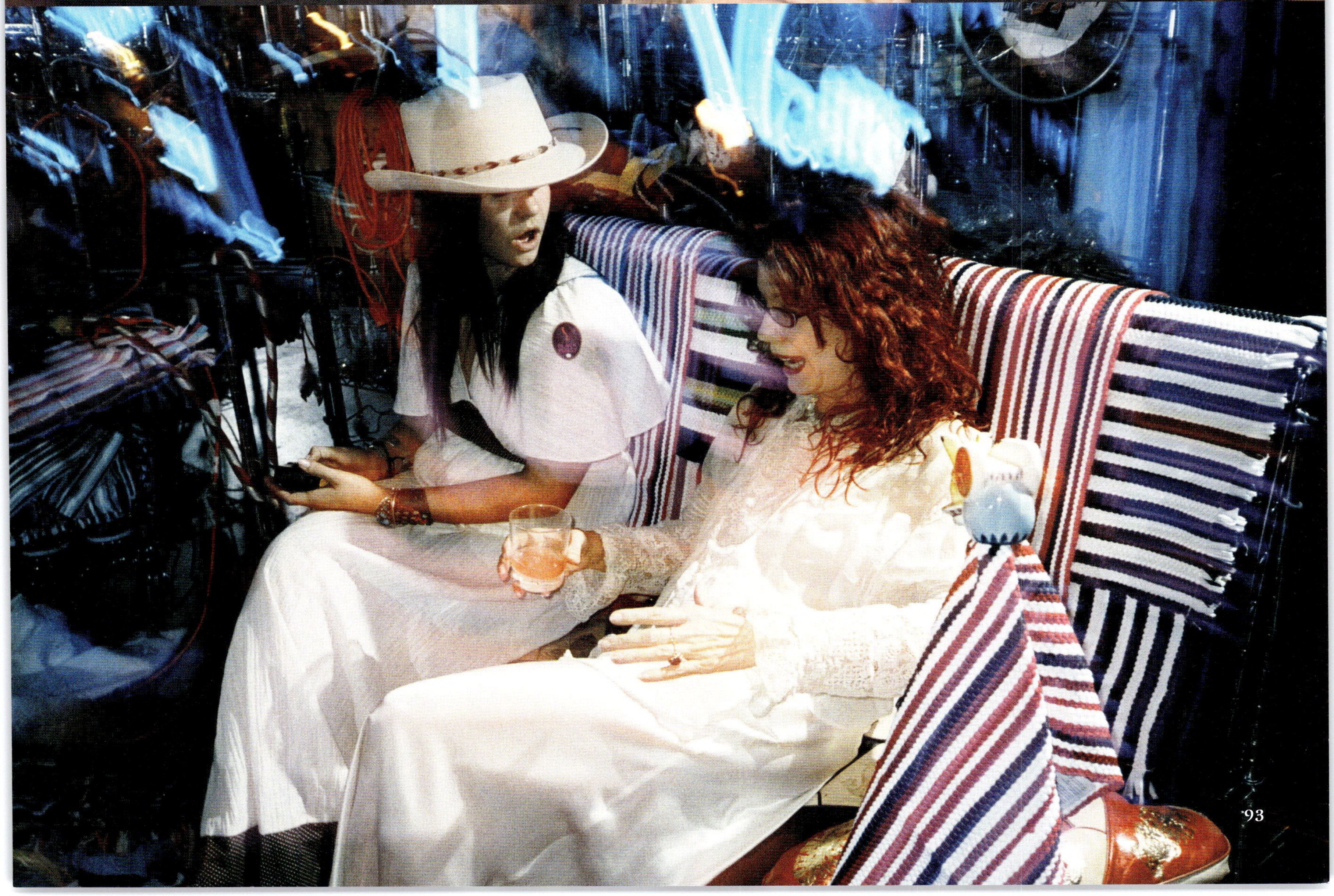

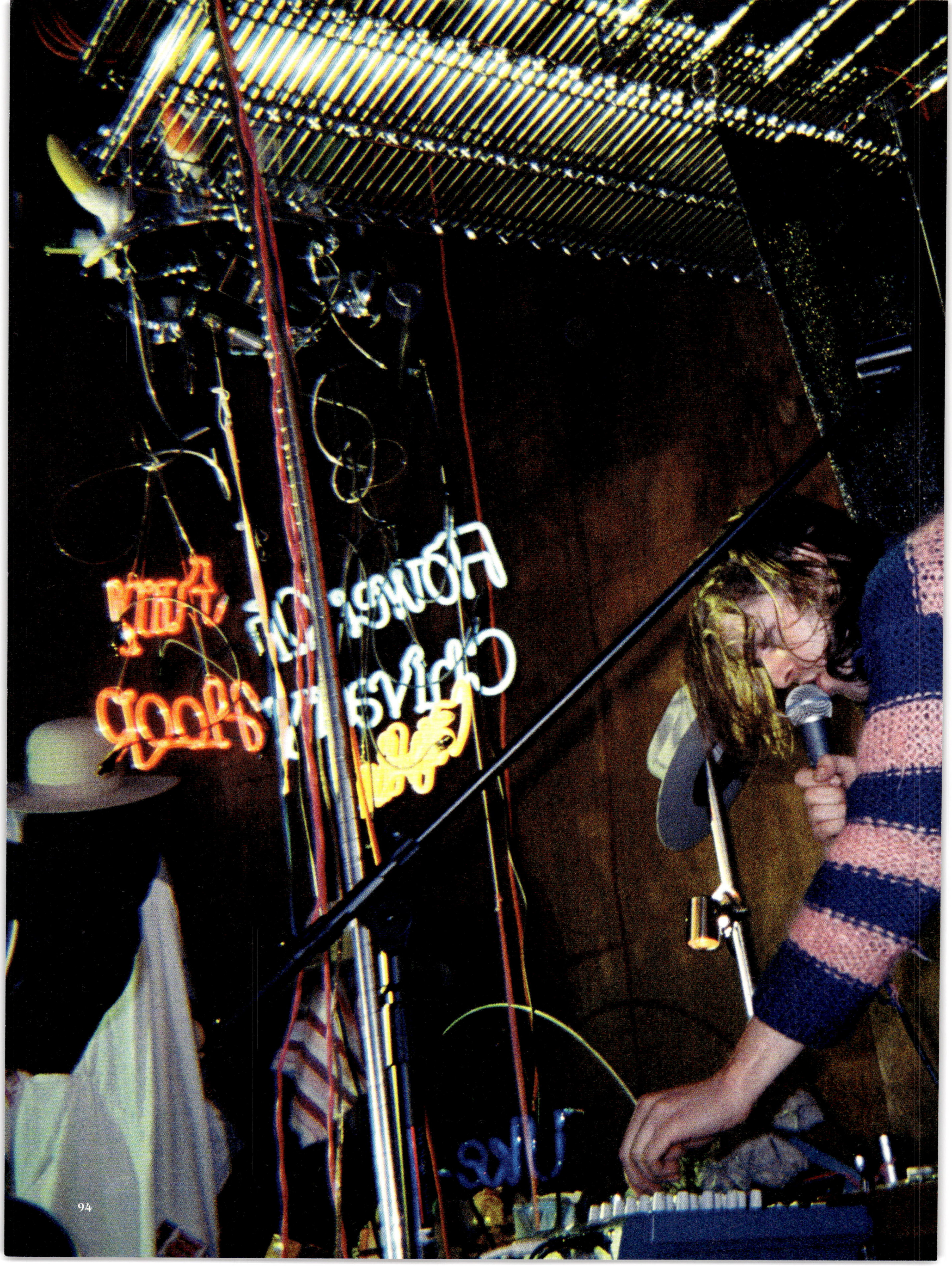

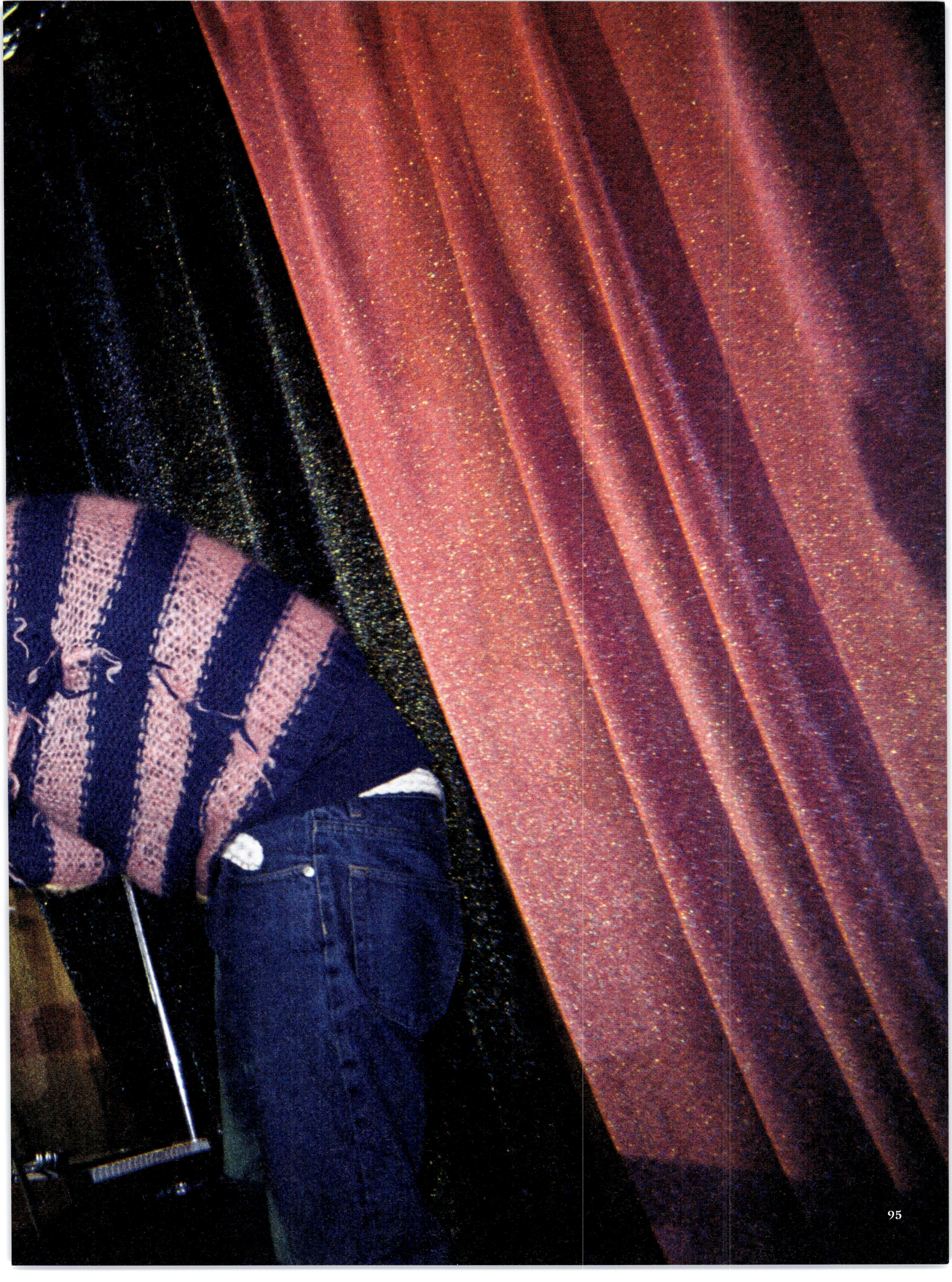

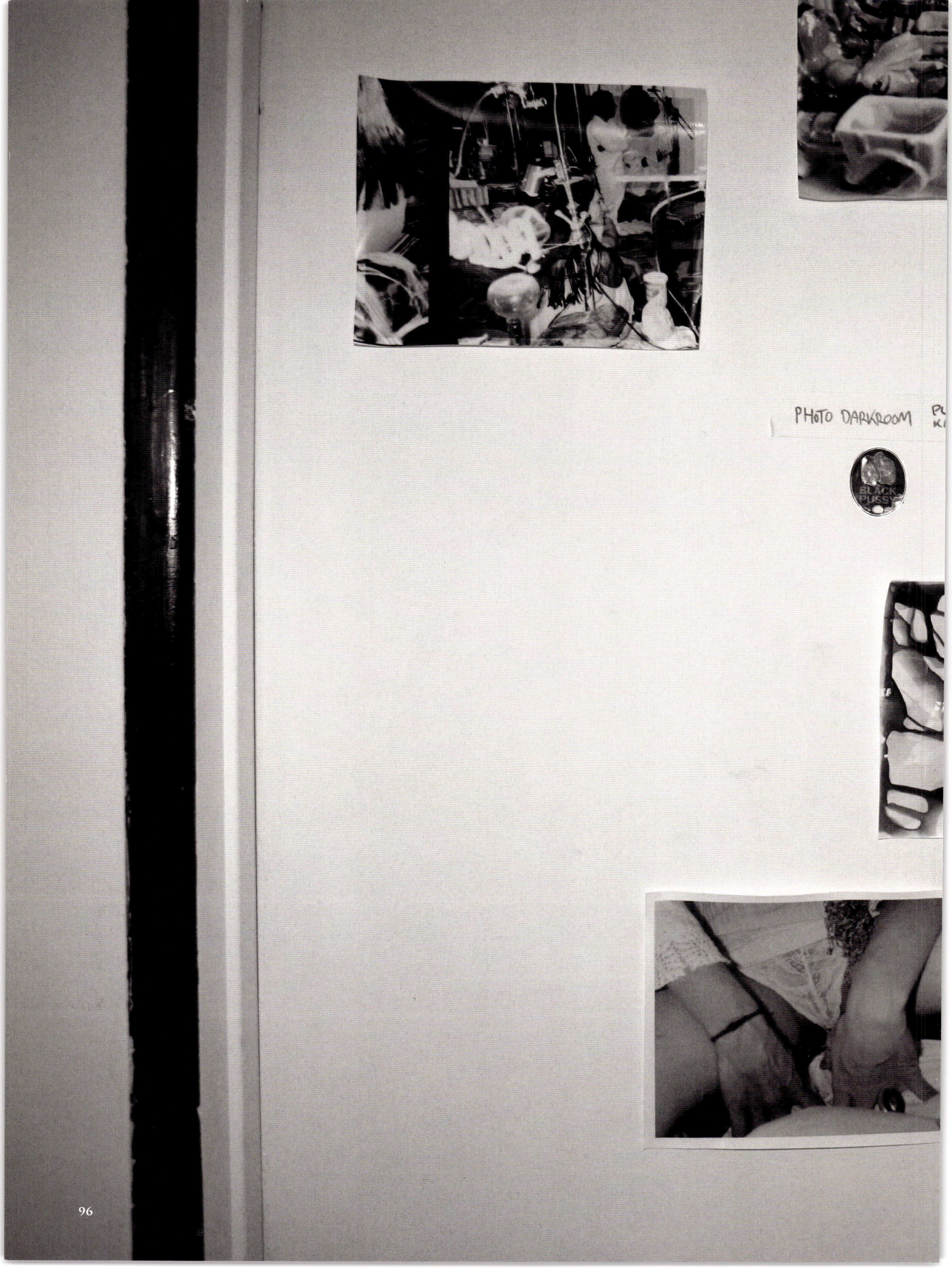
PHOTO DARKROOM
BLACK PUSSY

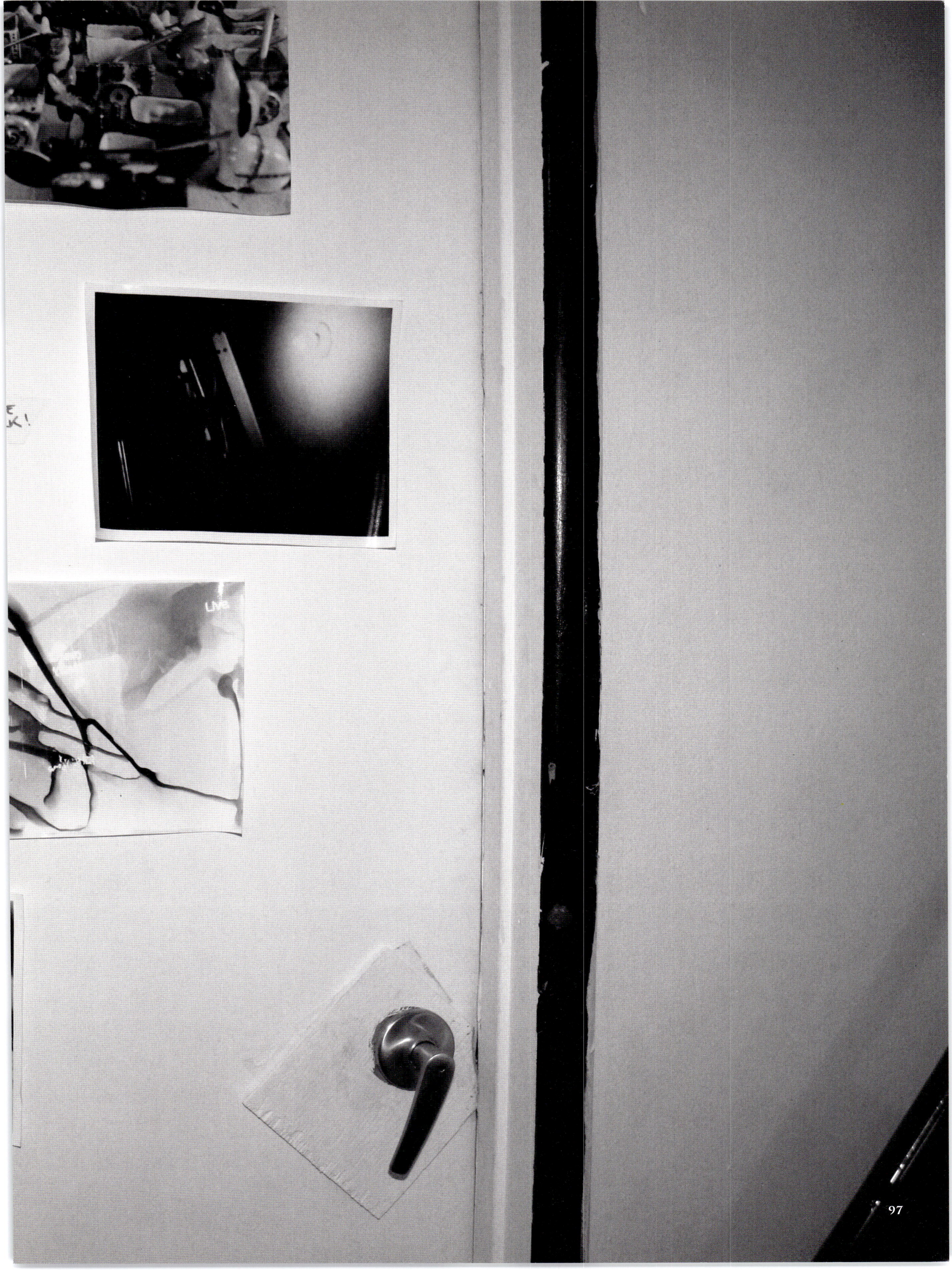

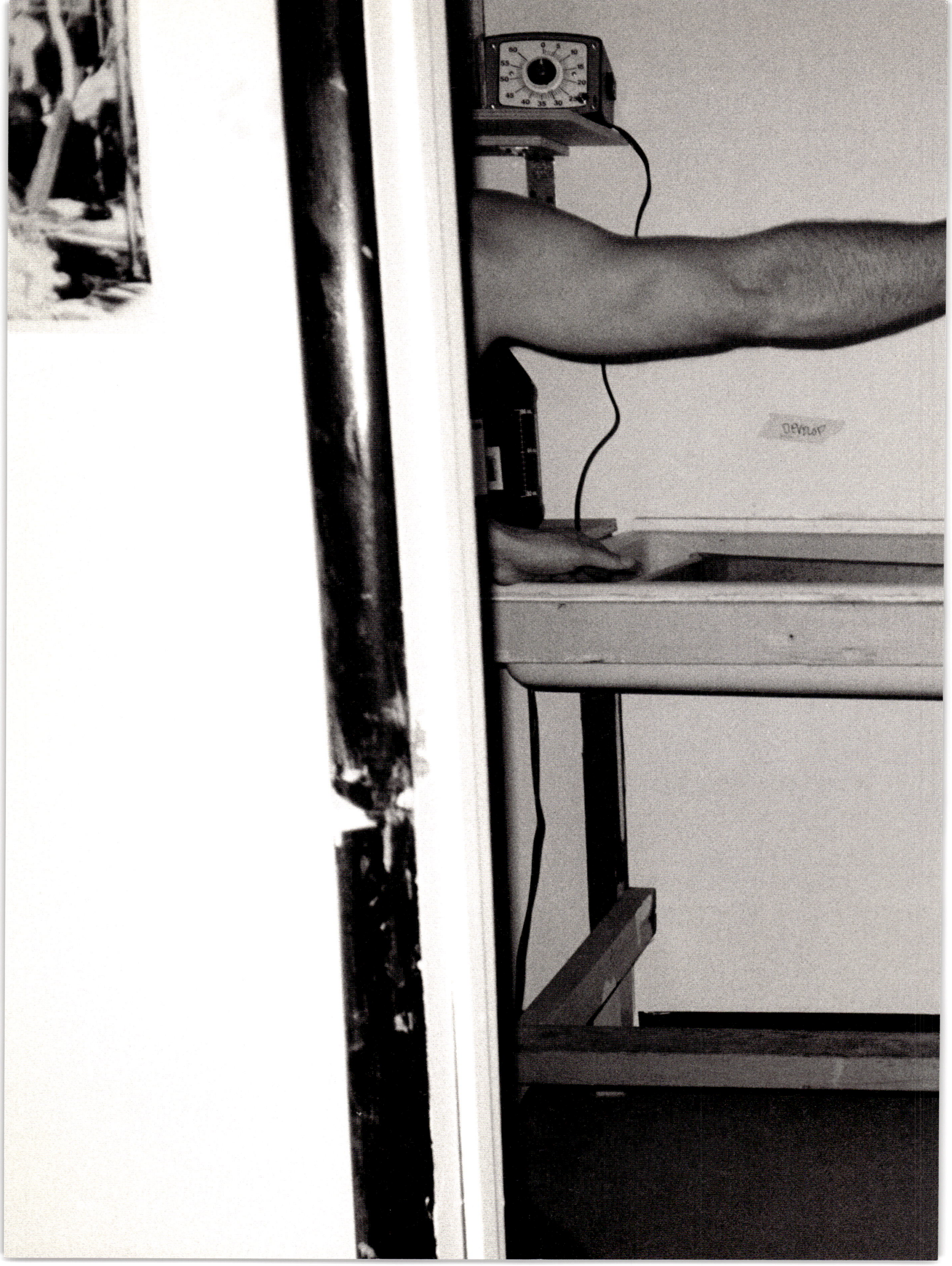

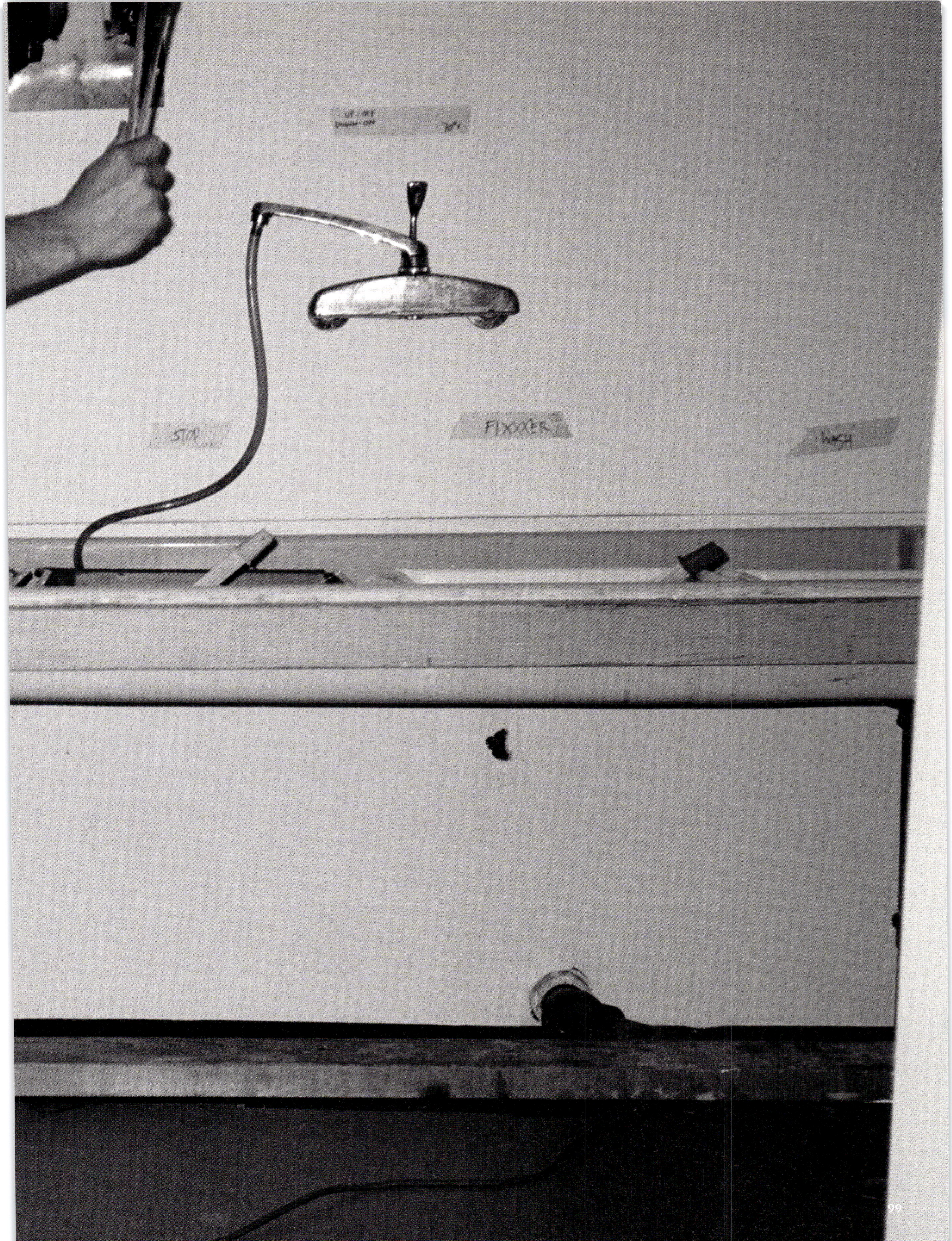
STOP
FIXXXER
WASH

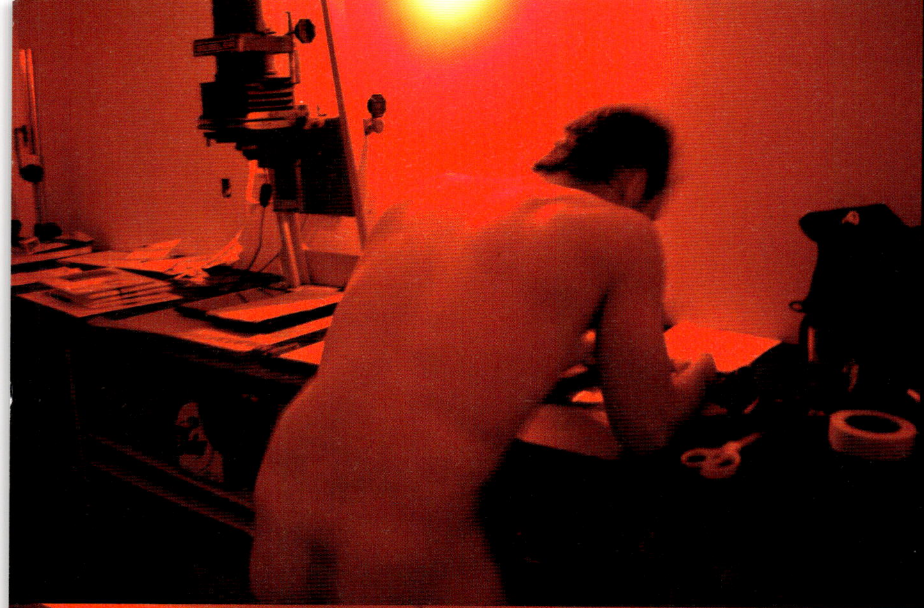

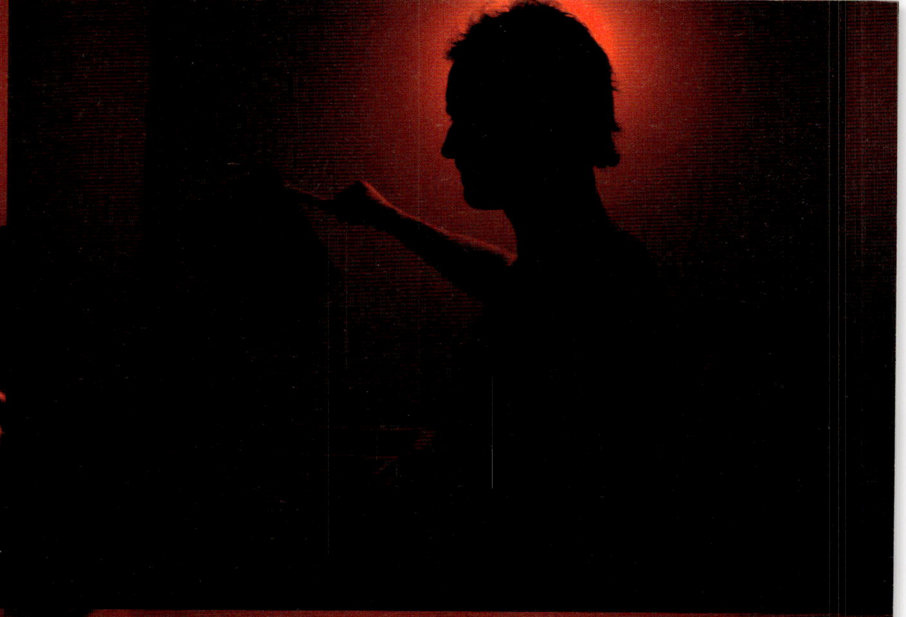

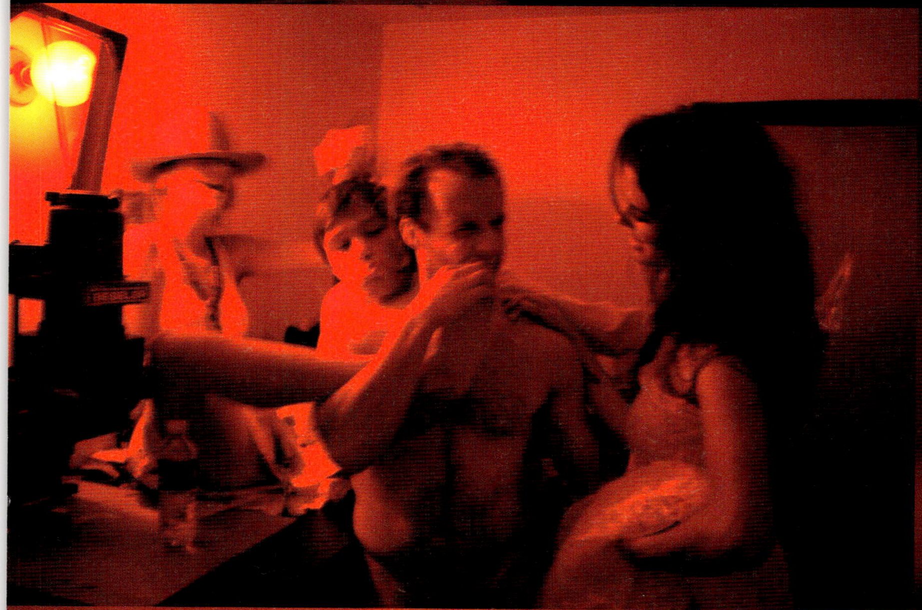

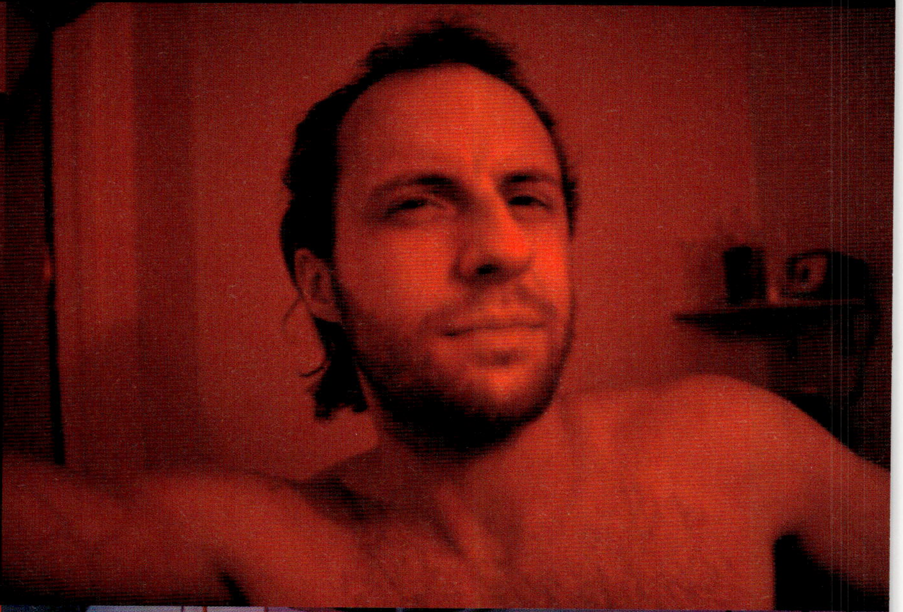

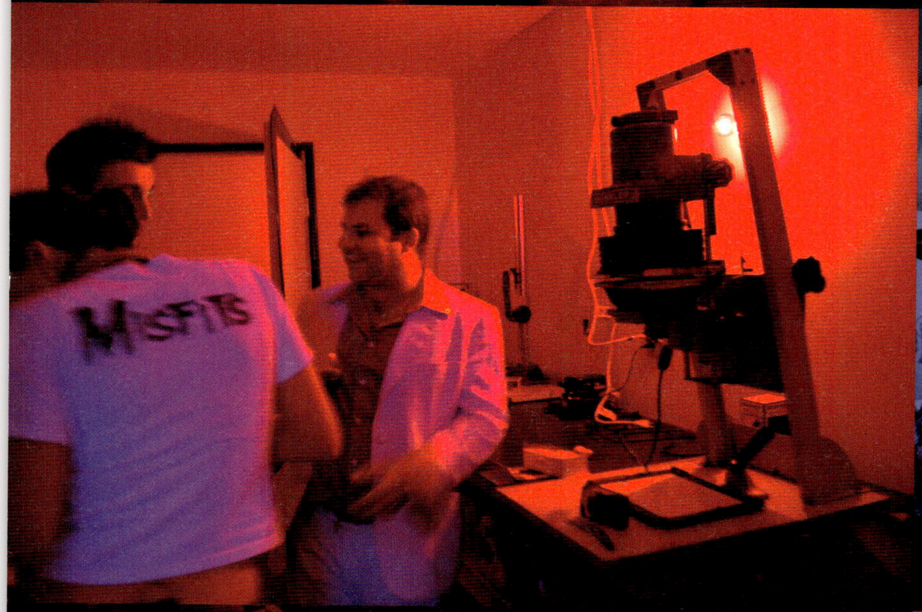
MISFITS

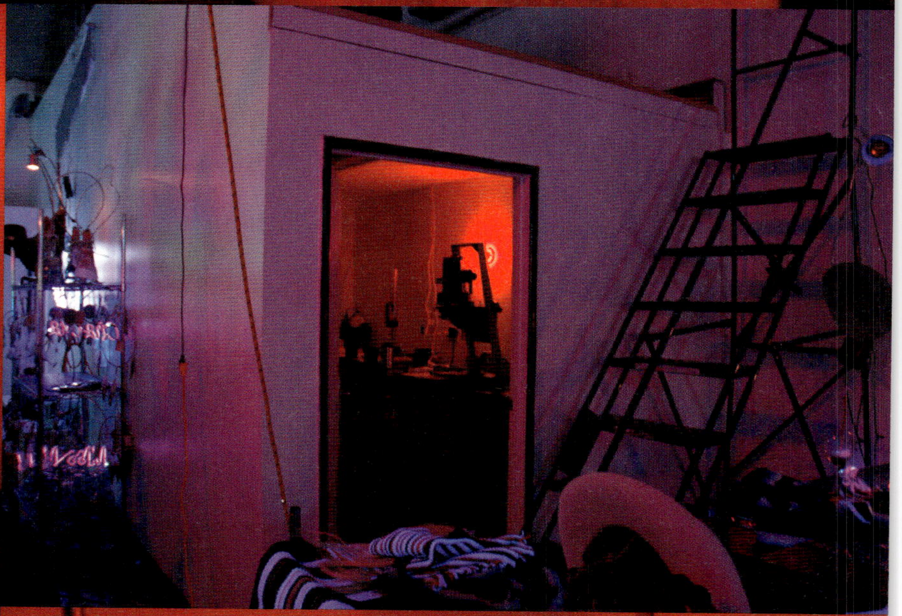

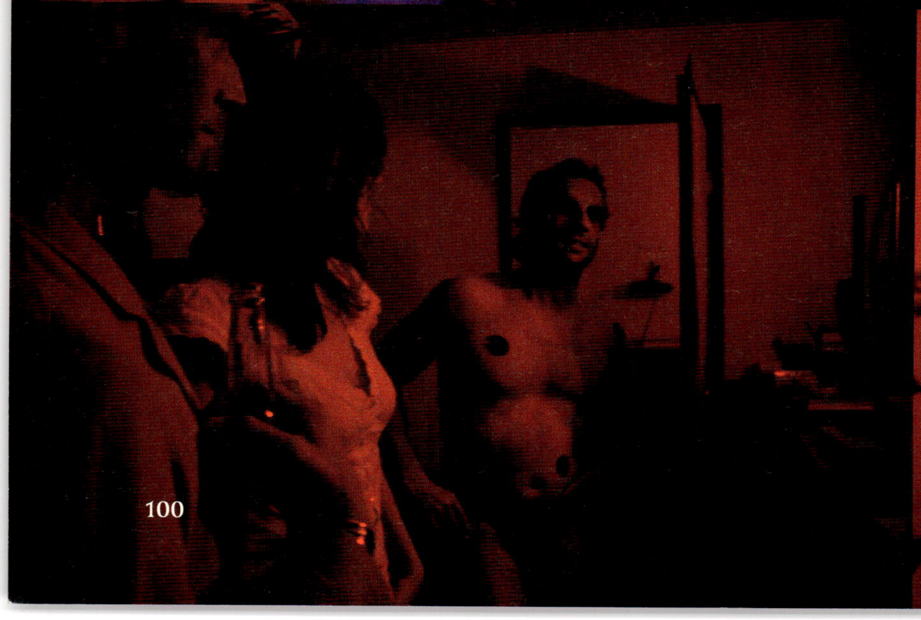

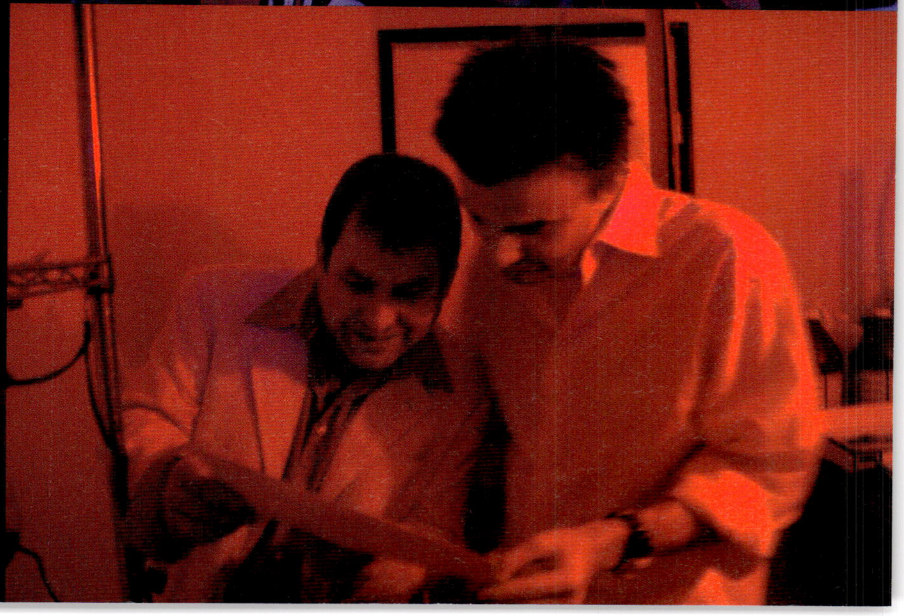

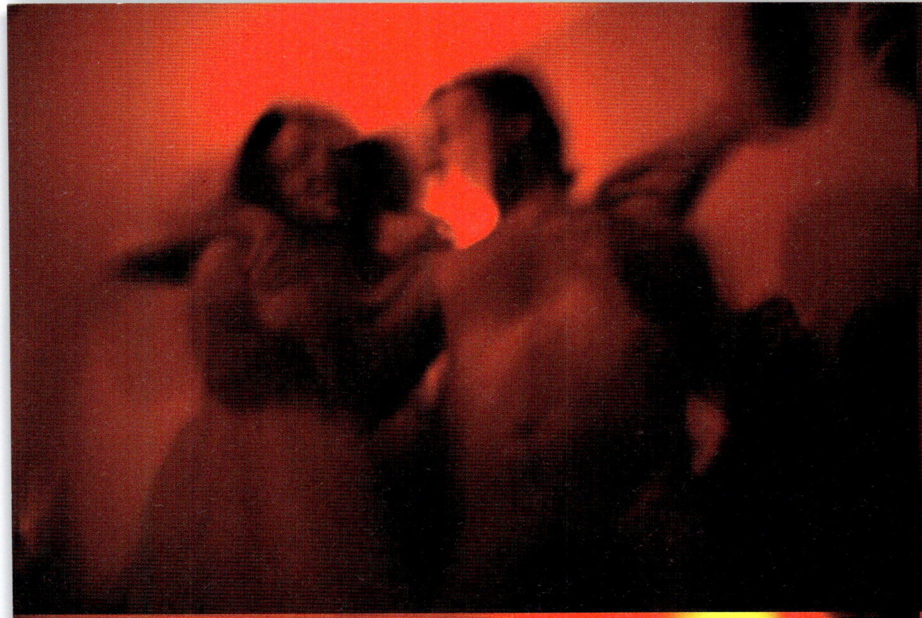
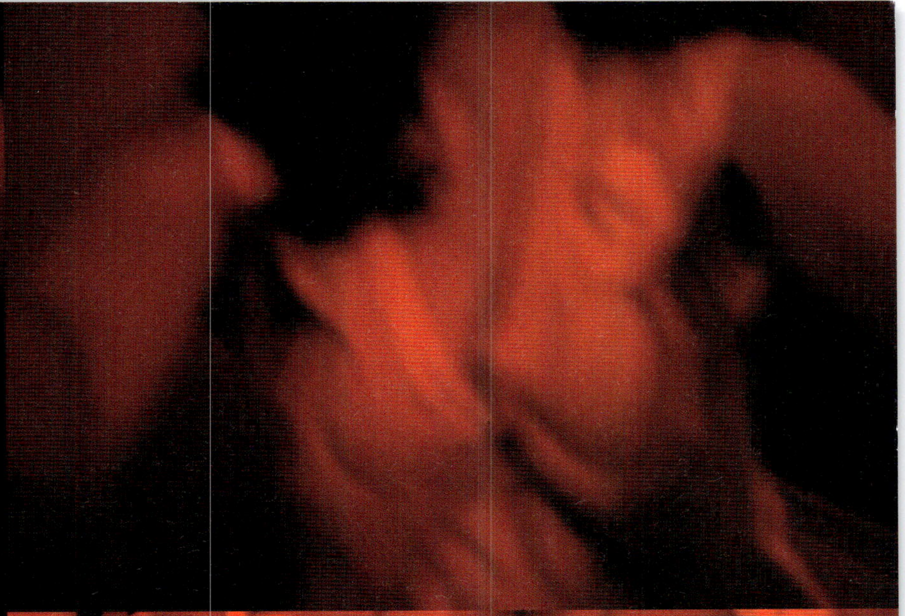
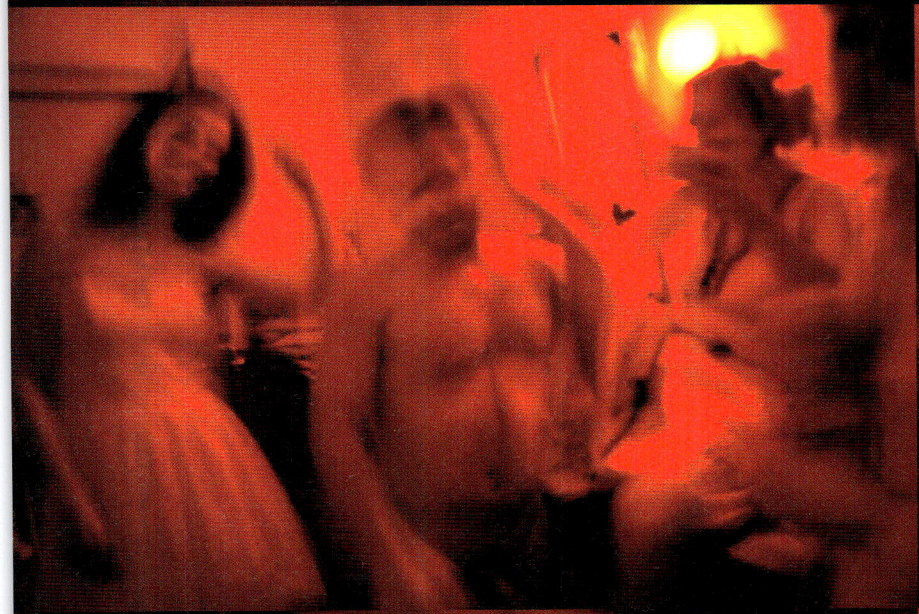
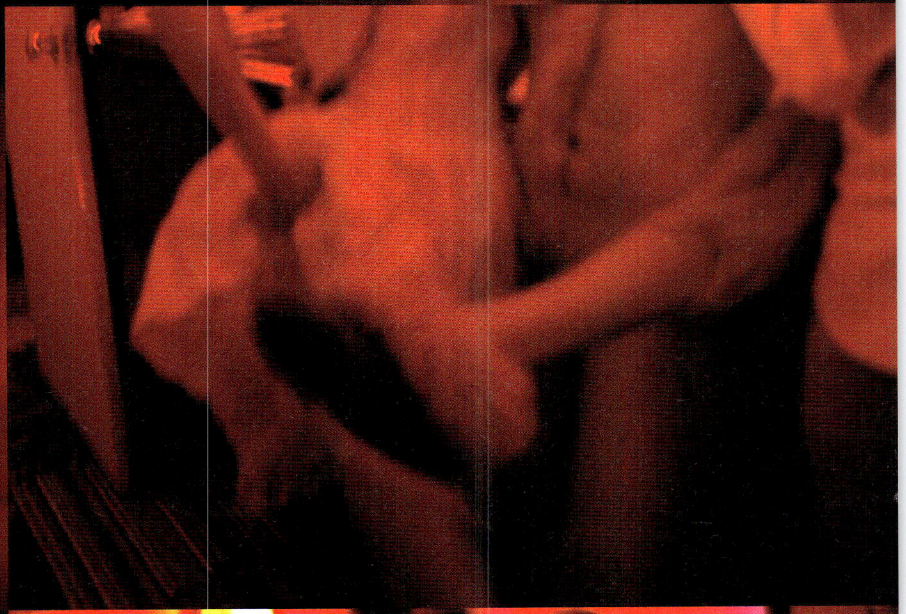
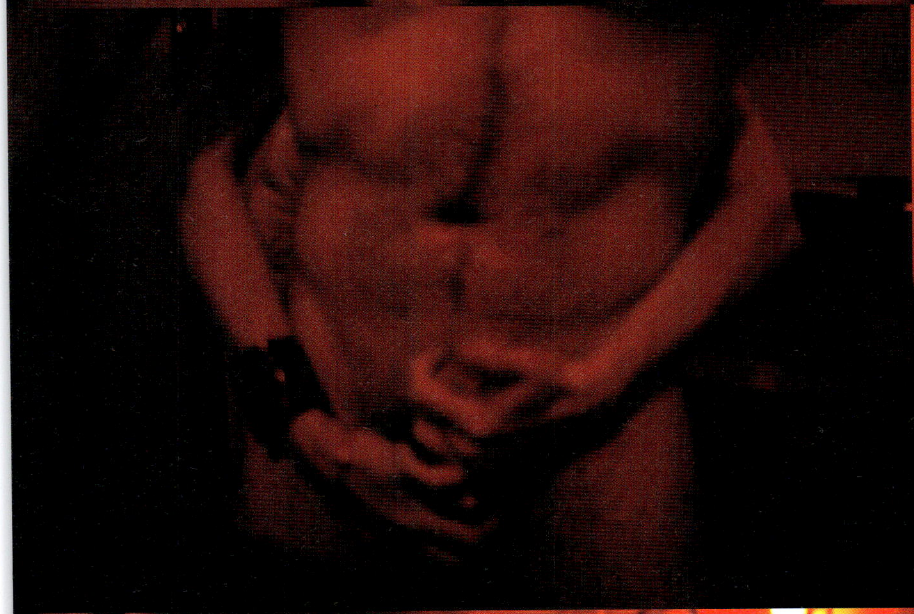
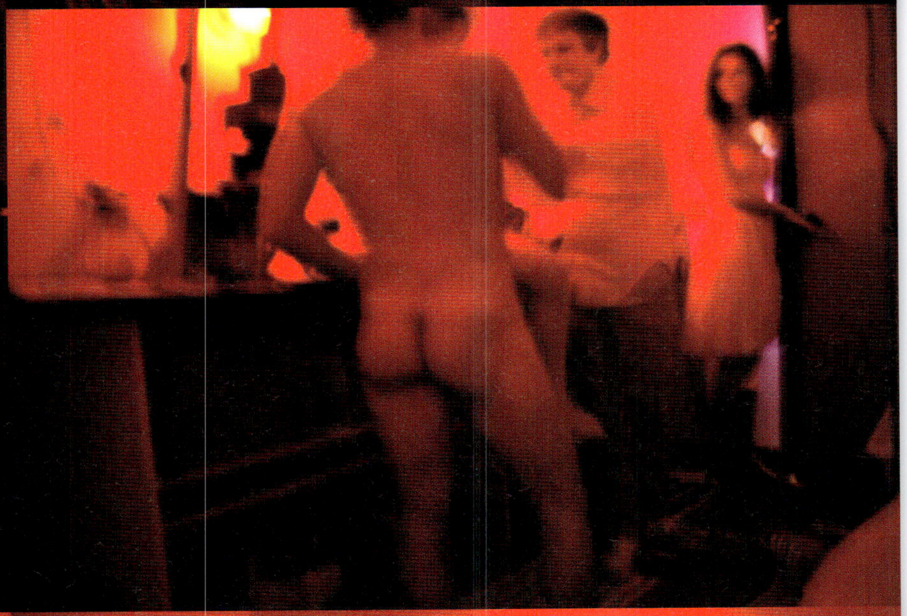
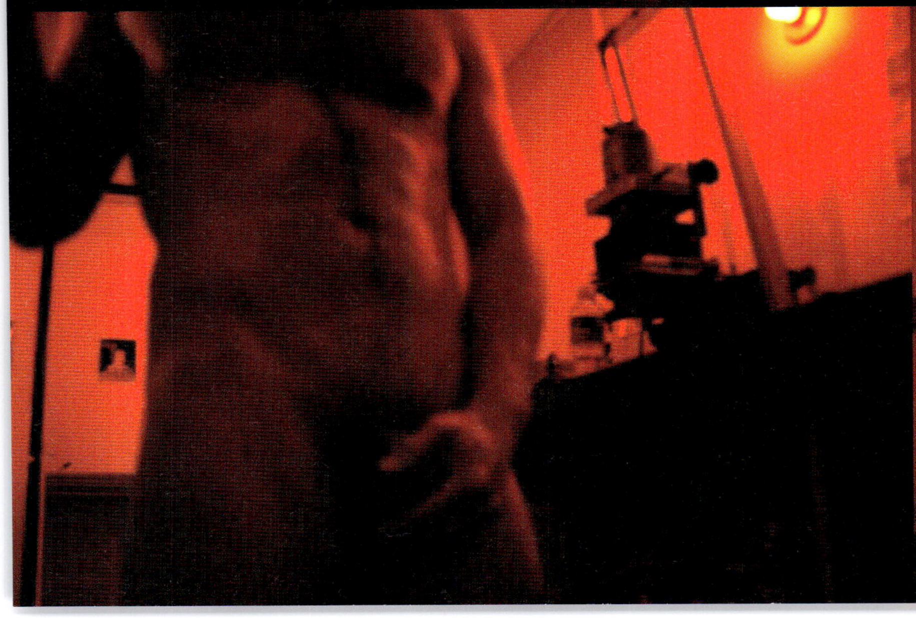
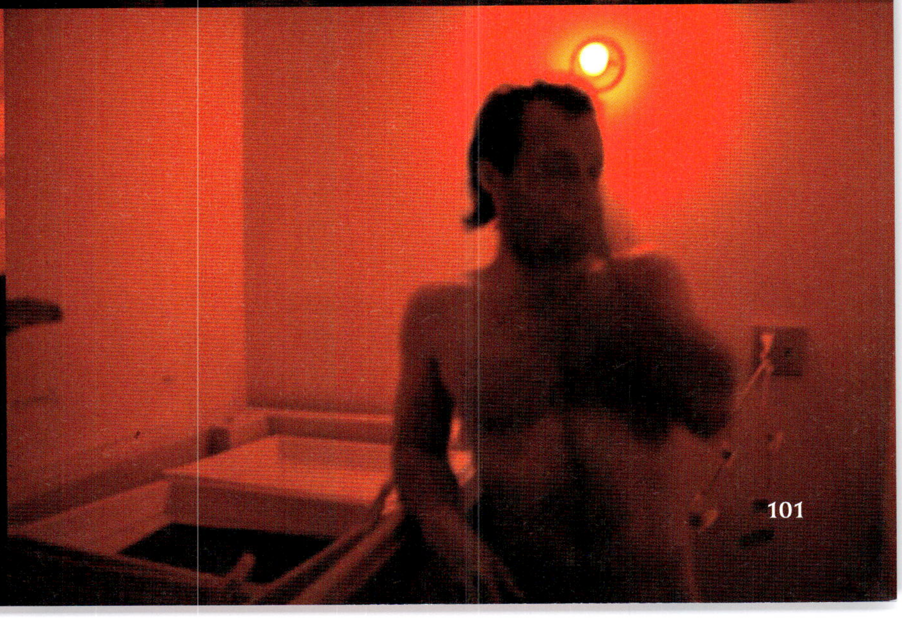

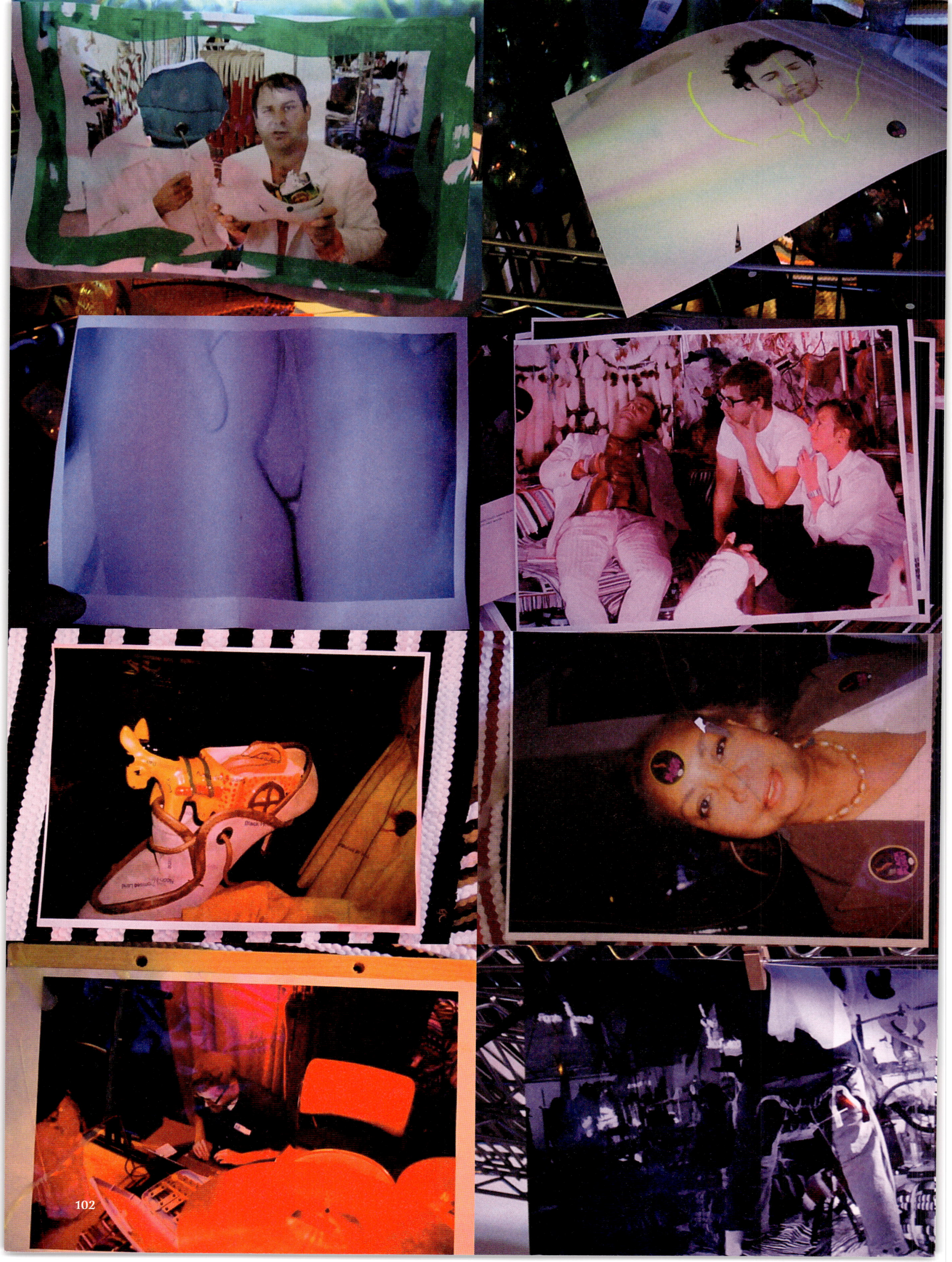

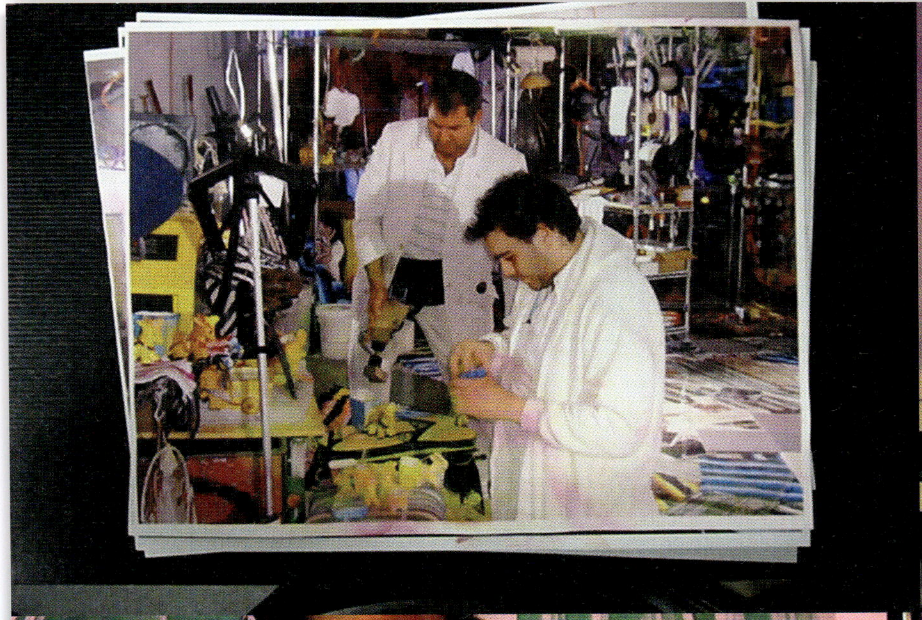

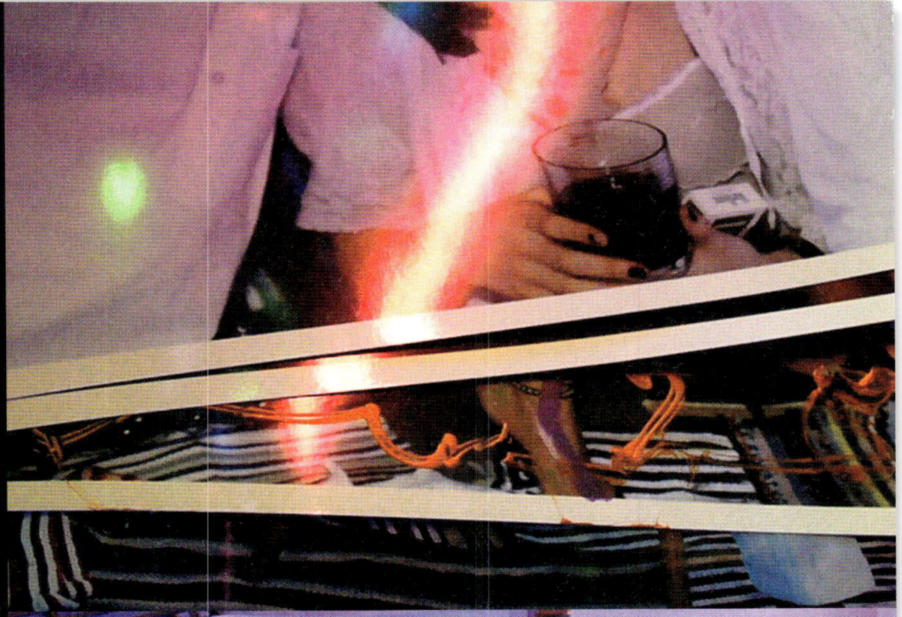

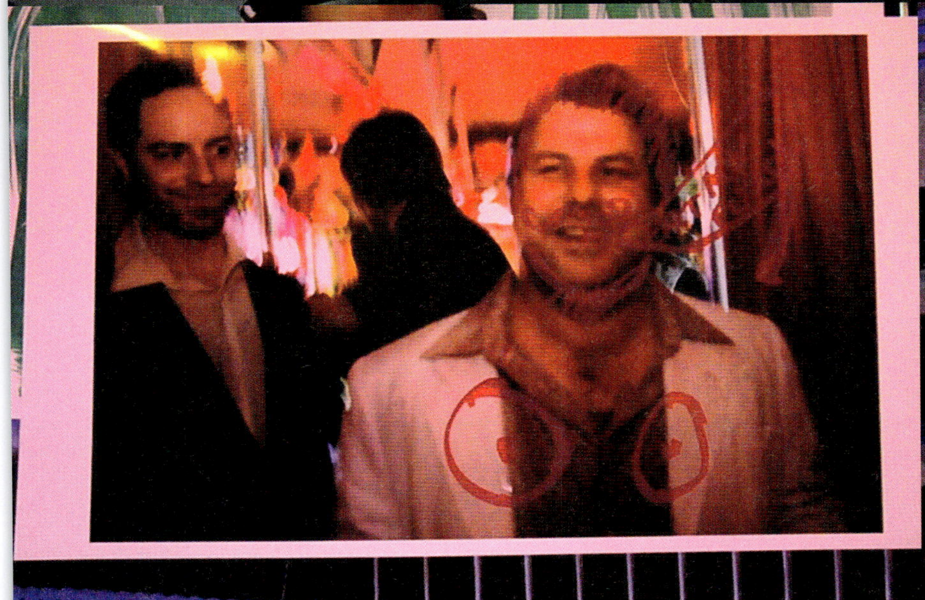

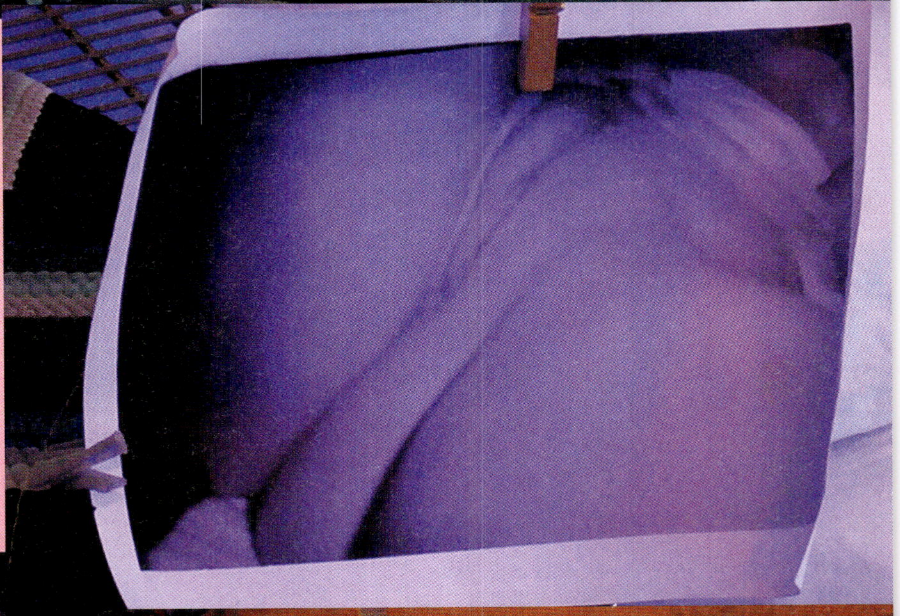

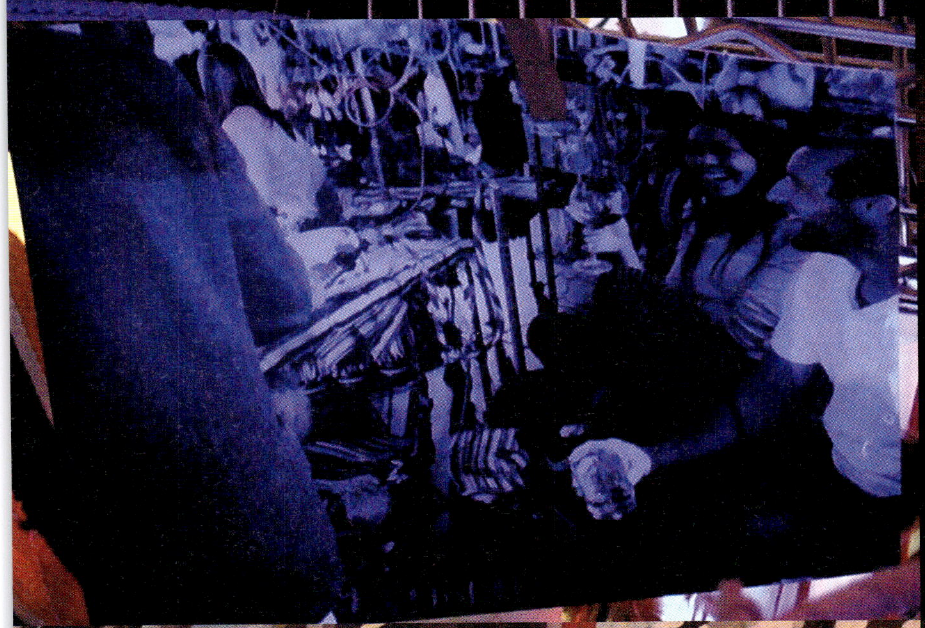

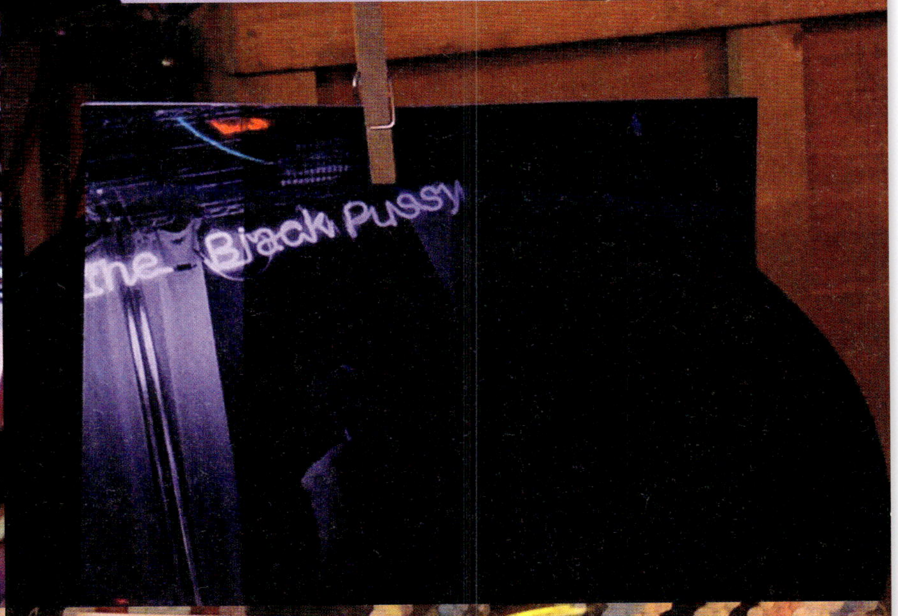
The Black Pussy

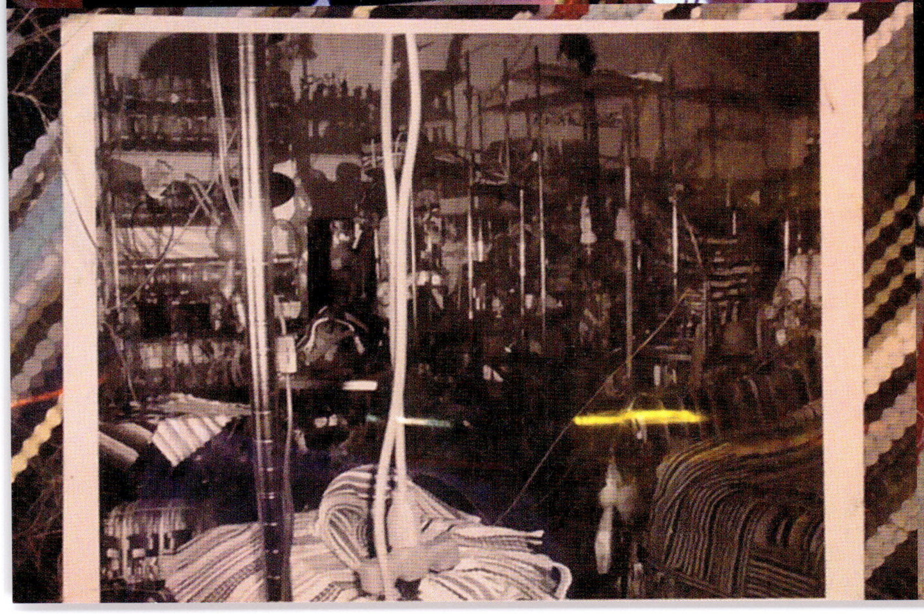

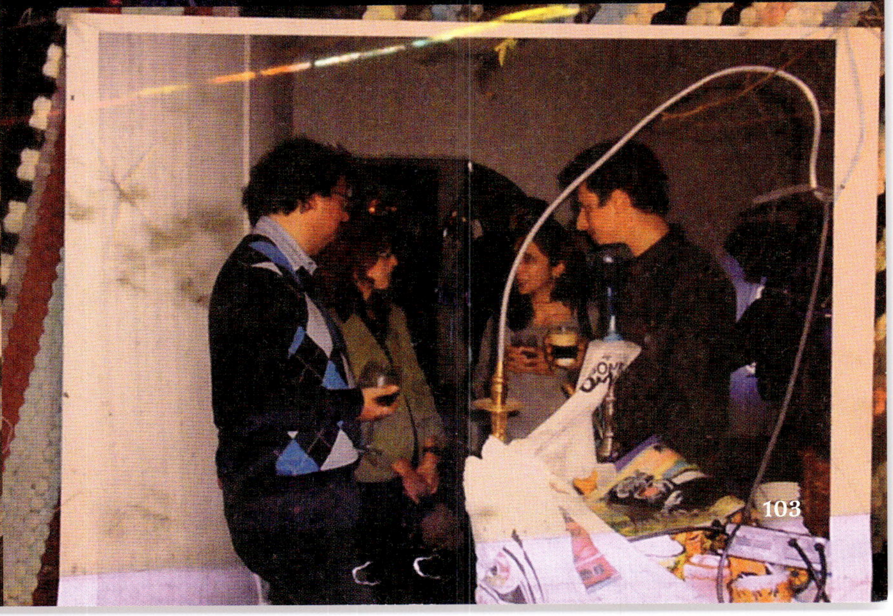

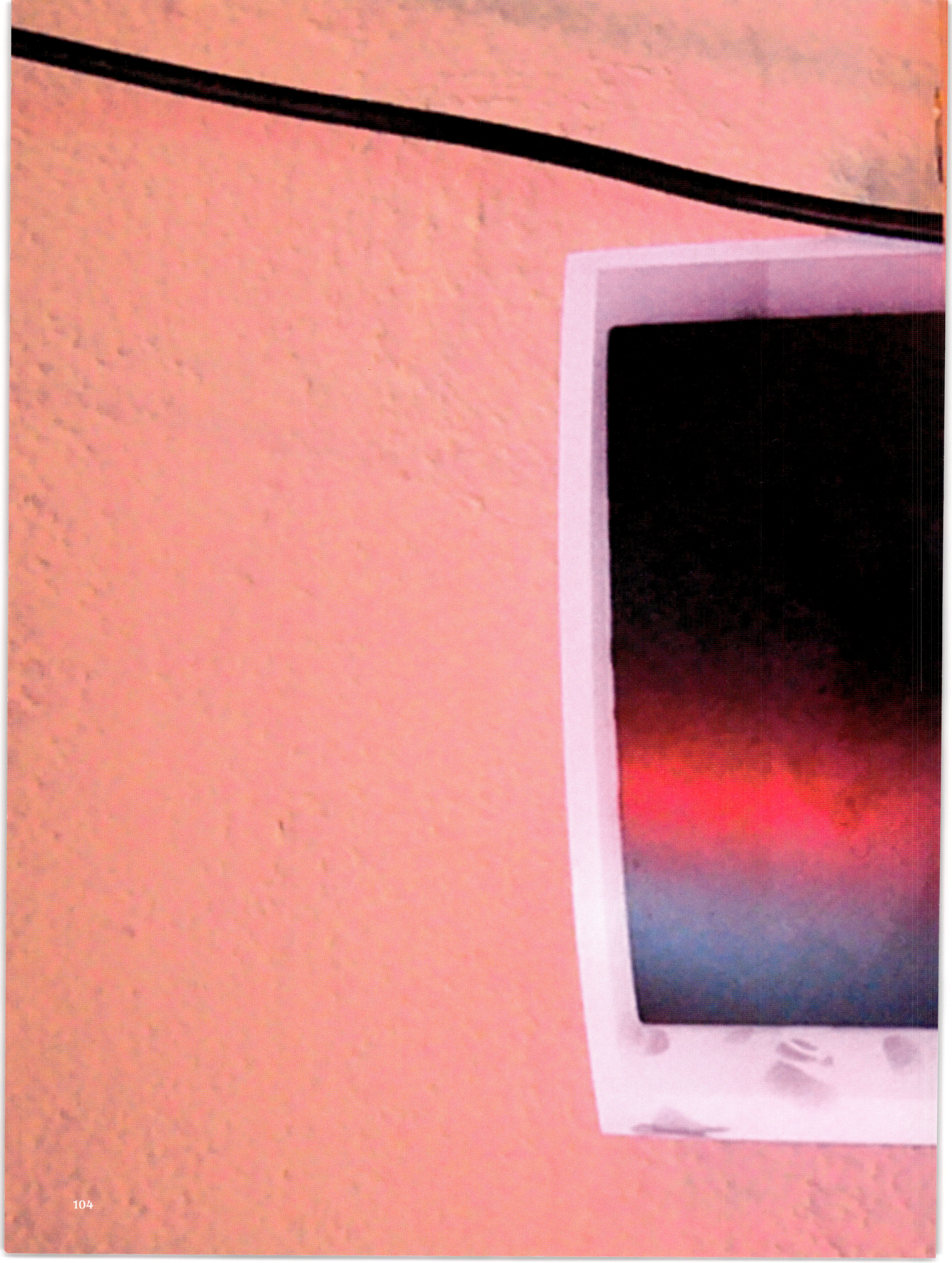

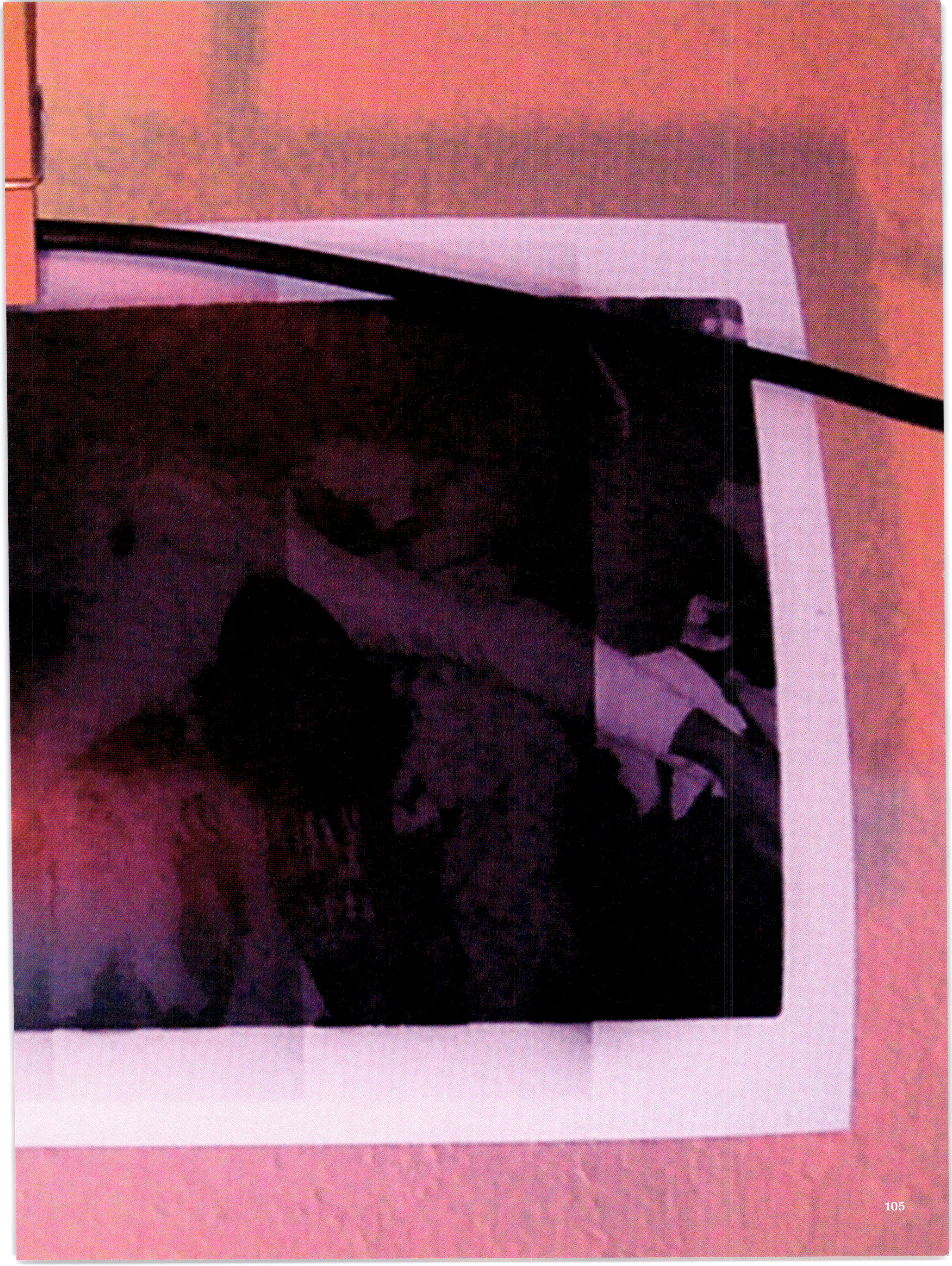

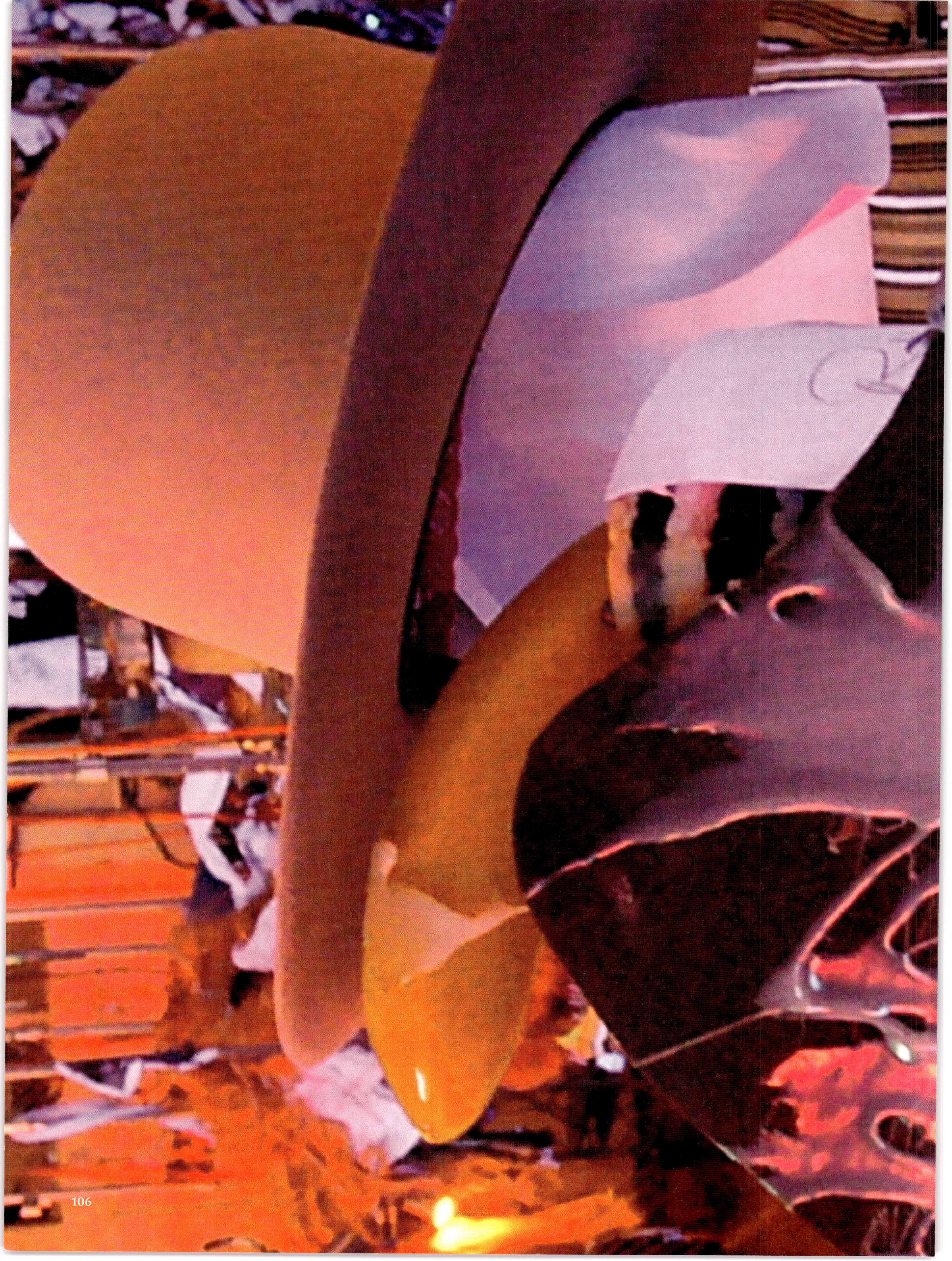

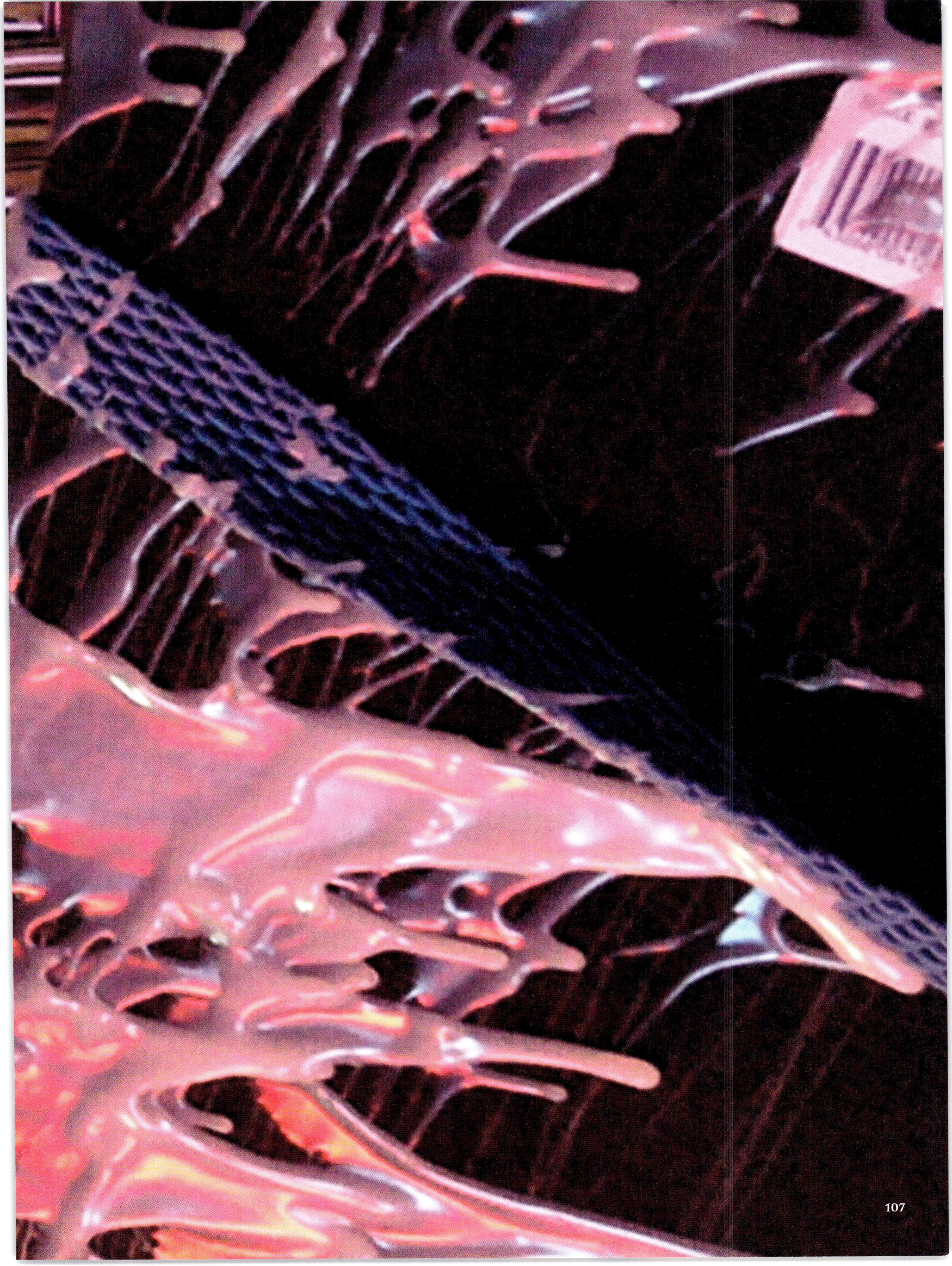

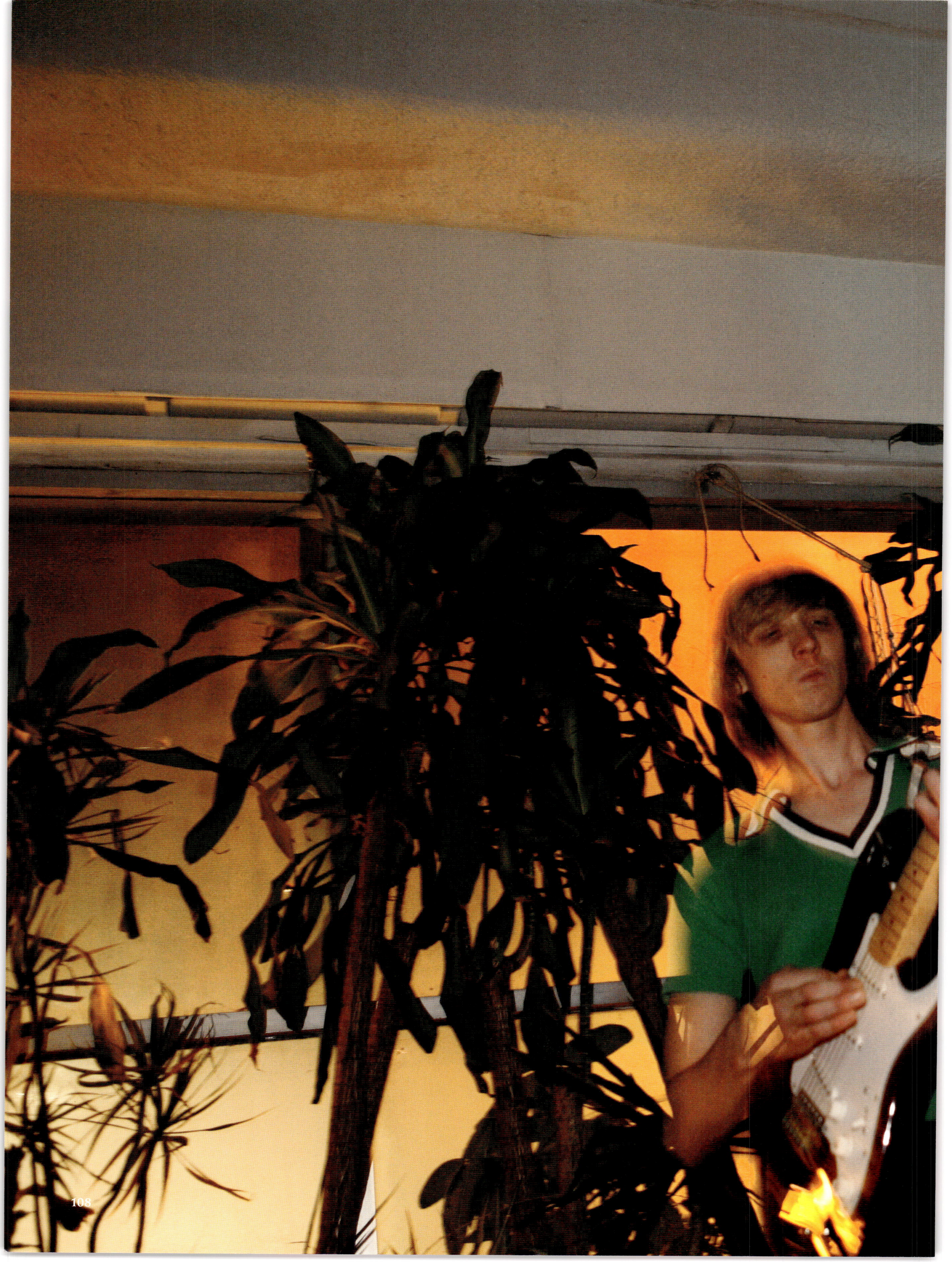

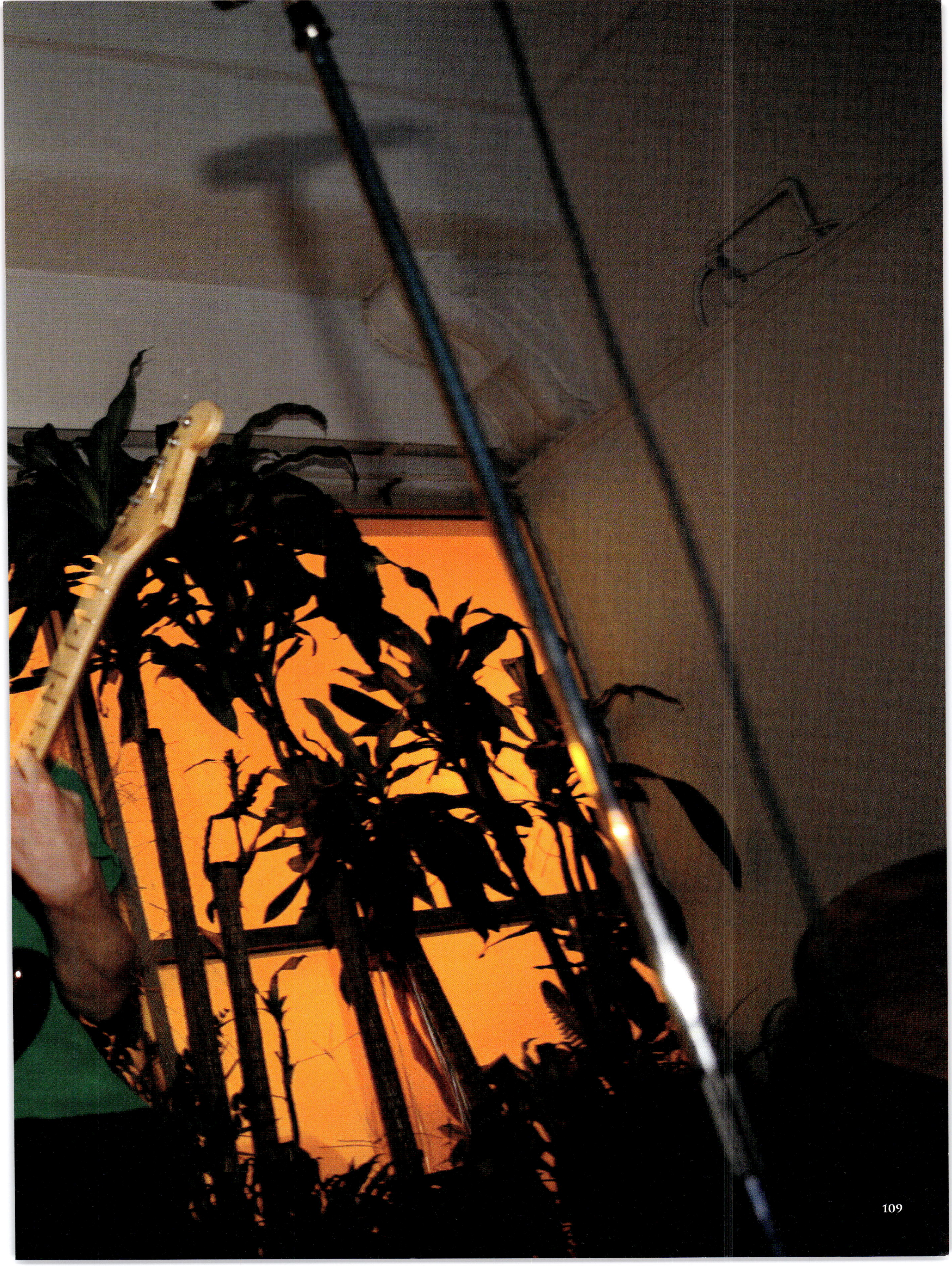

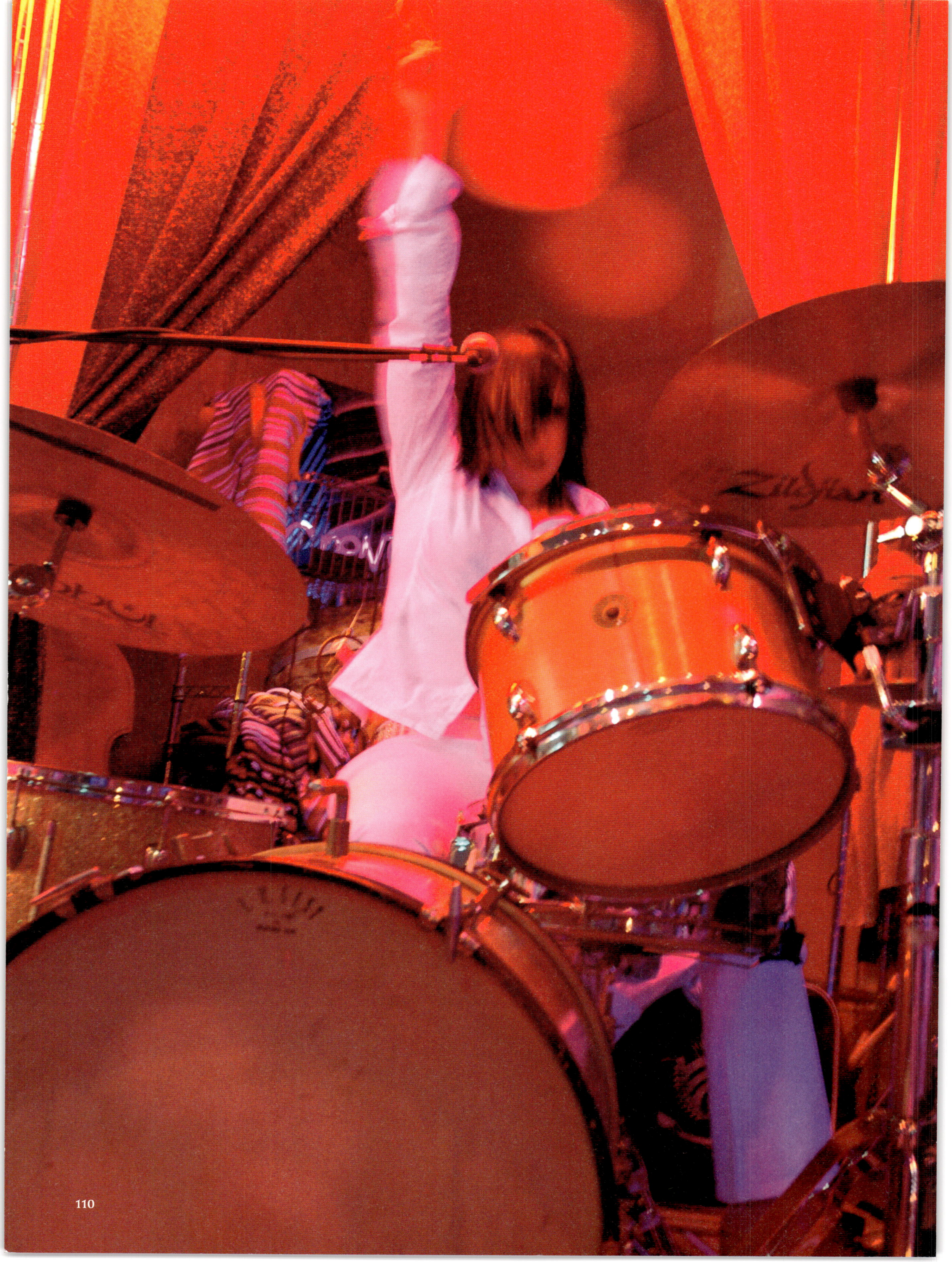
Zildjian

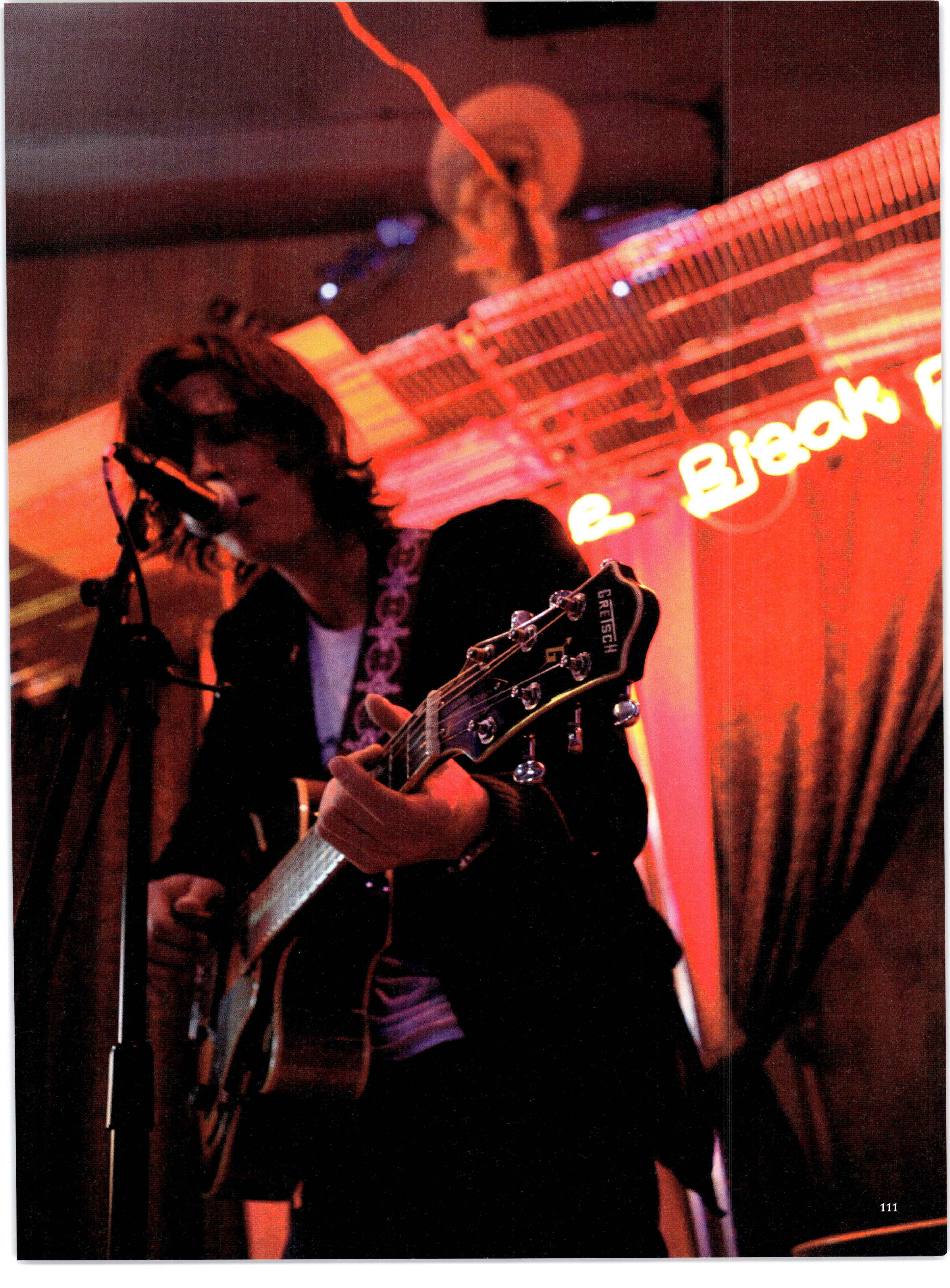
GRETSCH

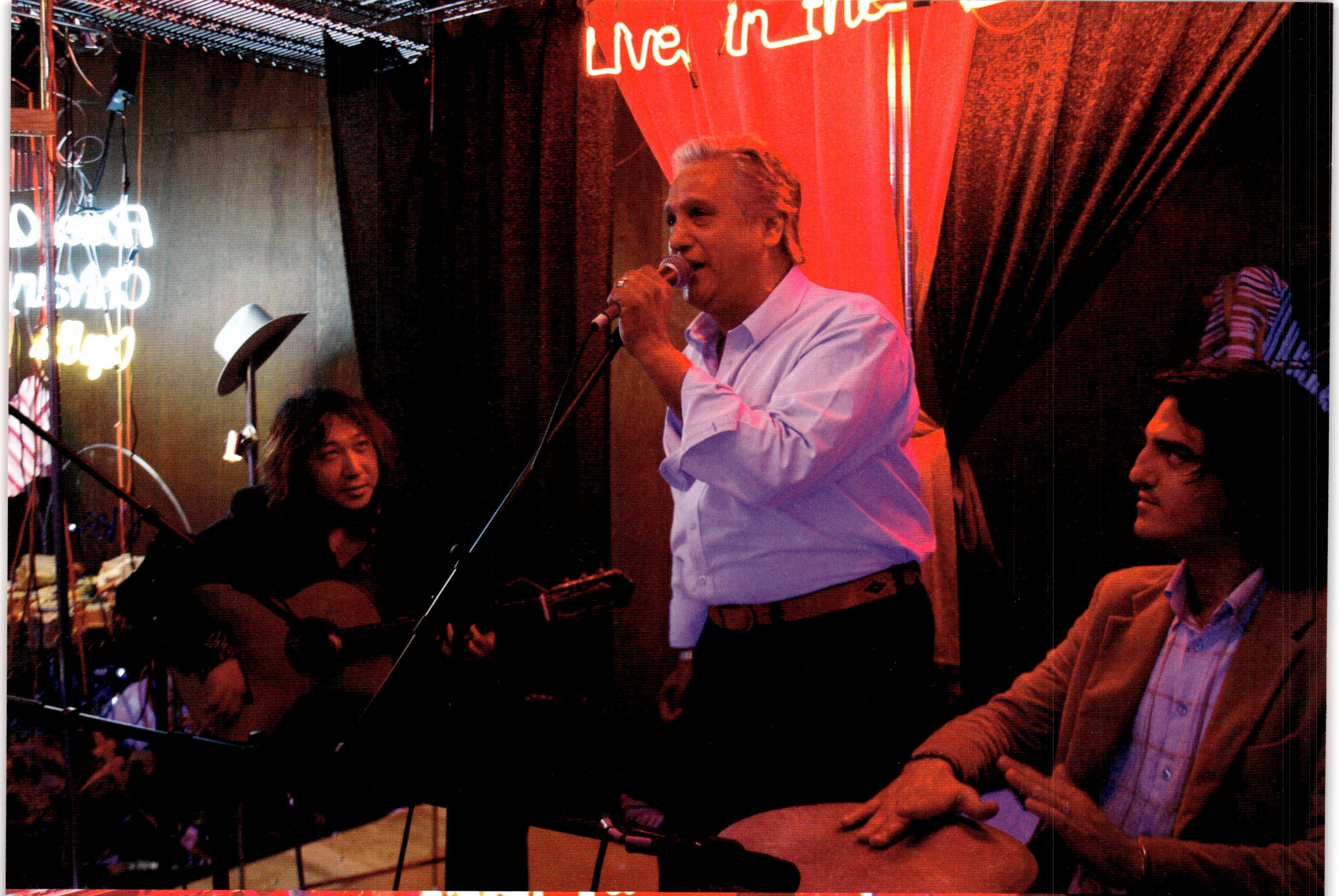

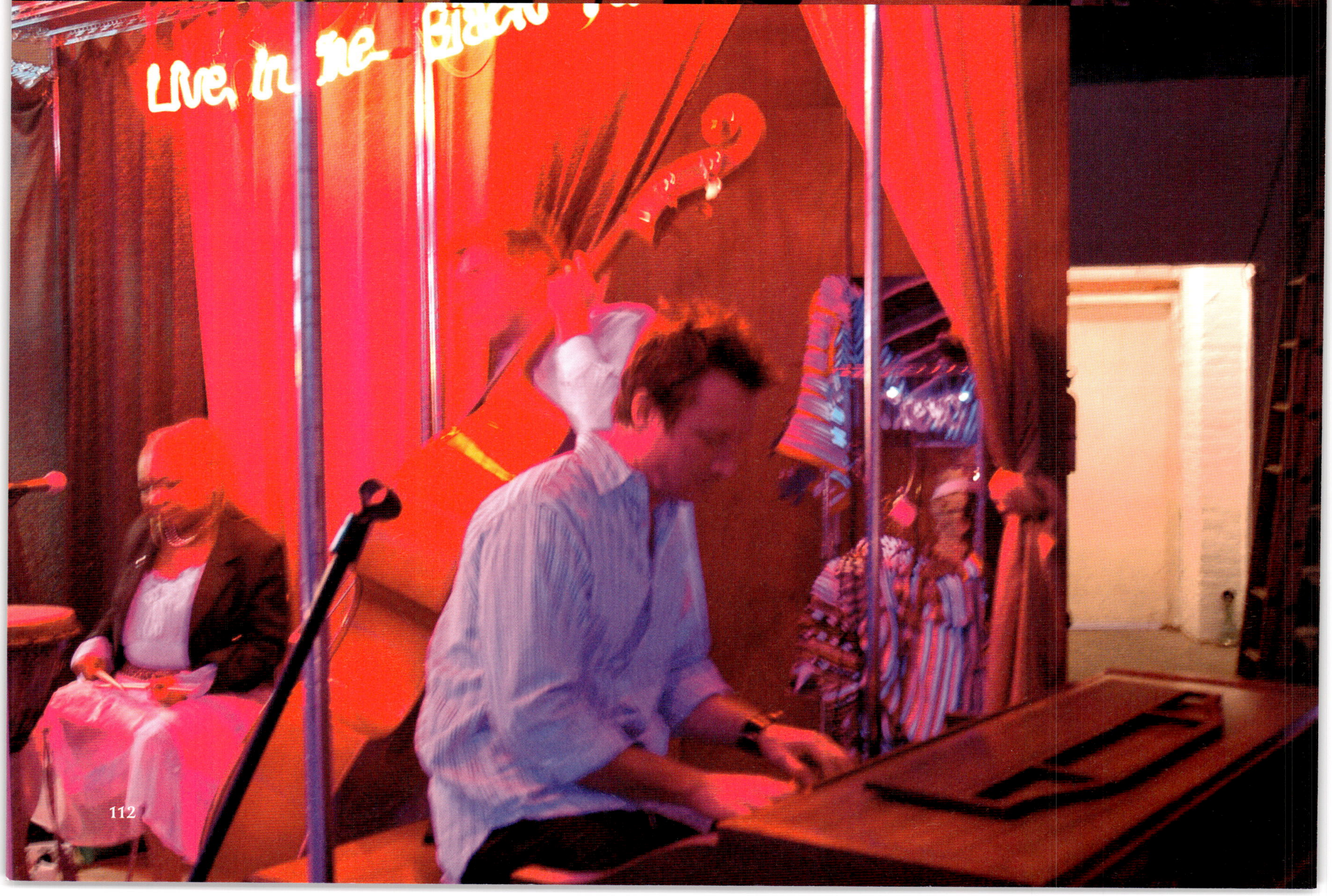
Live in the

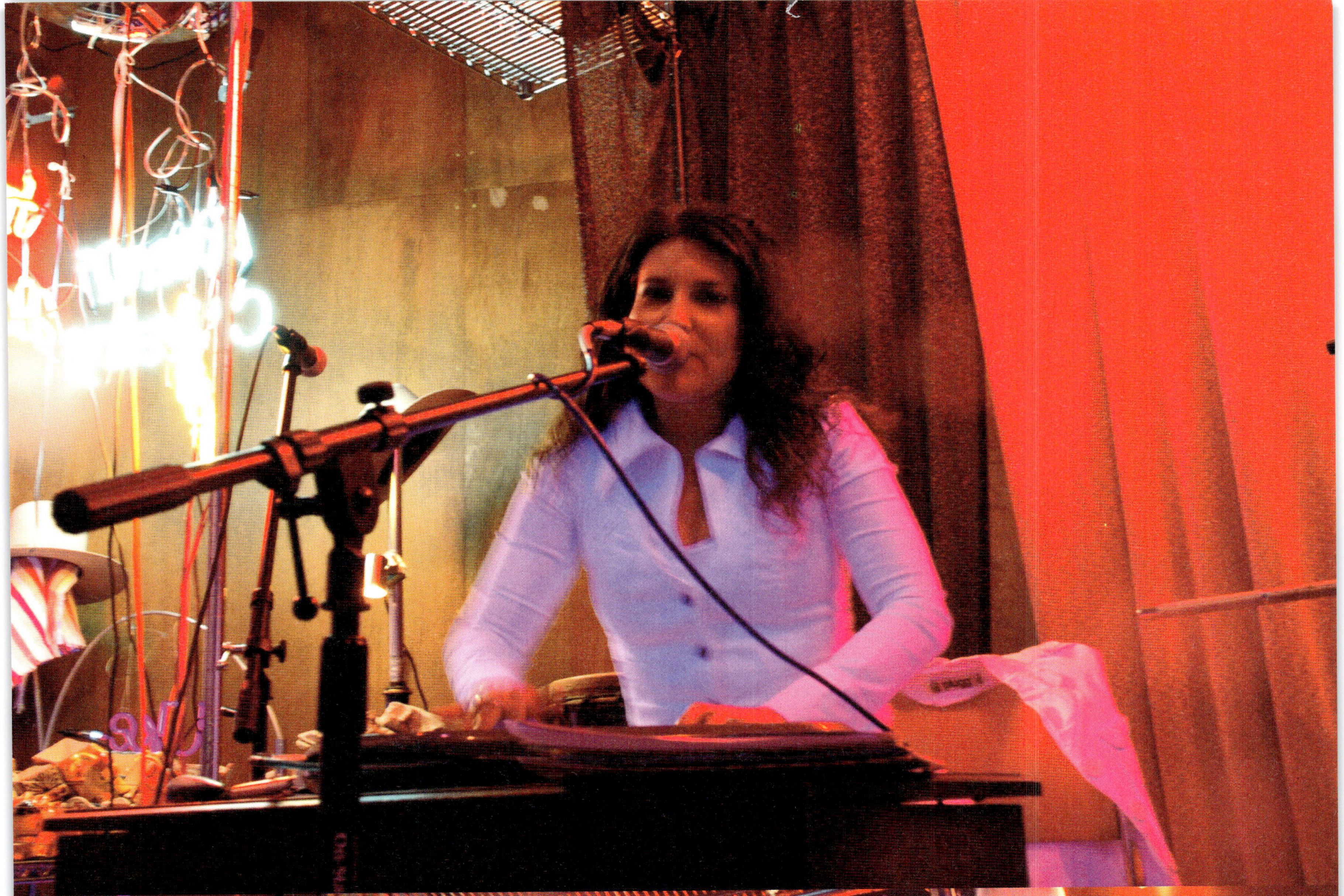

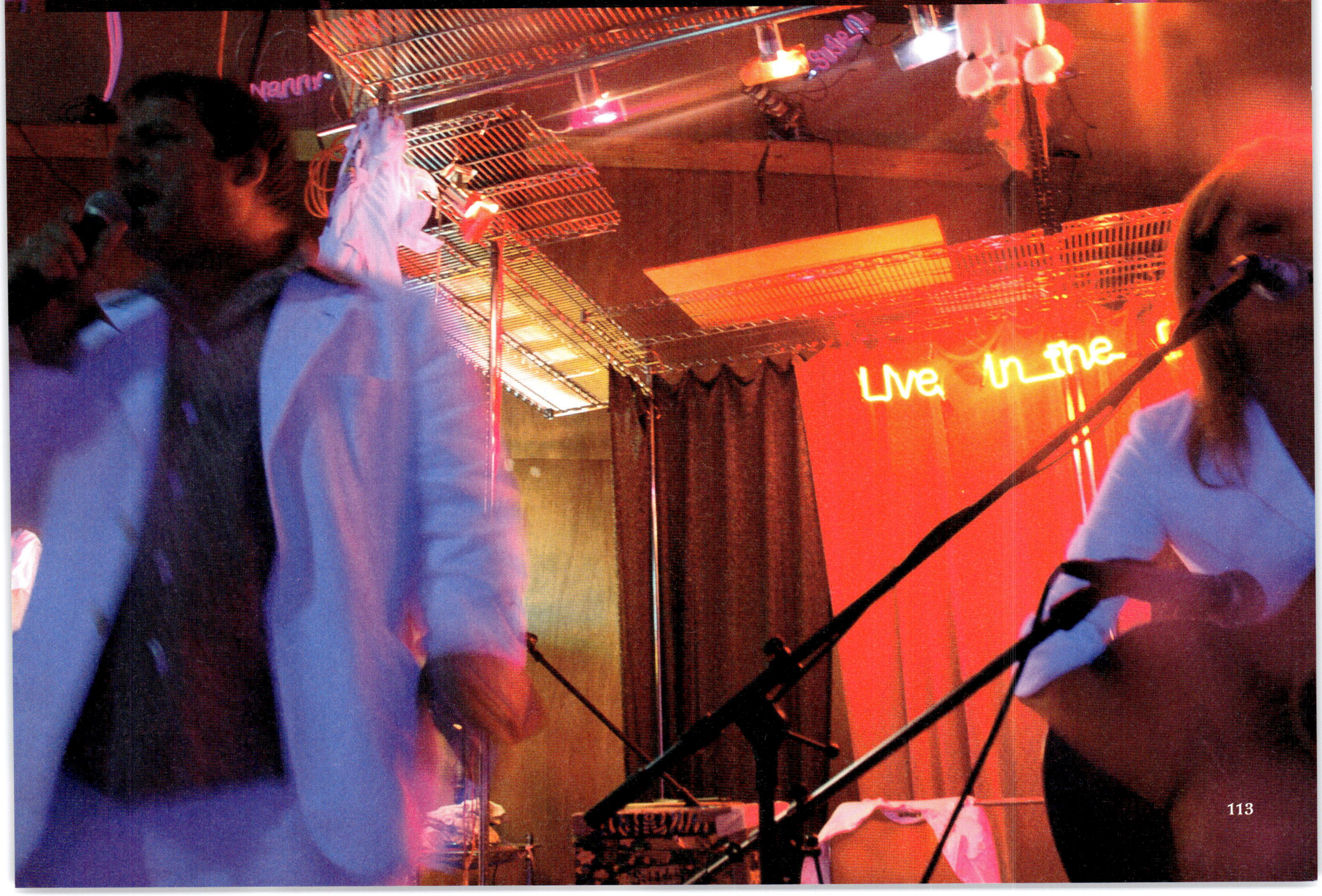
Live in the

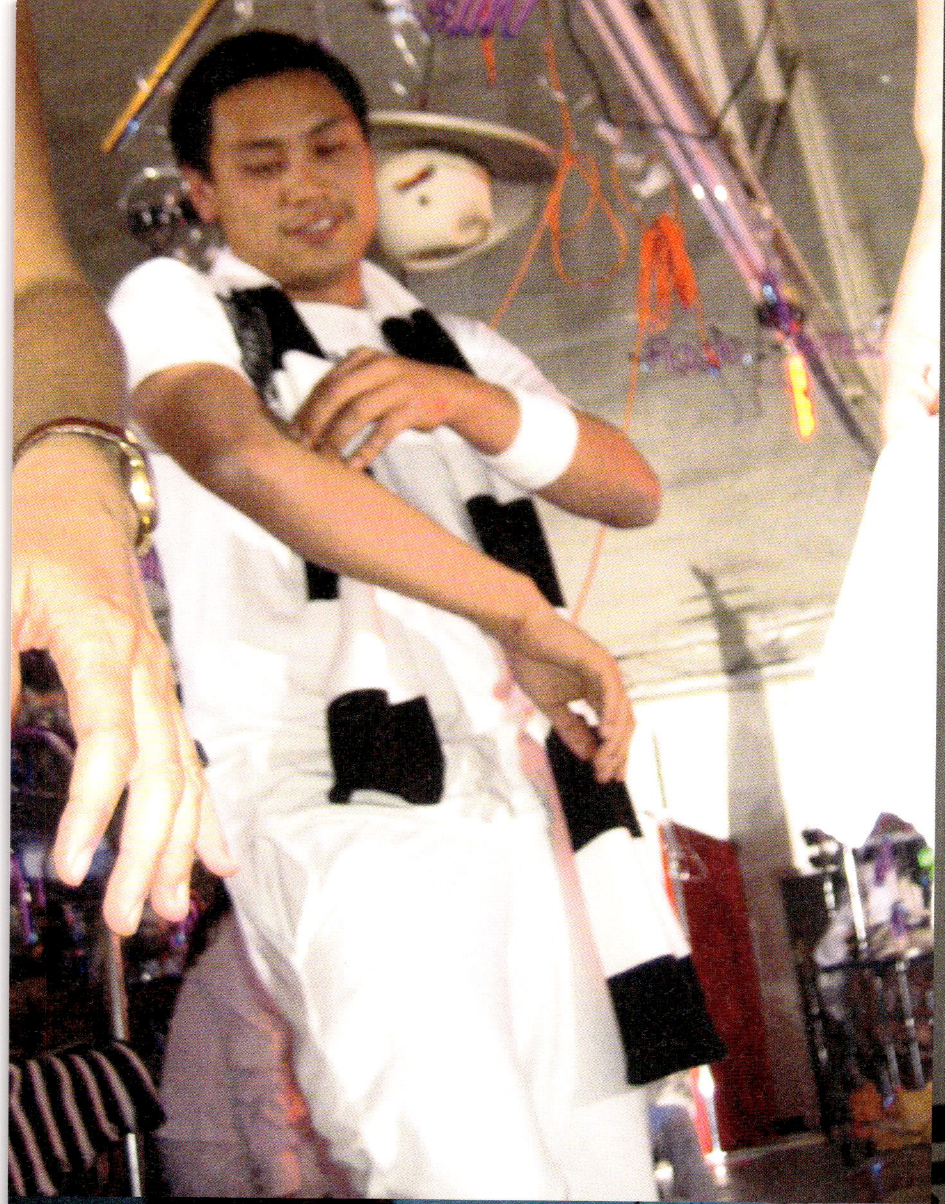

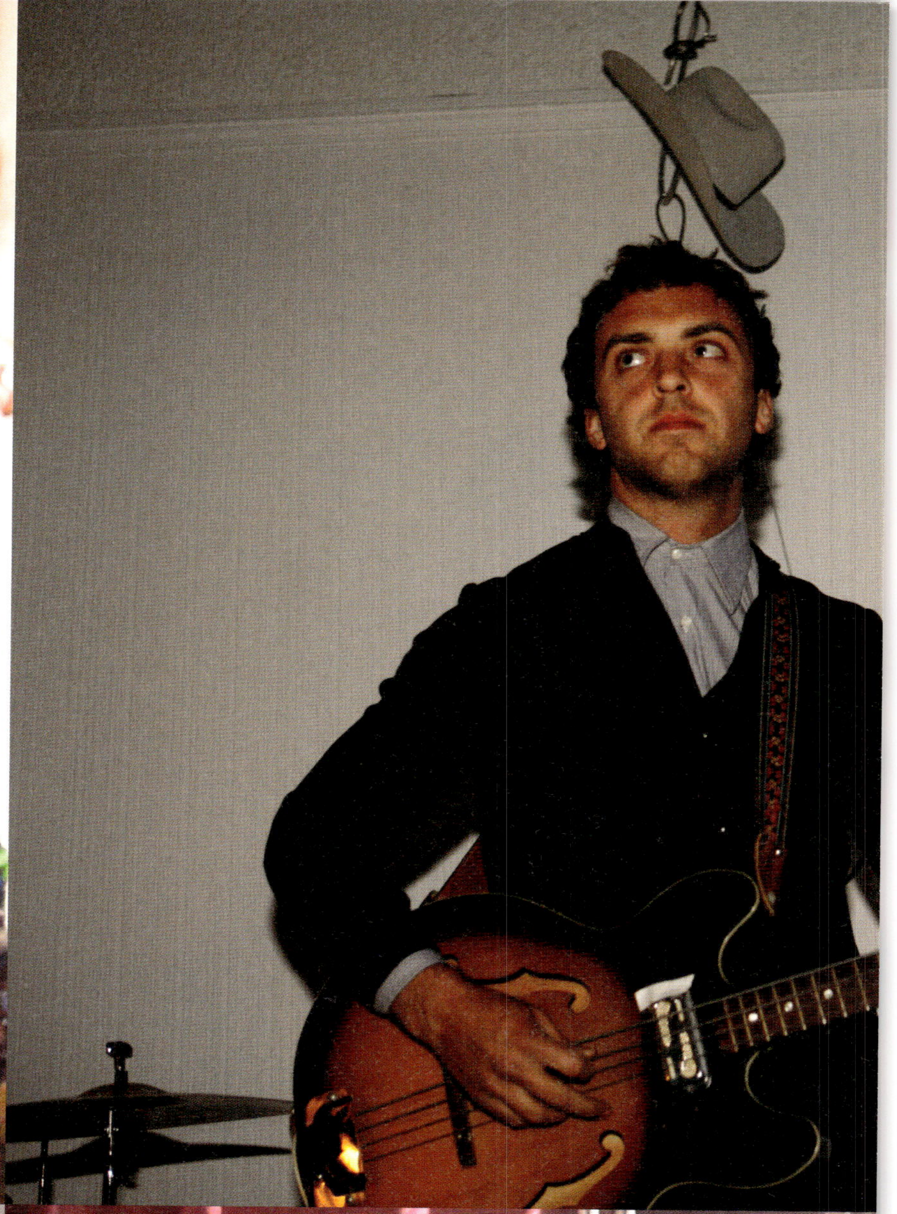

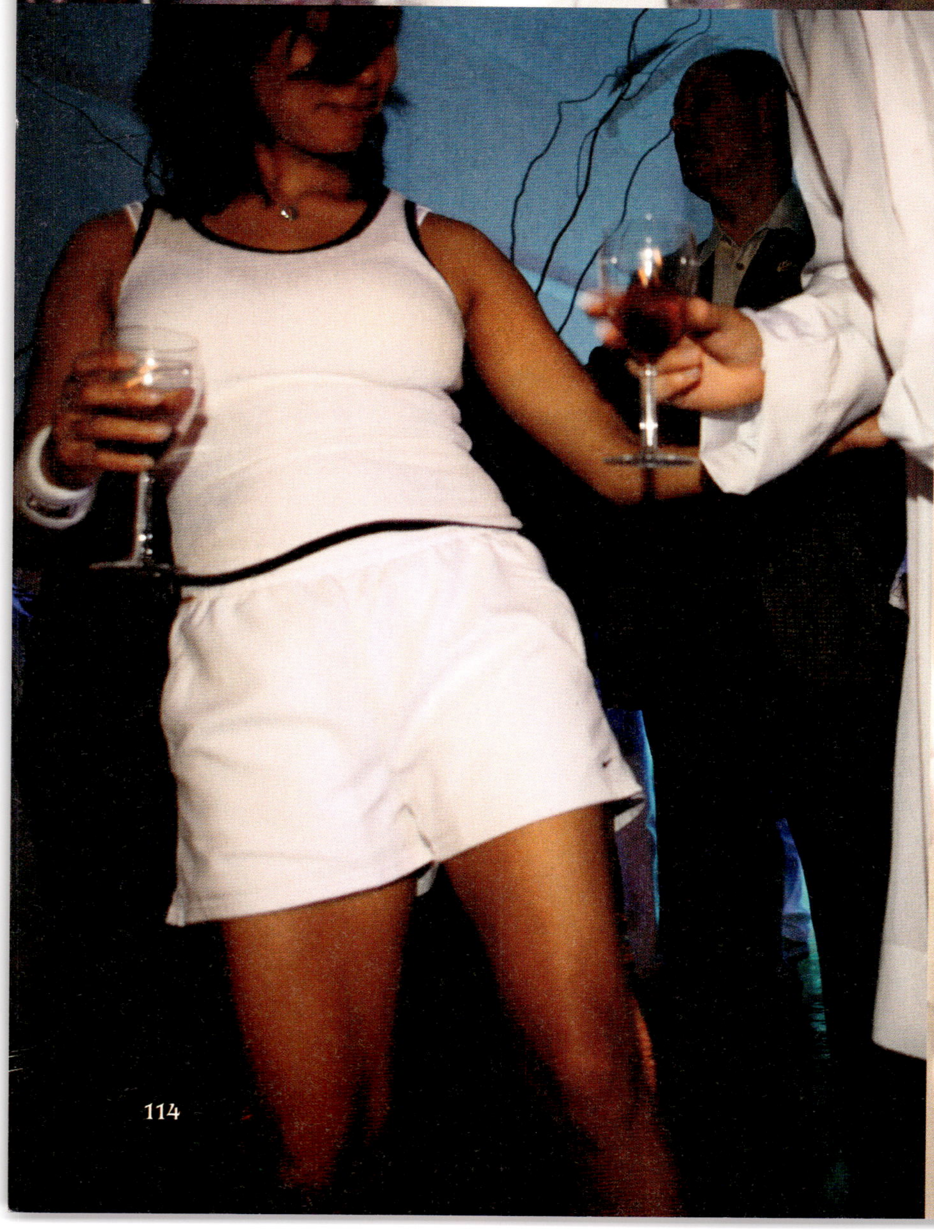

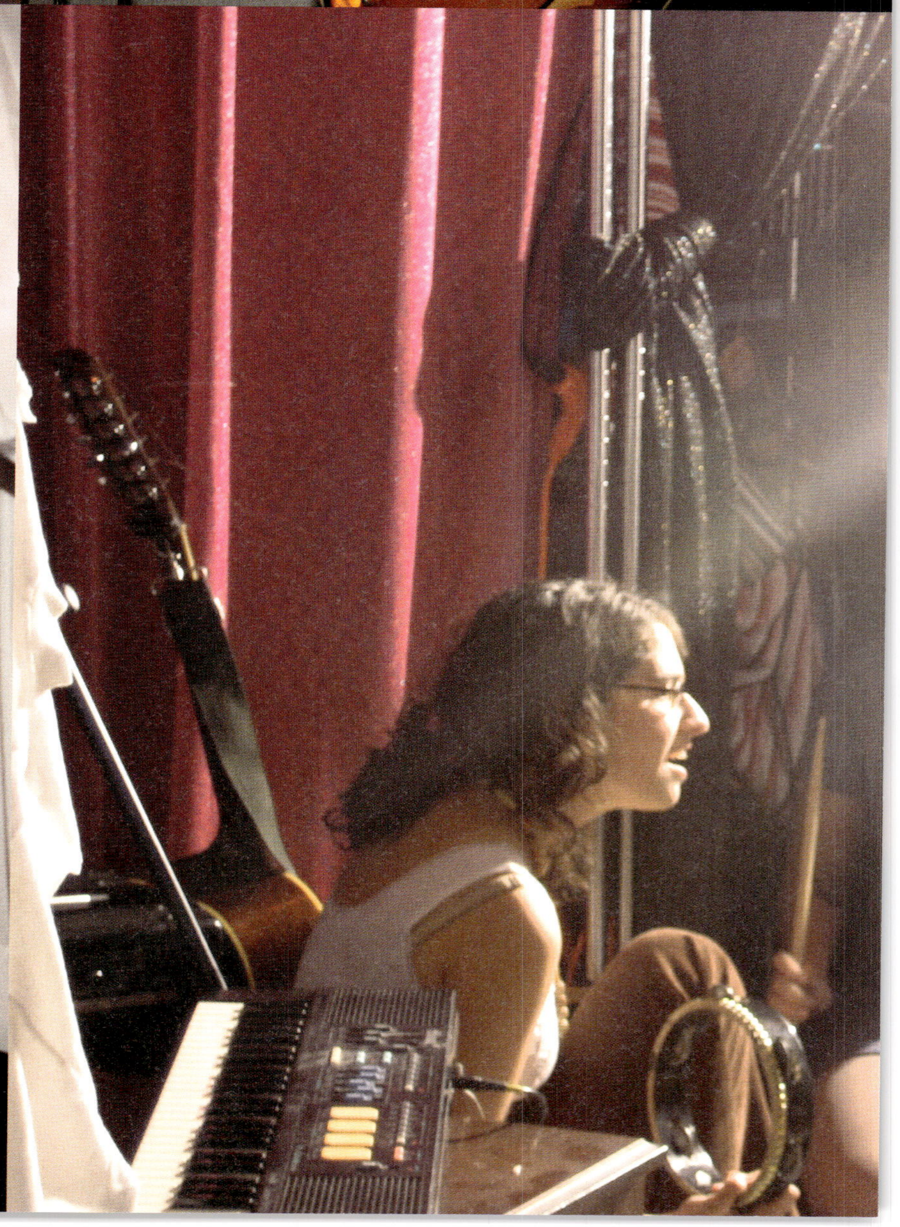

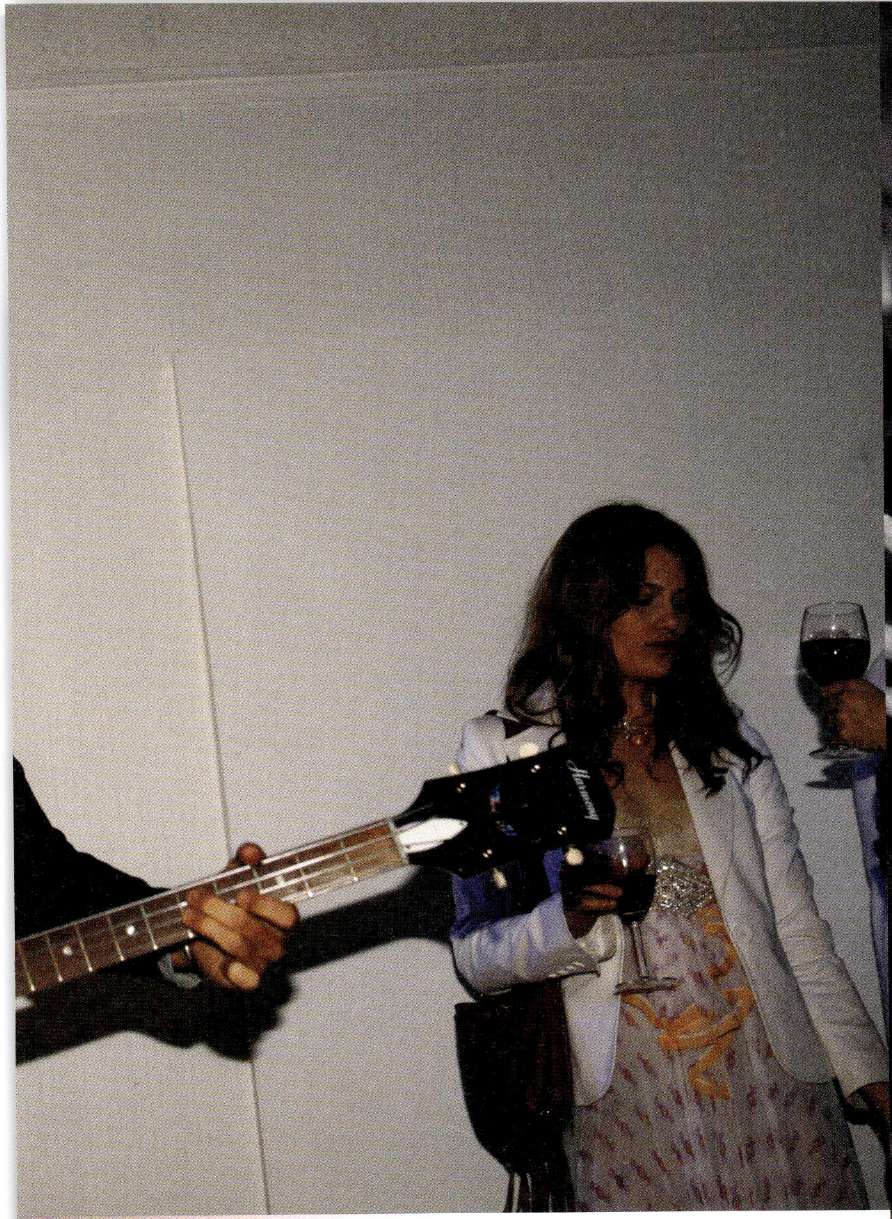
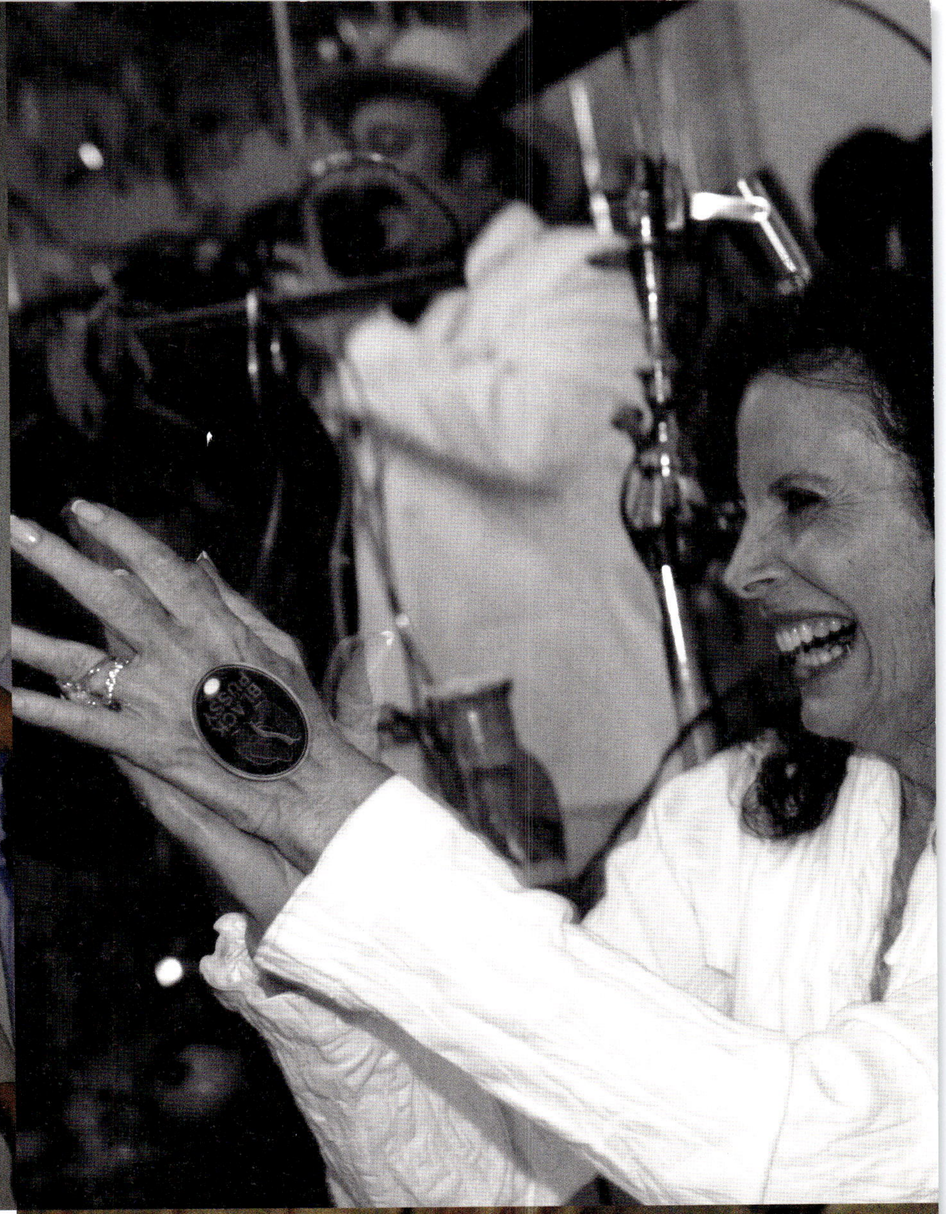
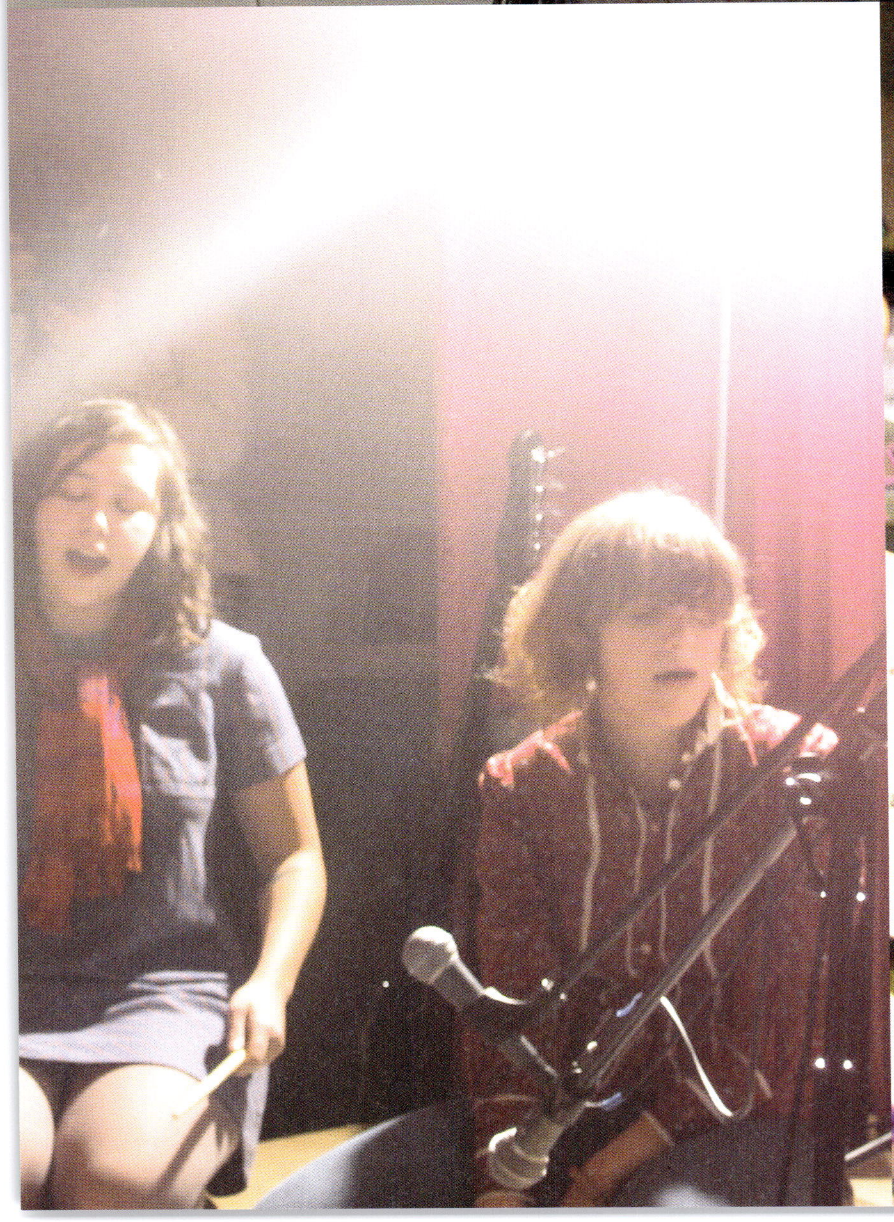
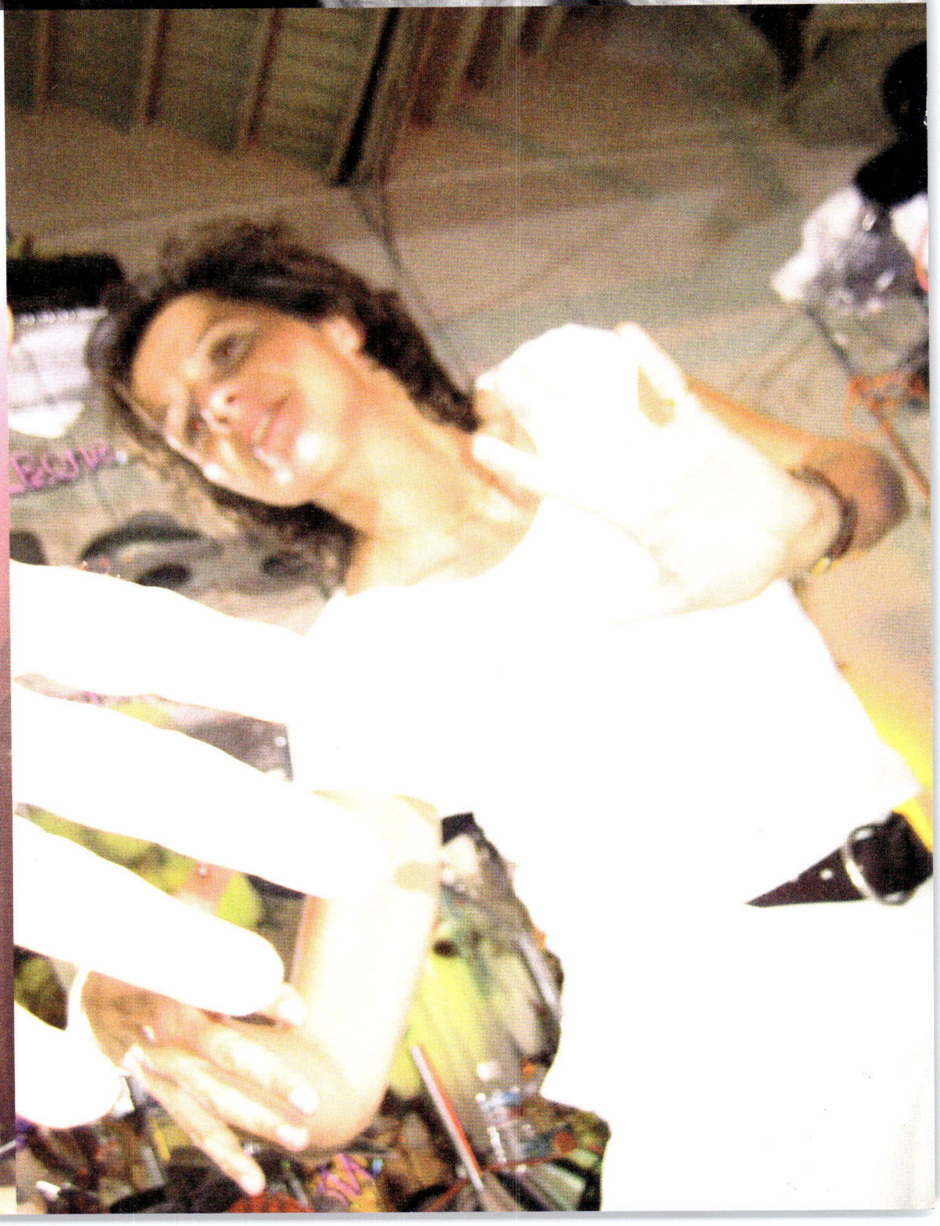

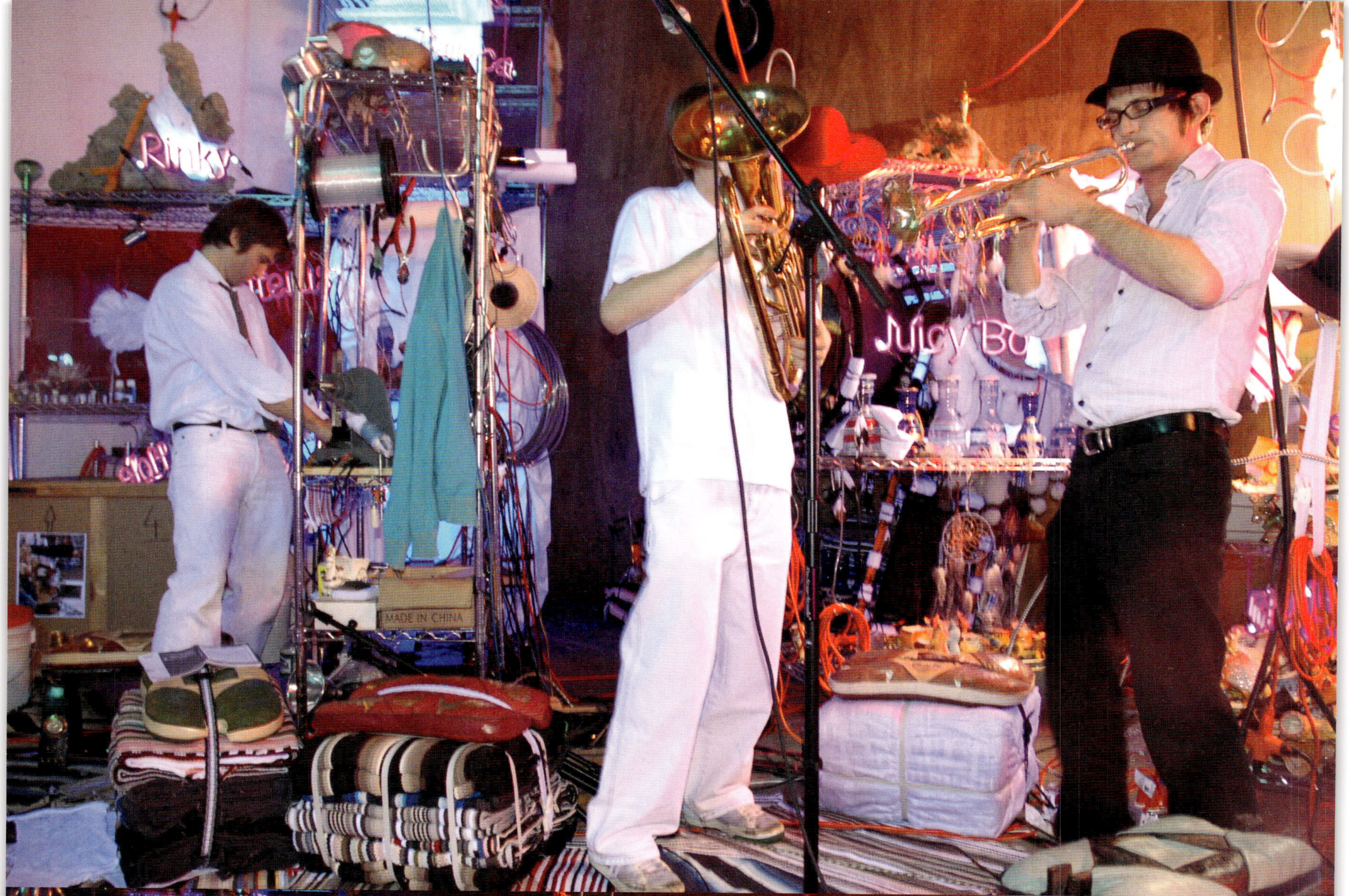
Rinky
Juicy Bo
MADE IN CHINA

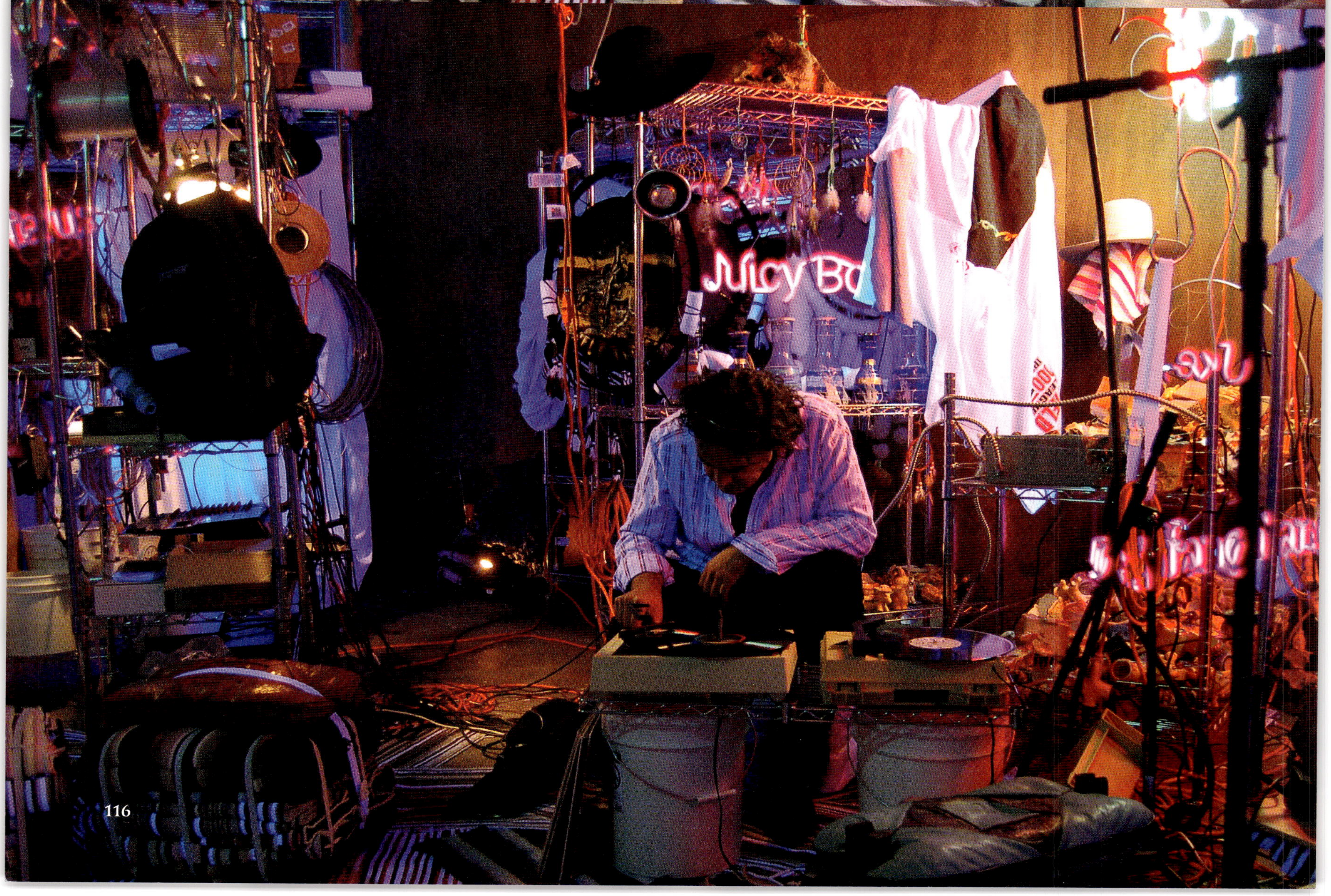
Juicy Bo

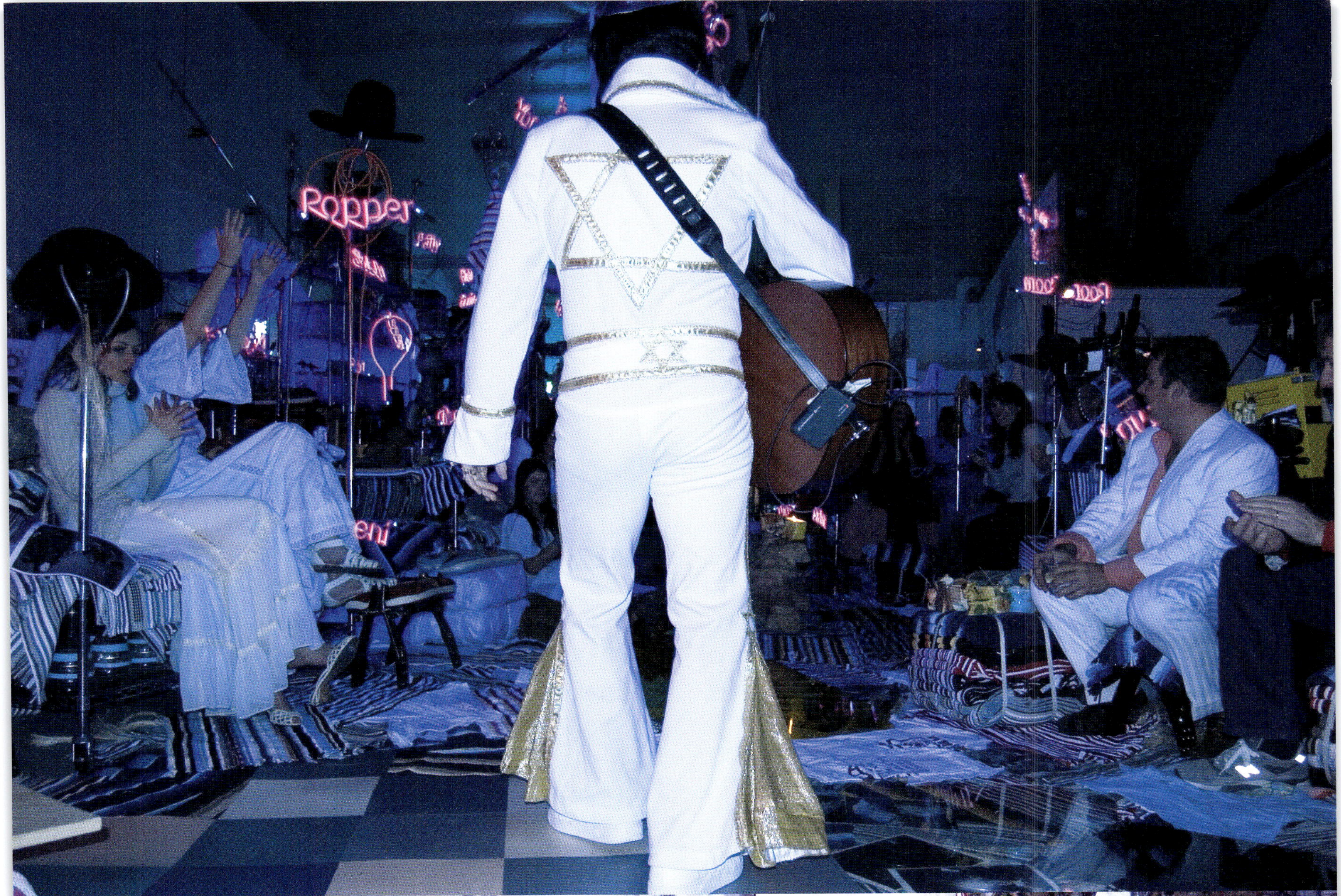

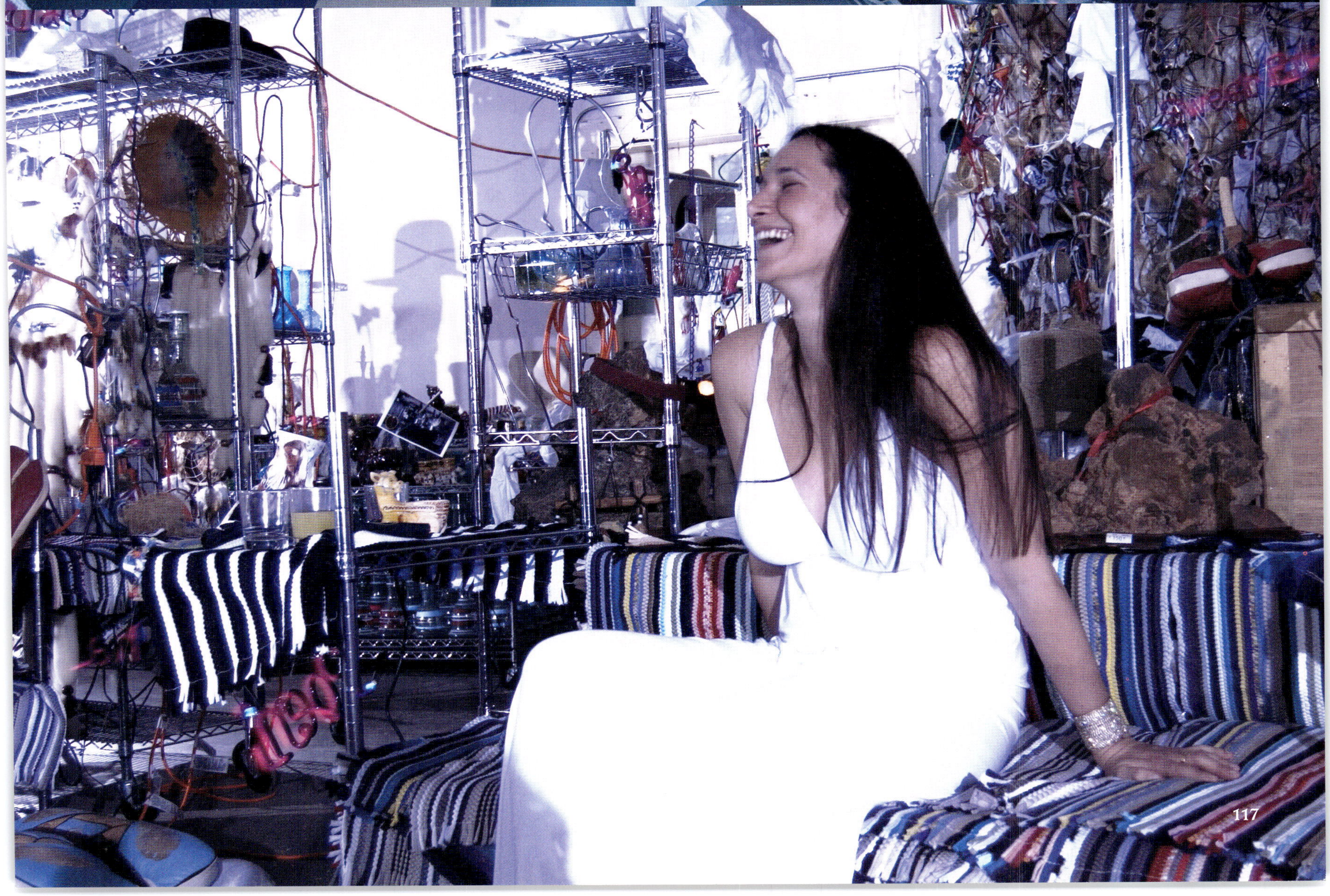

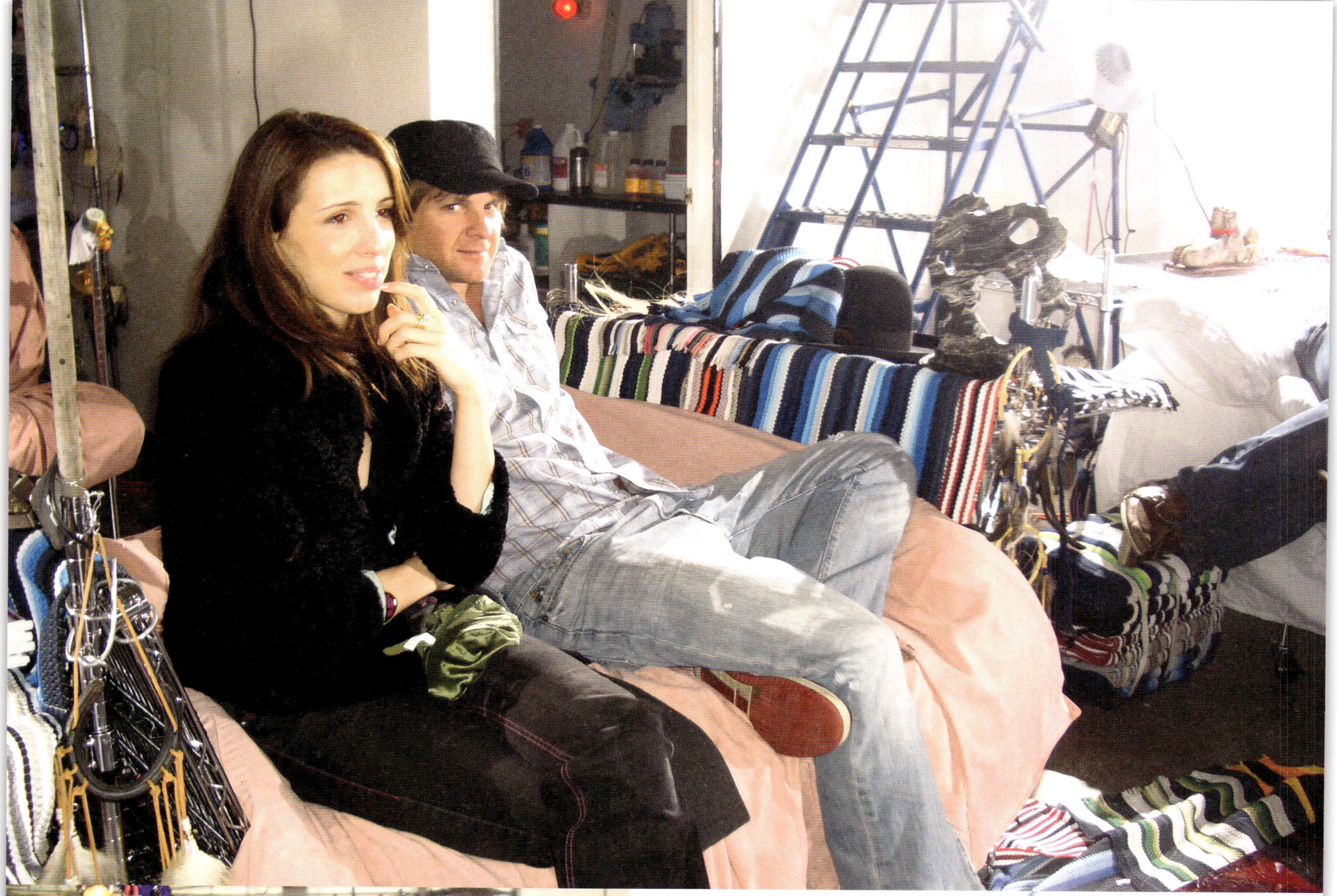

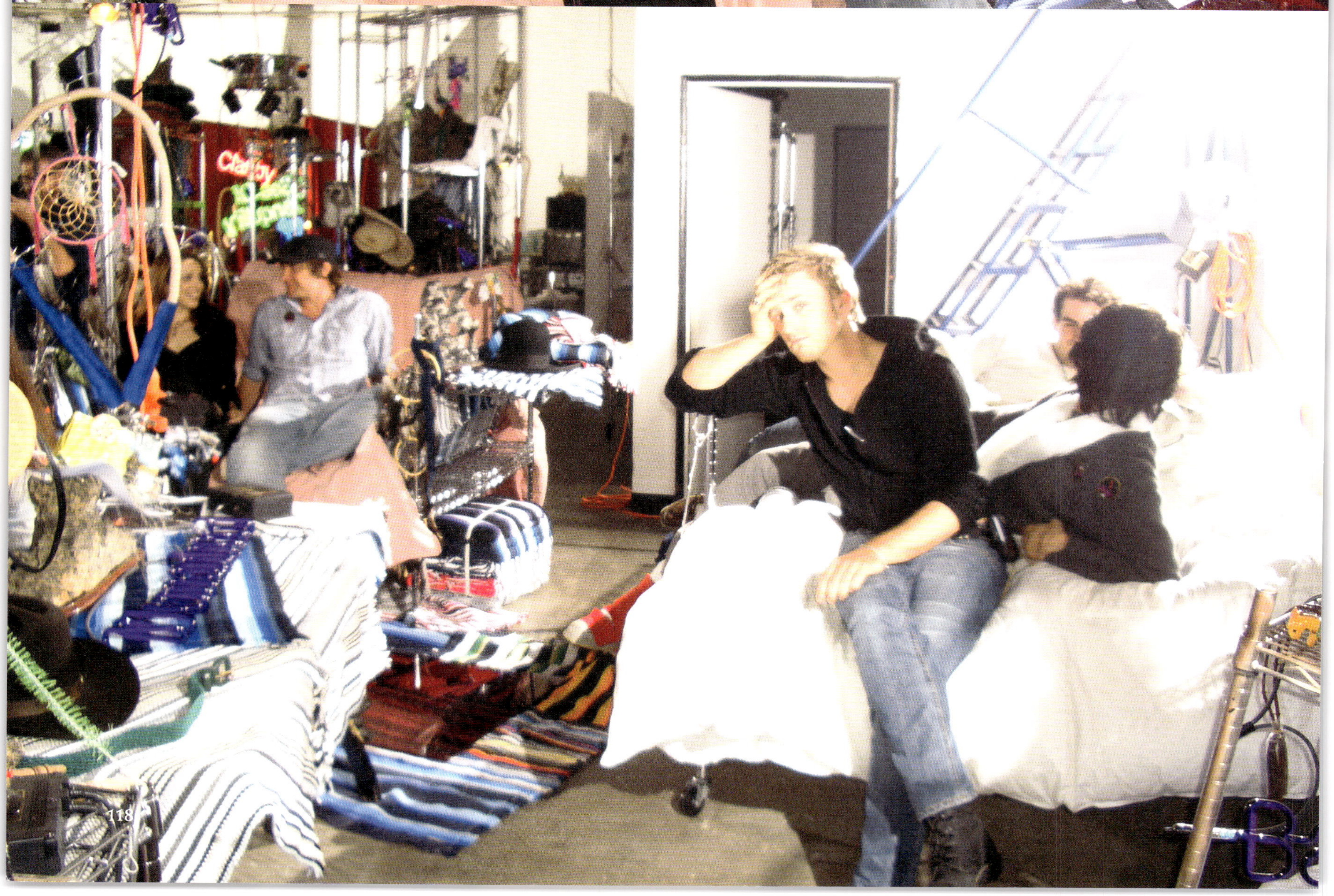

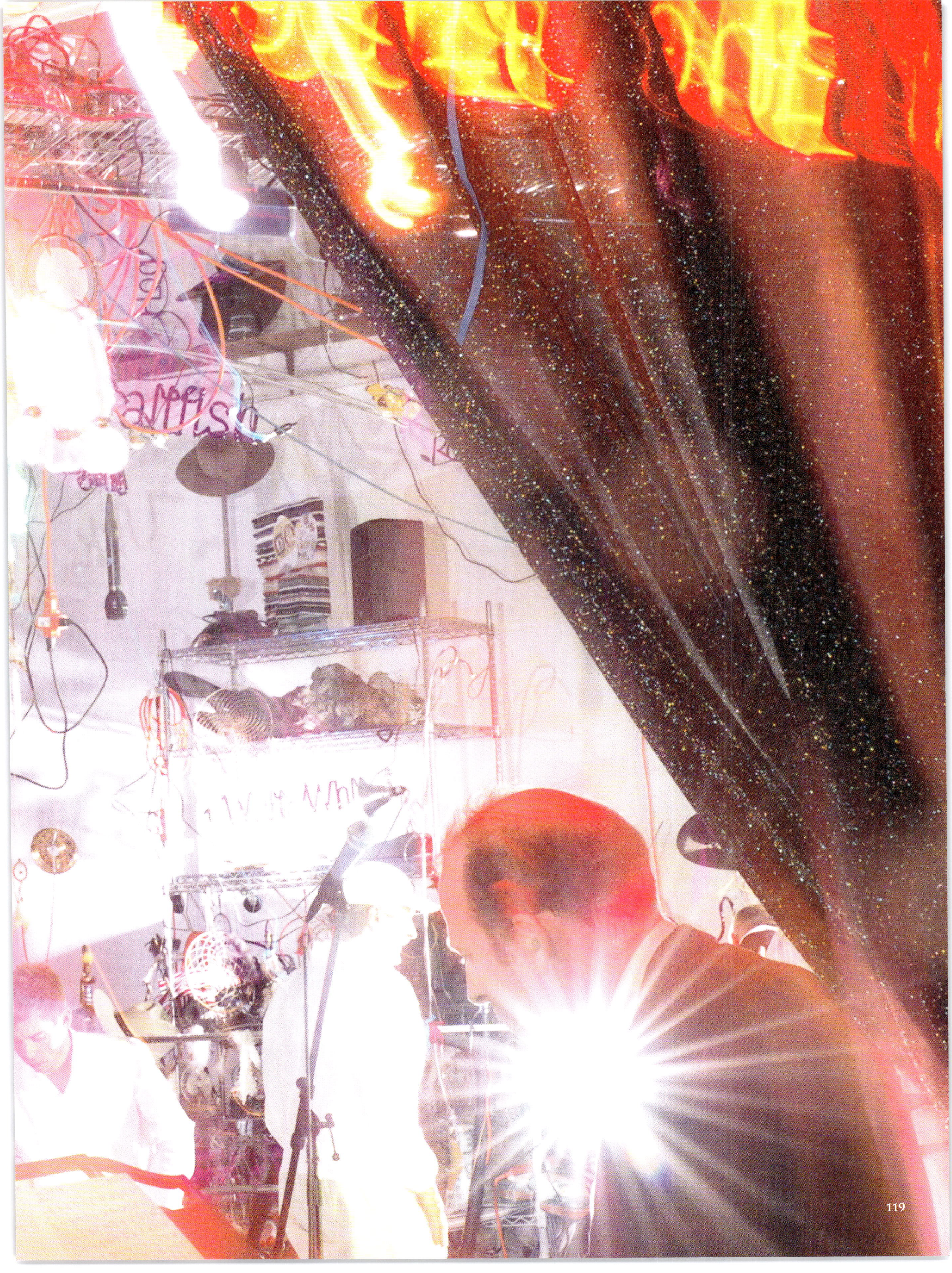

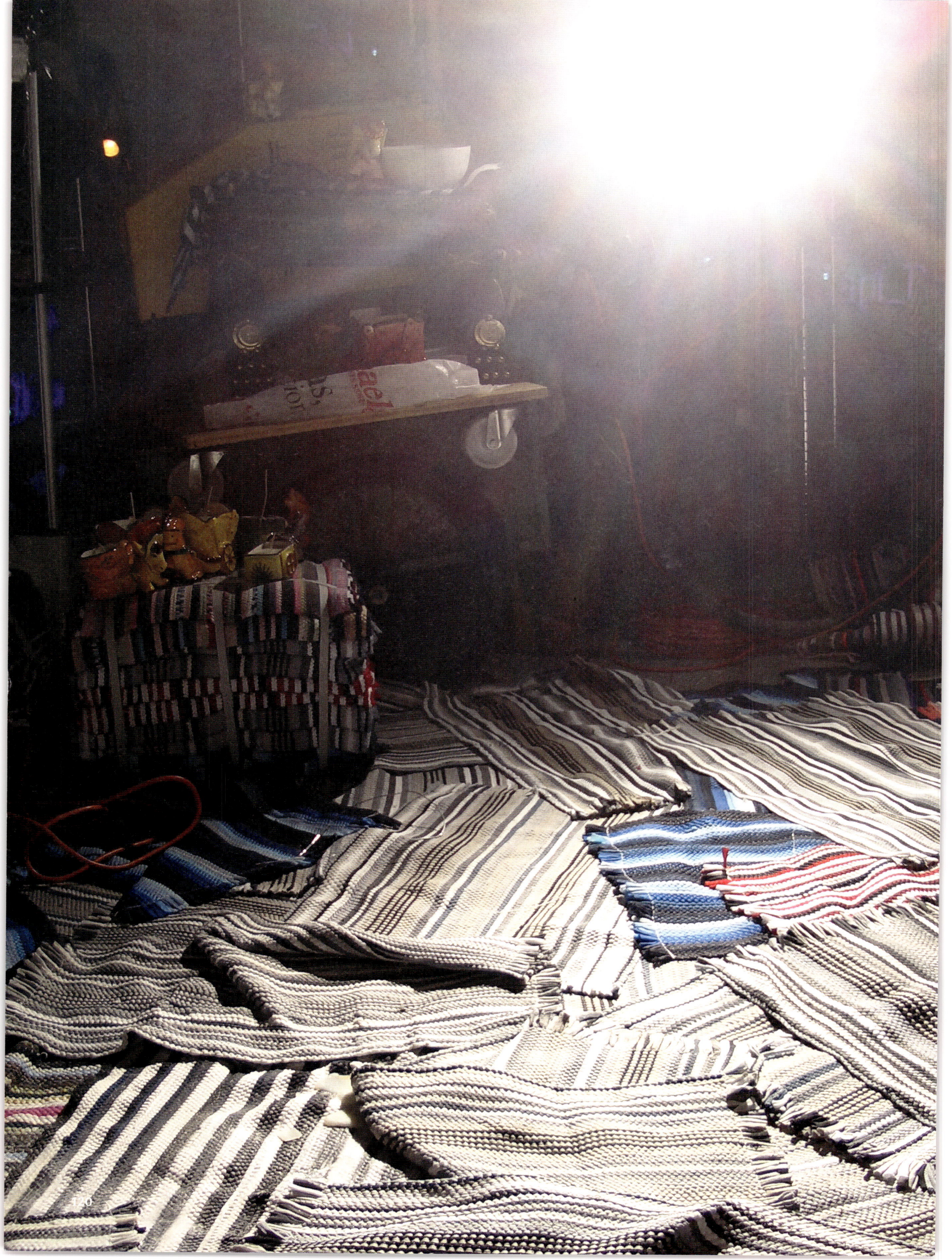

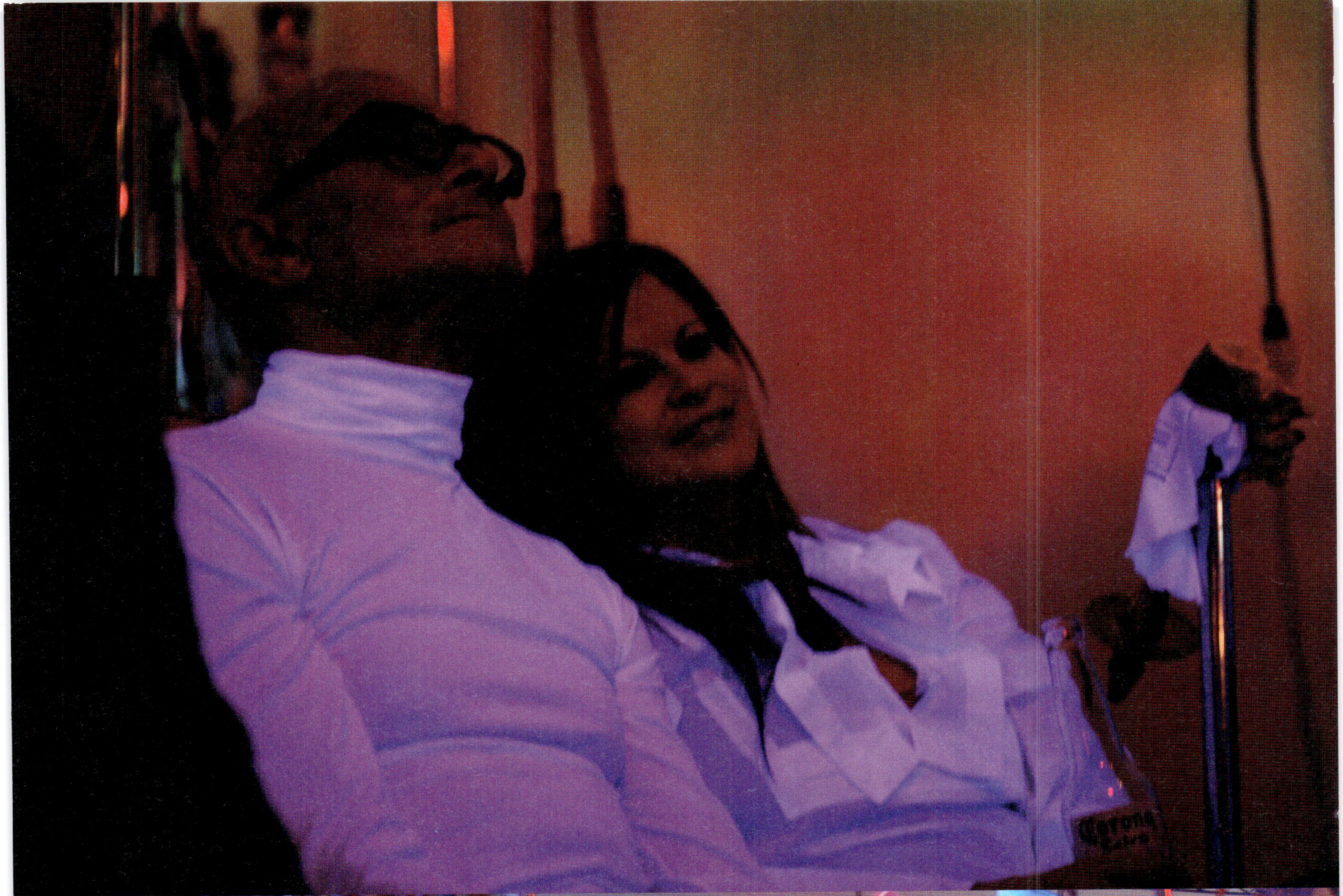

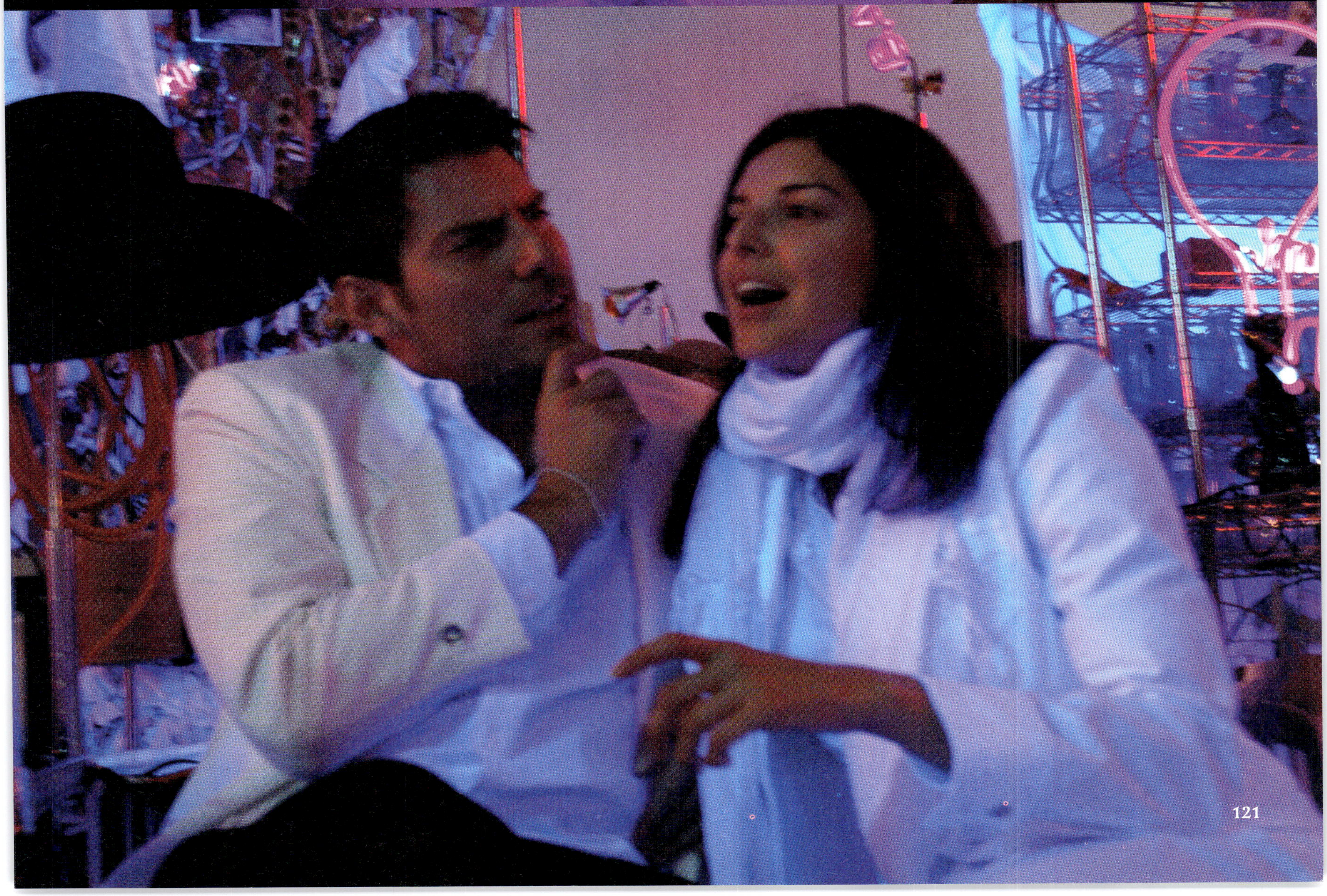

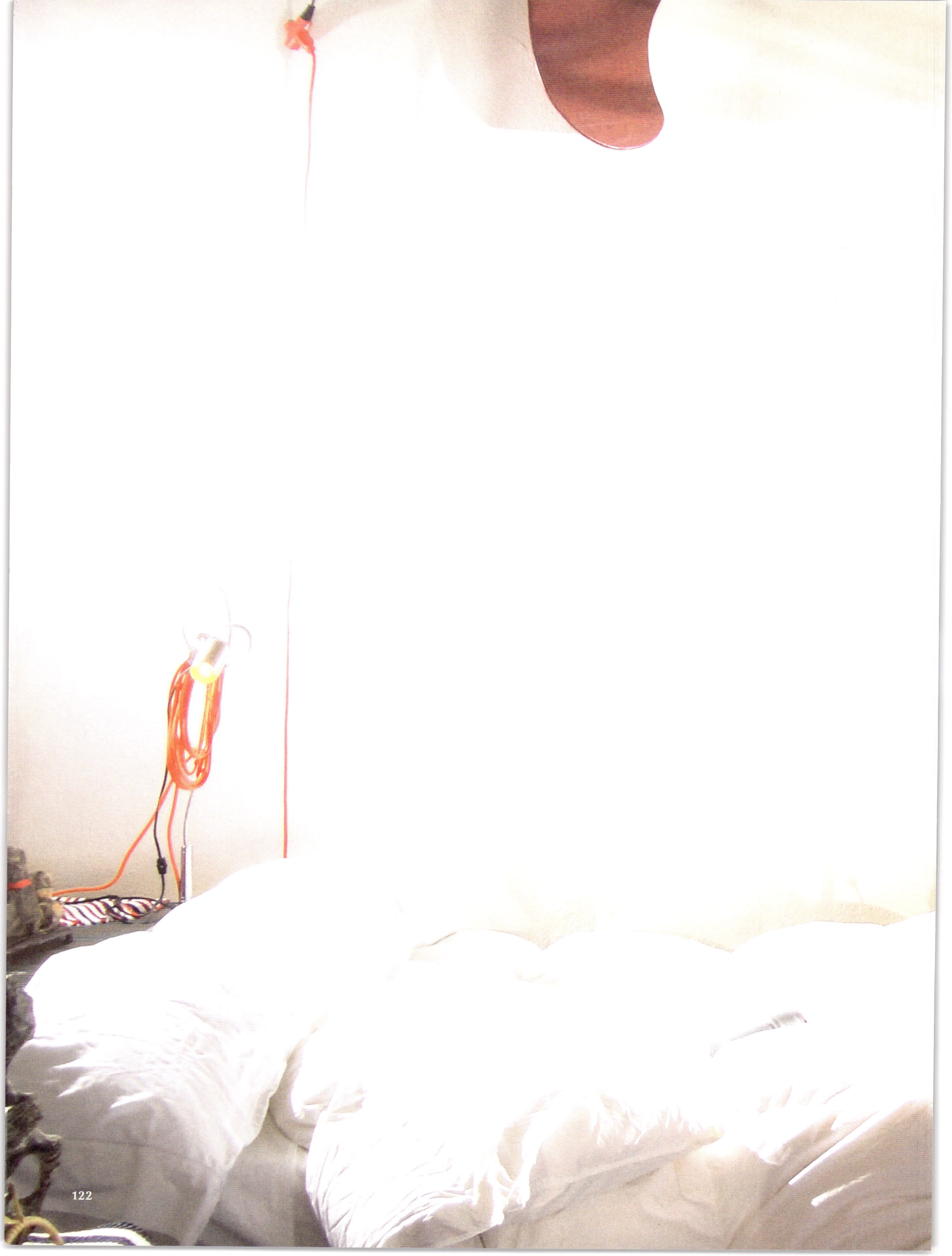

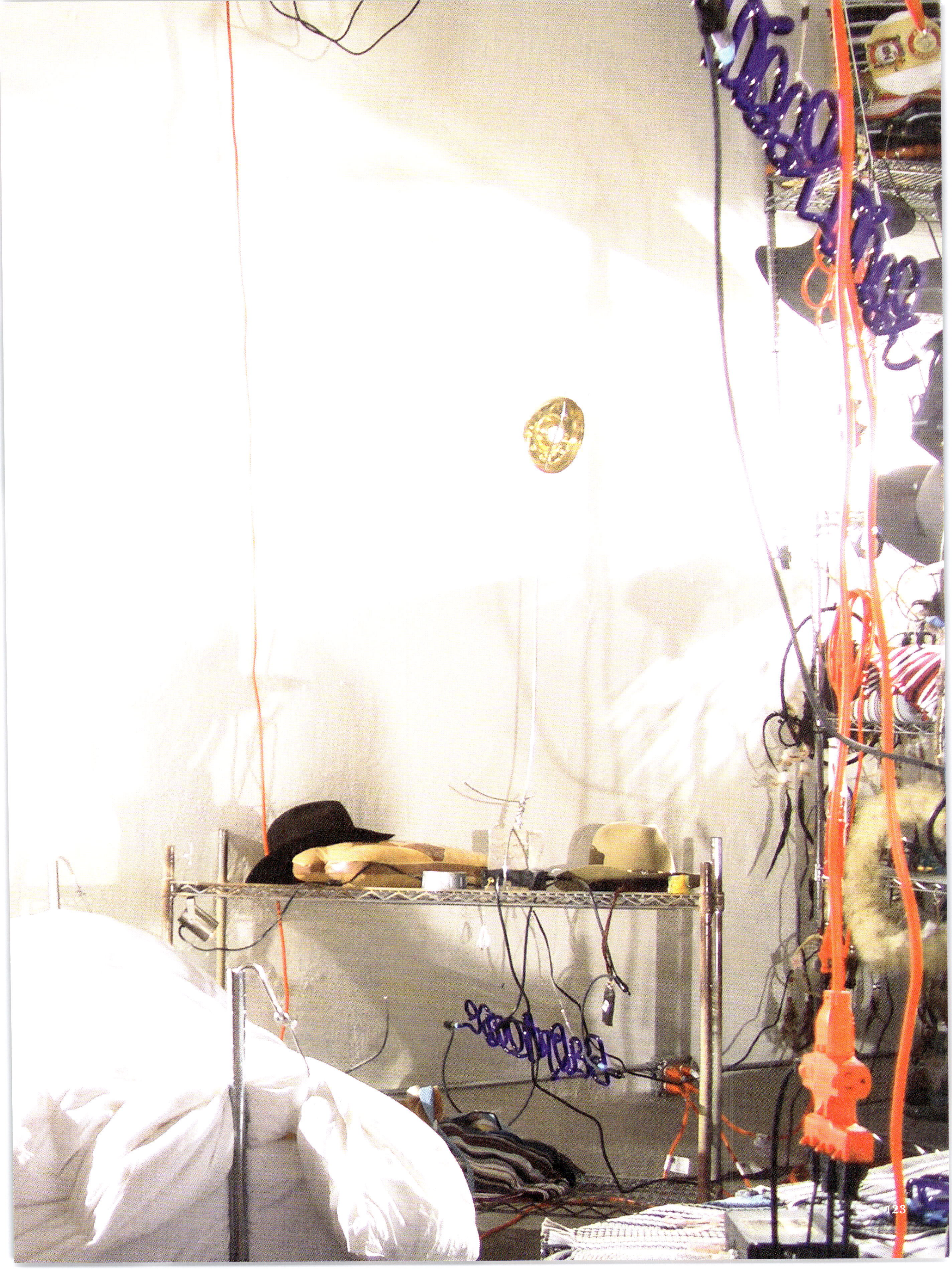

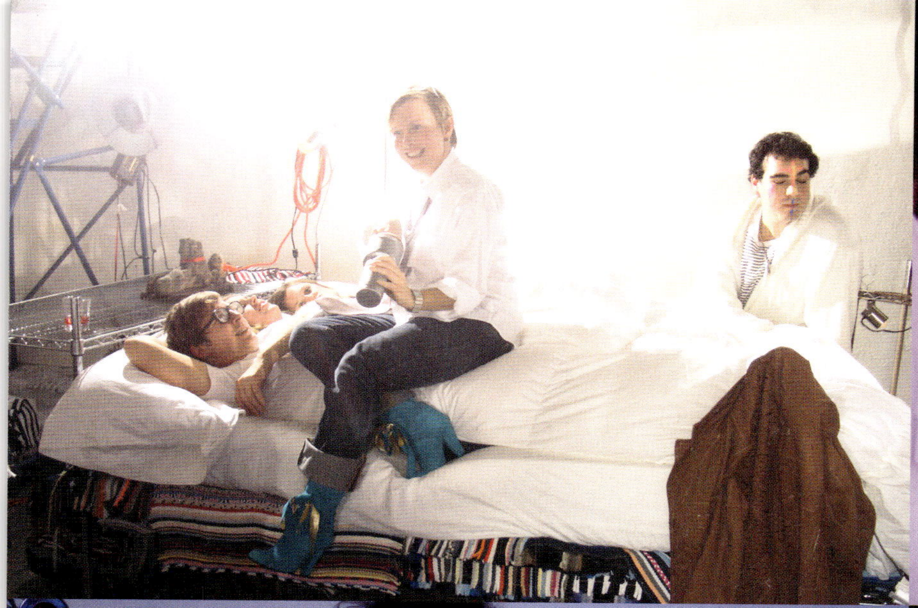

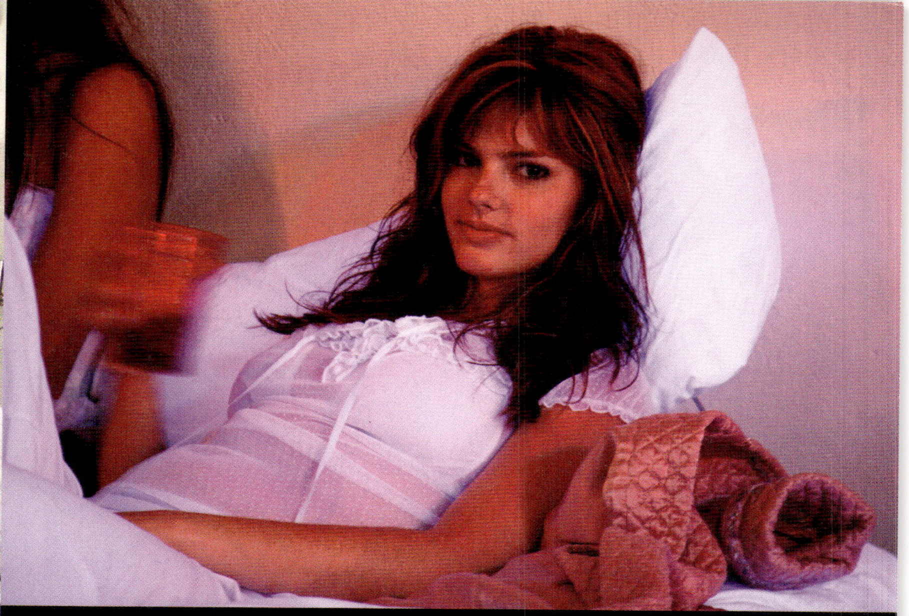

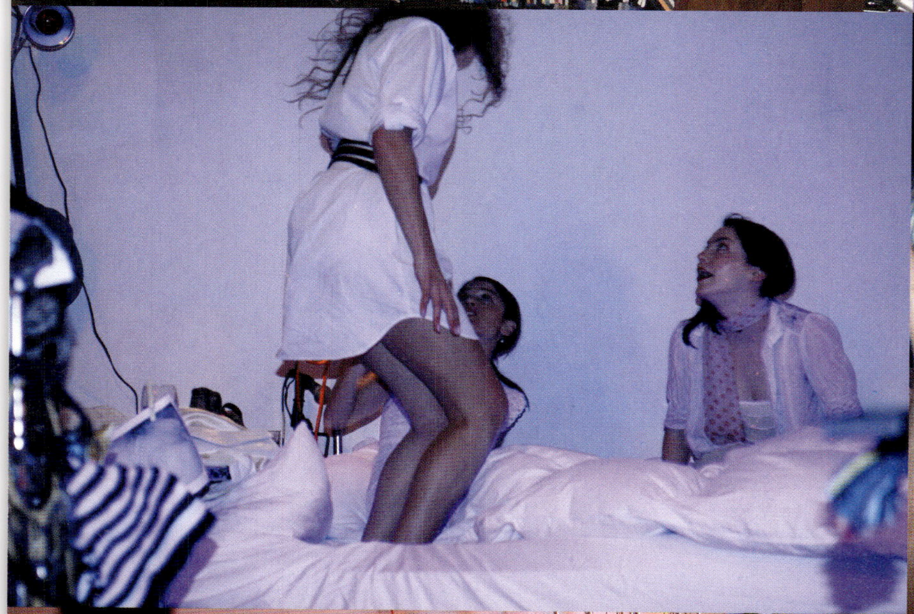

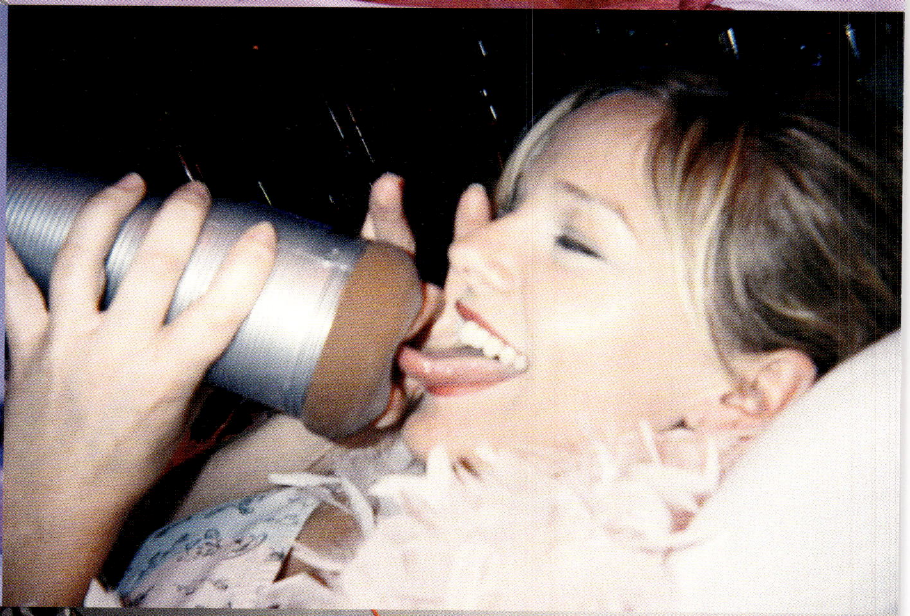

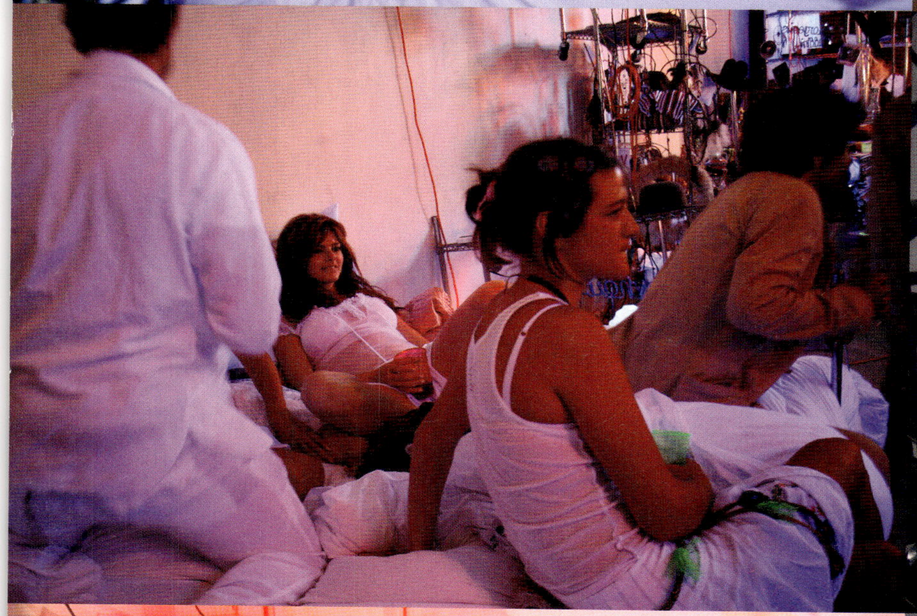

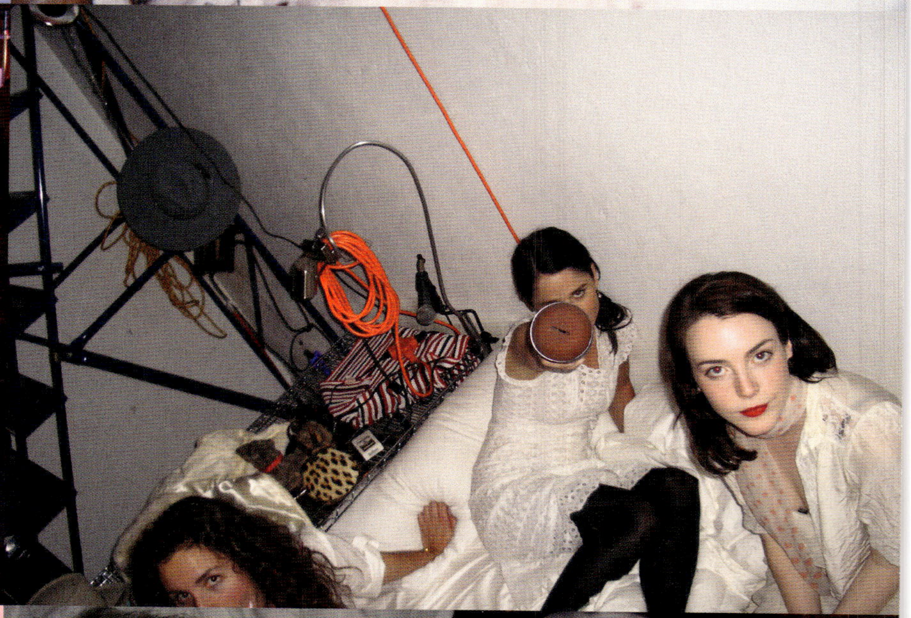

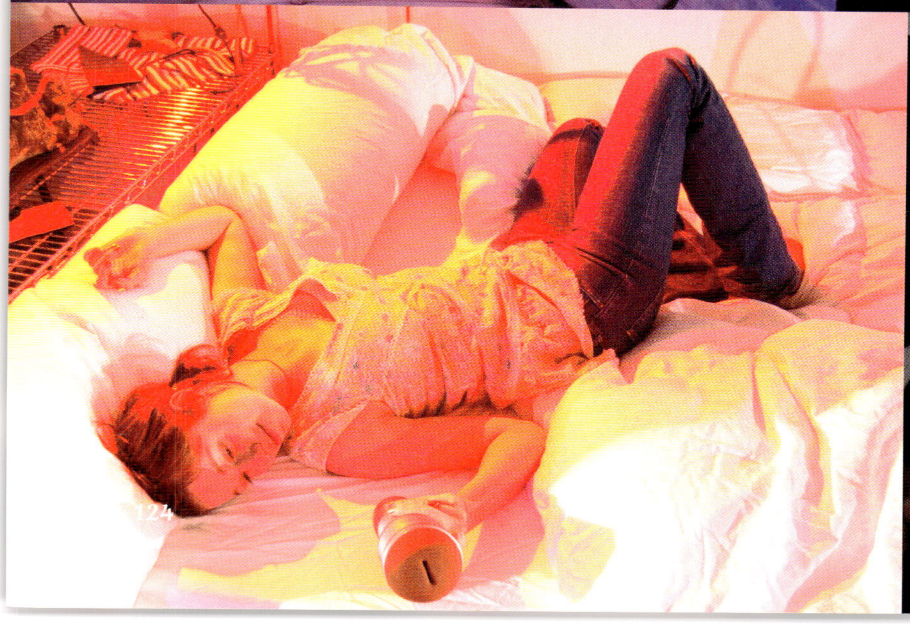

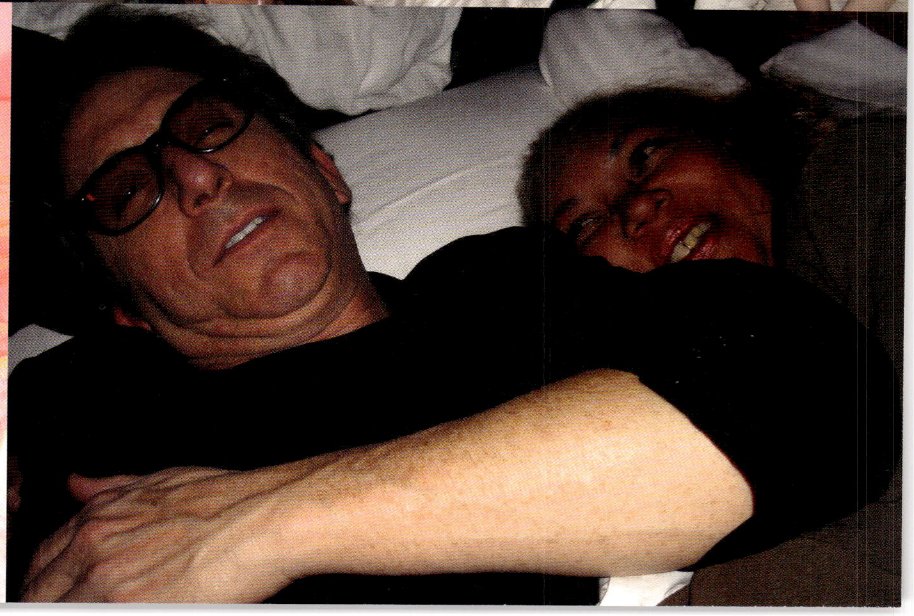

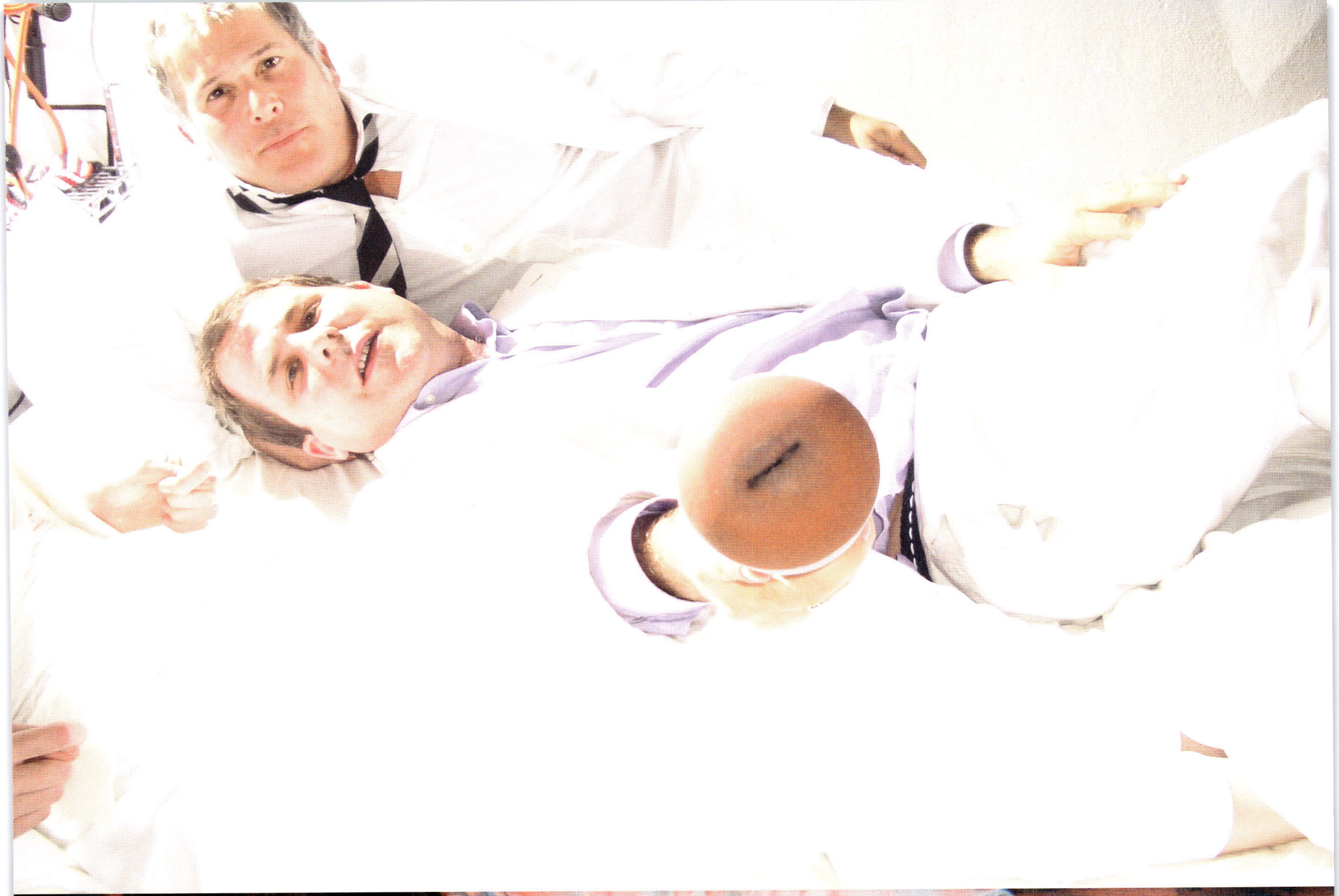

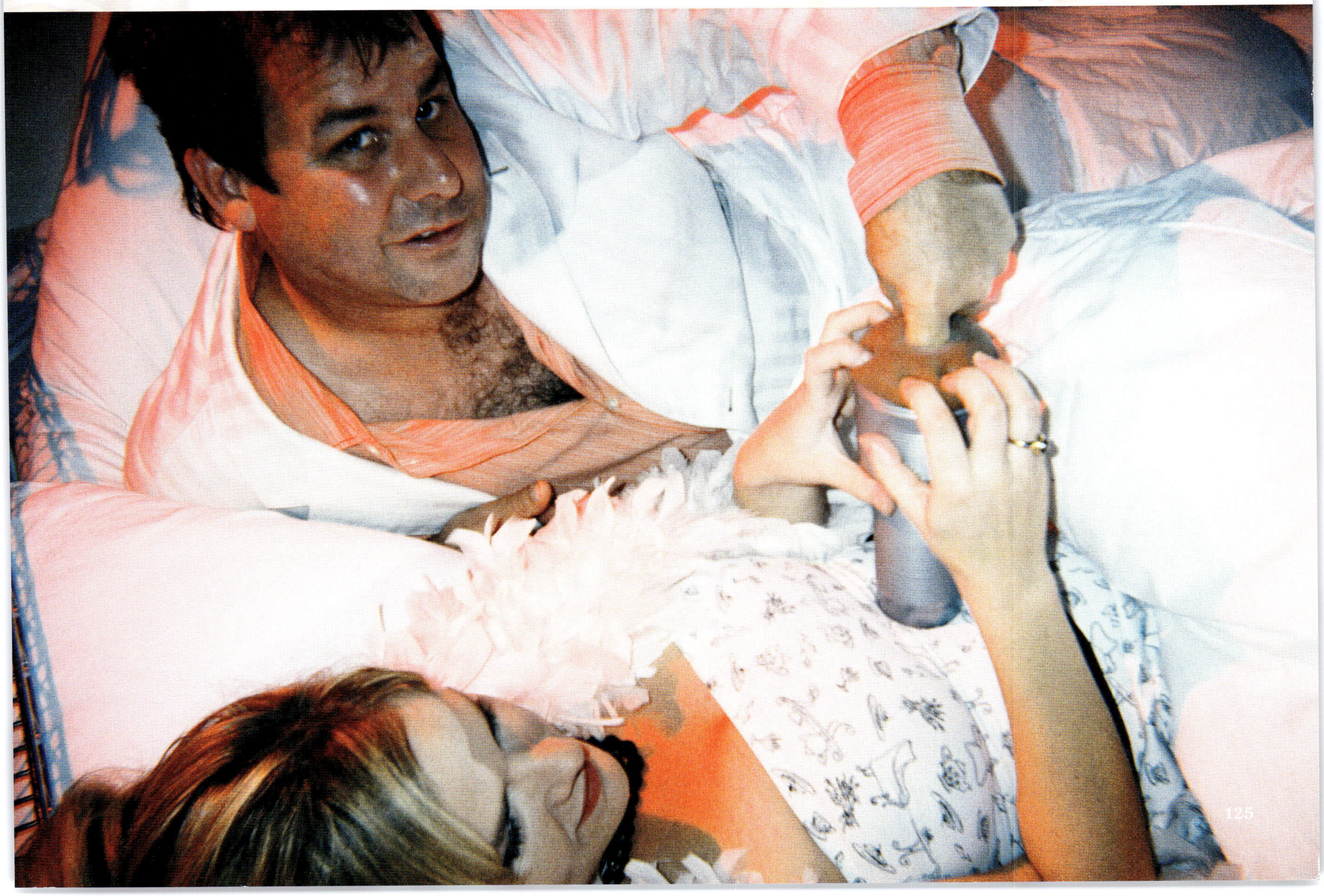

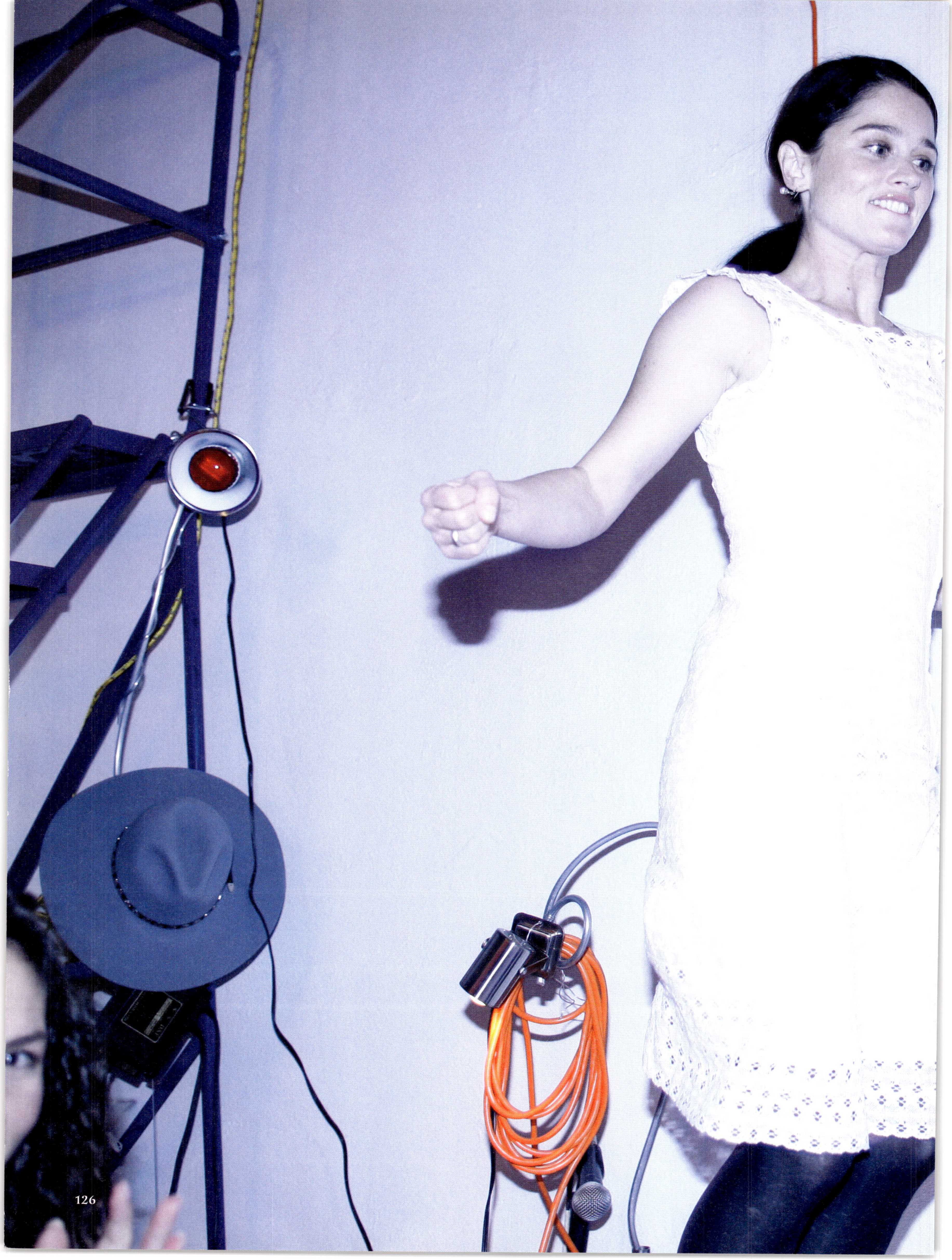

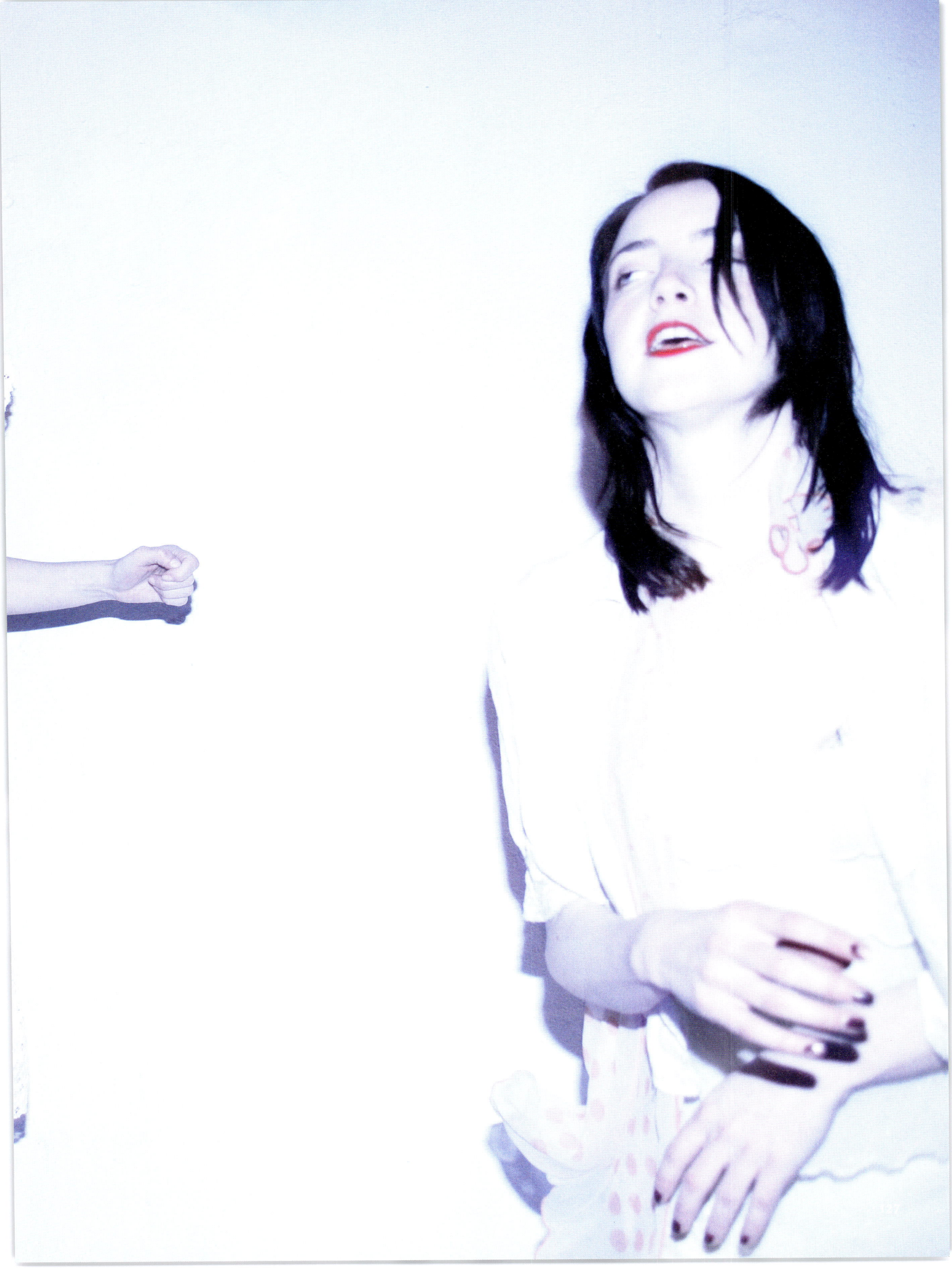

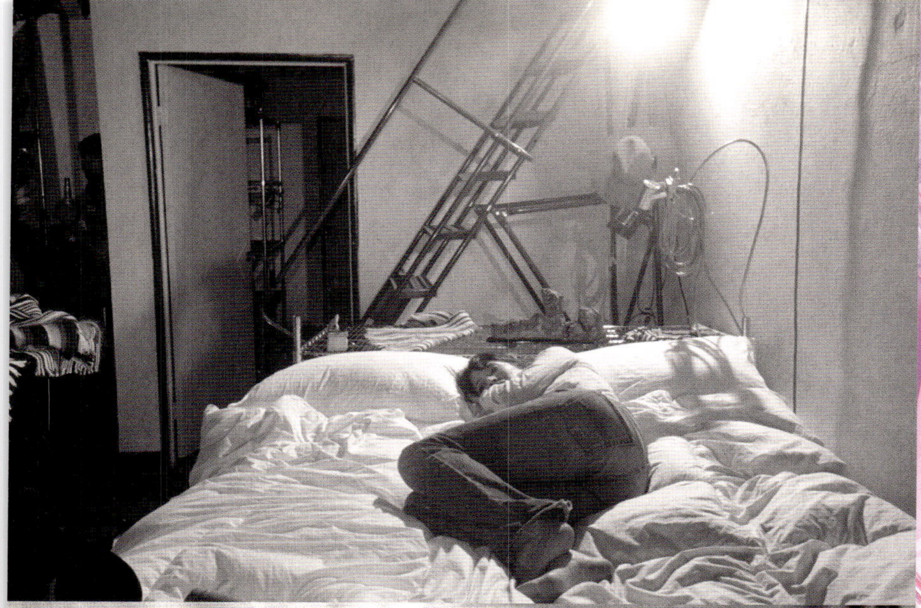
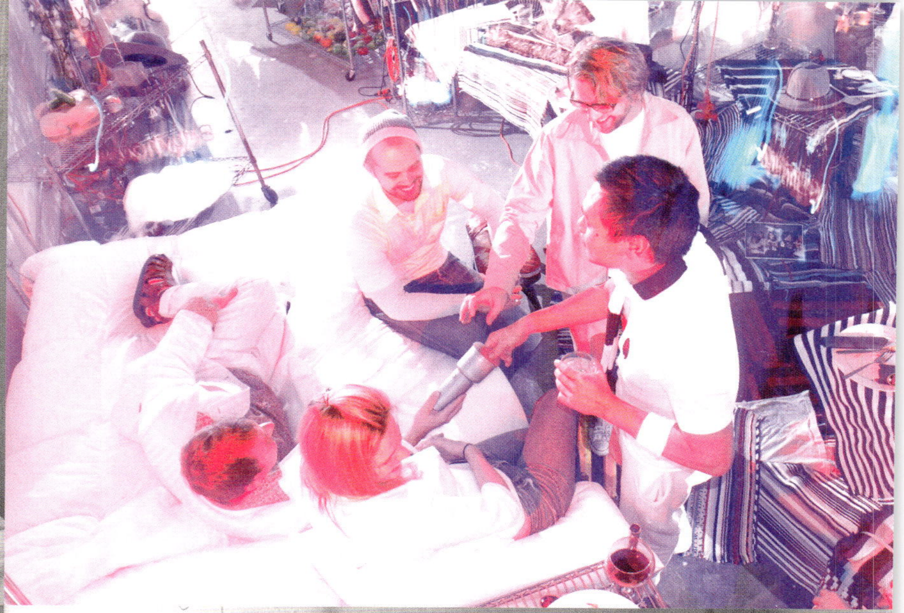
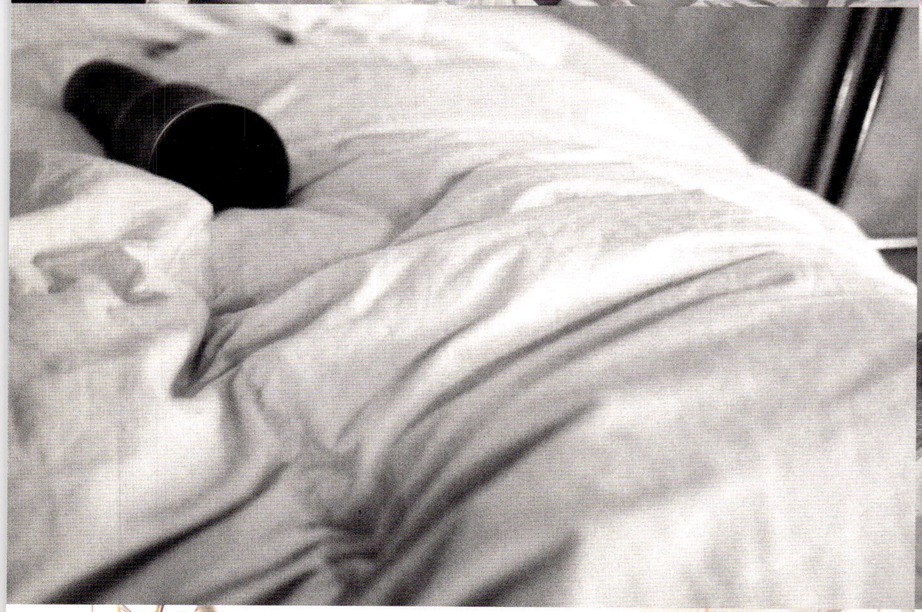
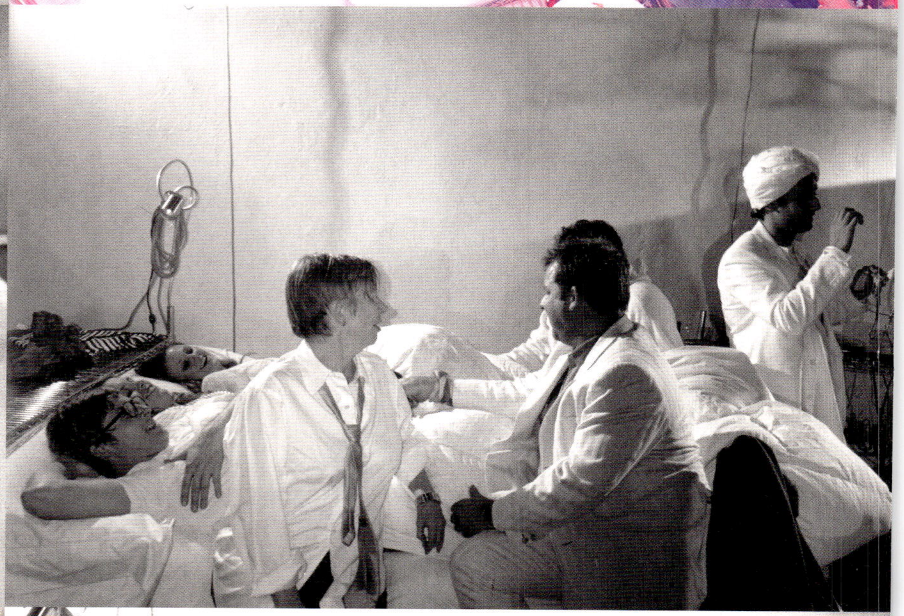
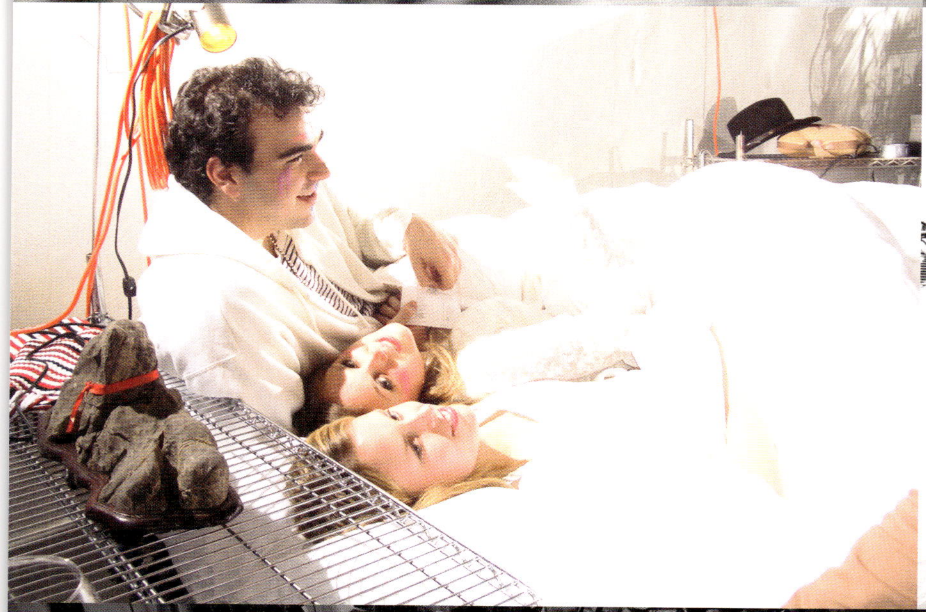
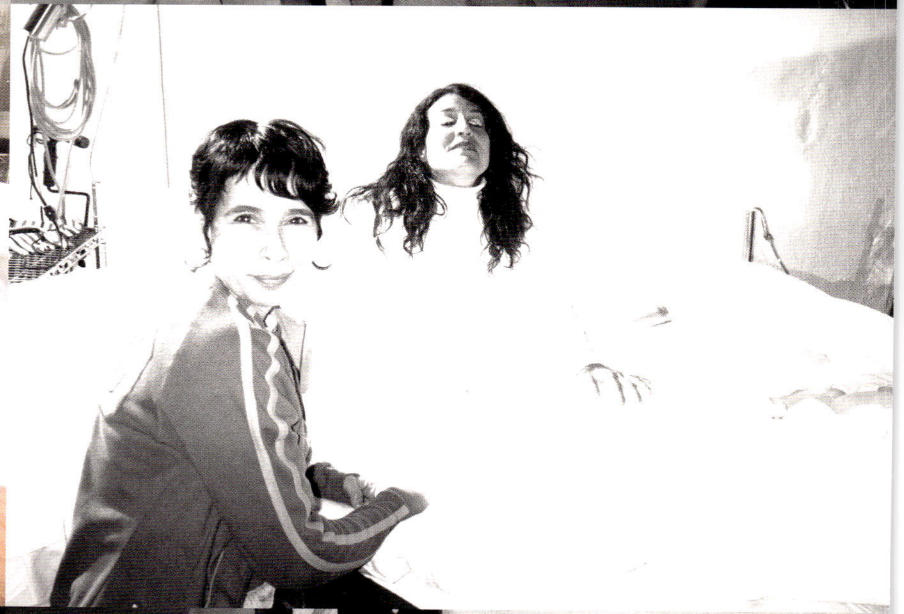
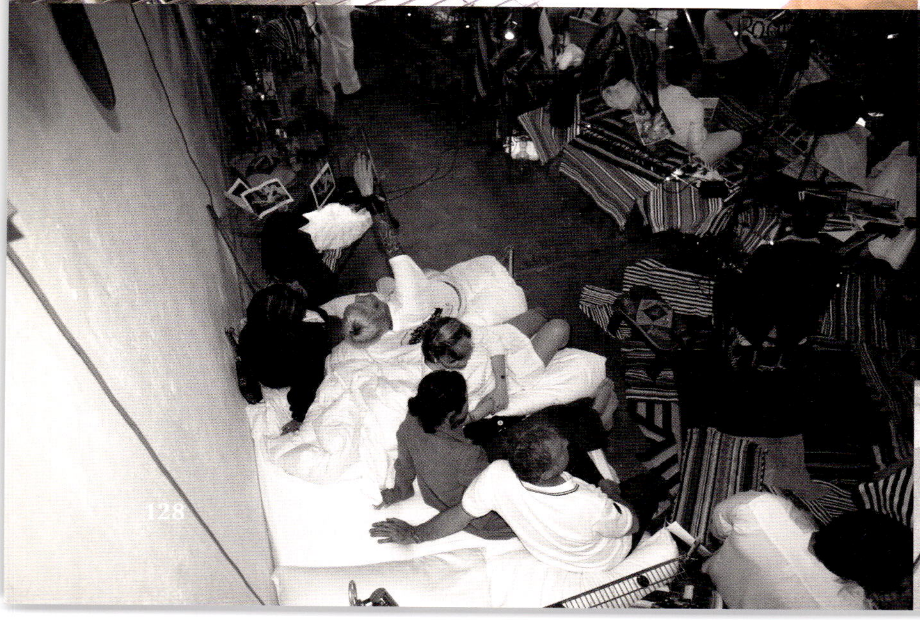
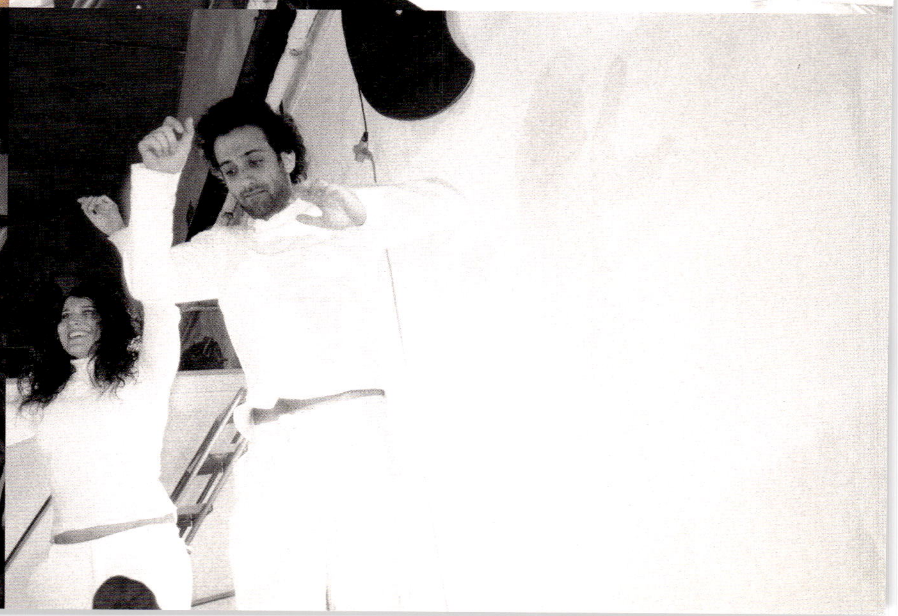

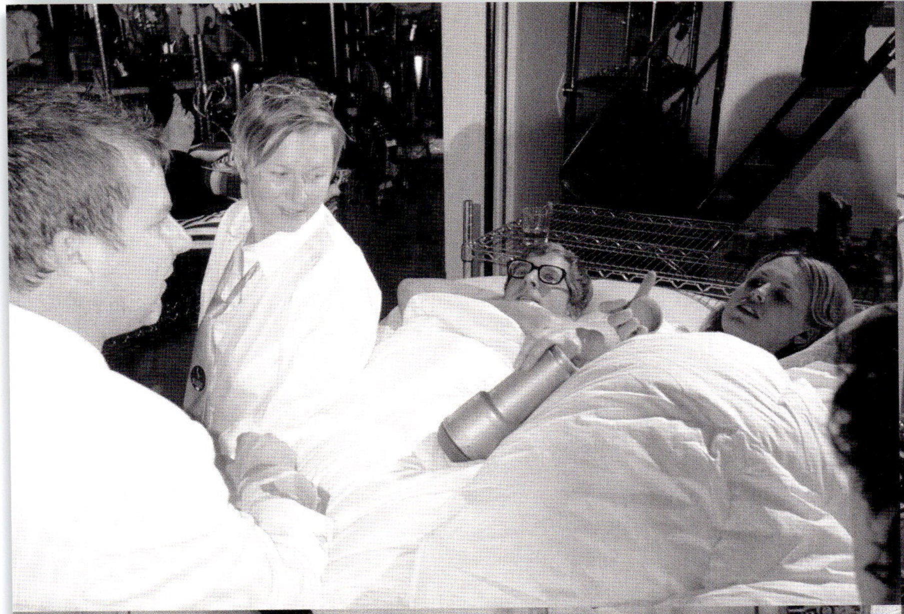
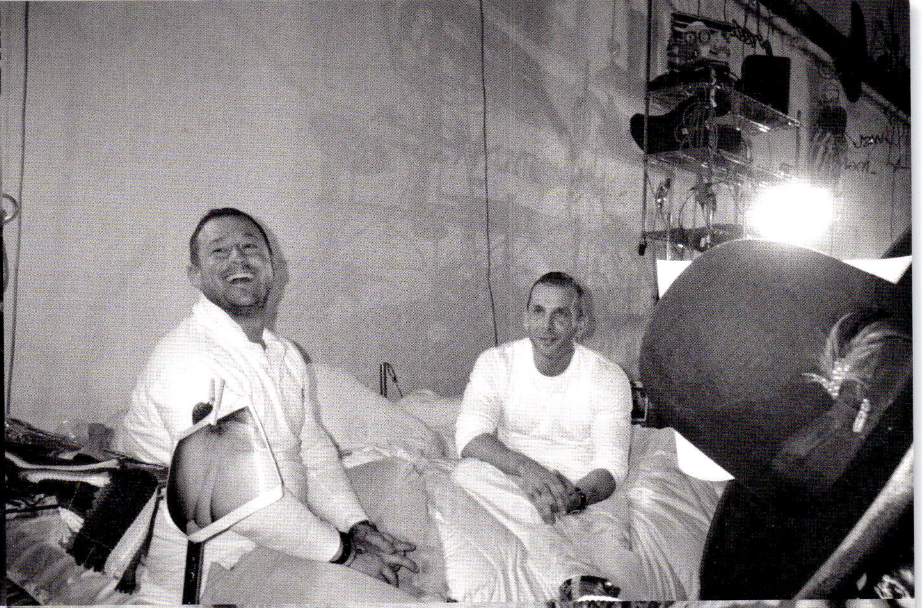
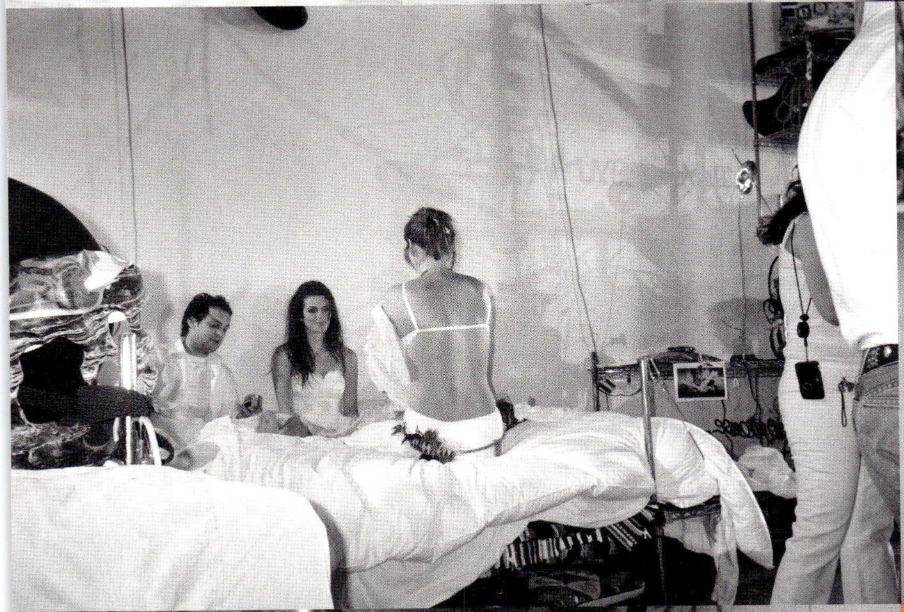
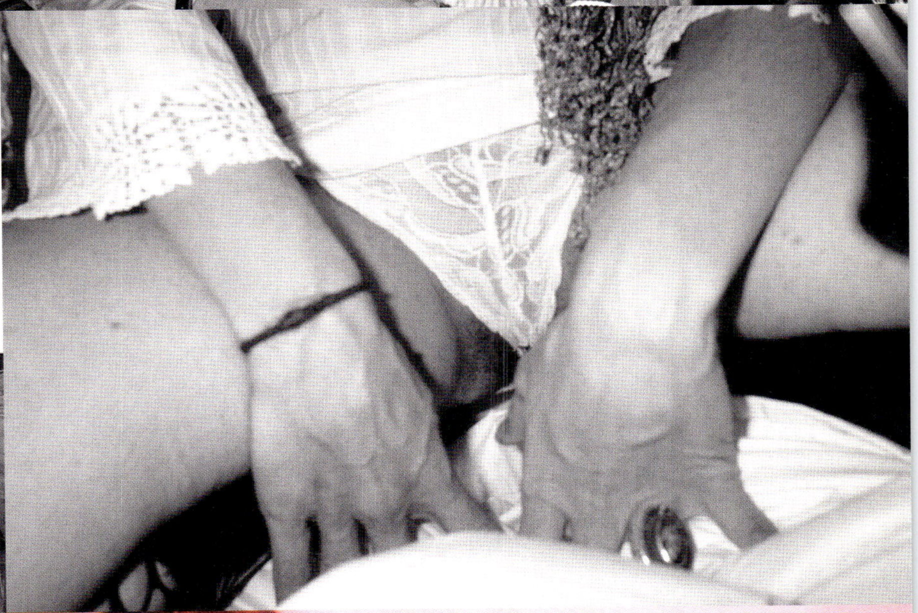
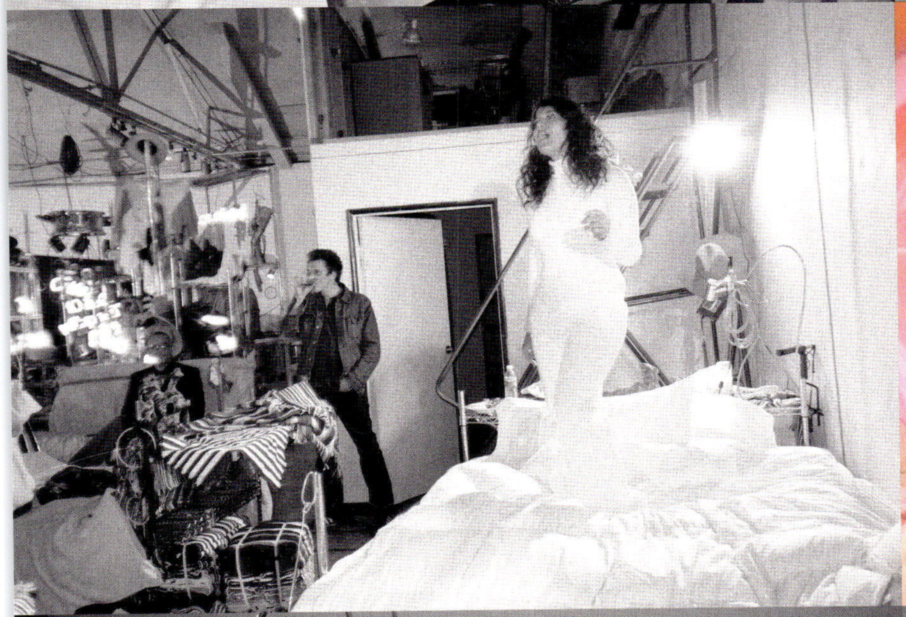
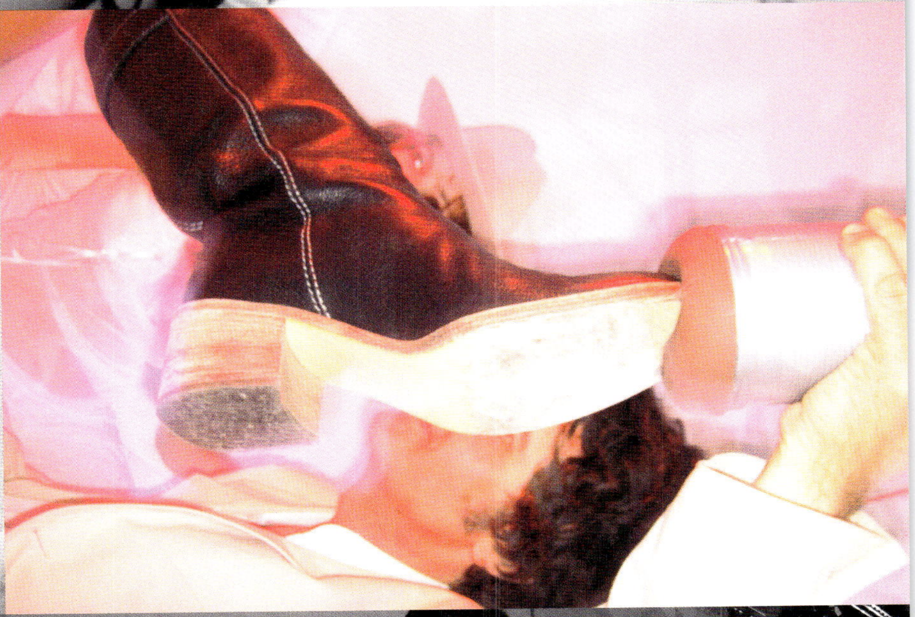
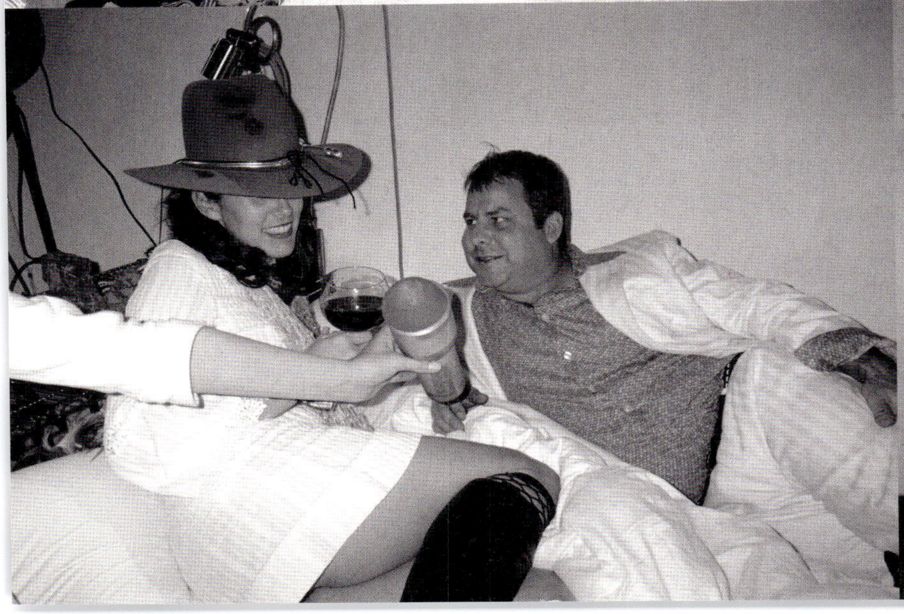
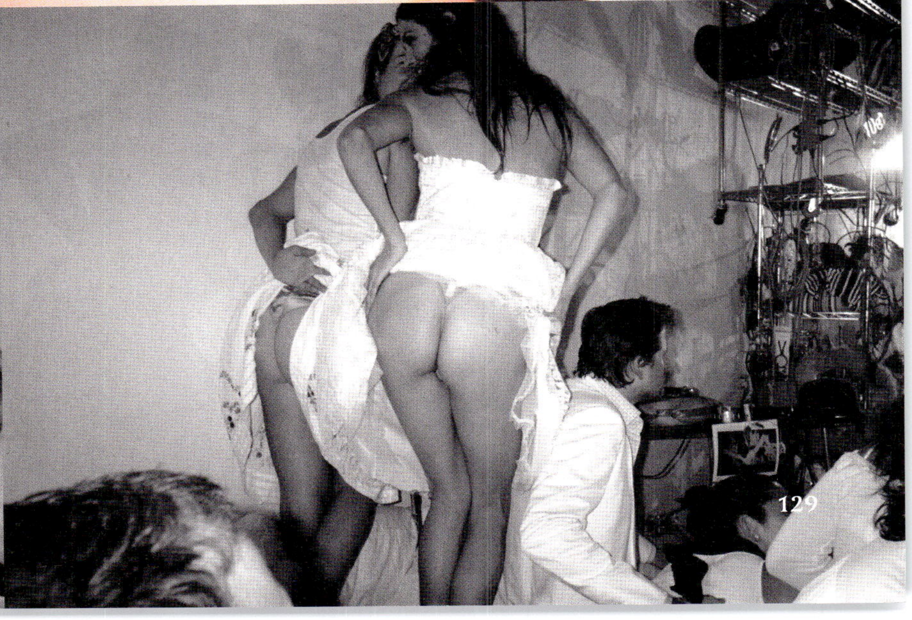

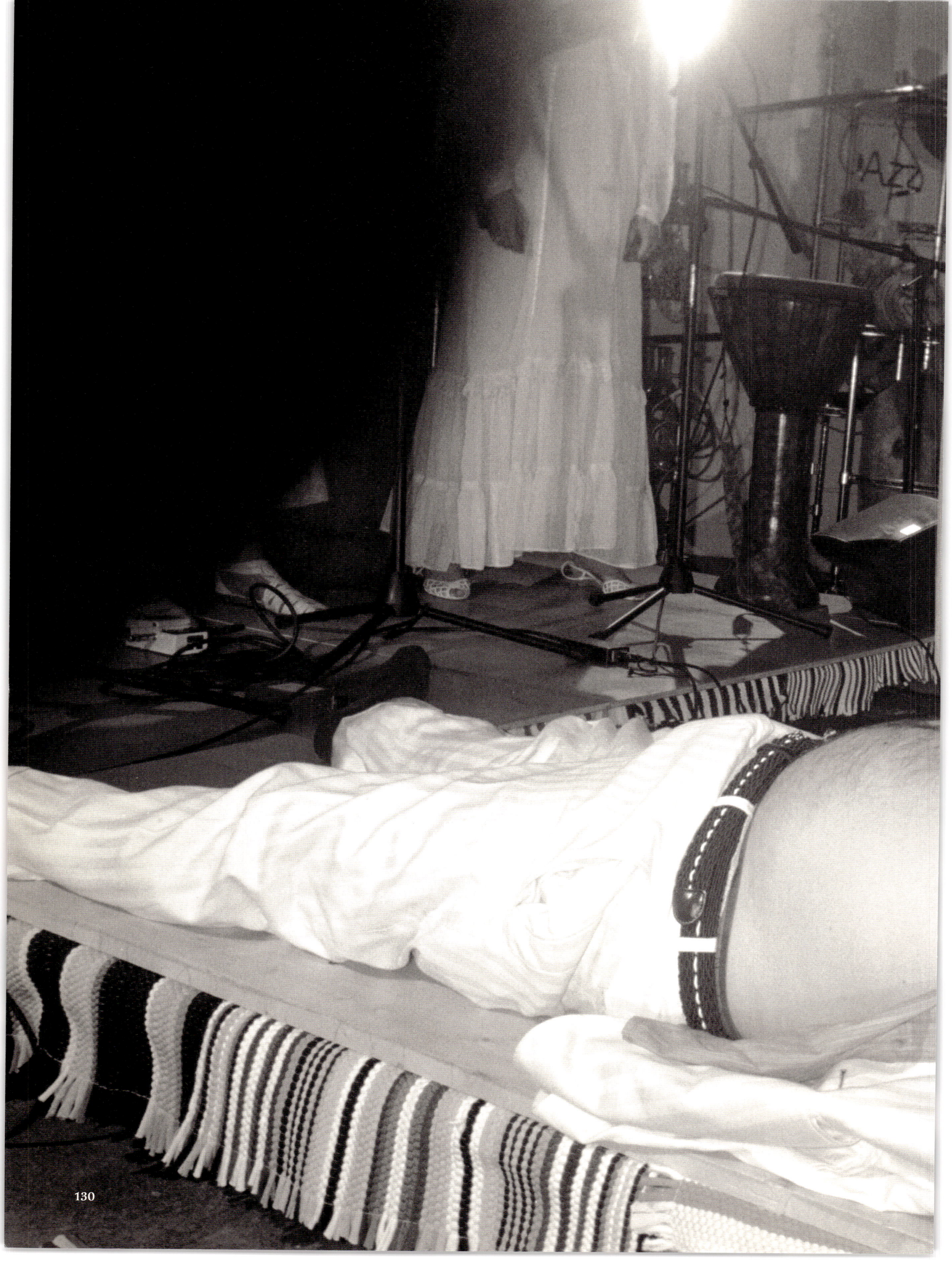

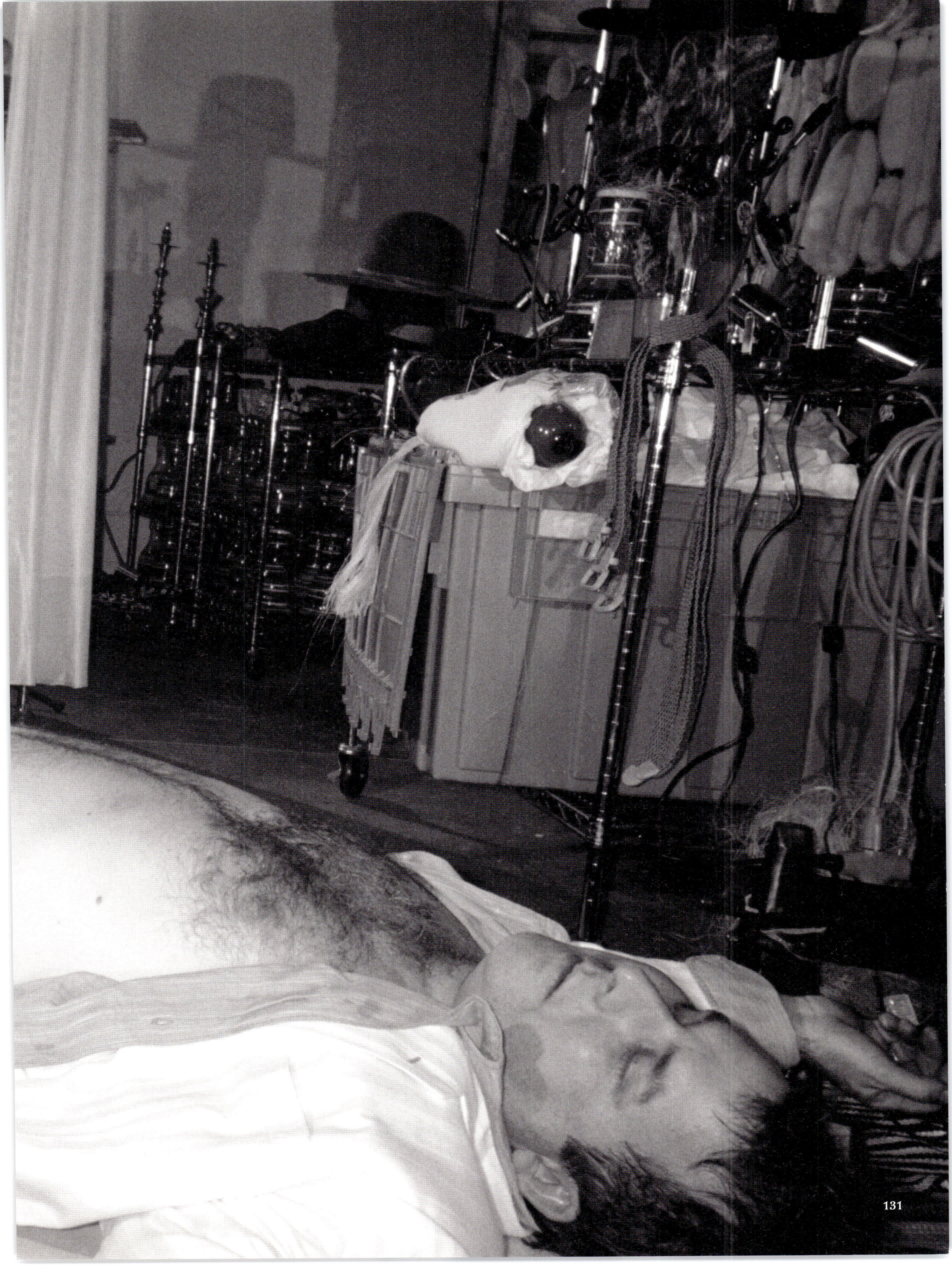

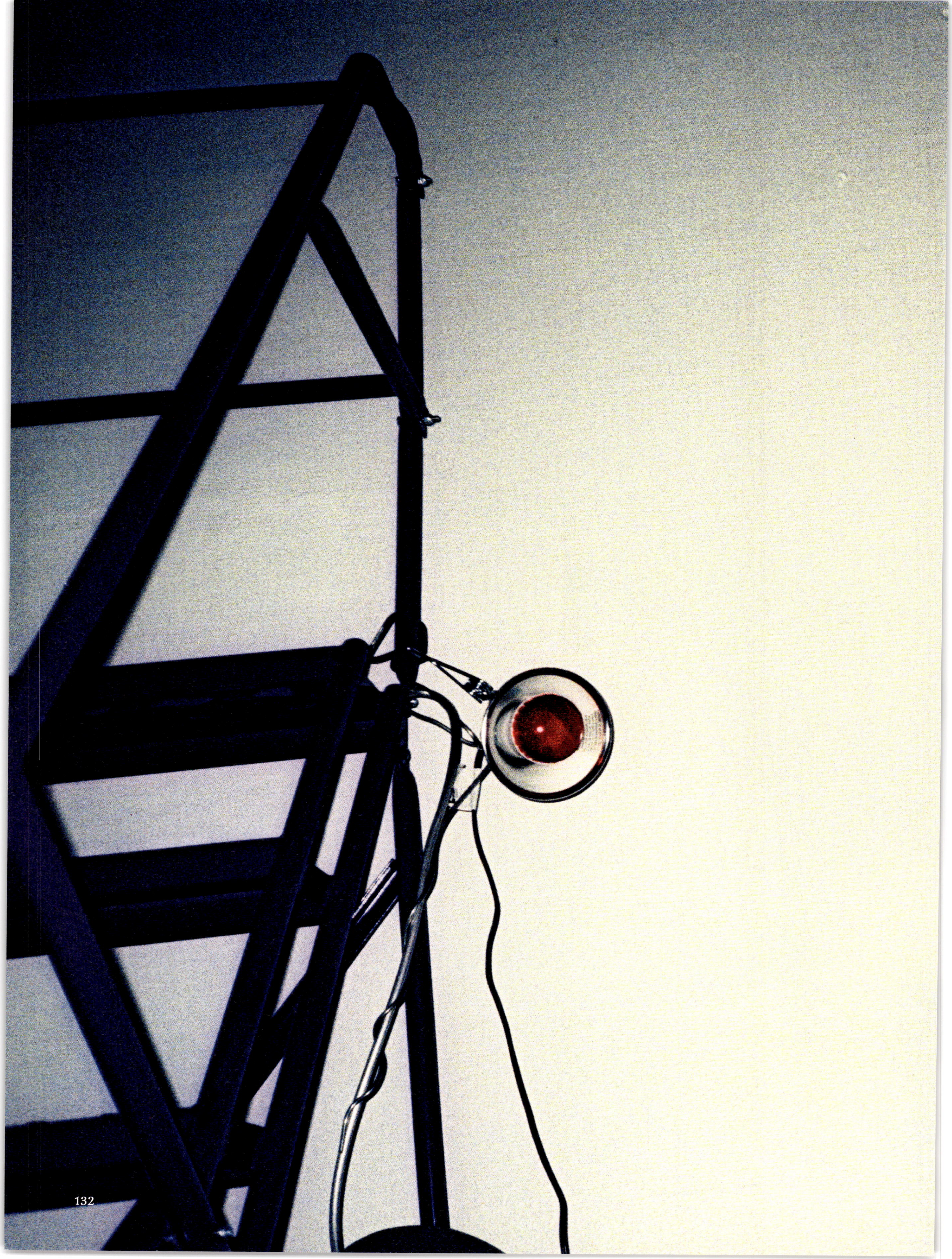

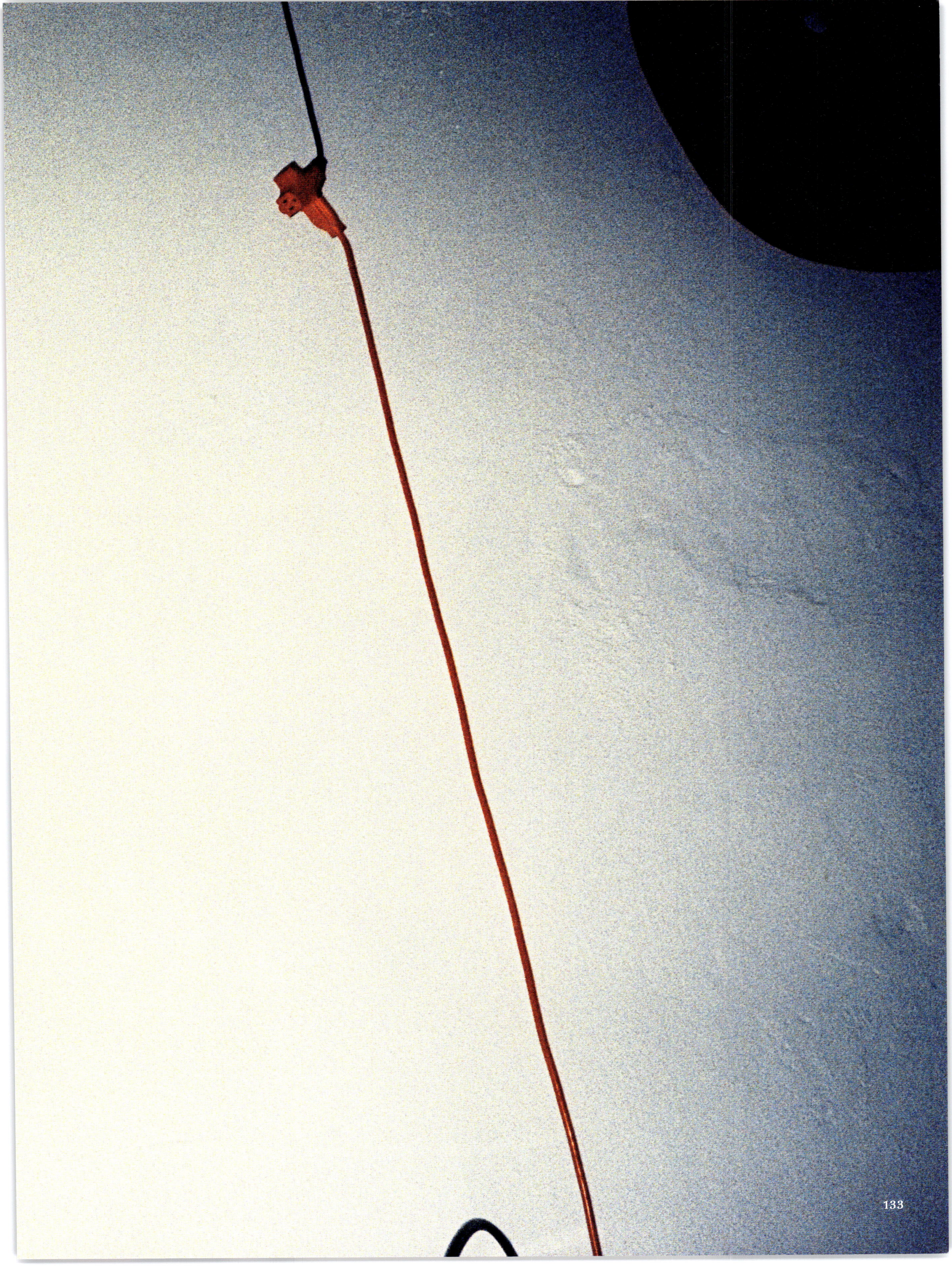

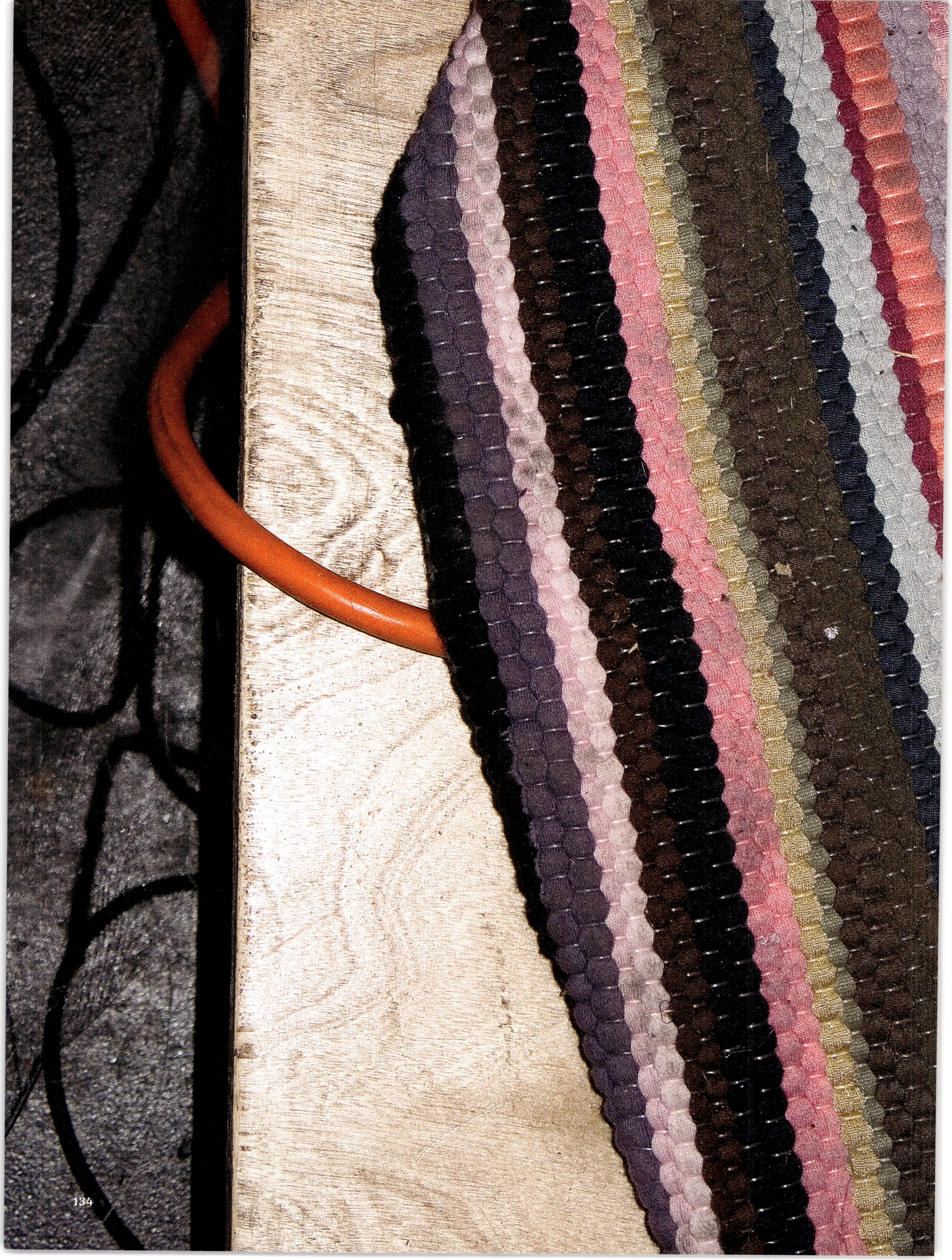

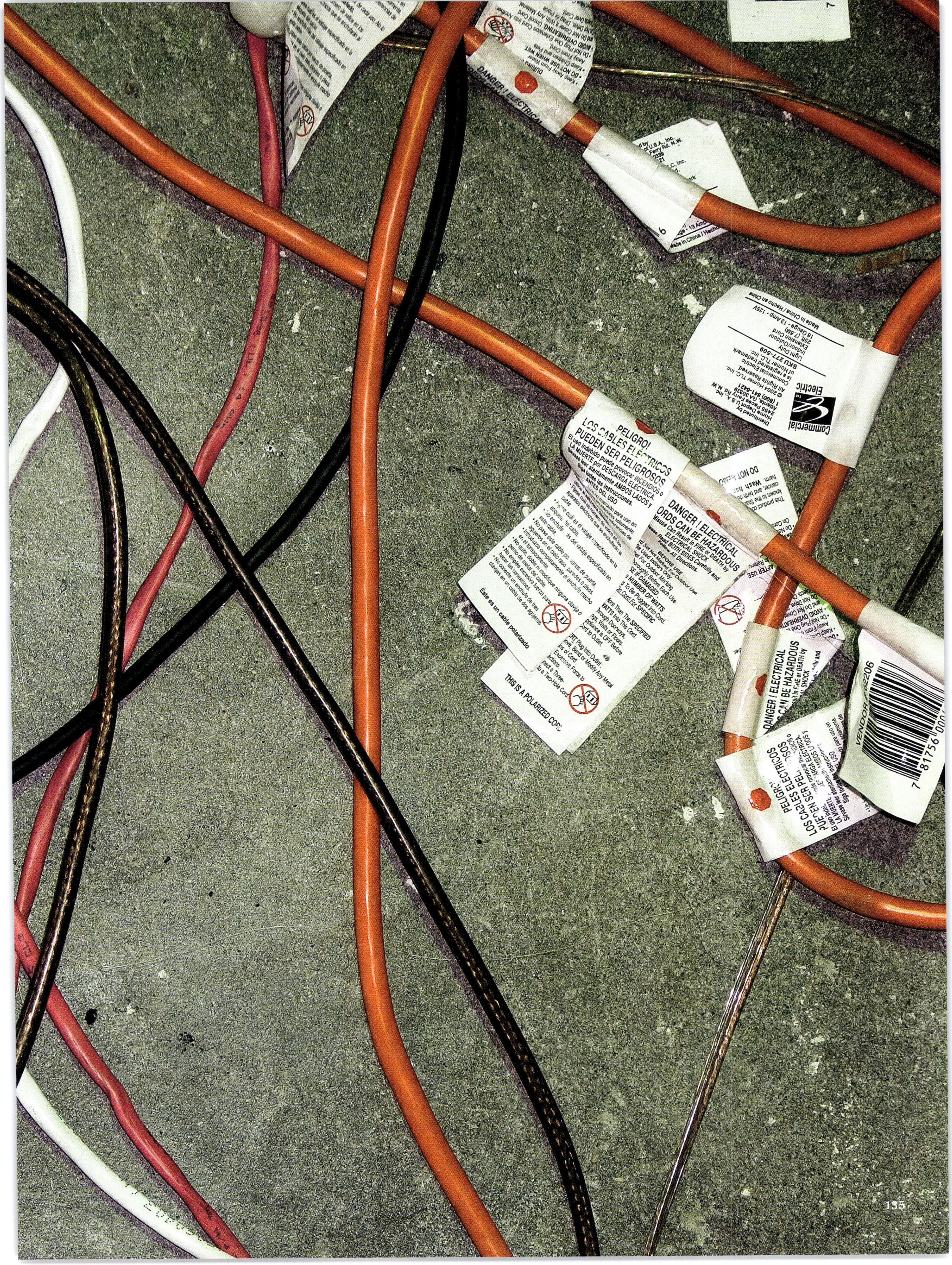
PELIGRO!
LOS CABLES ELECTRICOS
PUEDEN SER PELIGROSOS
DANGER | ELECTRICAL
CORDS CAN BE HAZARDOUS
THIS IS A POLARIZED CORD
Este es un cable polarizado

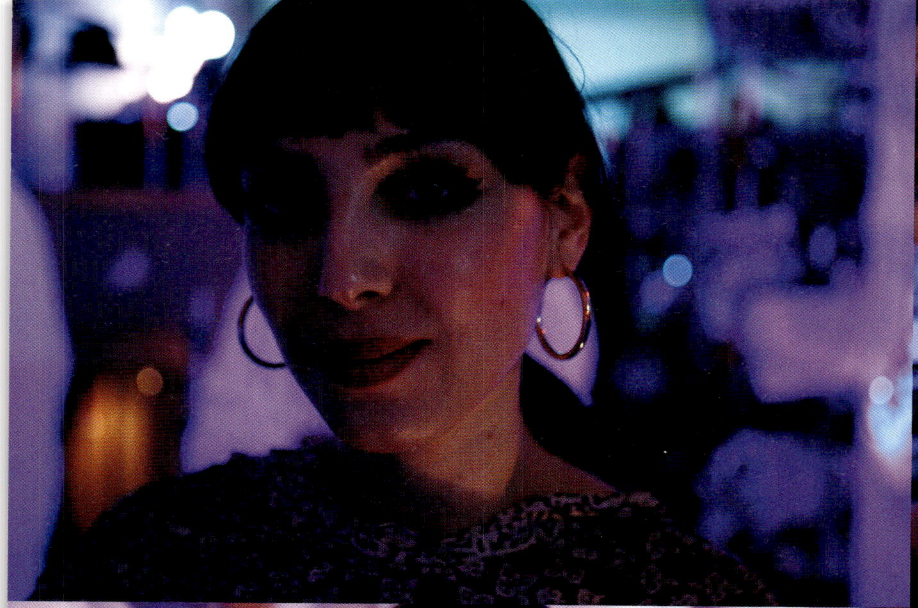

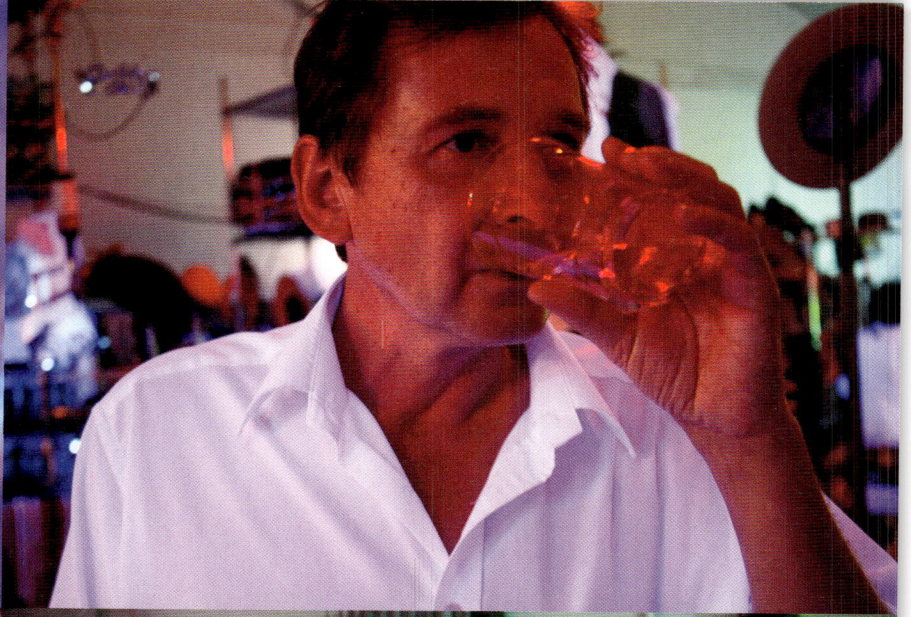

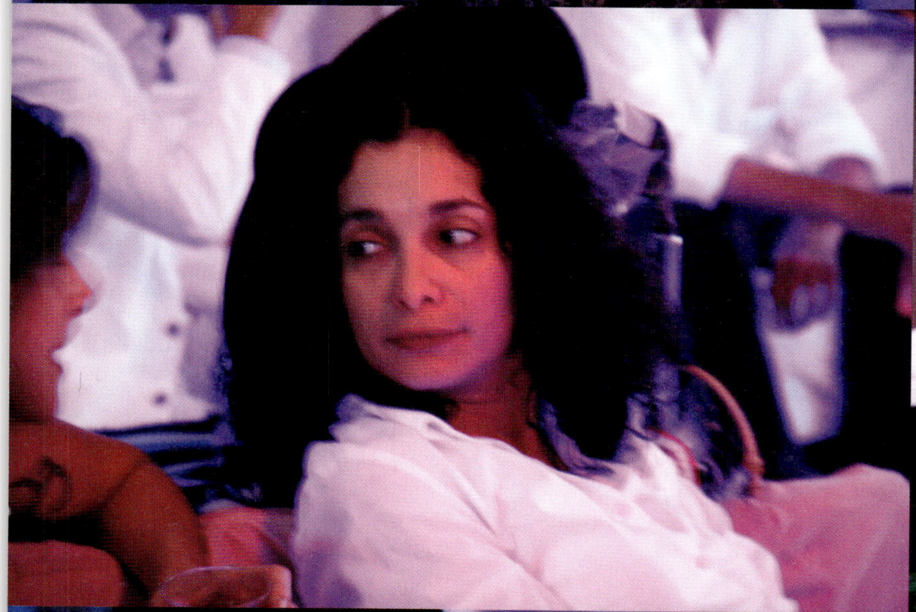

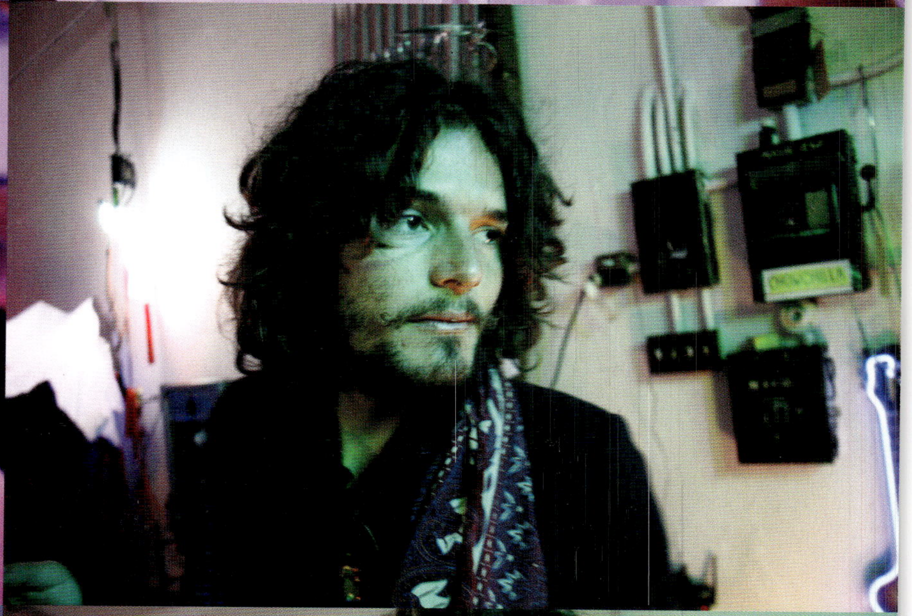

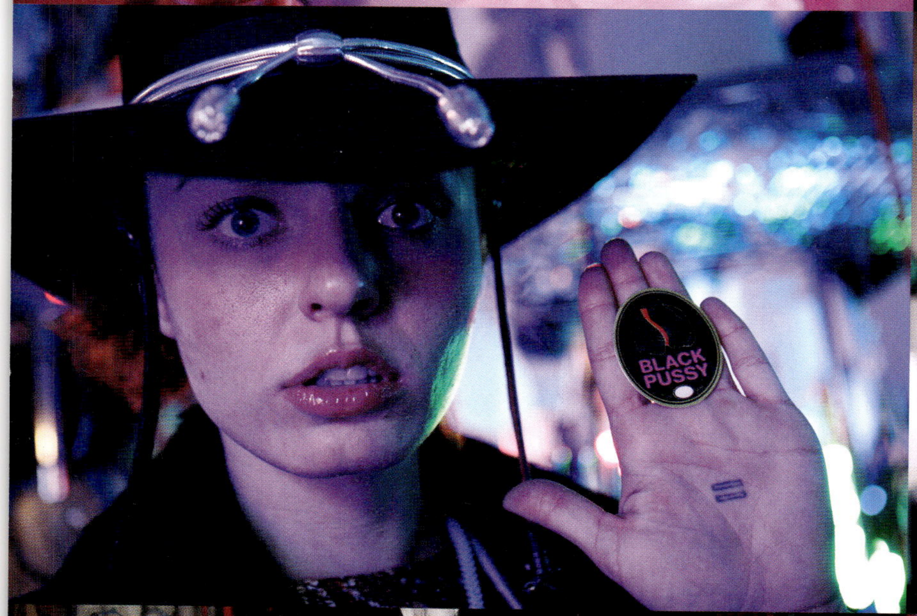
BLACK PUSSY

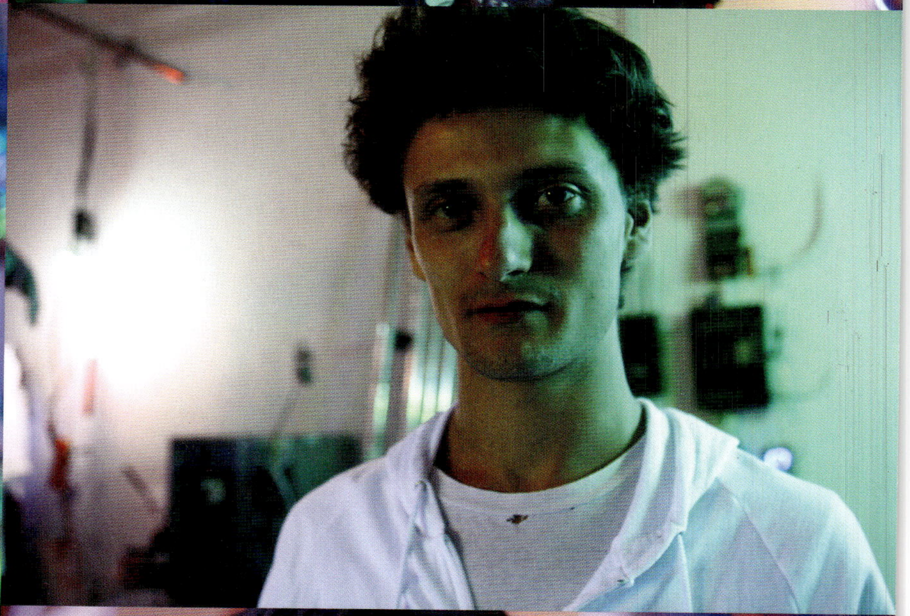

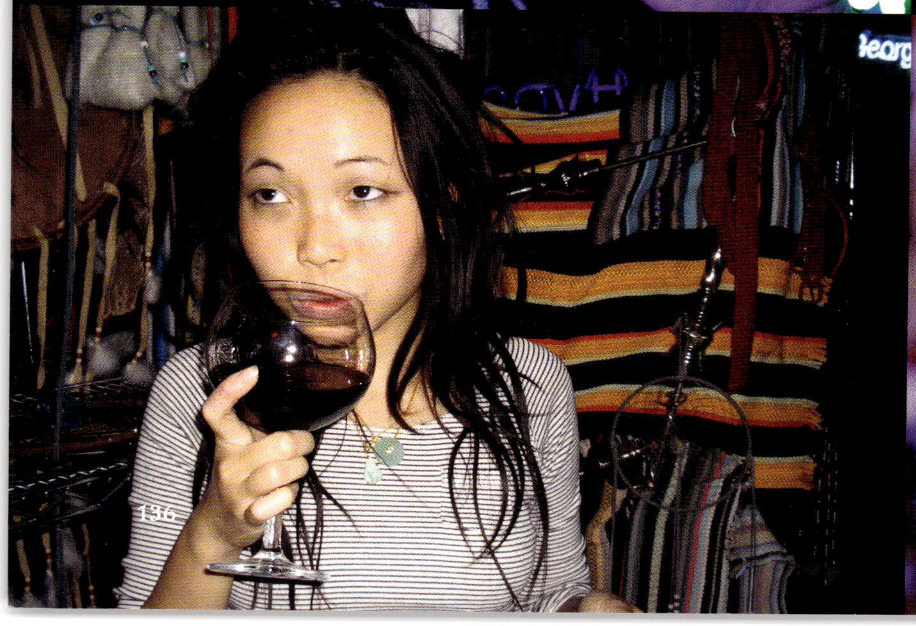

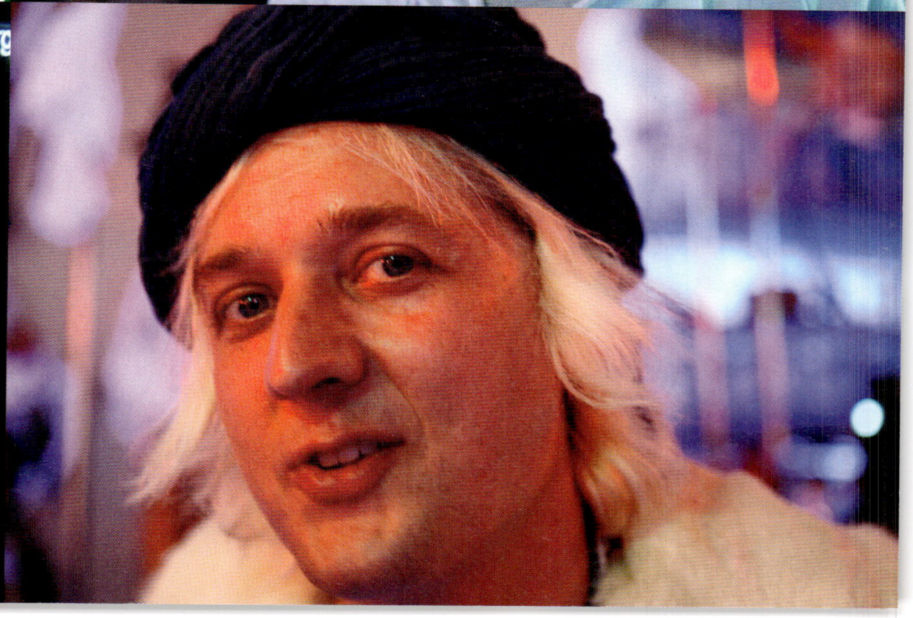

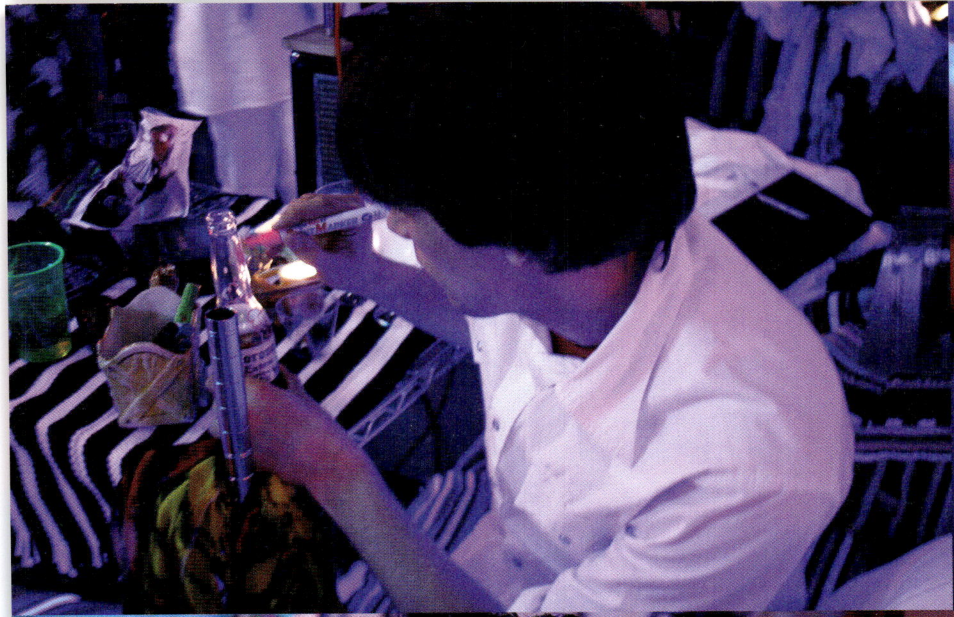

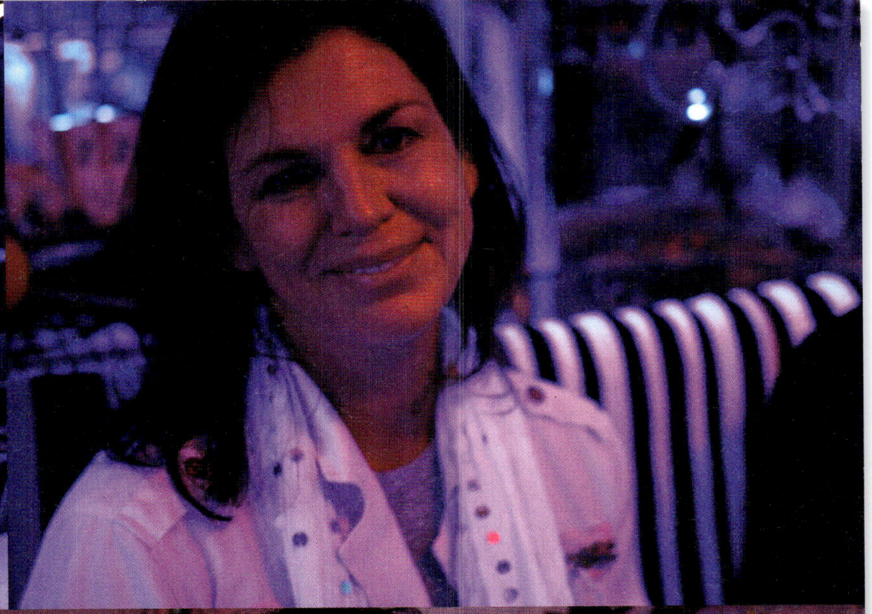

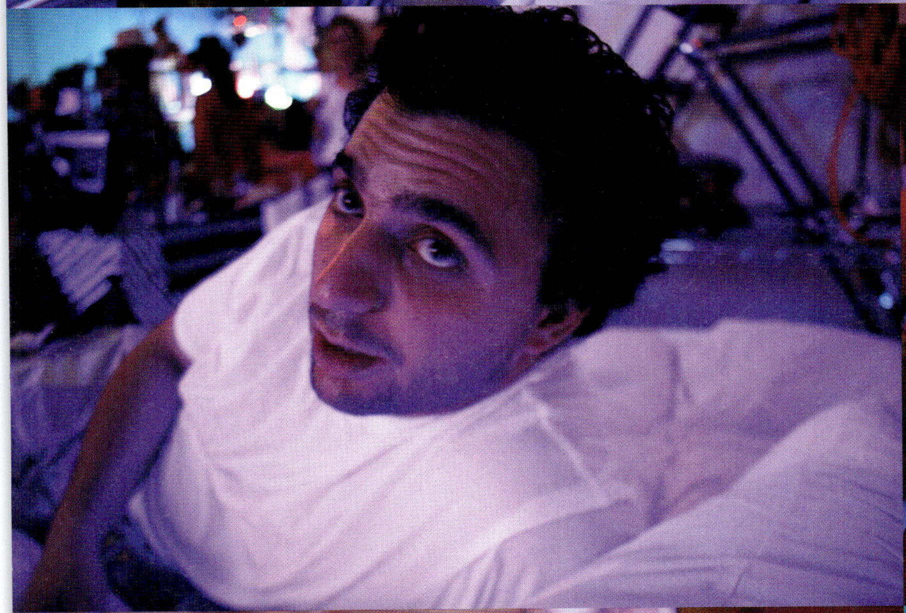

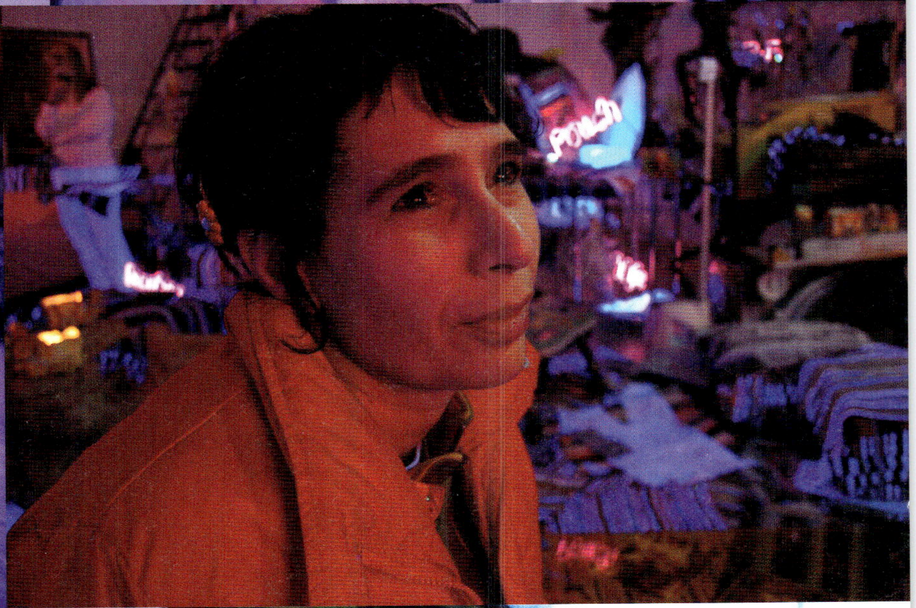

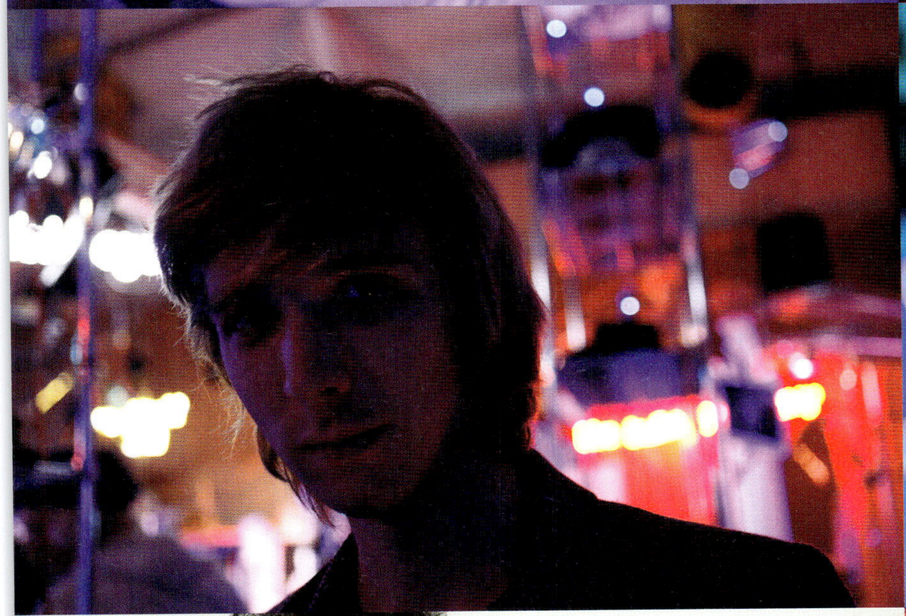

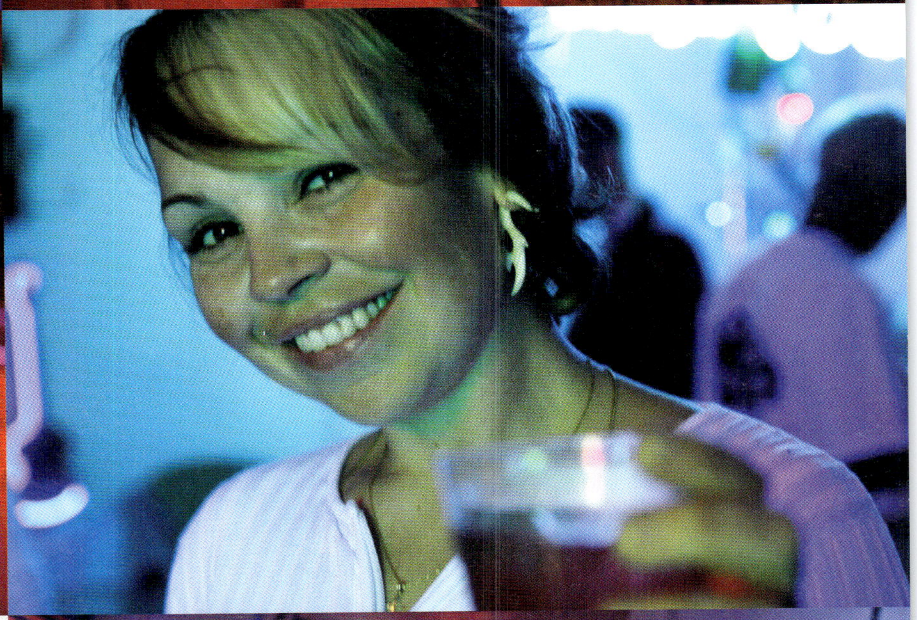

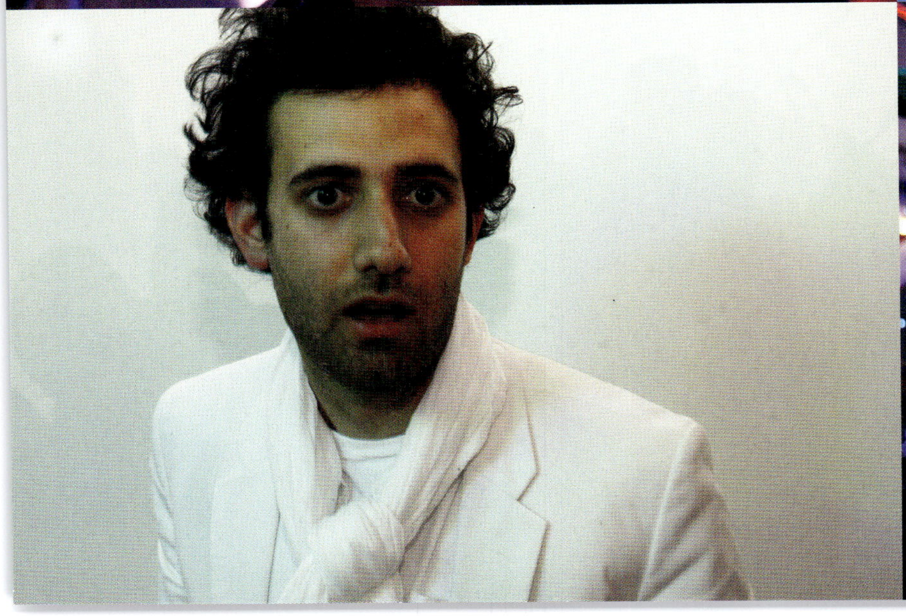

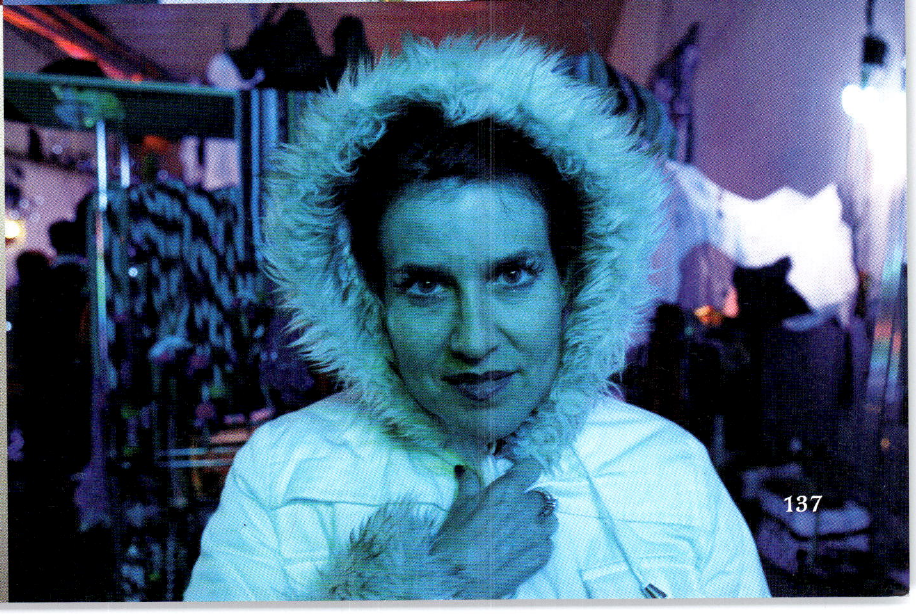

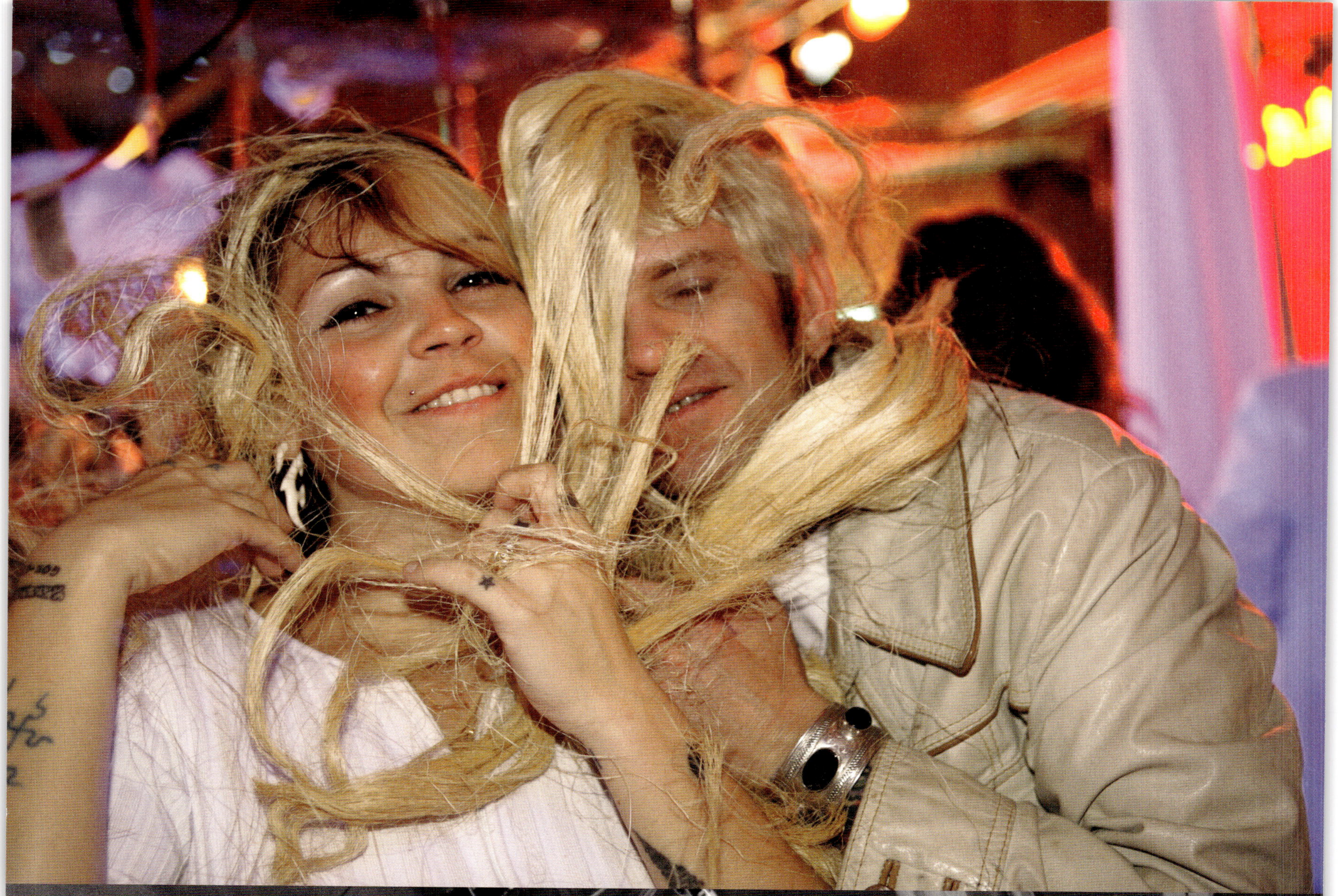

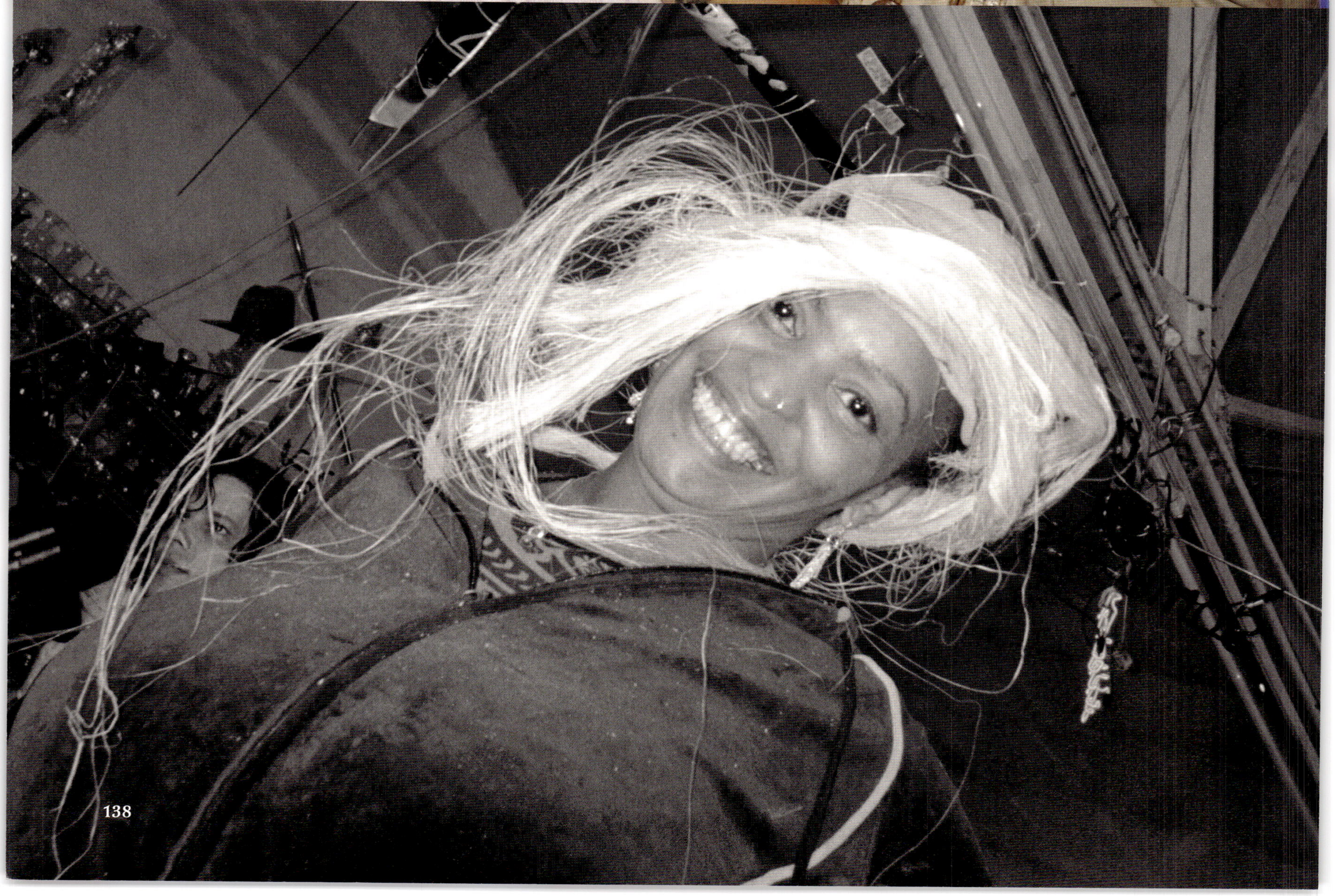

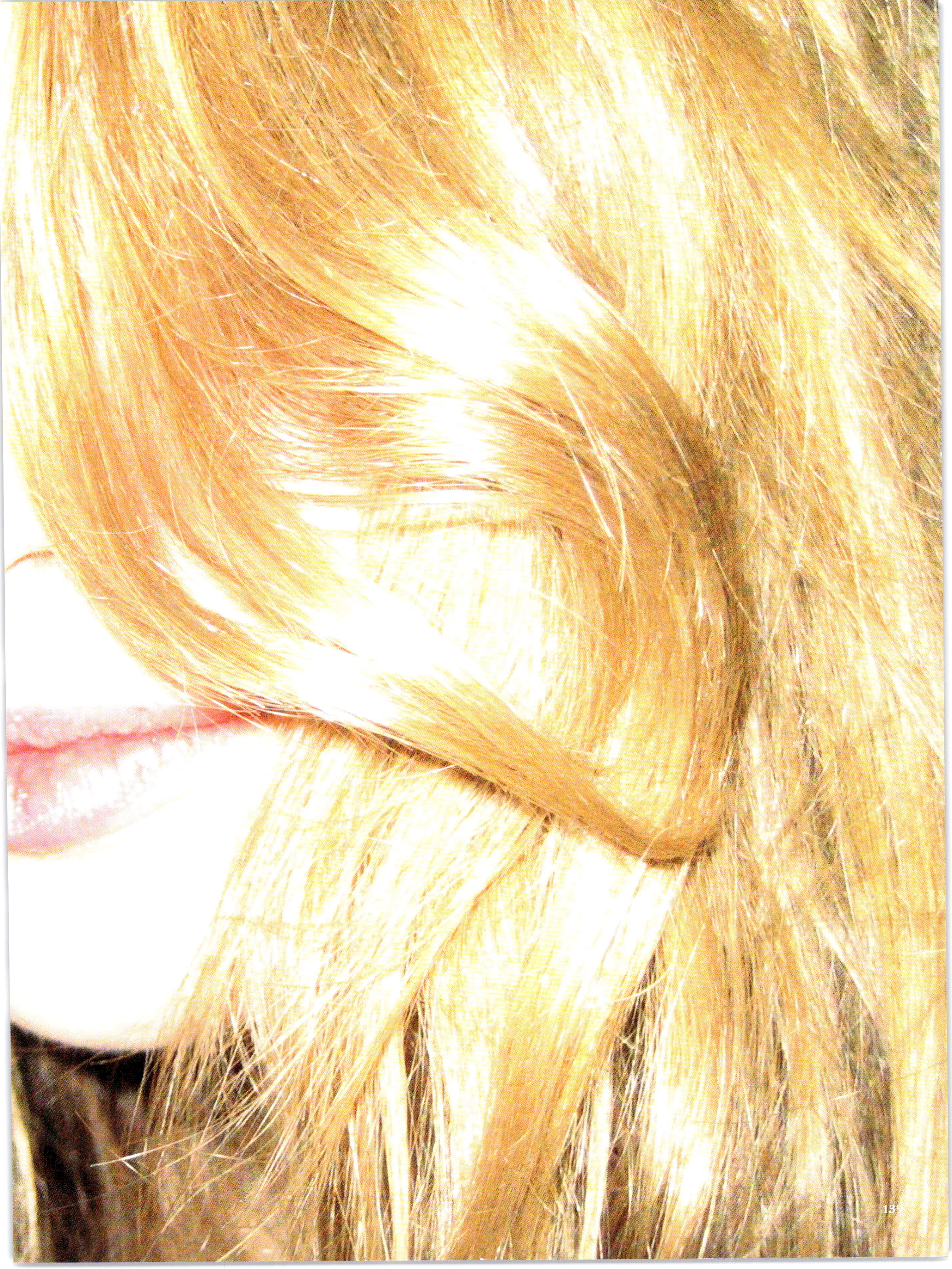

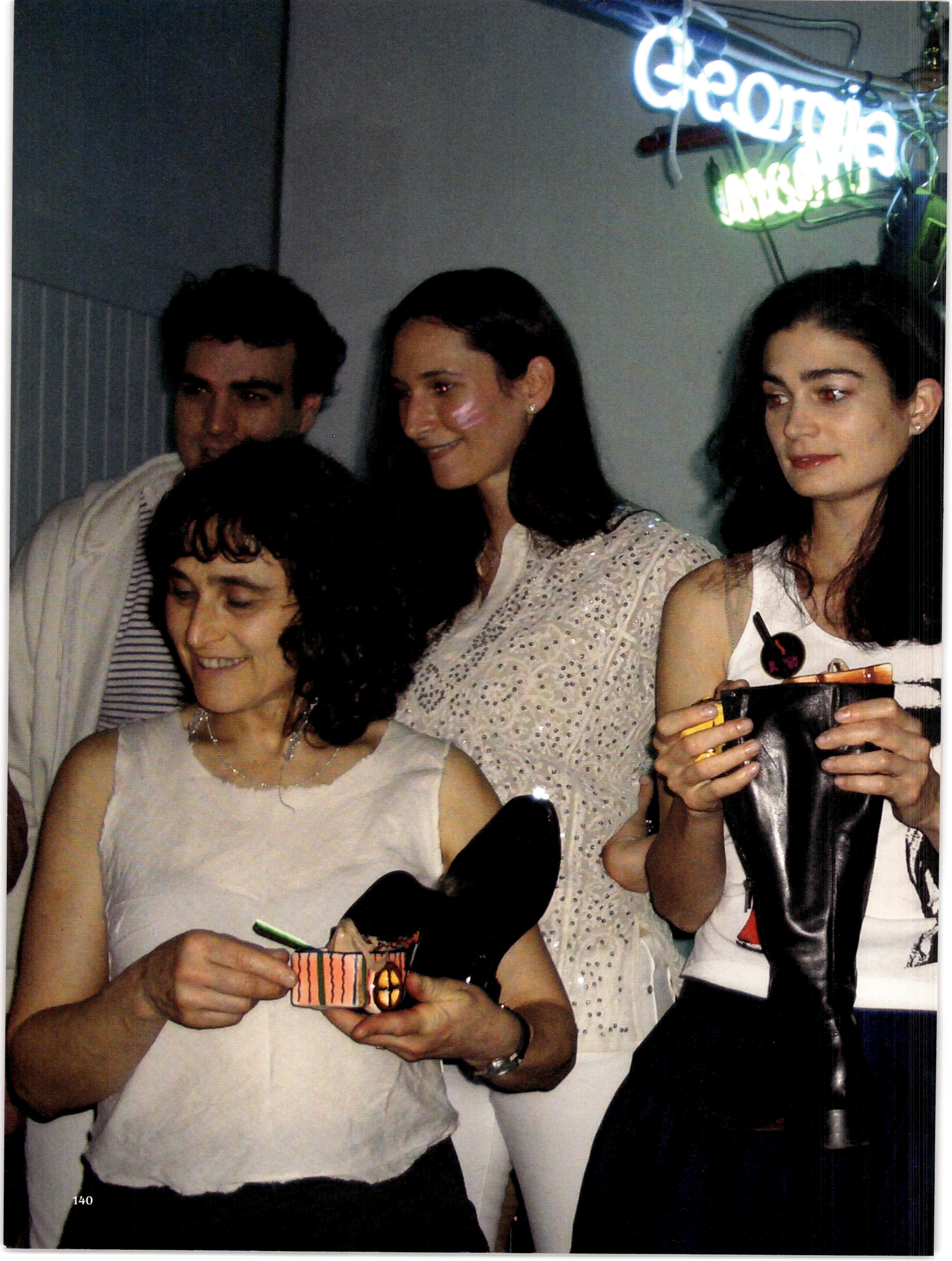
Georgia

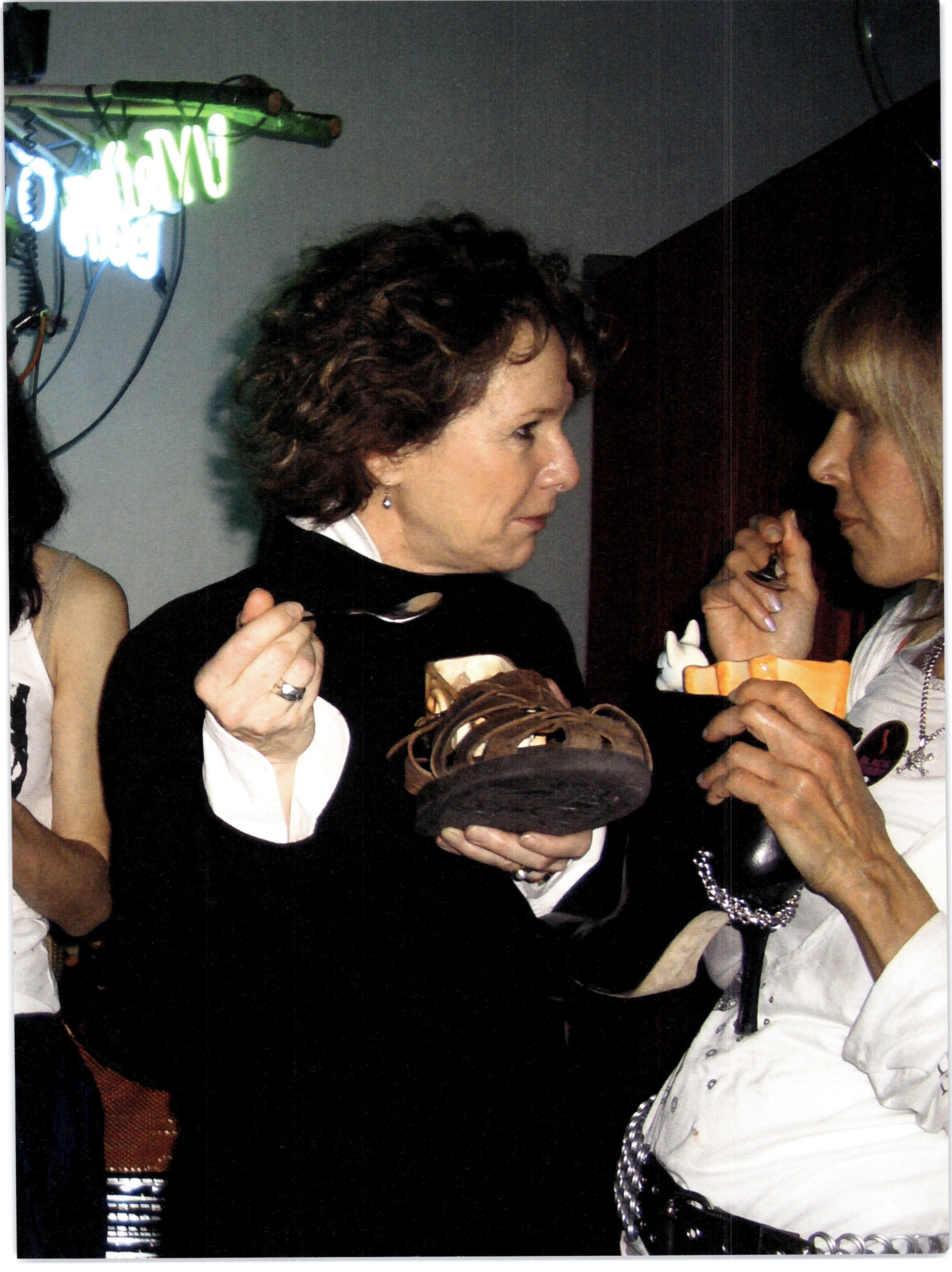

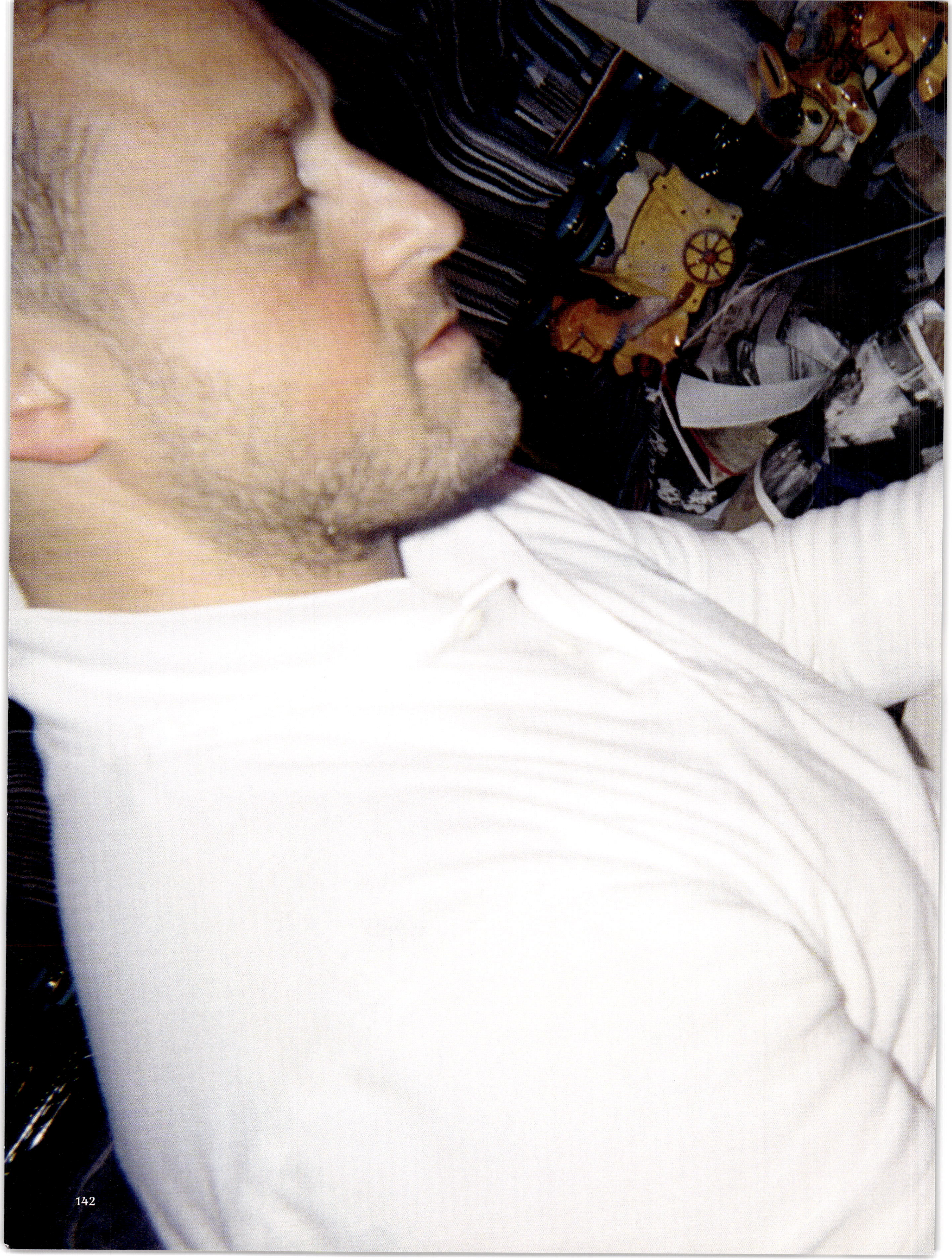

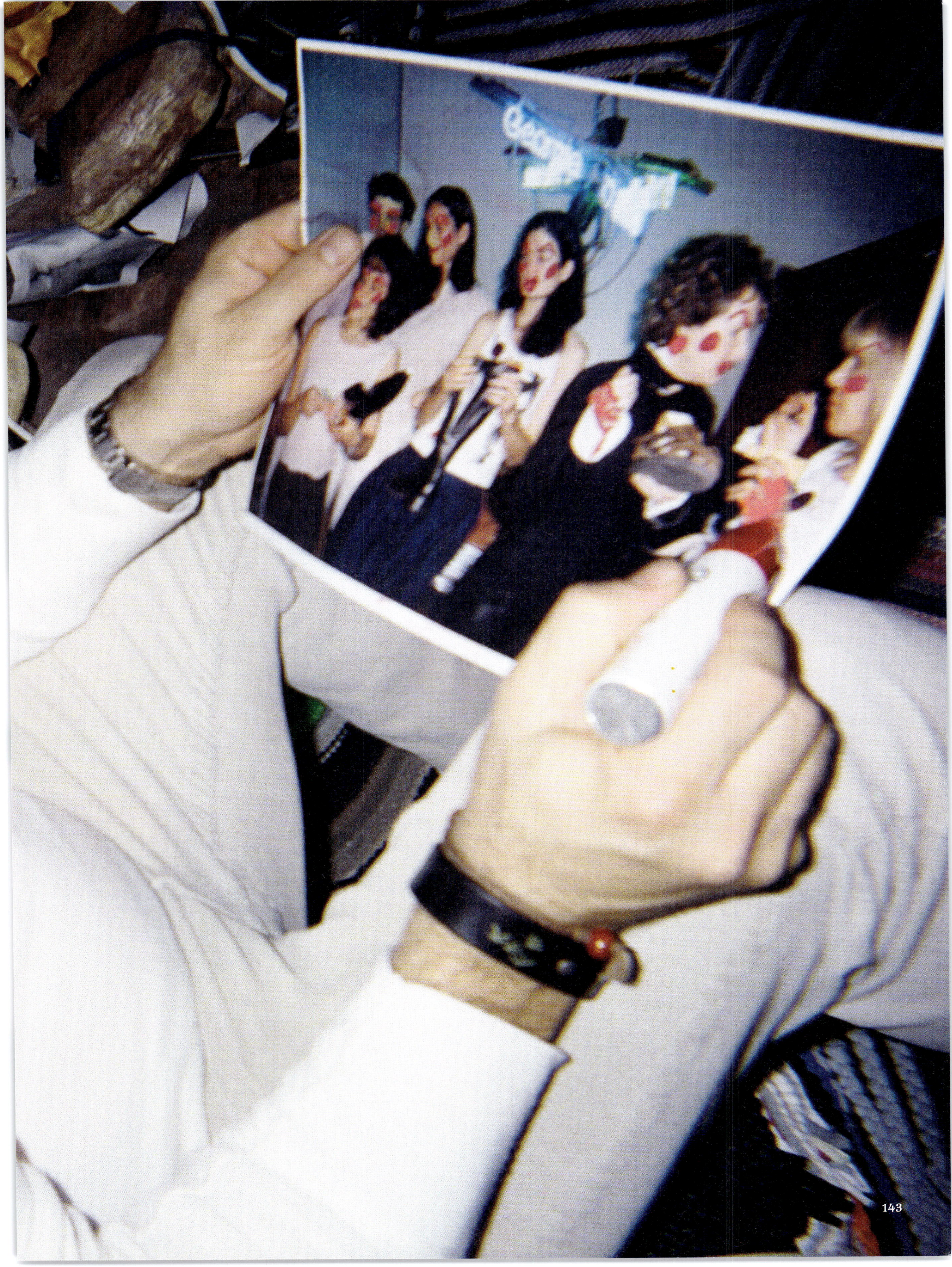

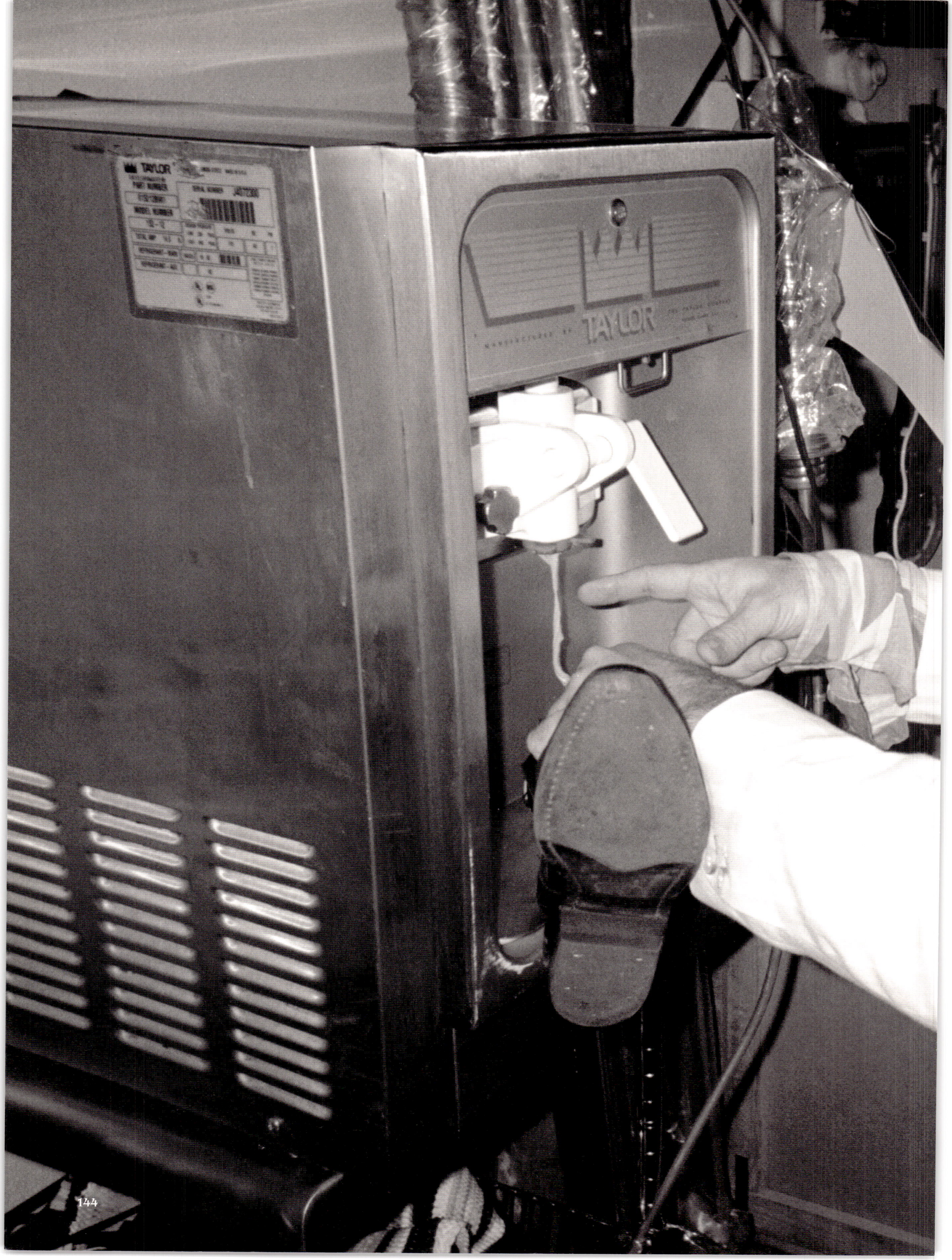
TAYLOR

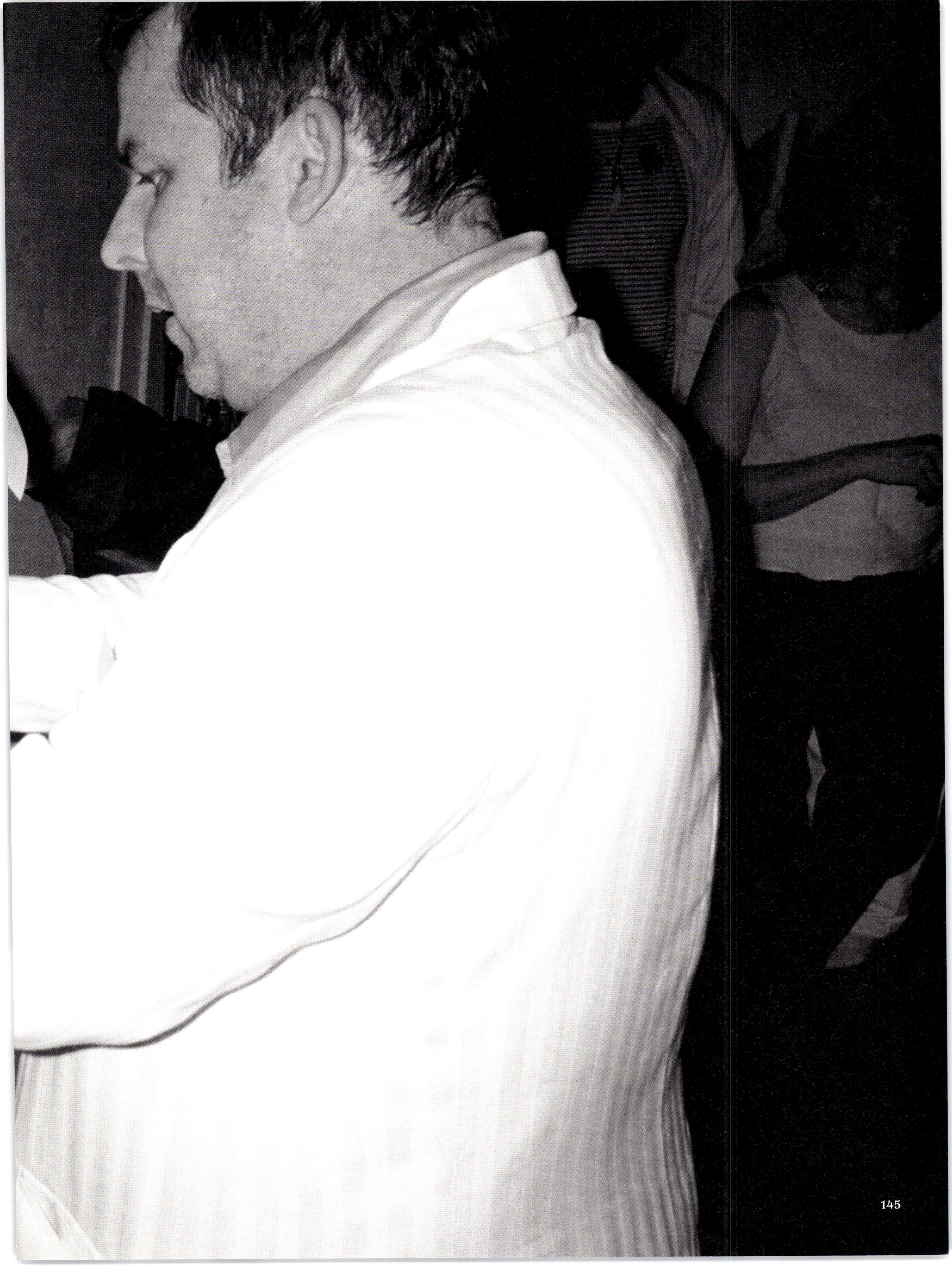

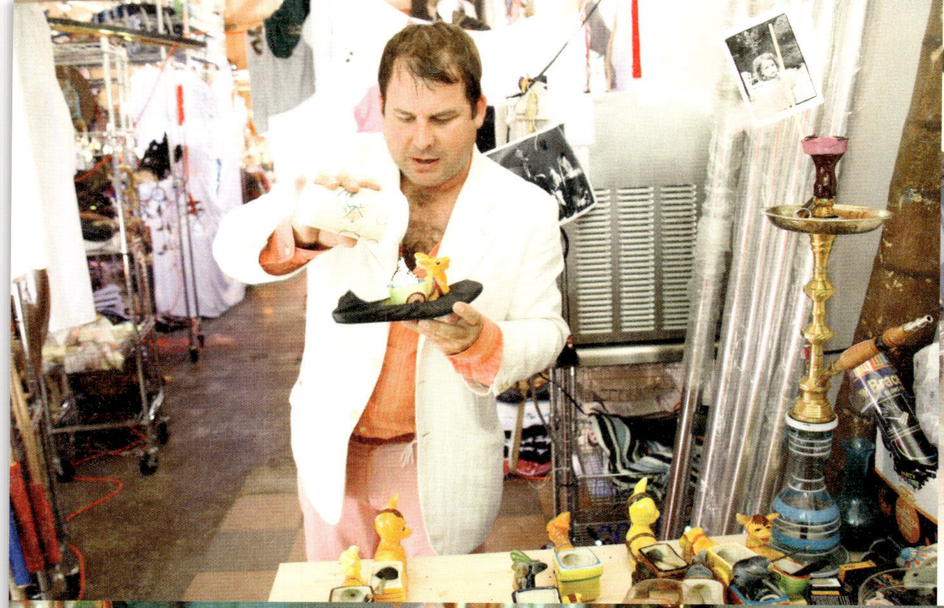
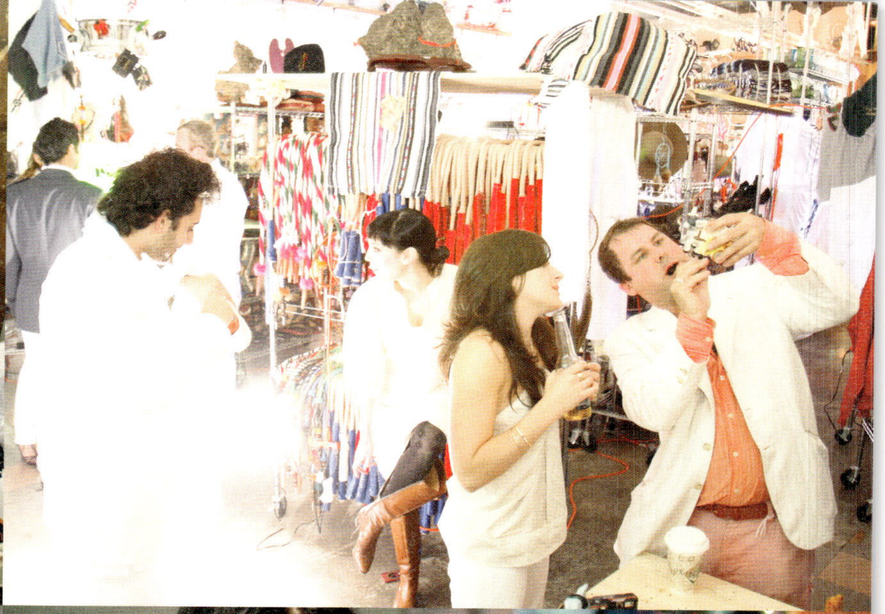
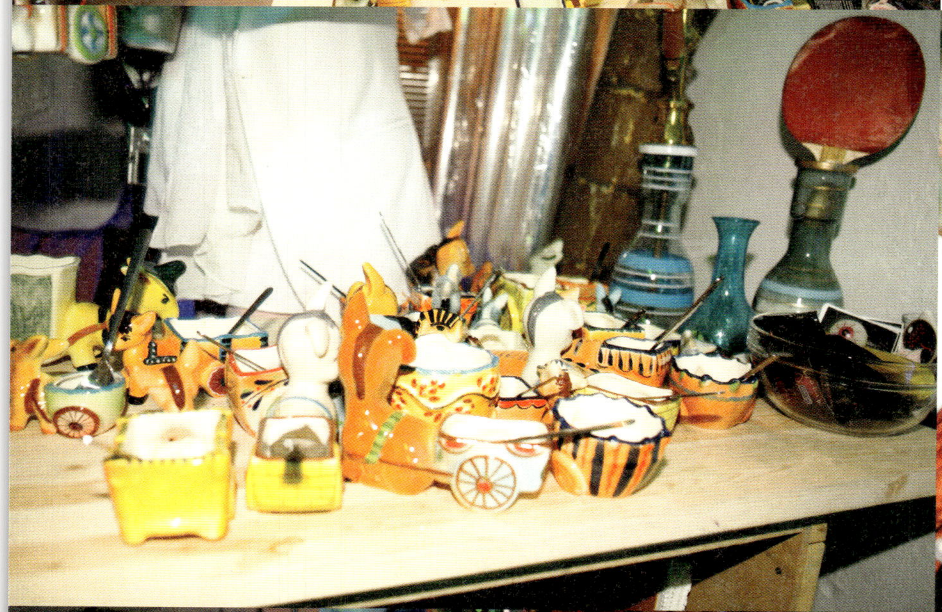
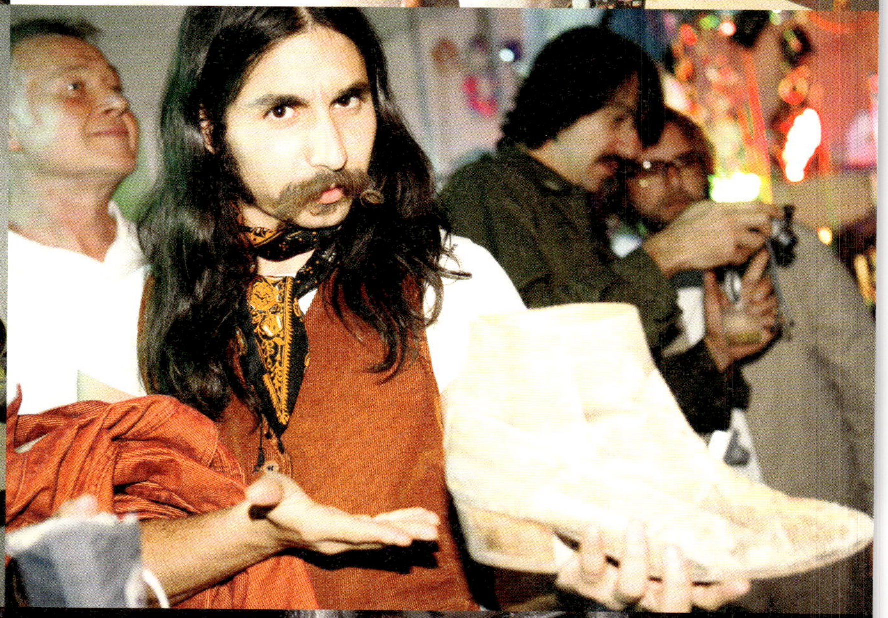
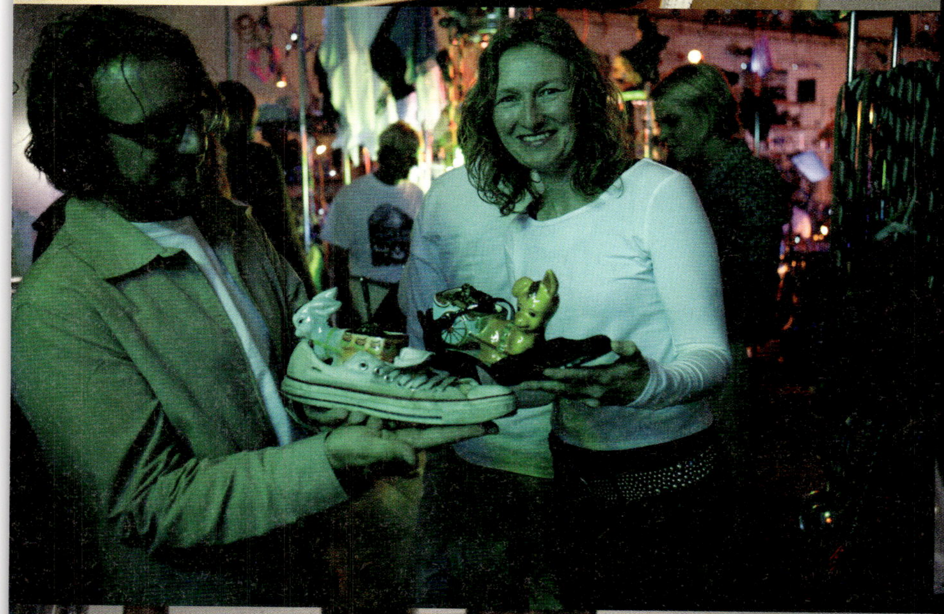
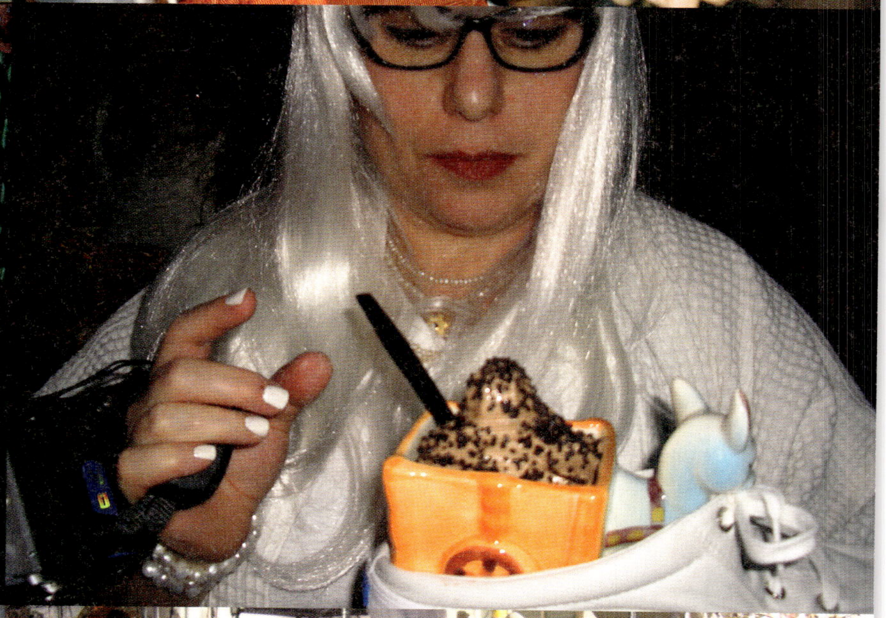
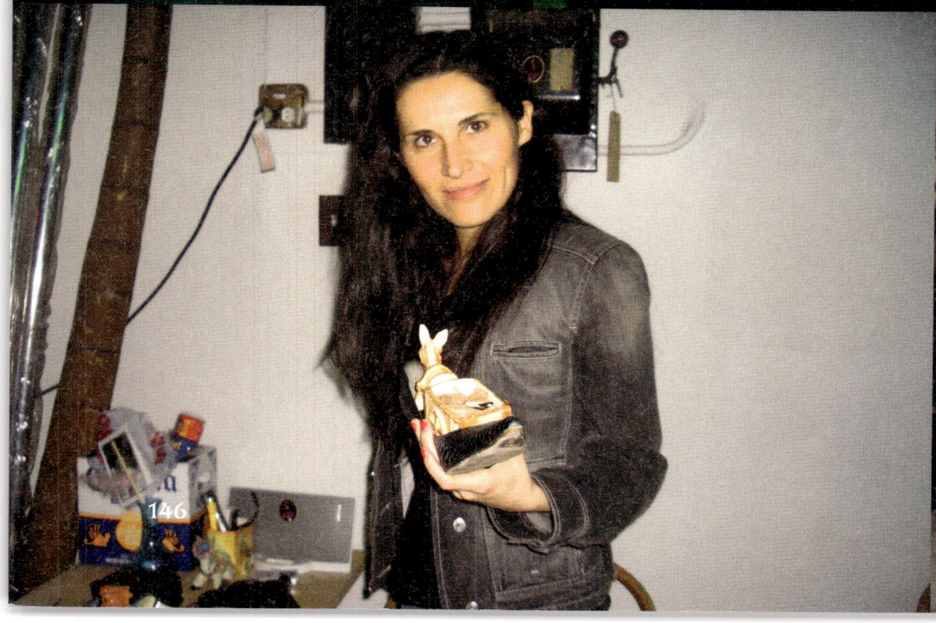
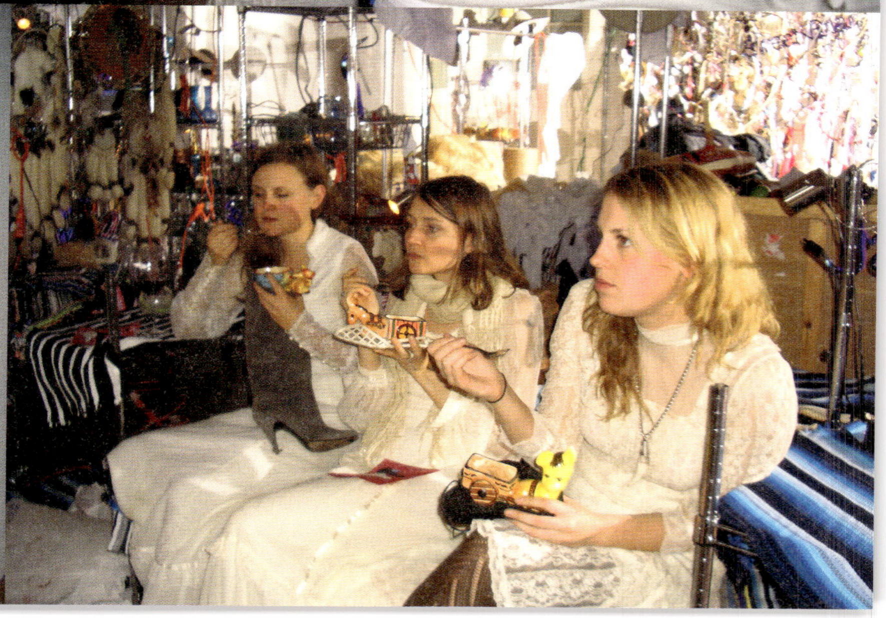

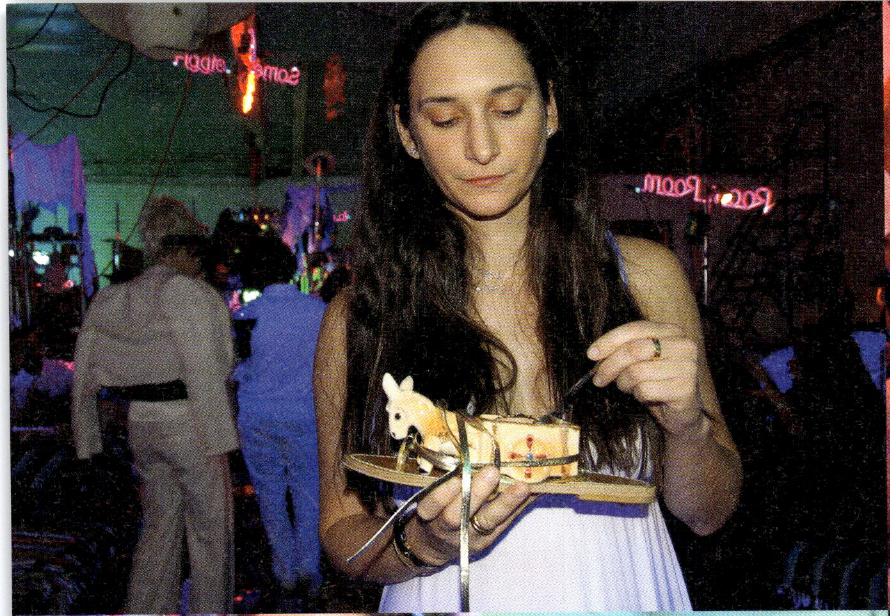
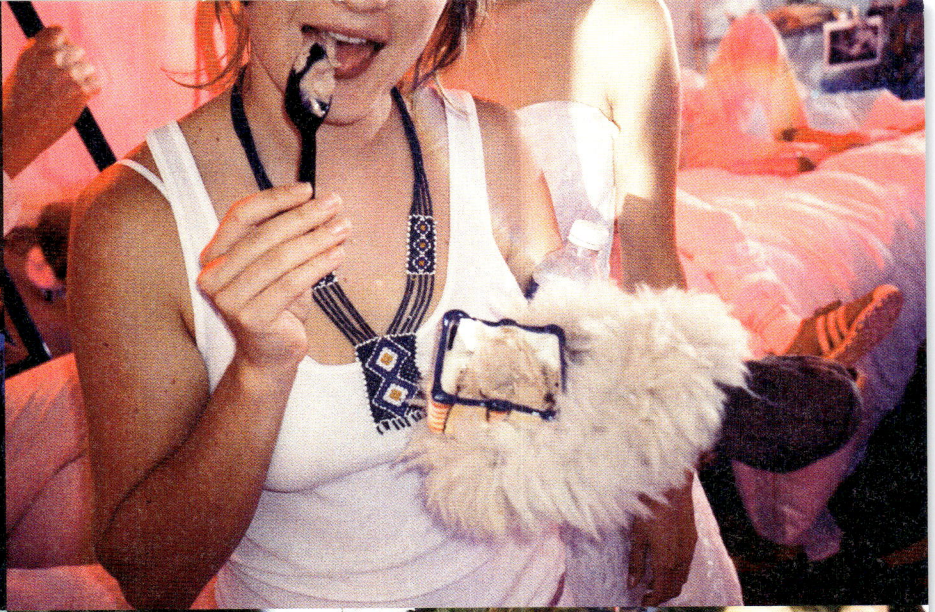
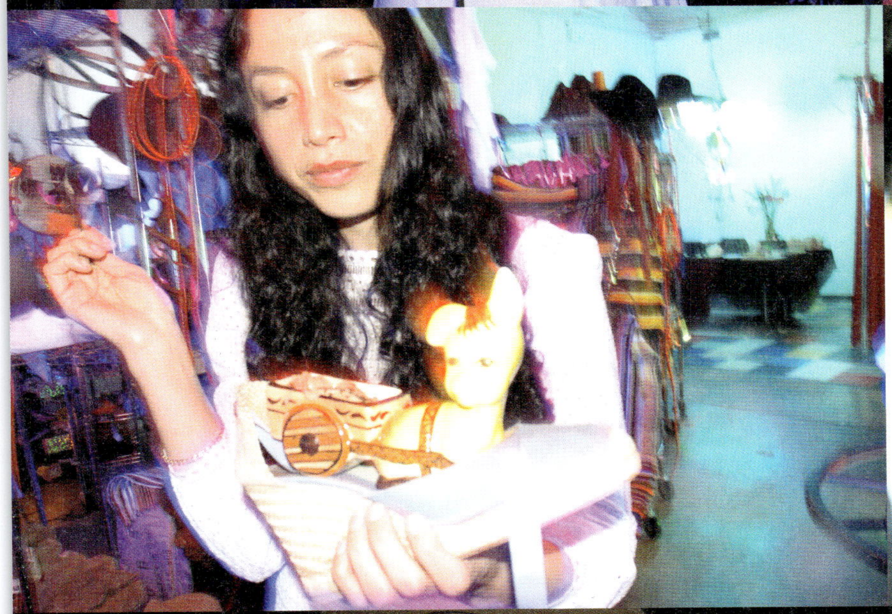
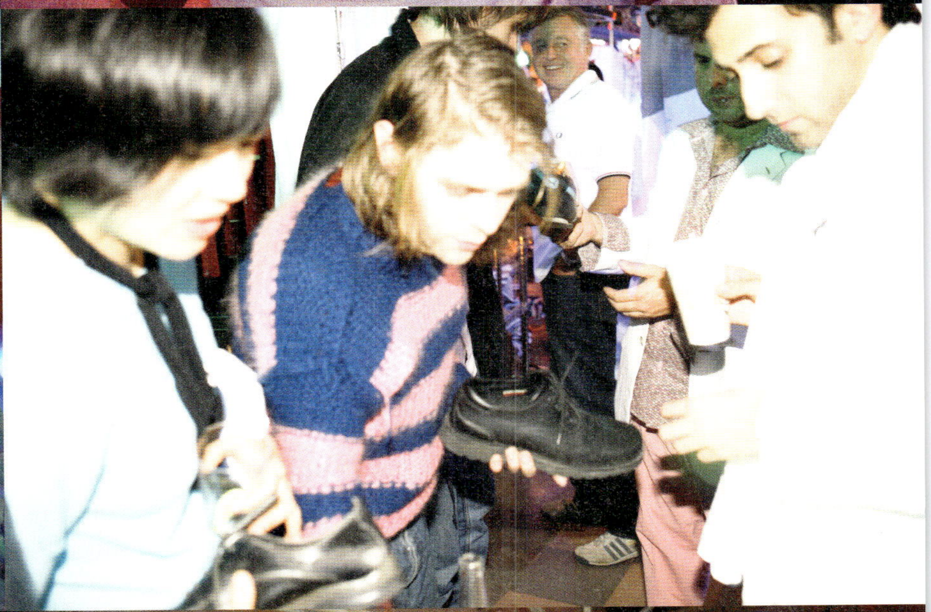
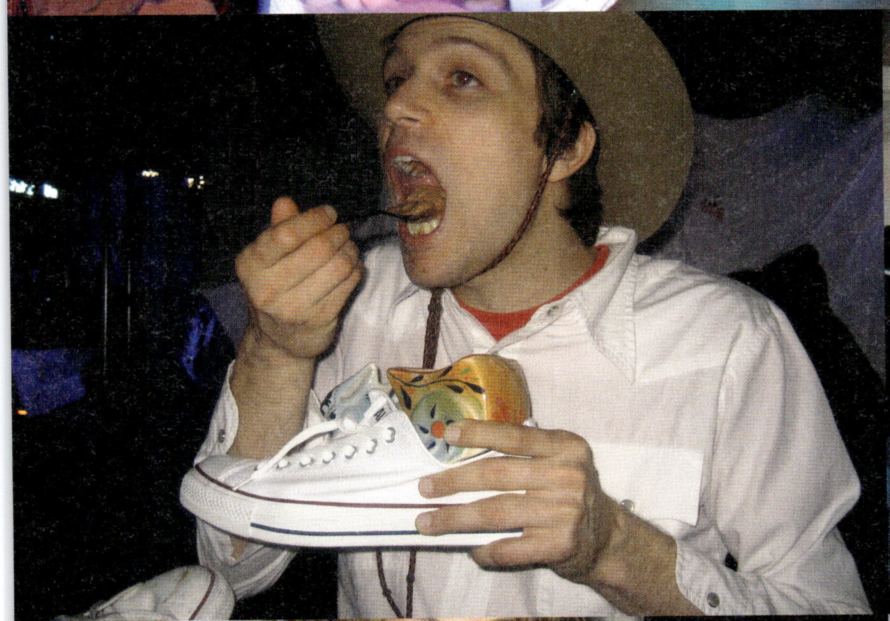
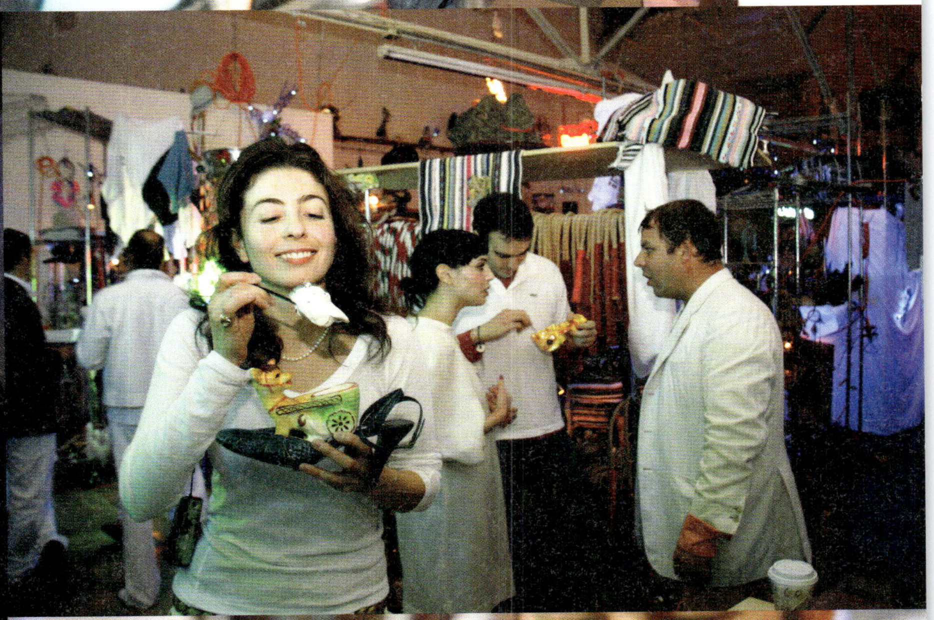
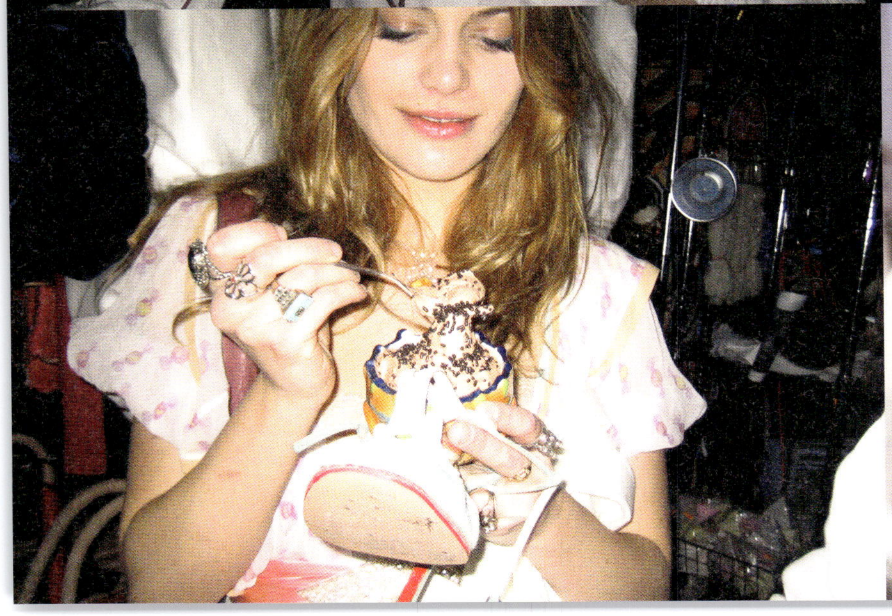
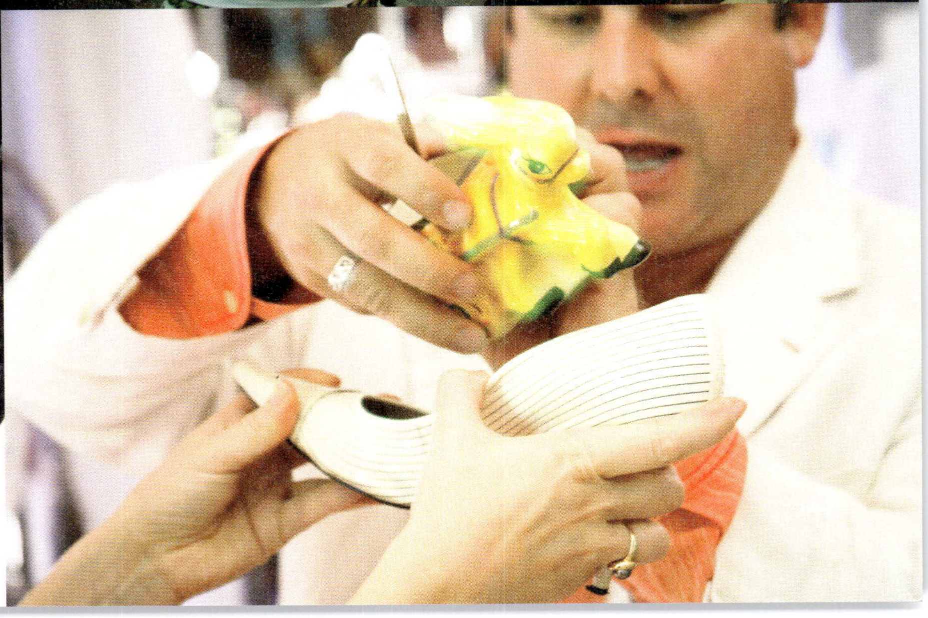

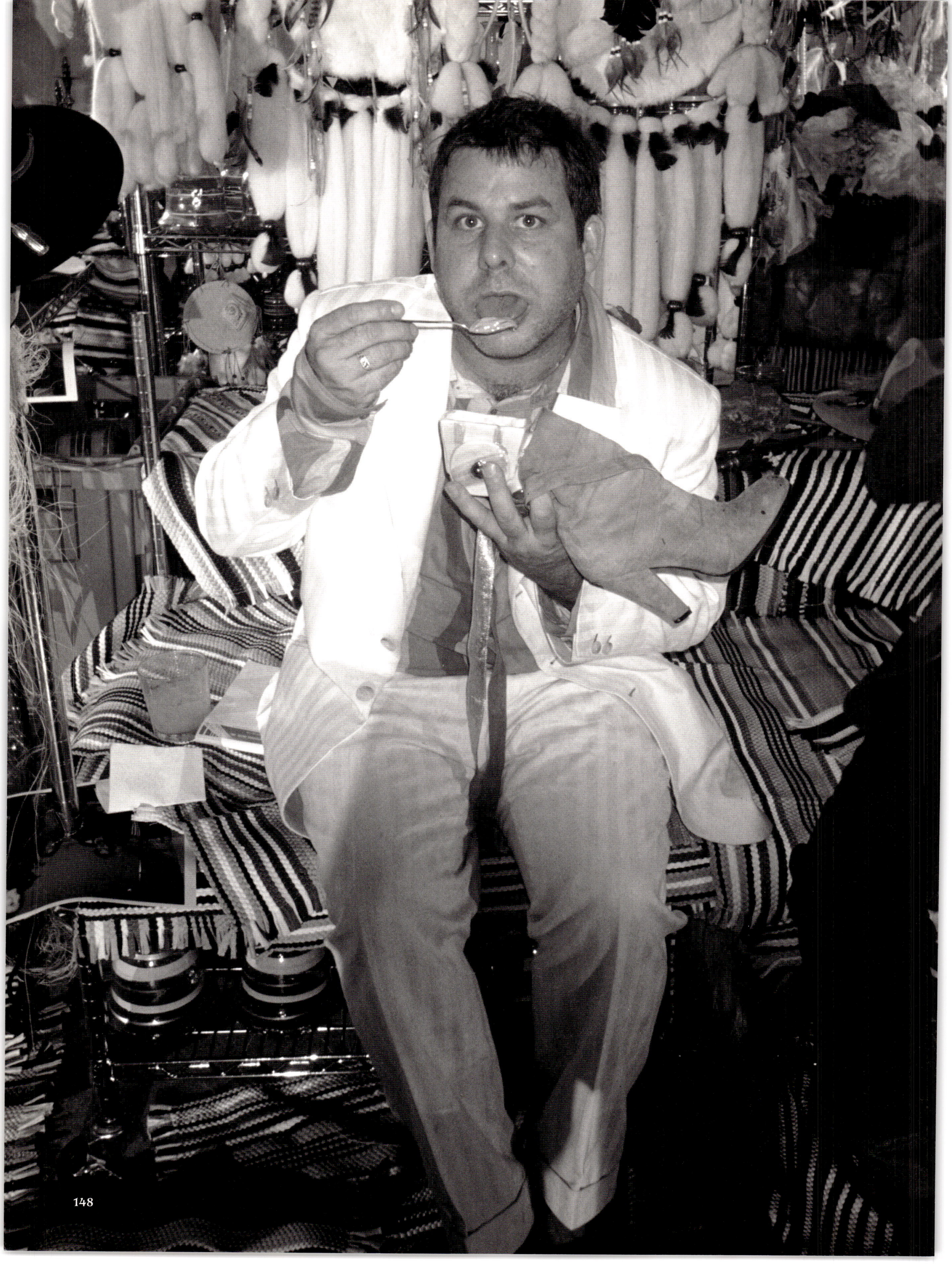

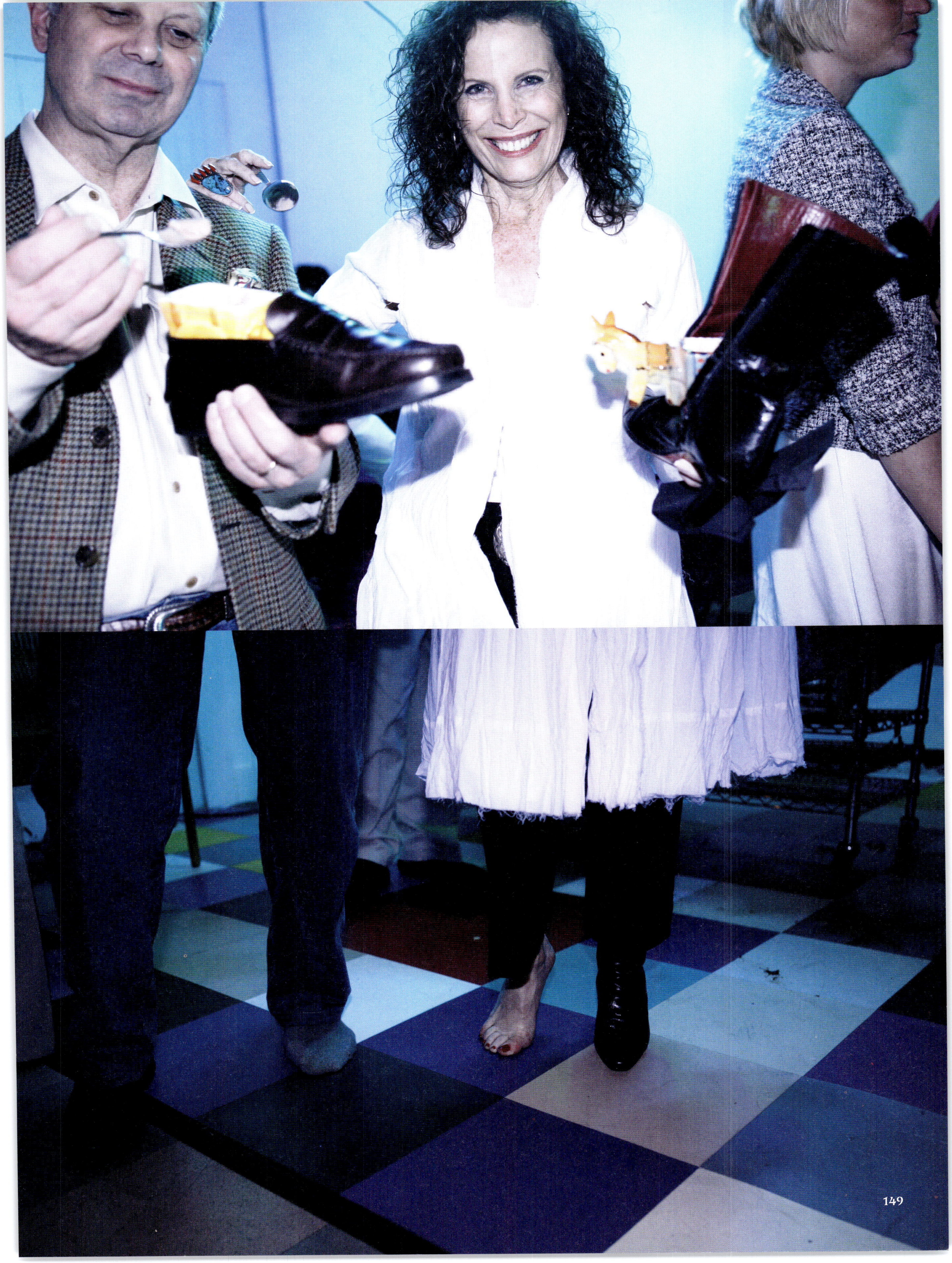

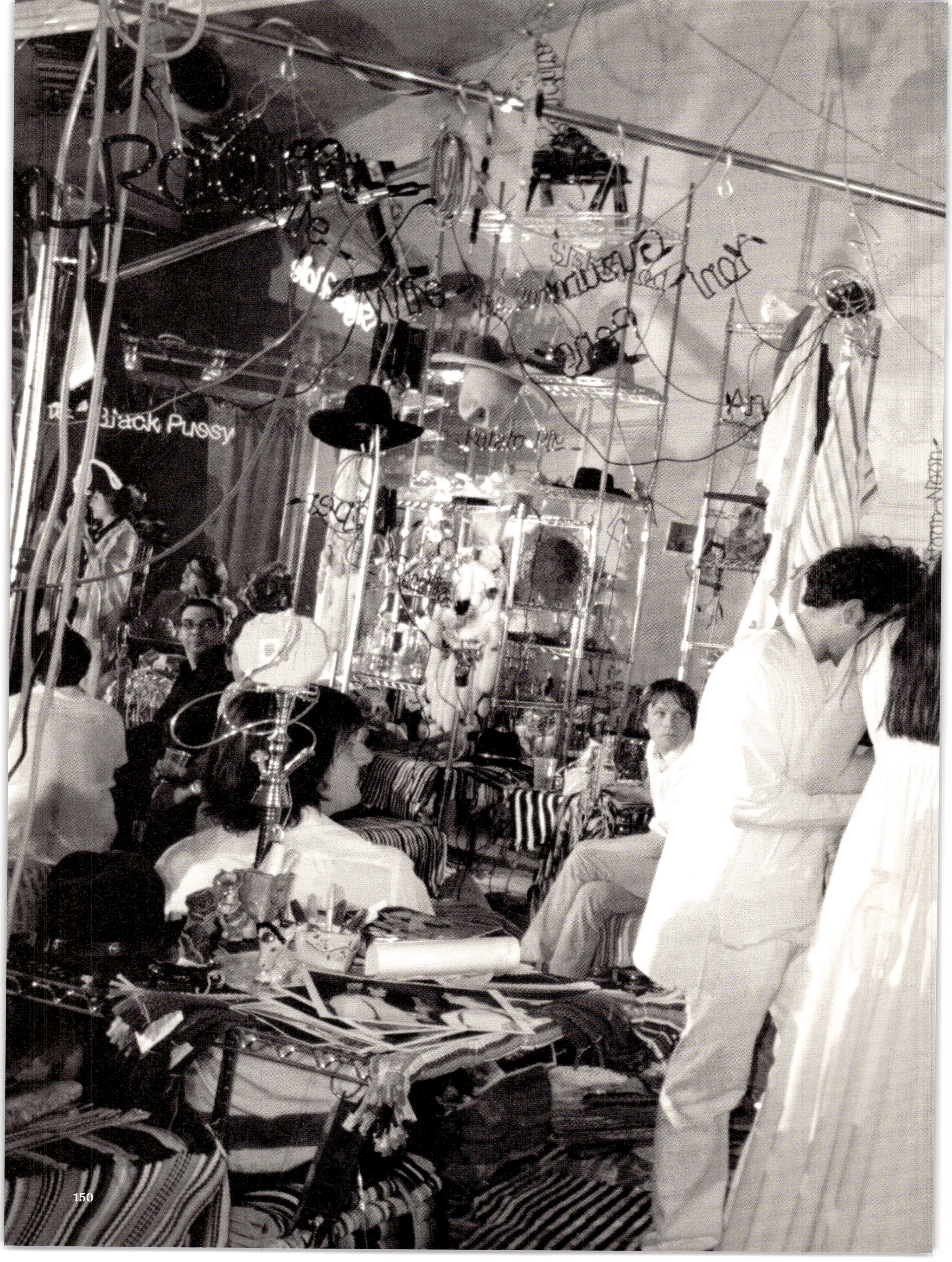
Black Pussy

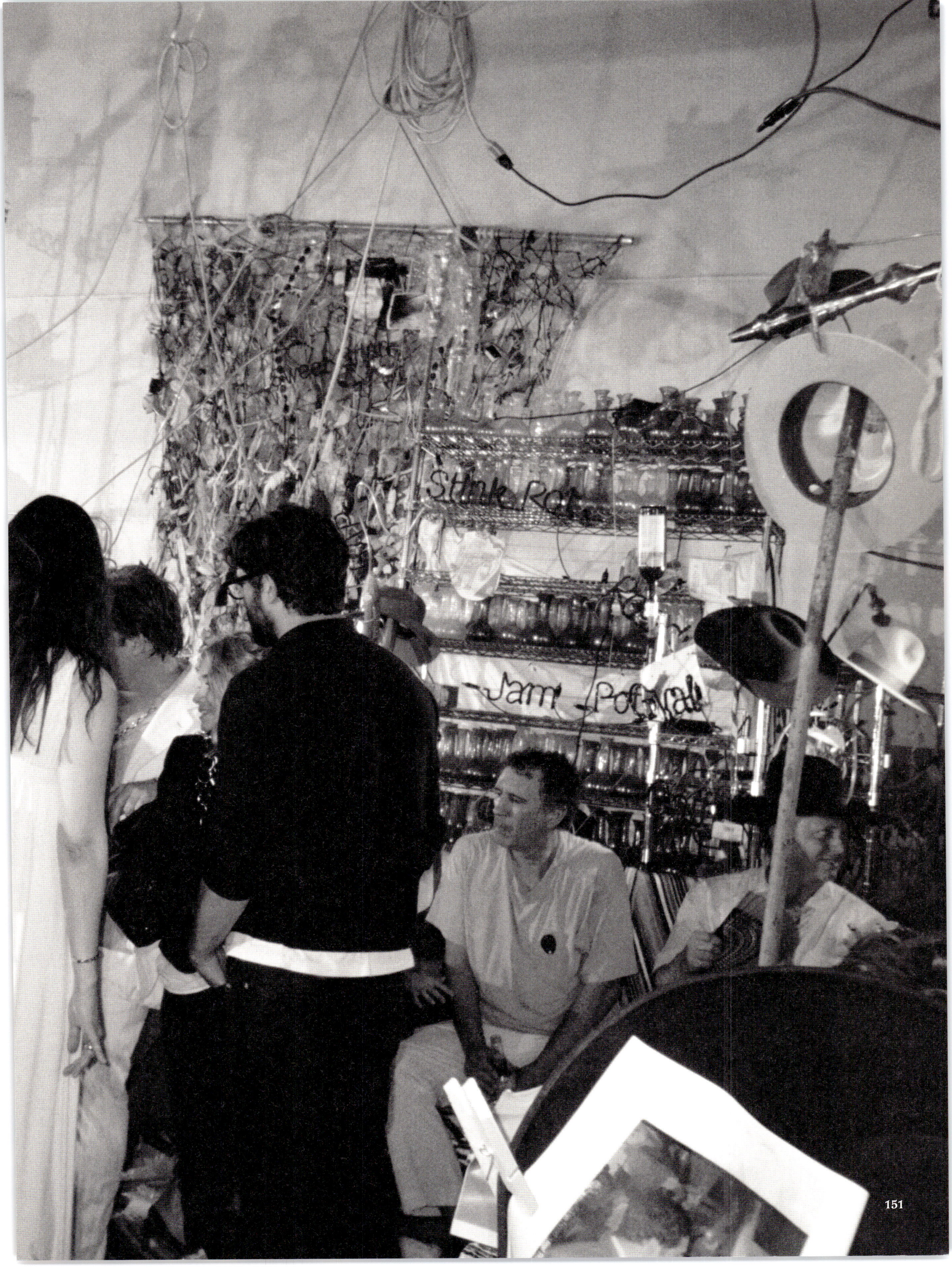
Stink Rat
Jam

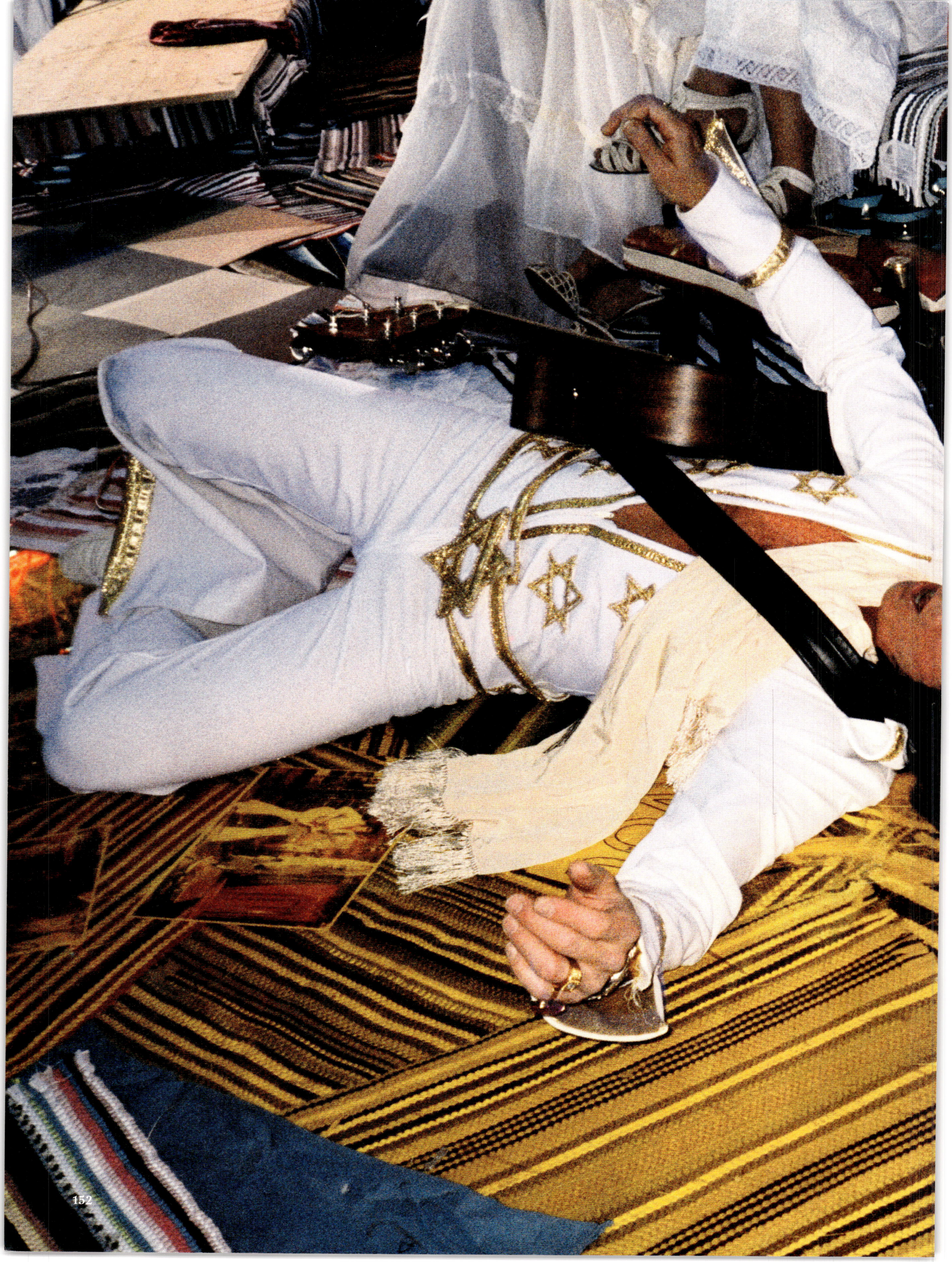

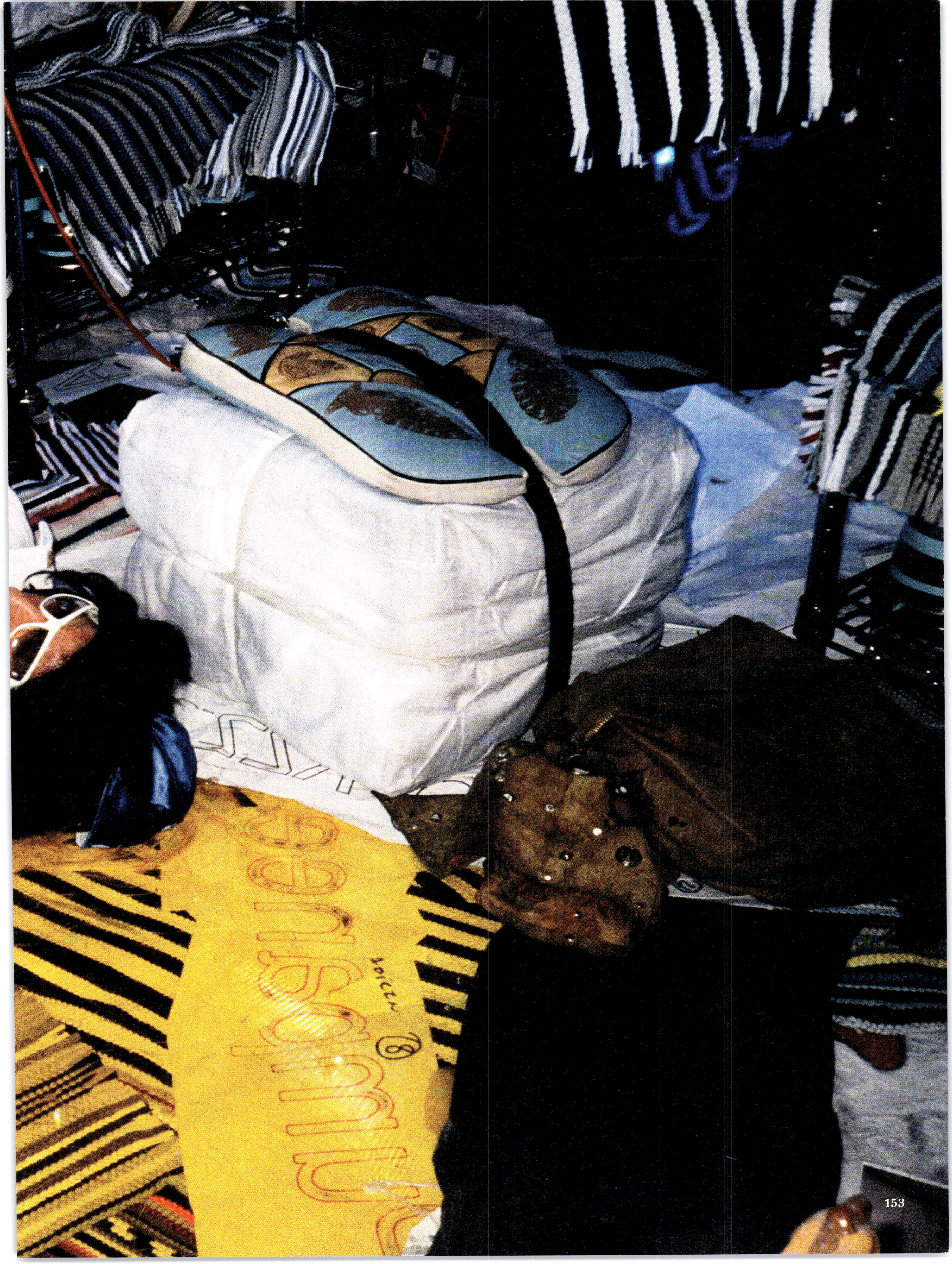

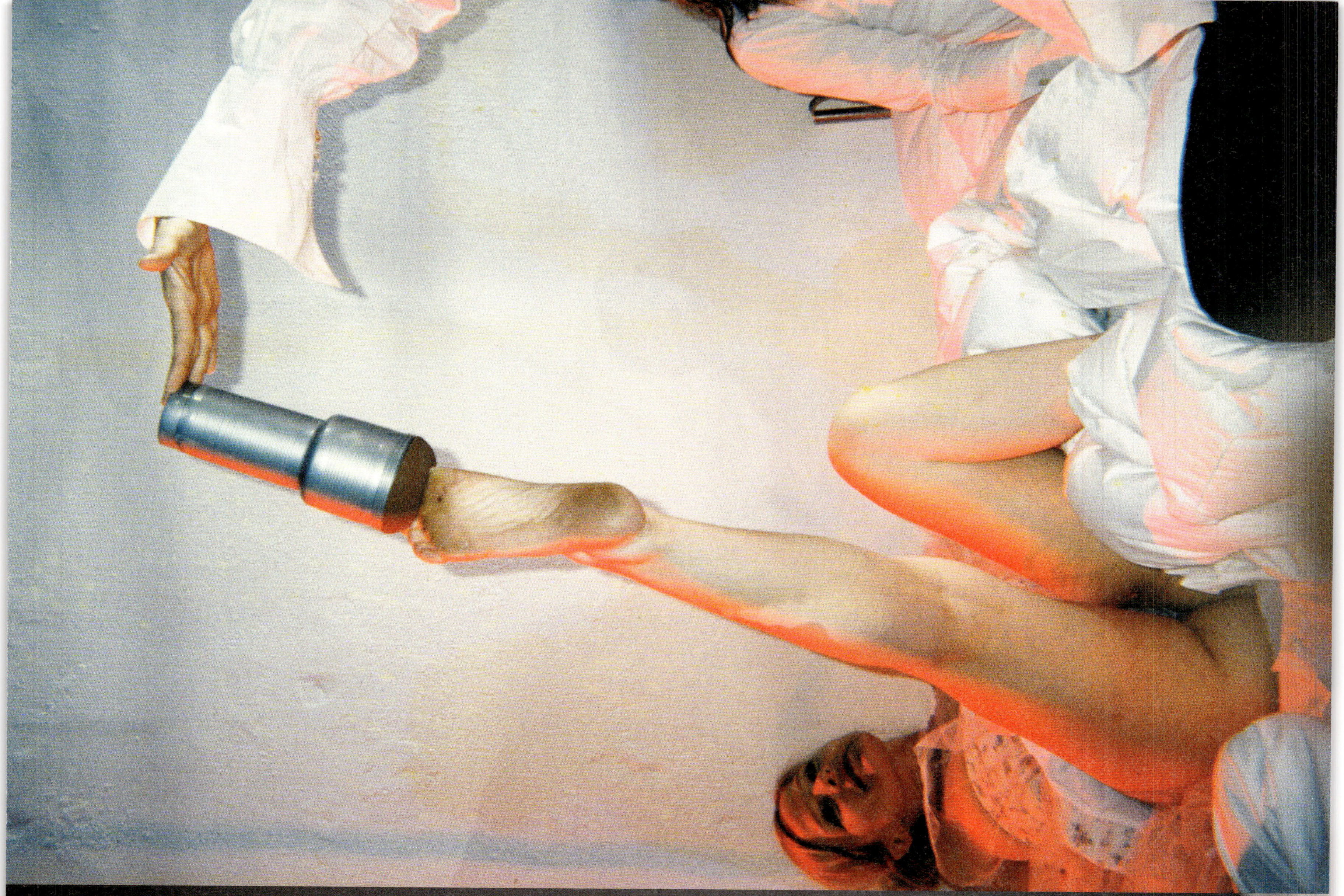

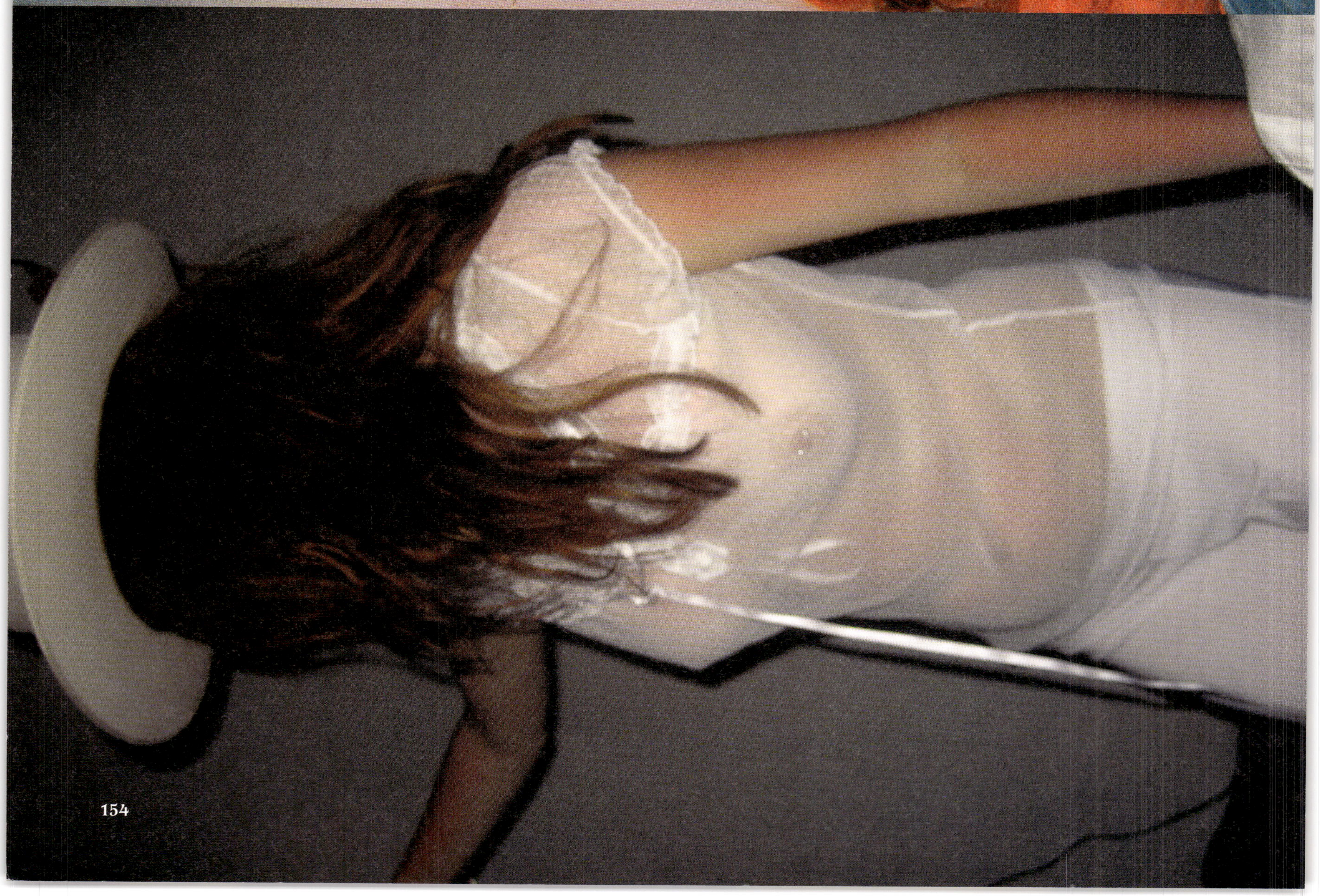

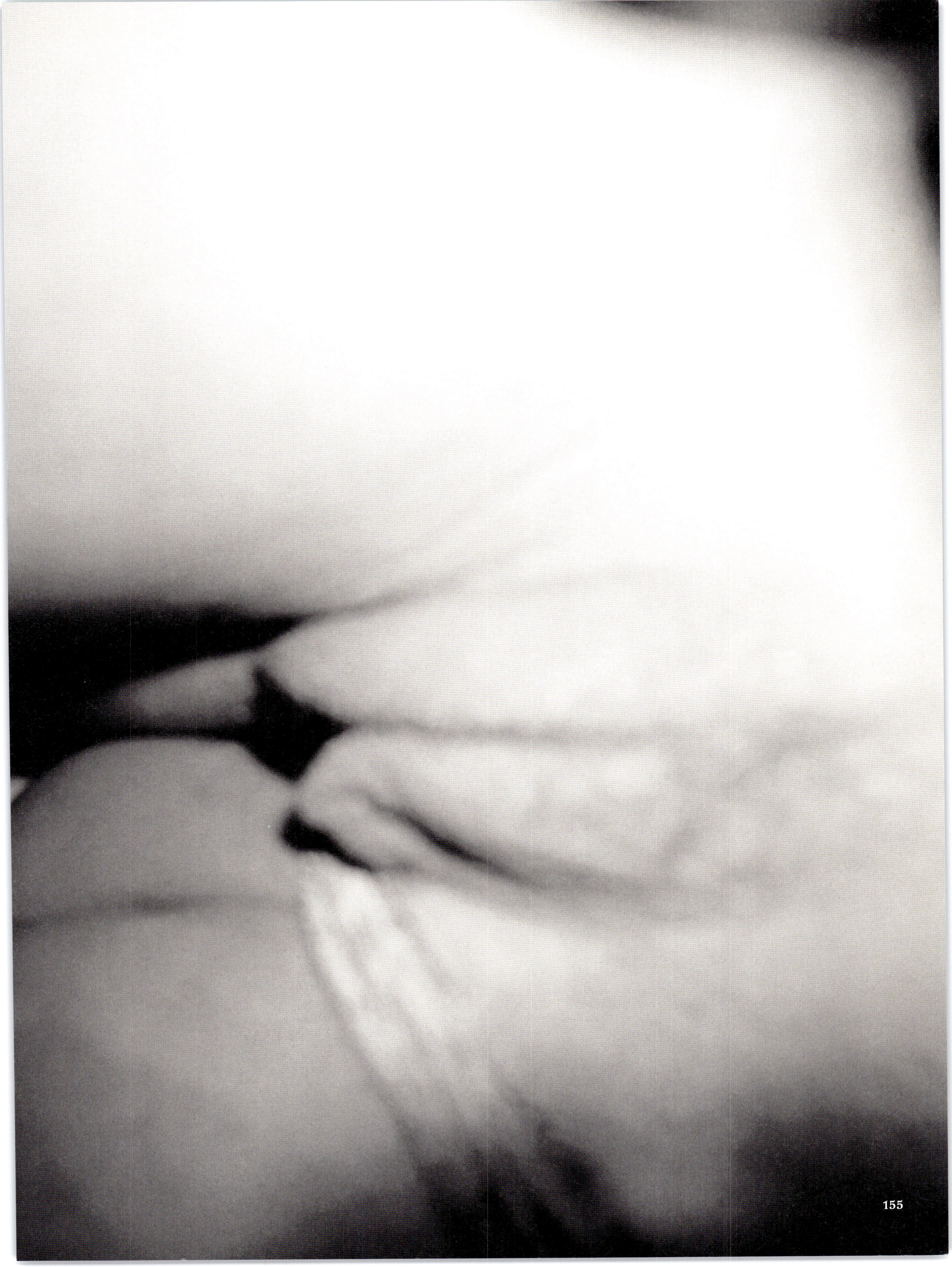

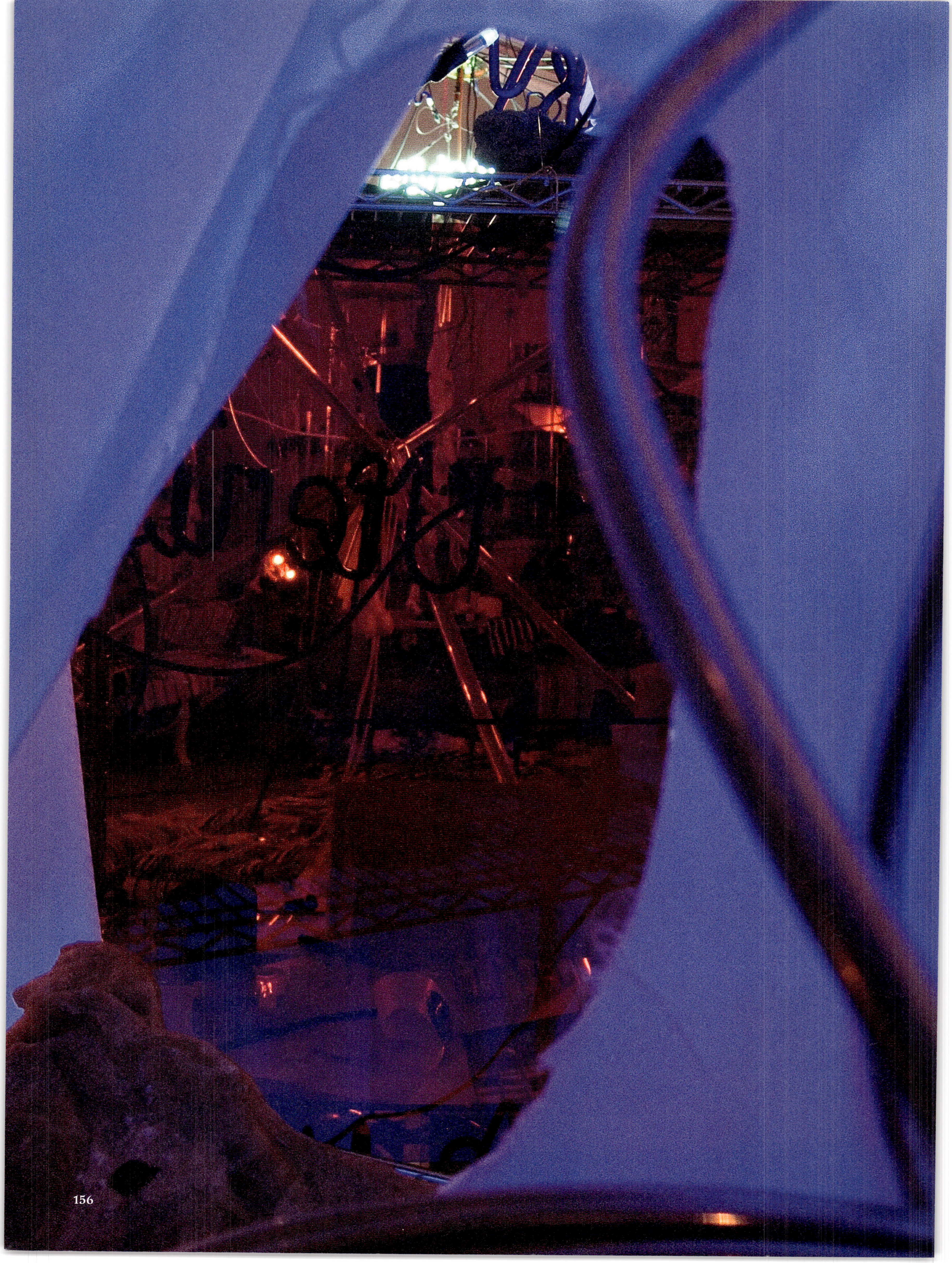

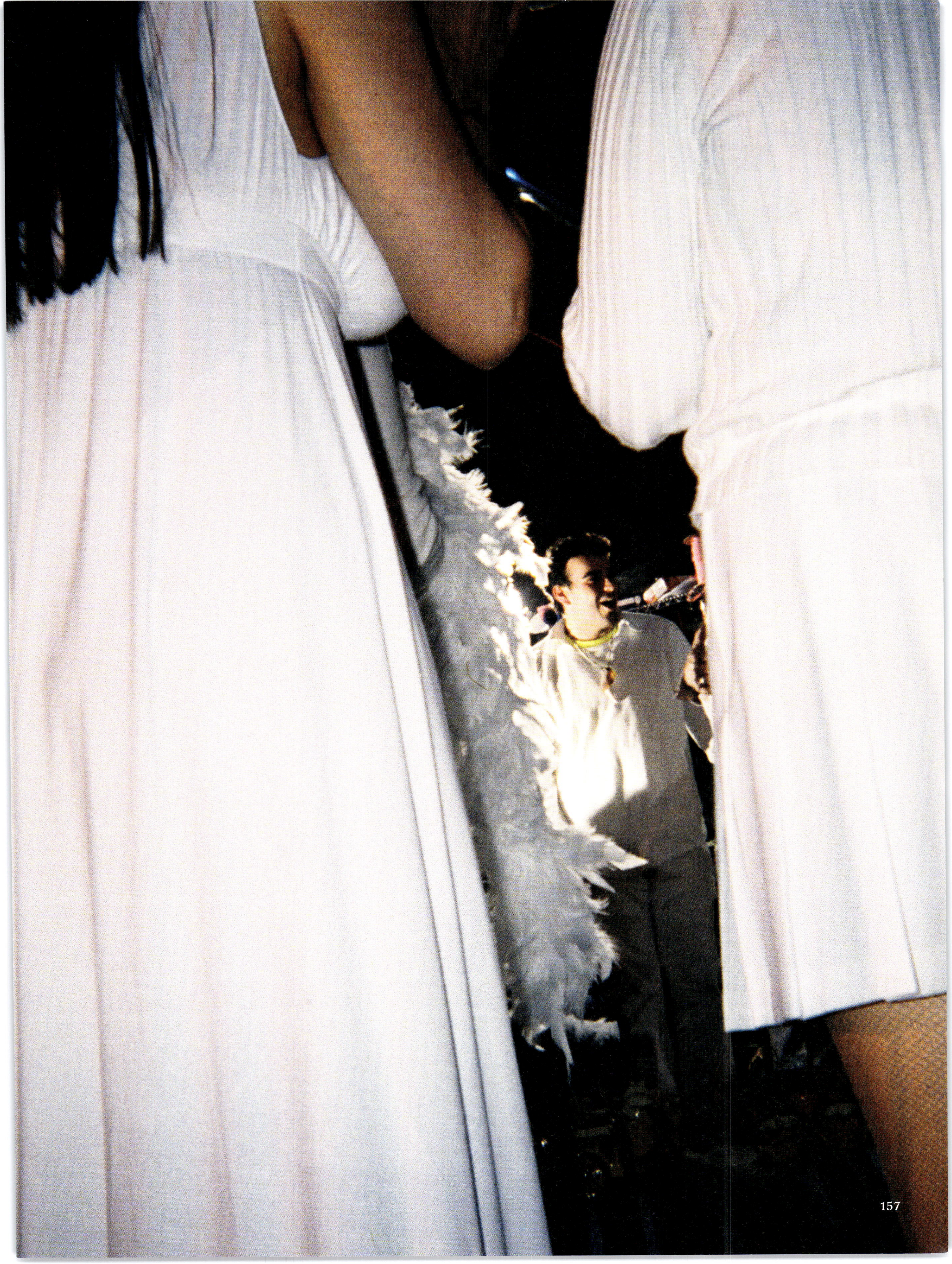

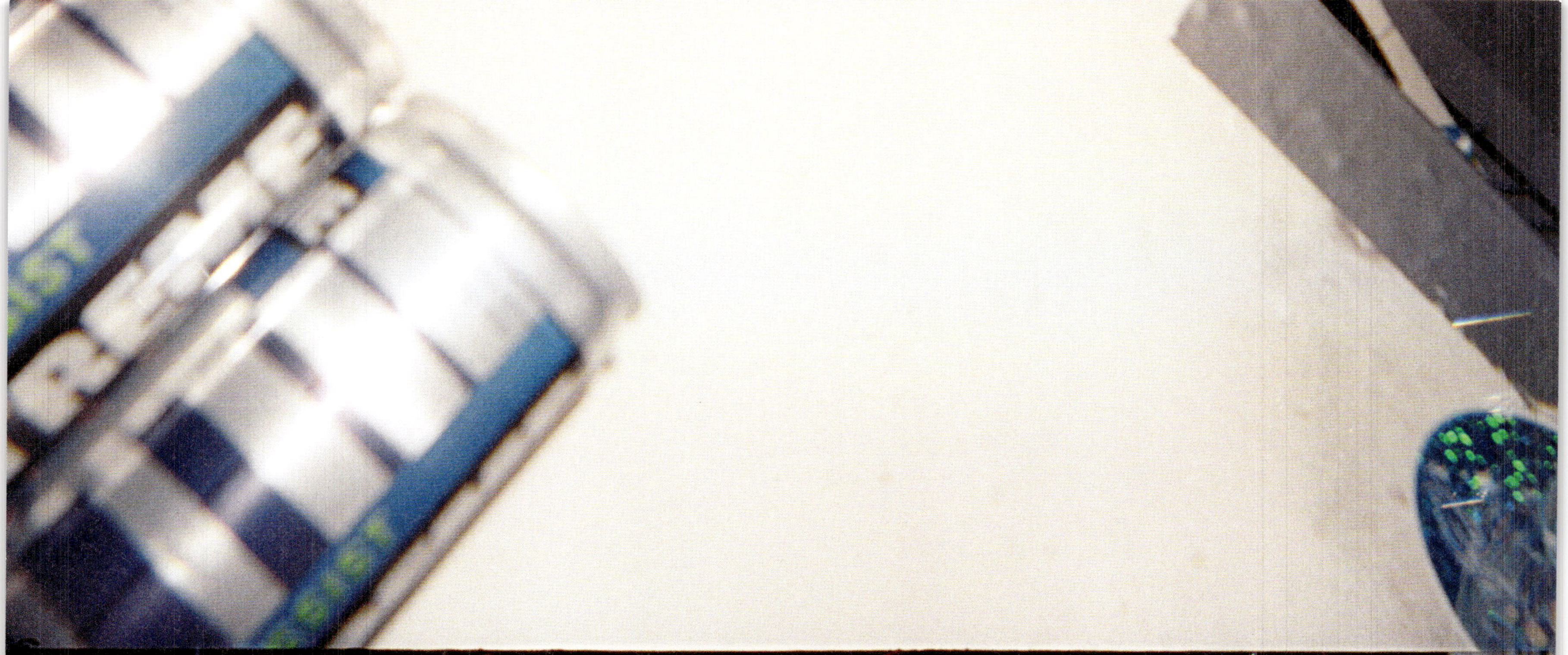

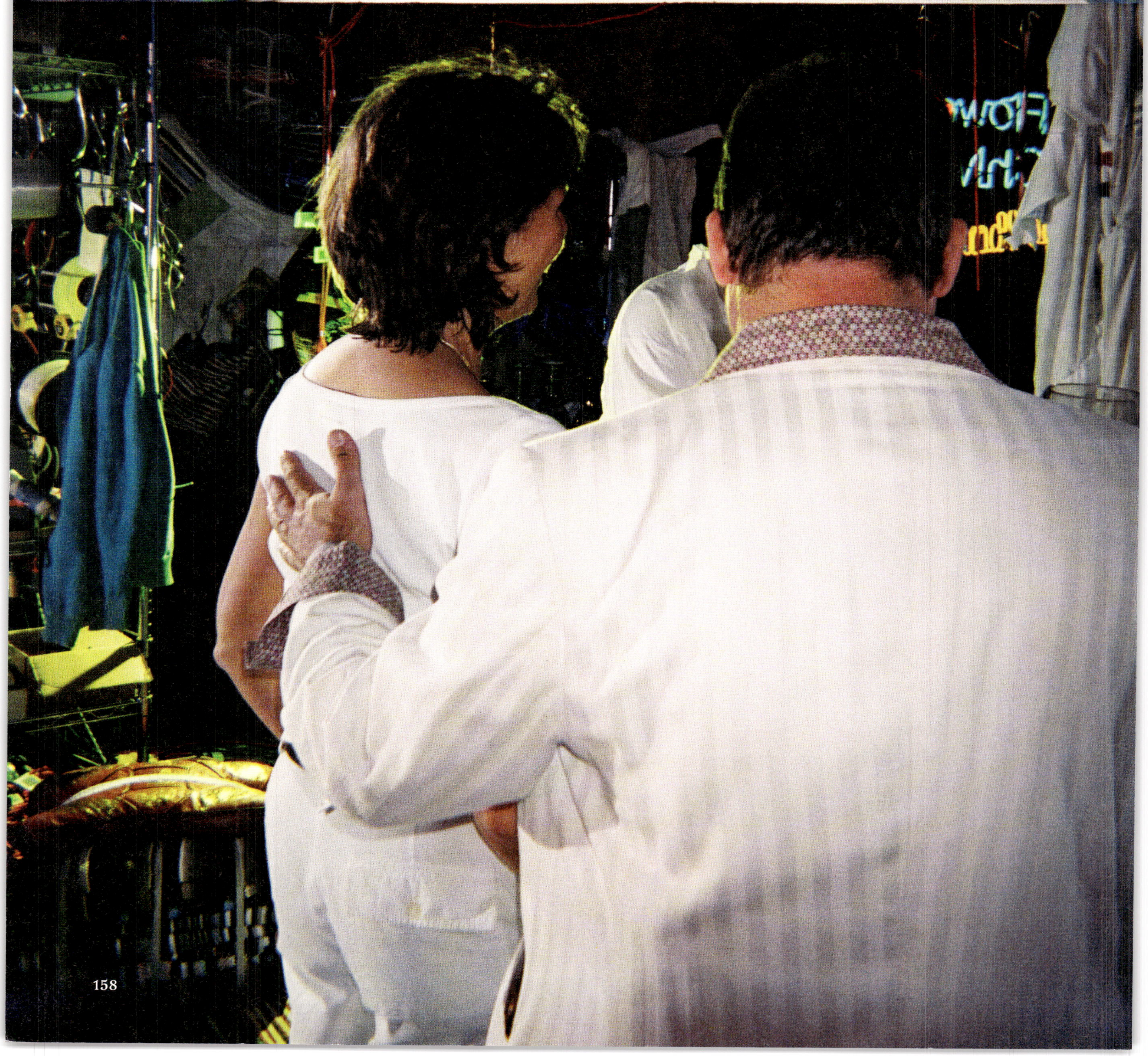

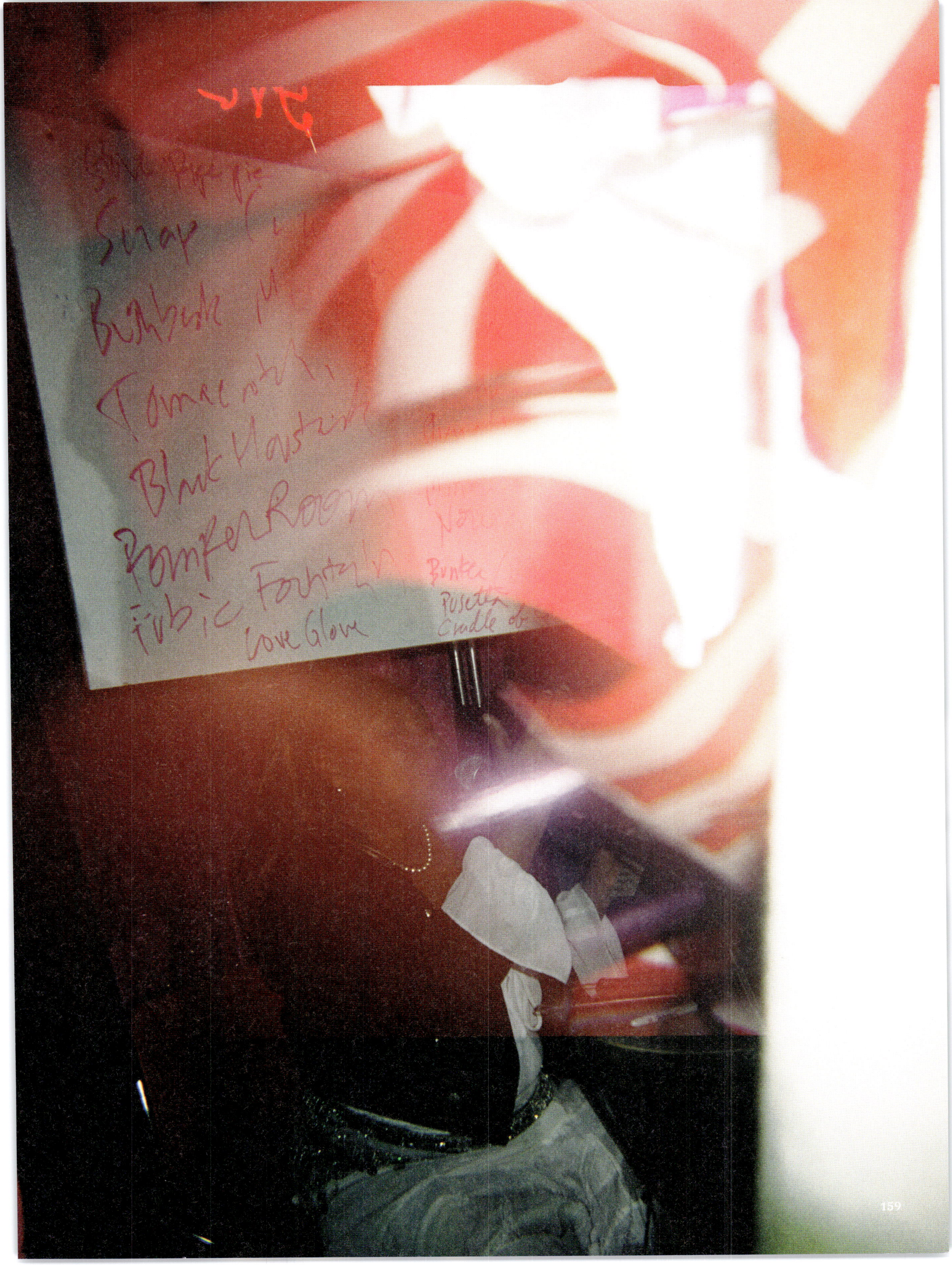
Love Glove

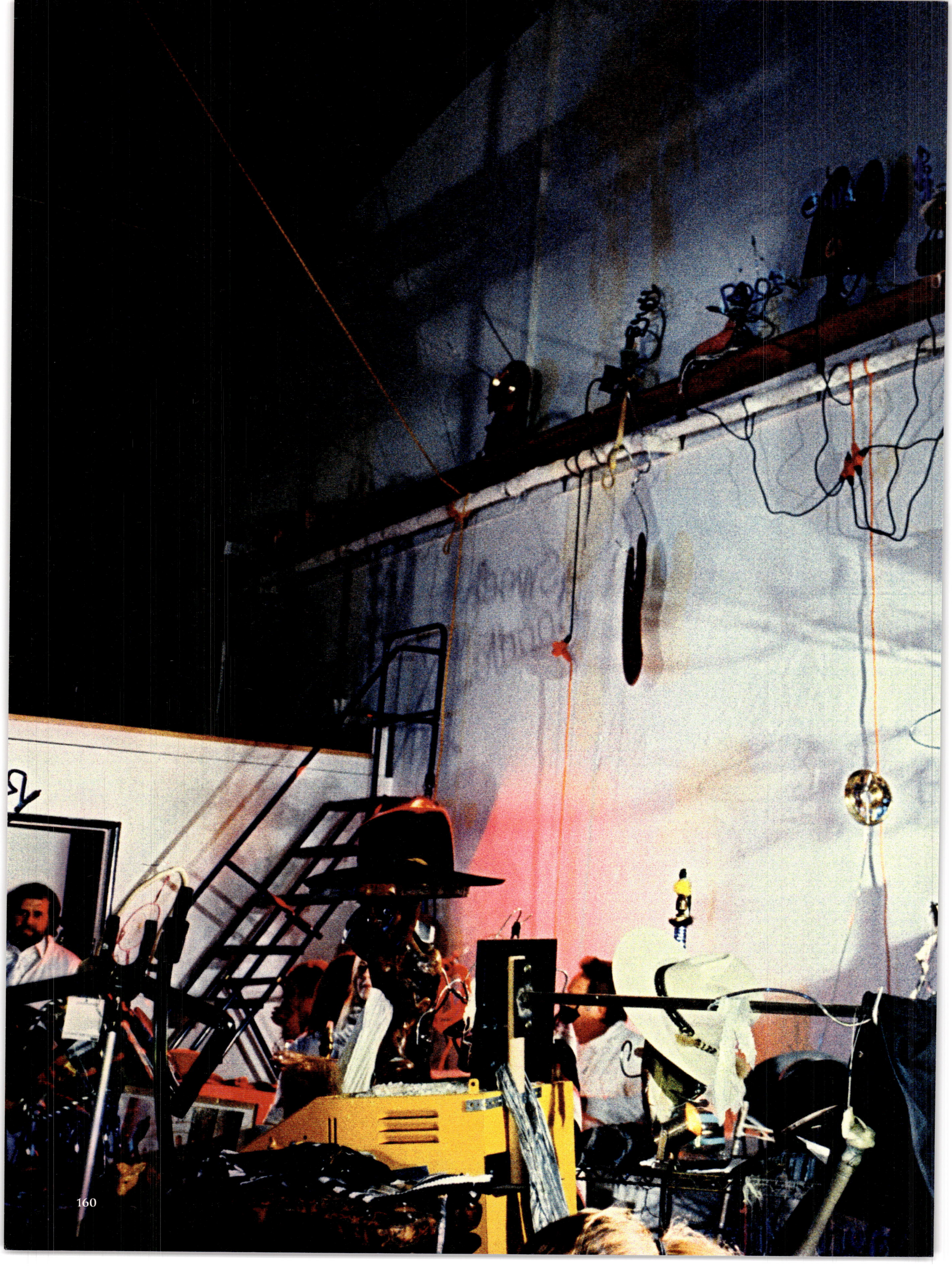

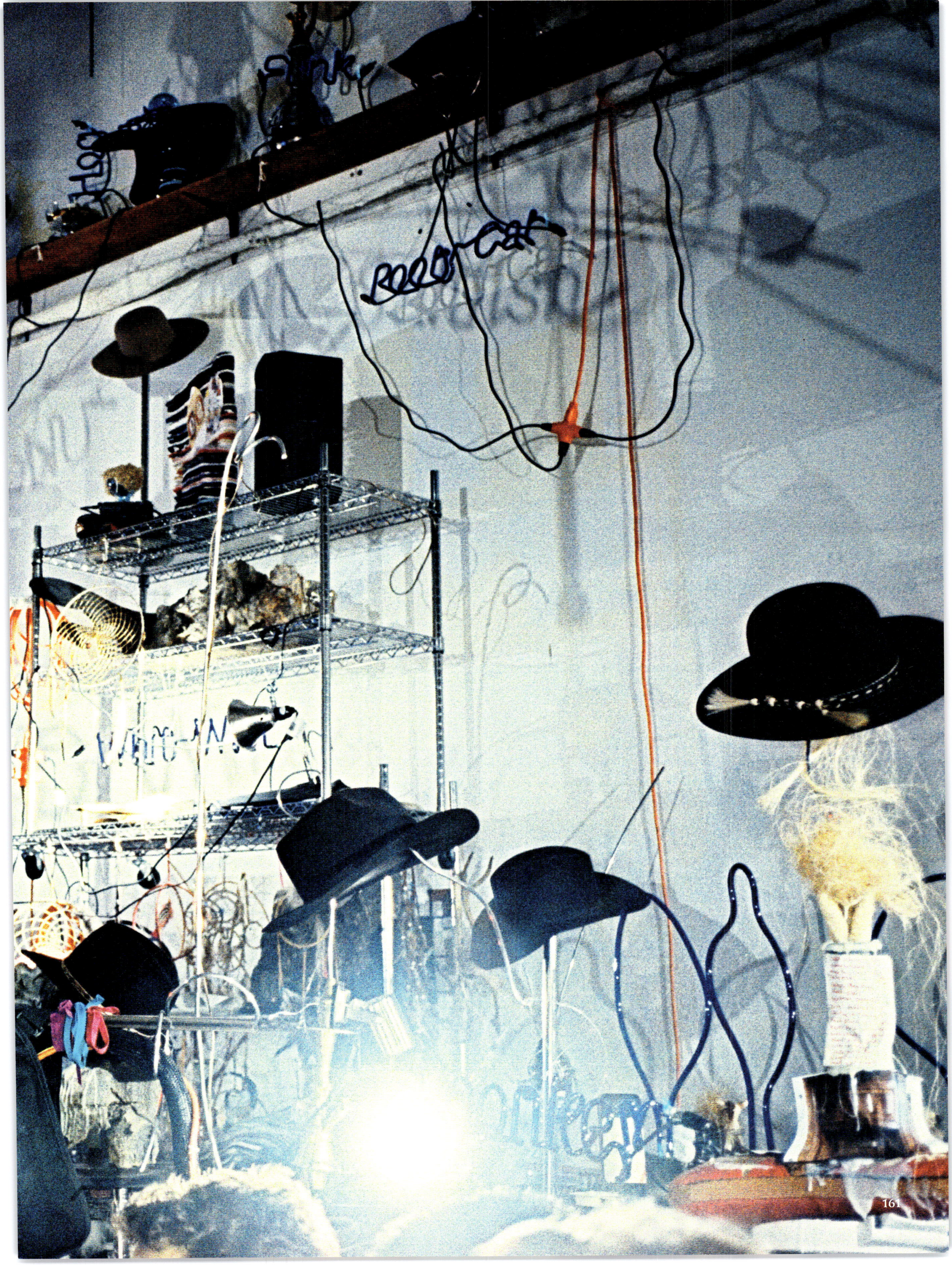

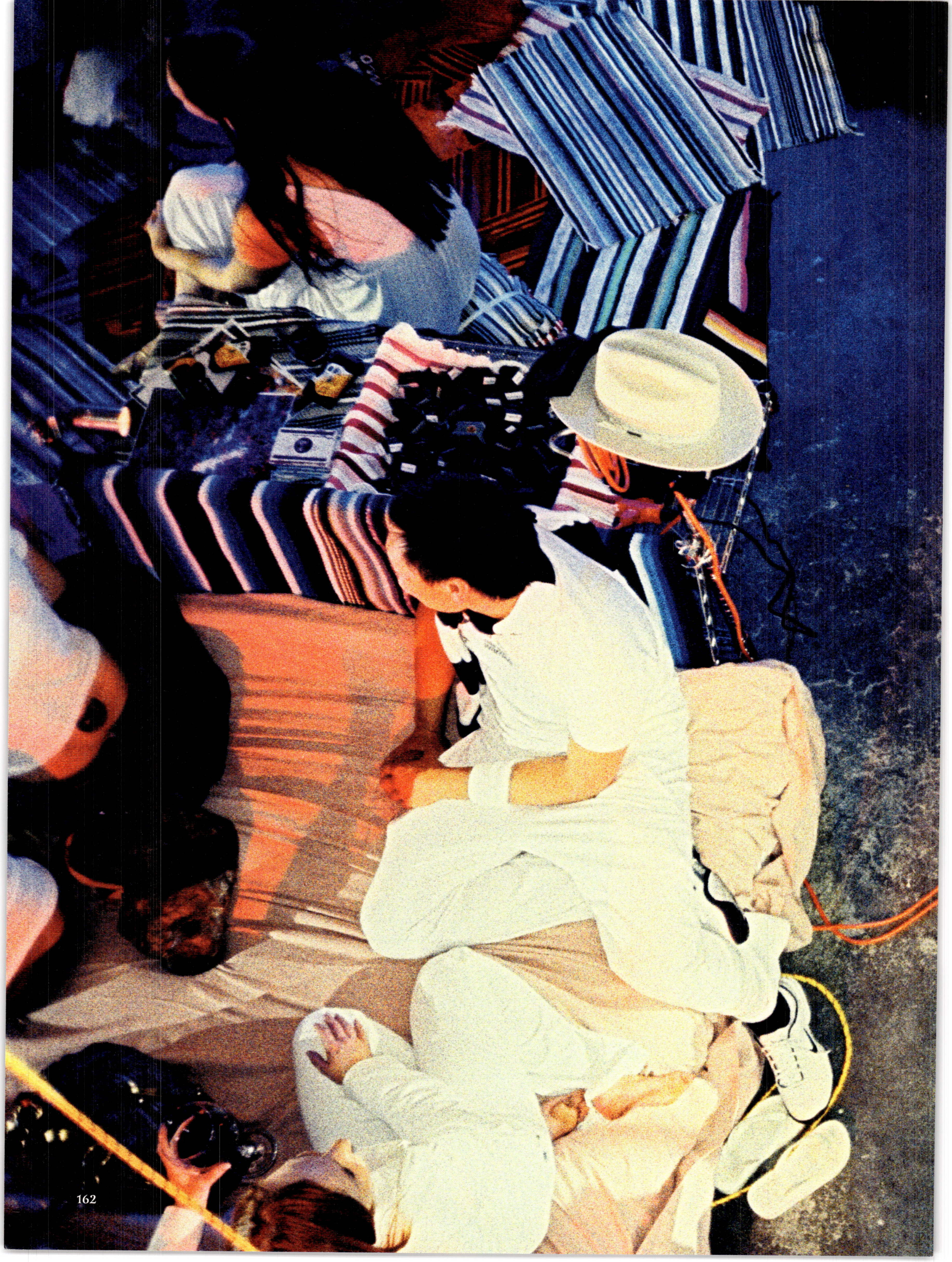

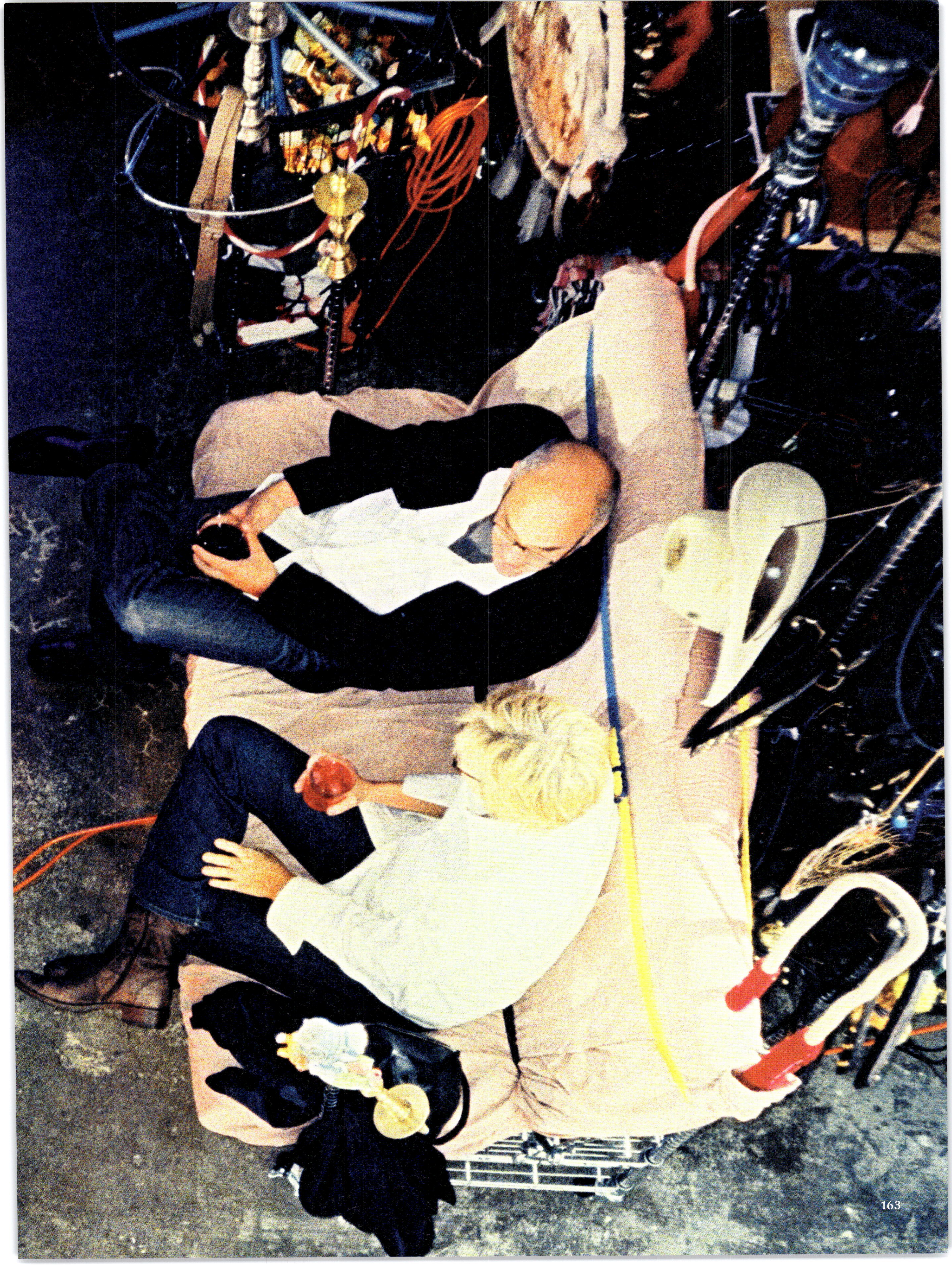

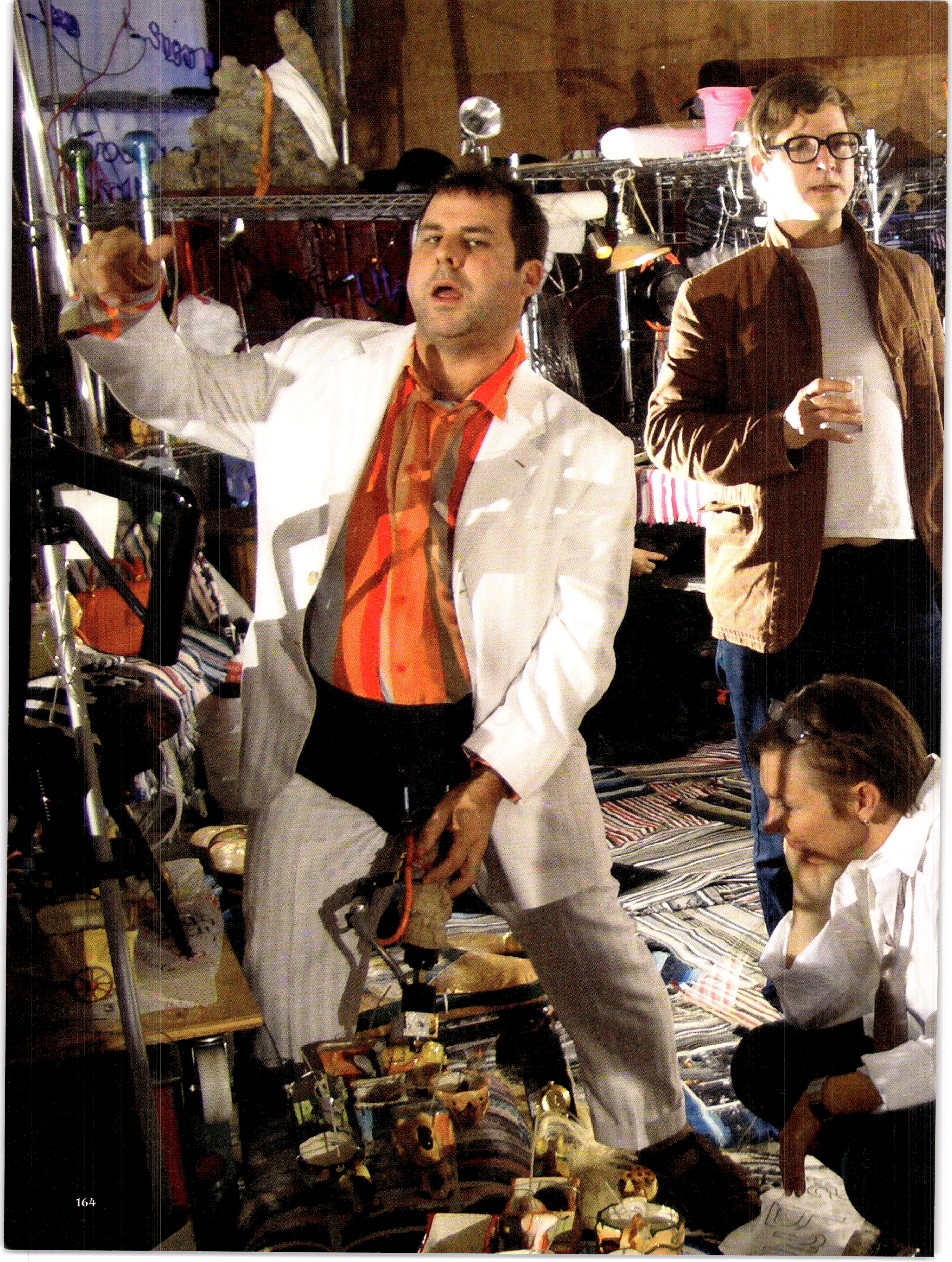

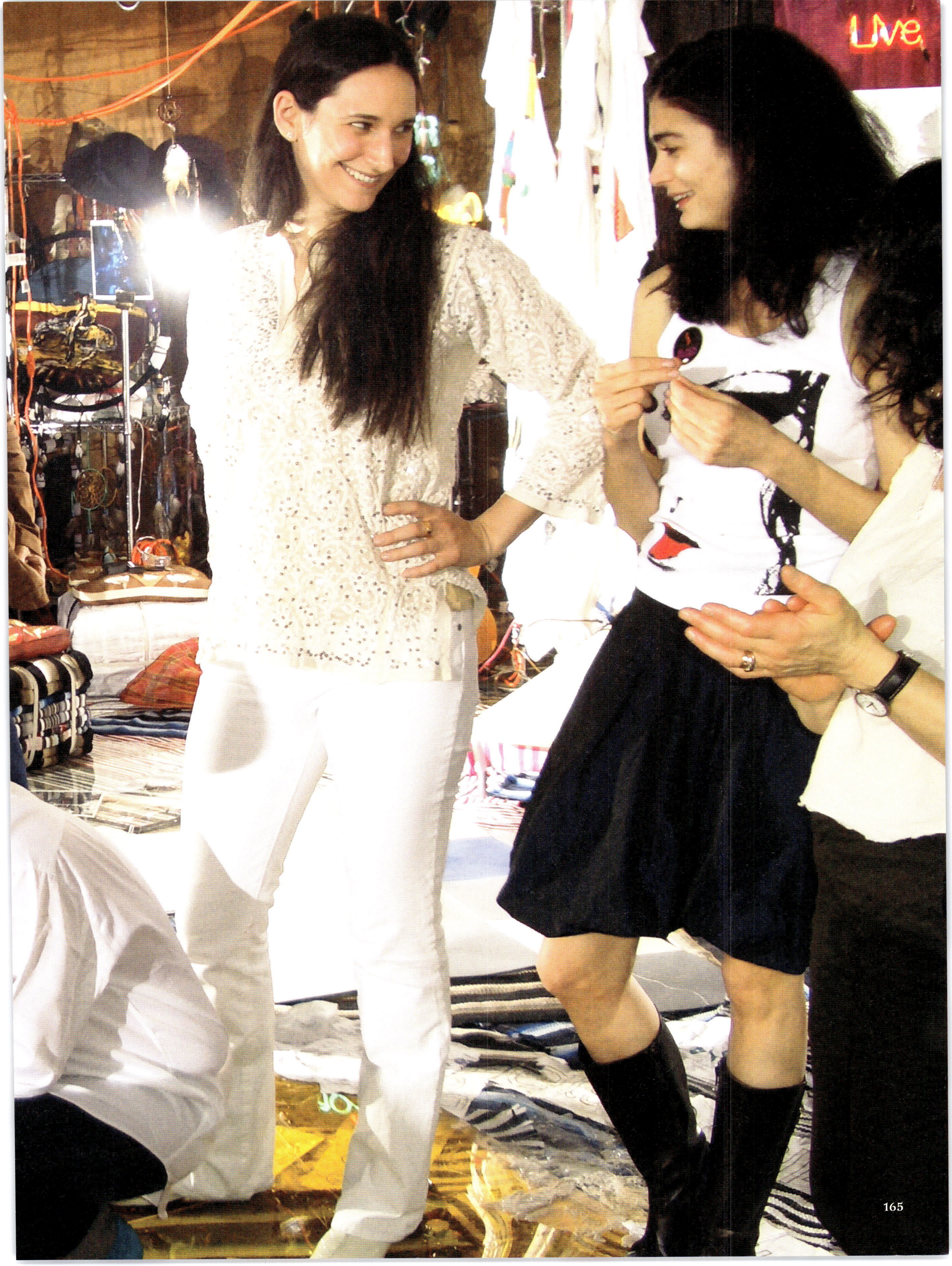
Live

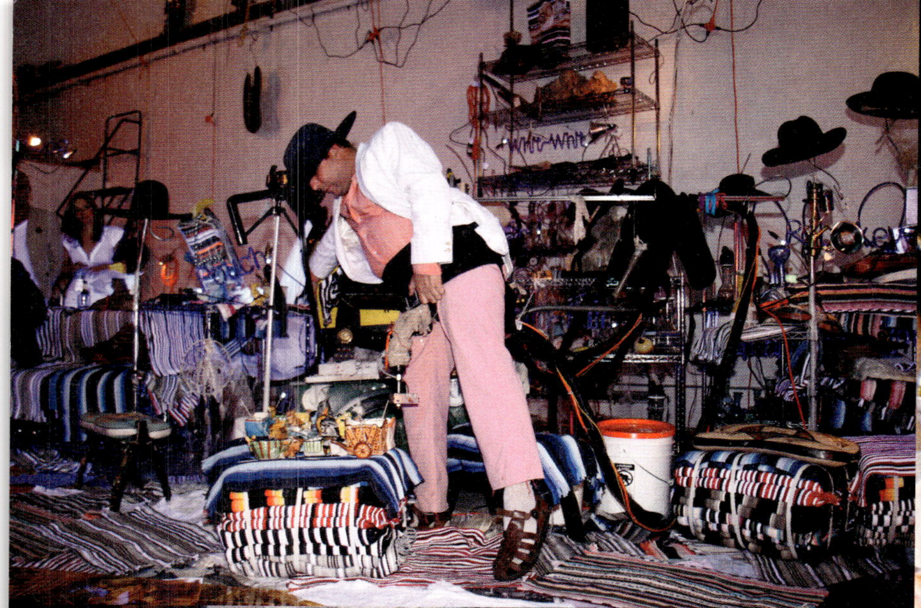

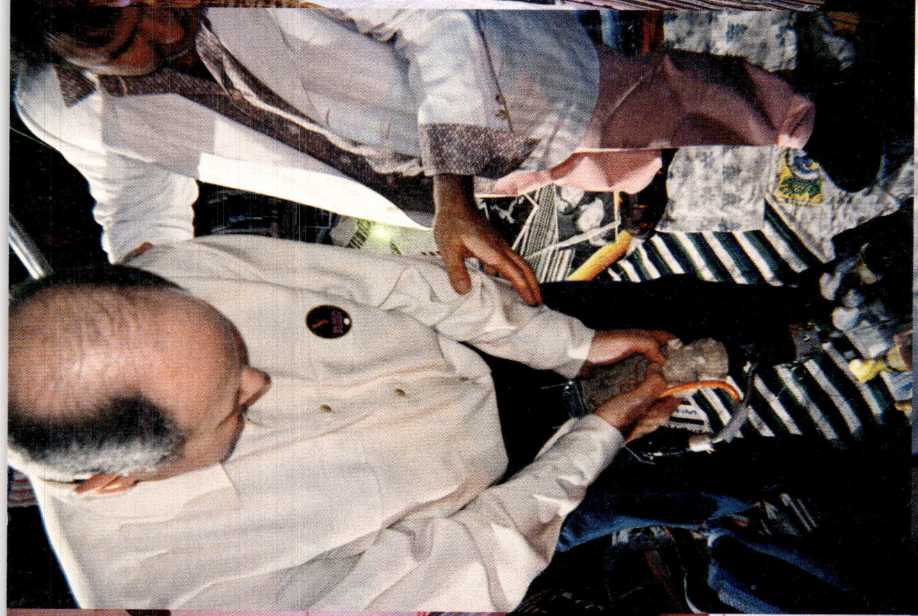

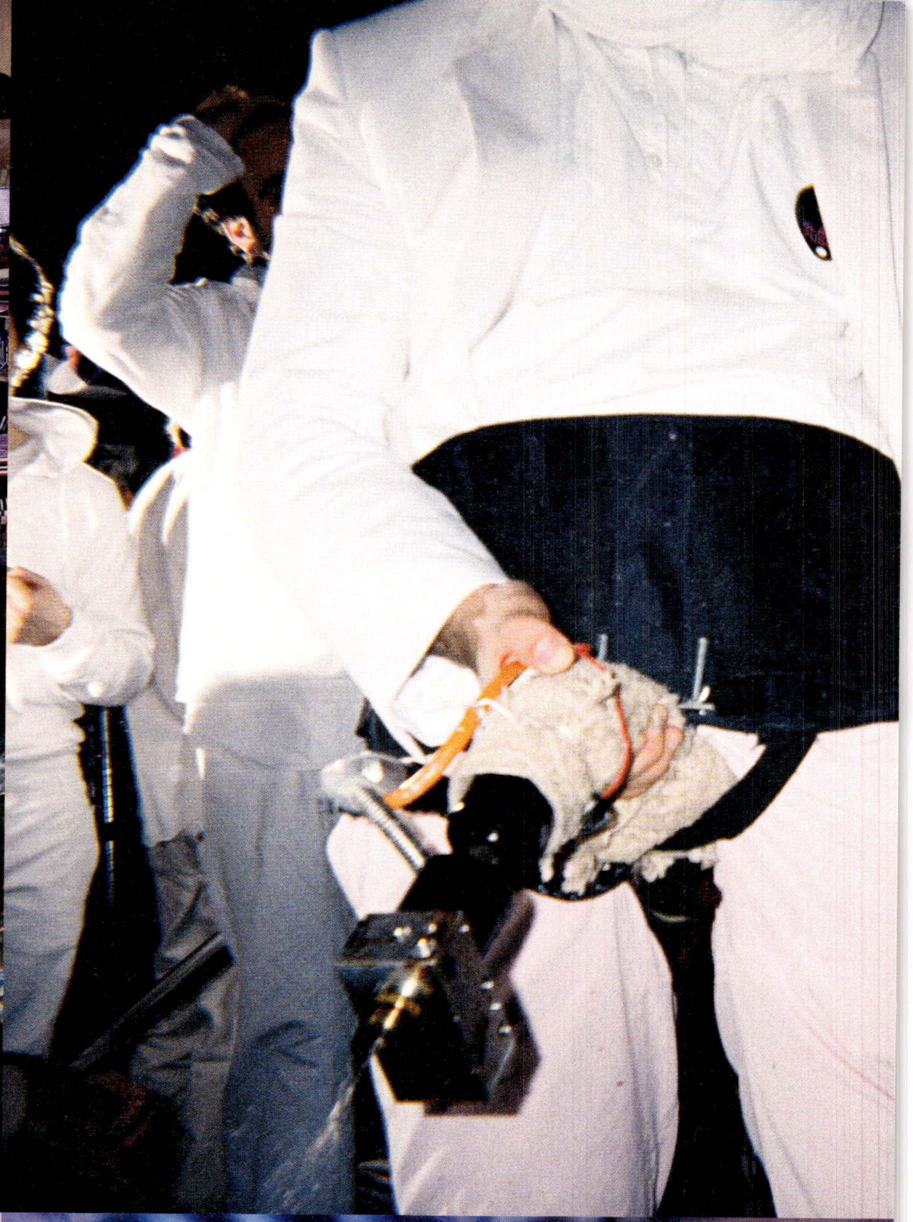

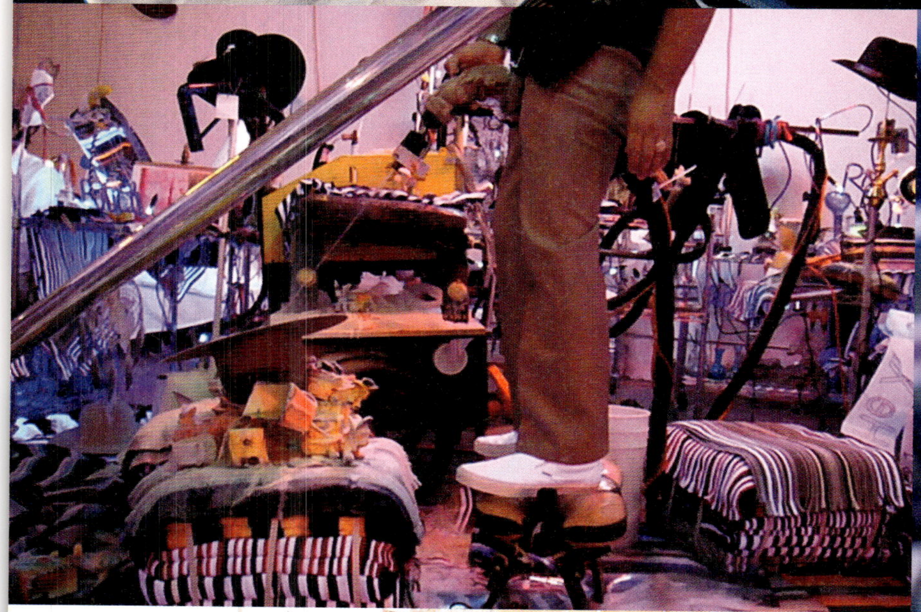

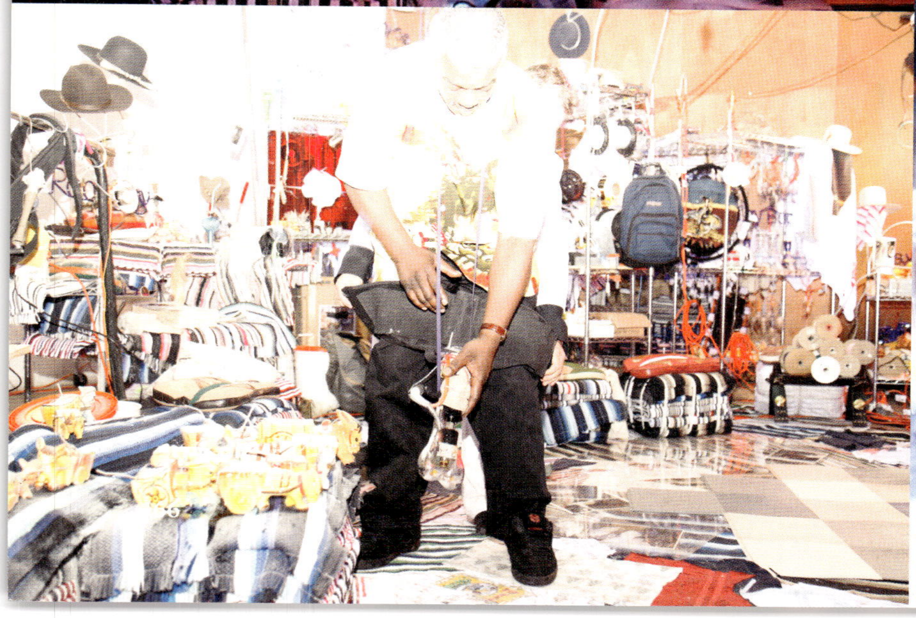

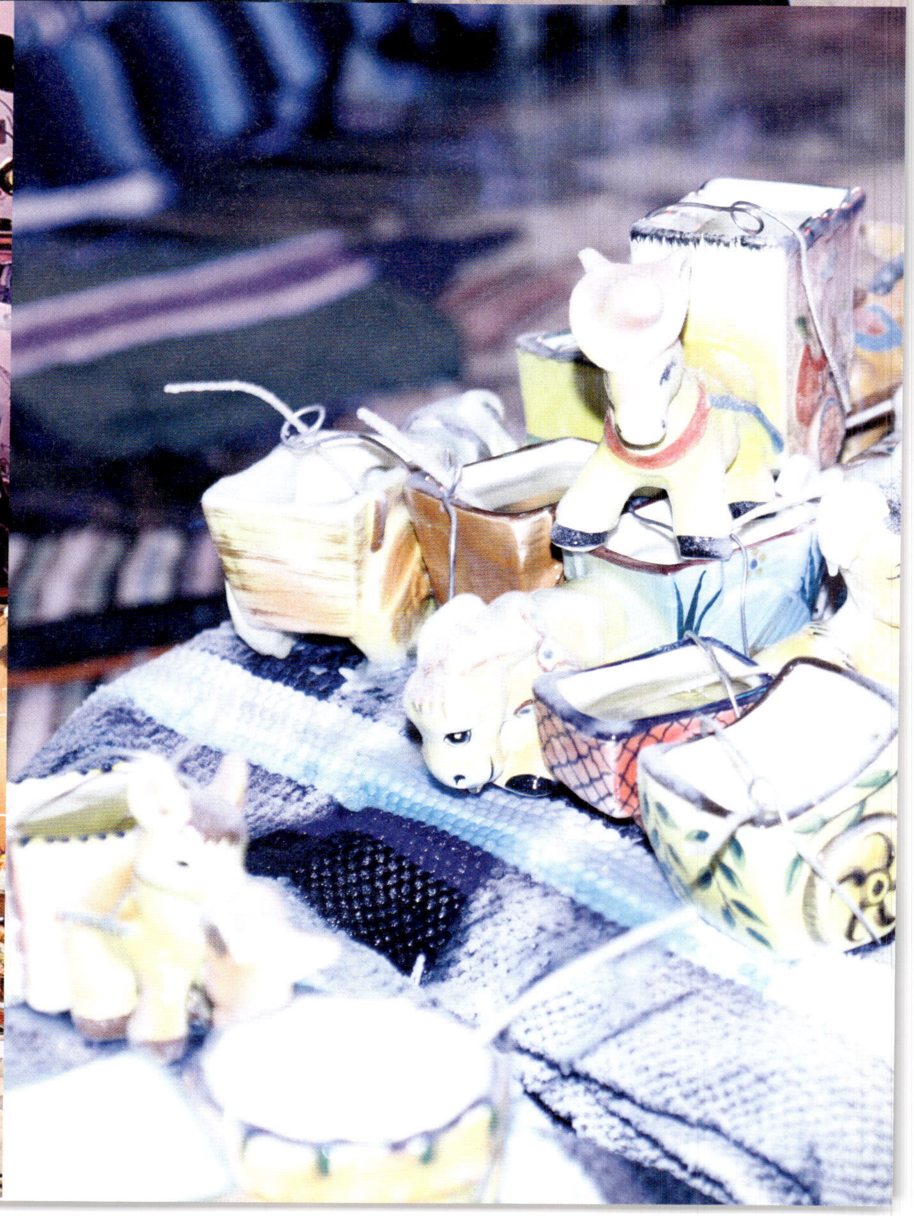

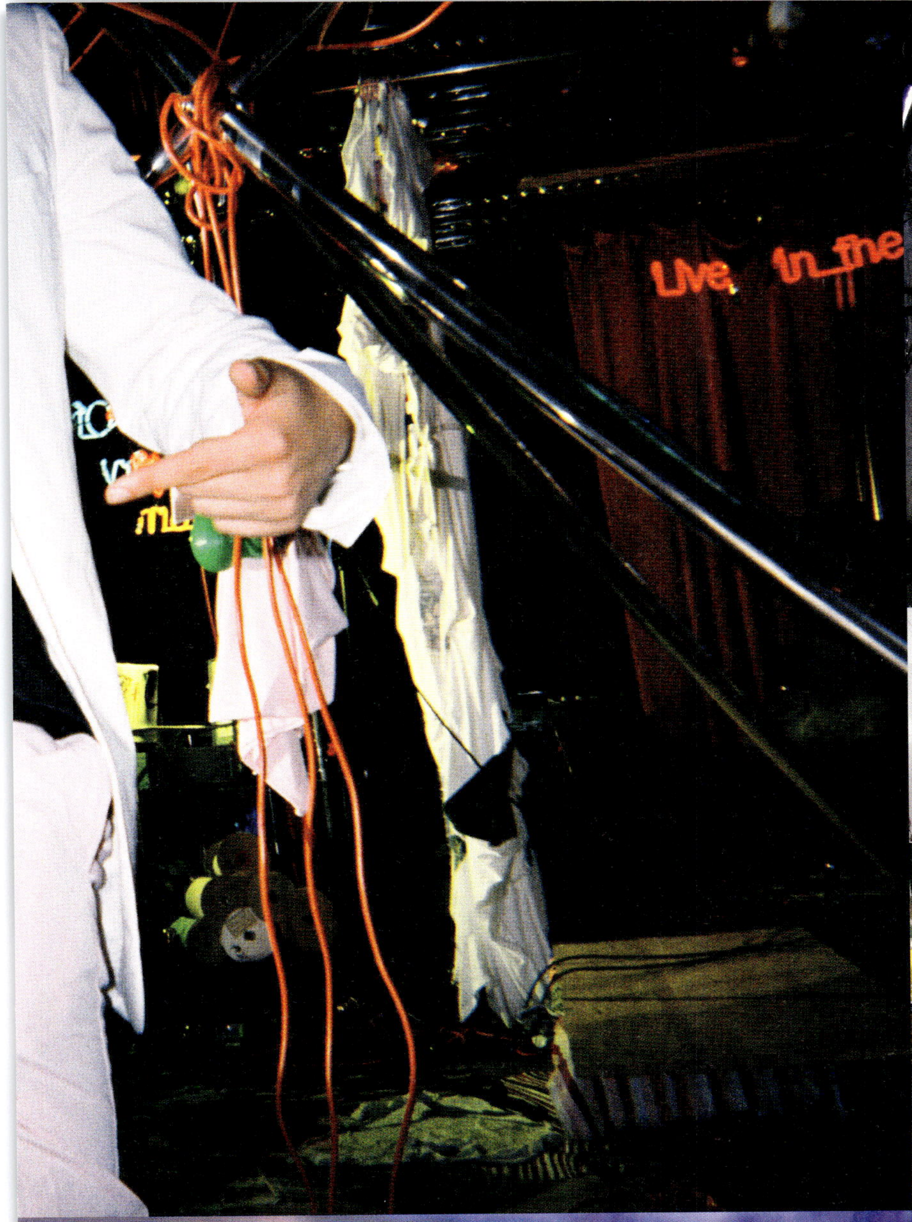
Live in the
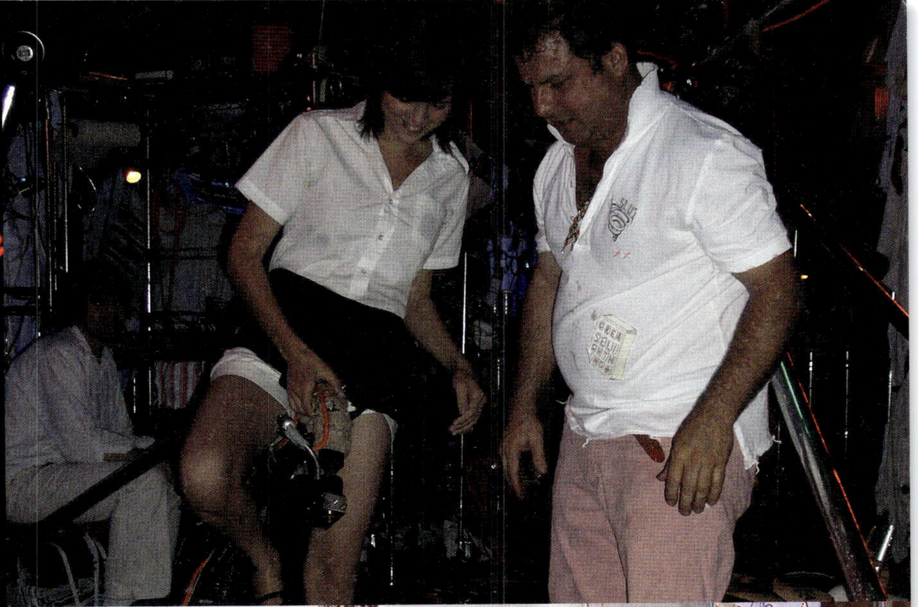
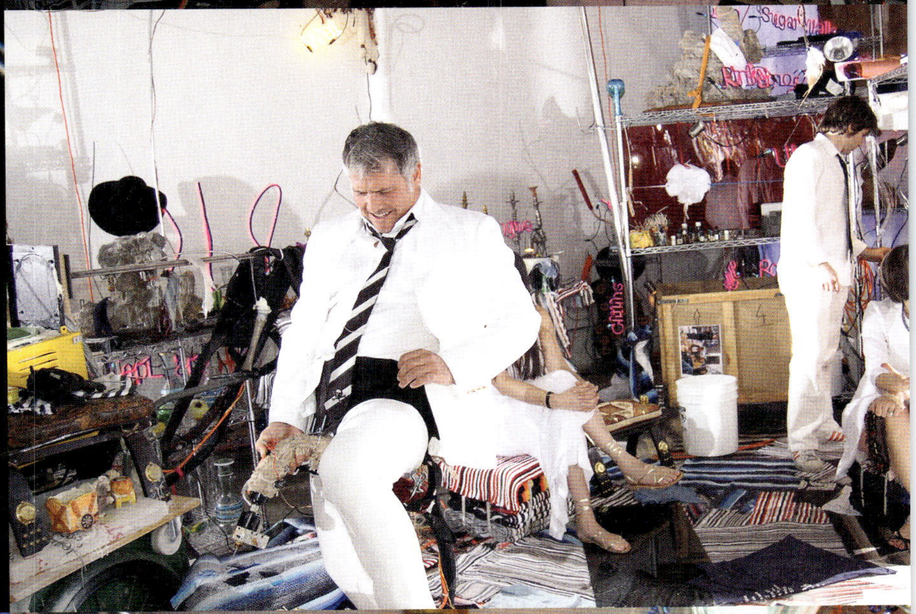
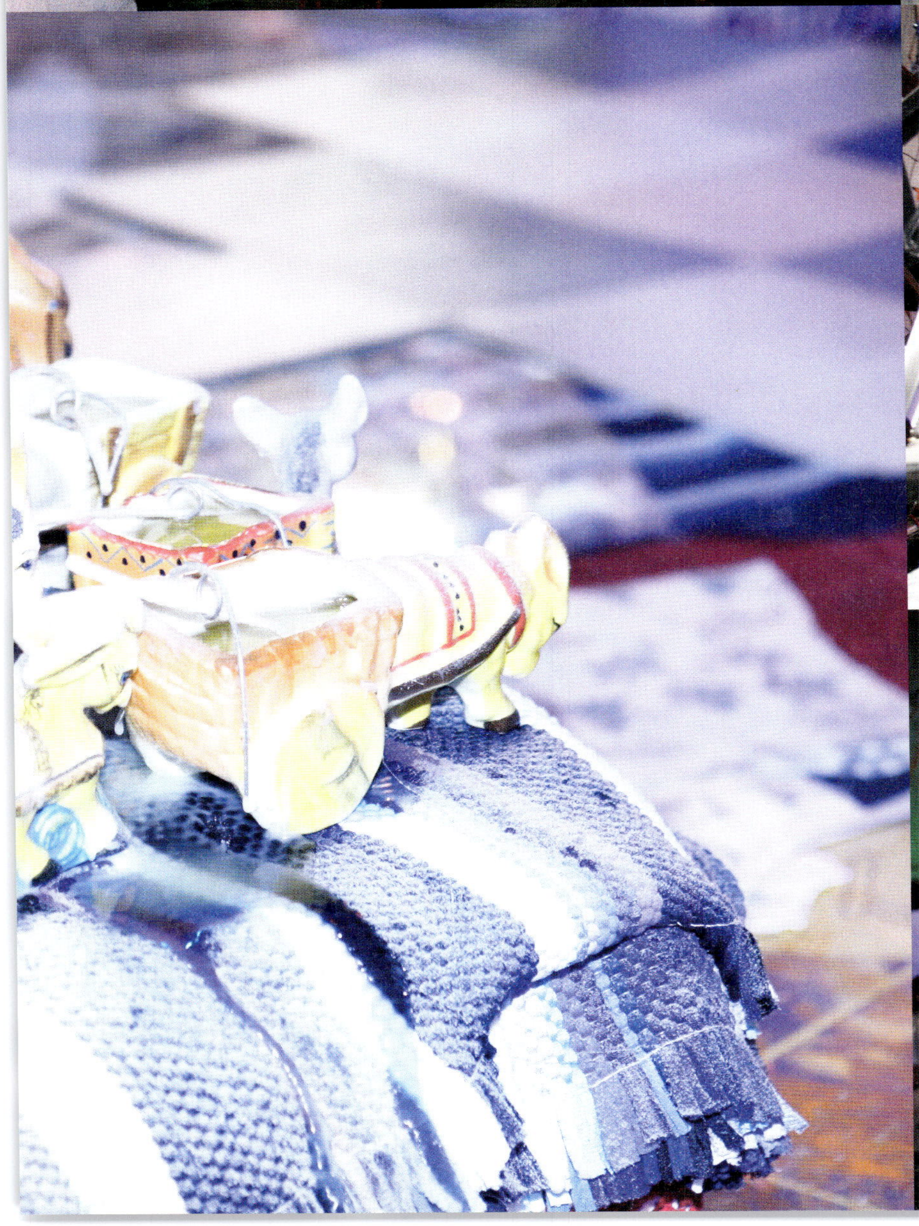
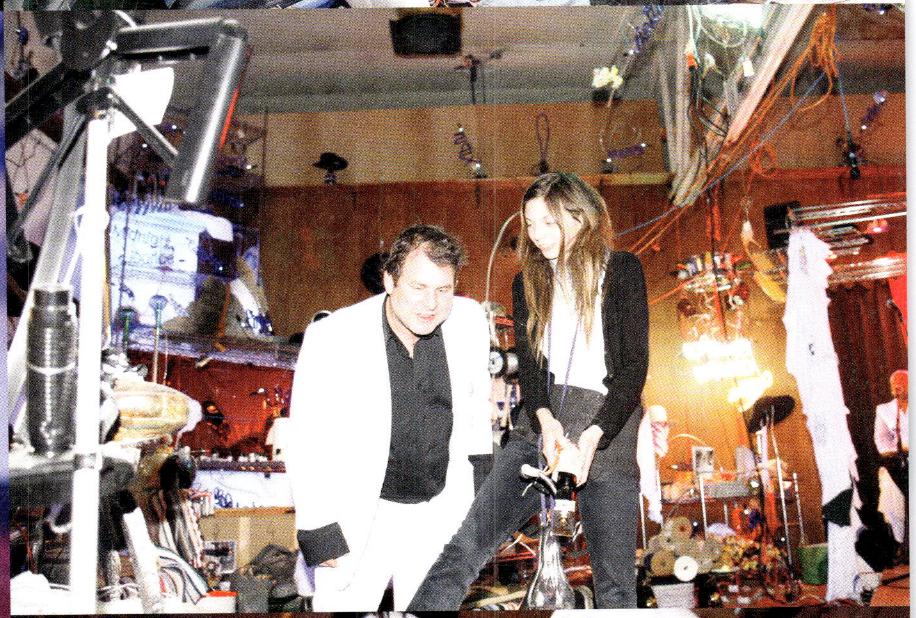
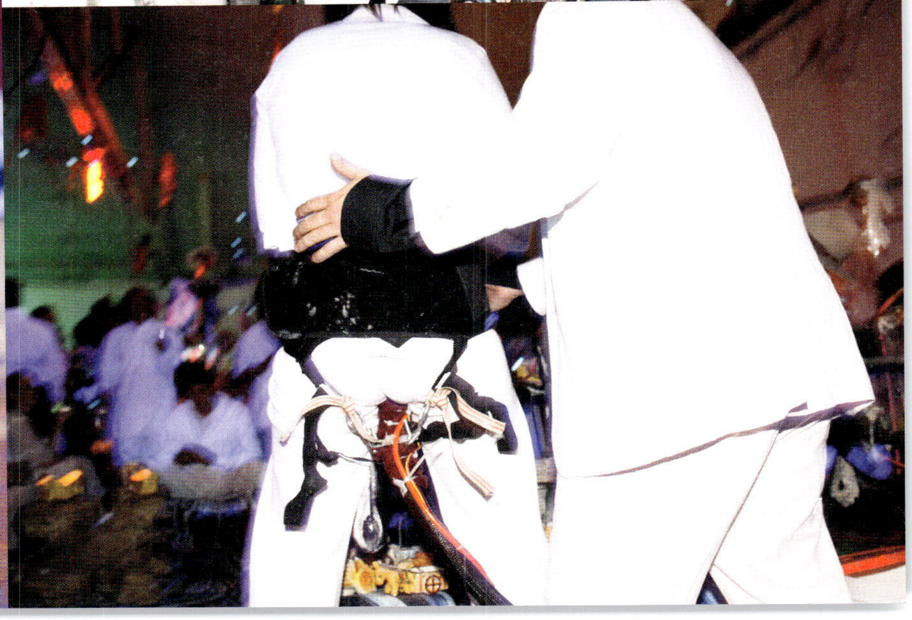

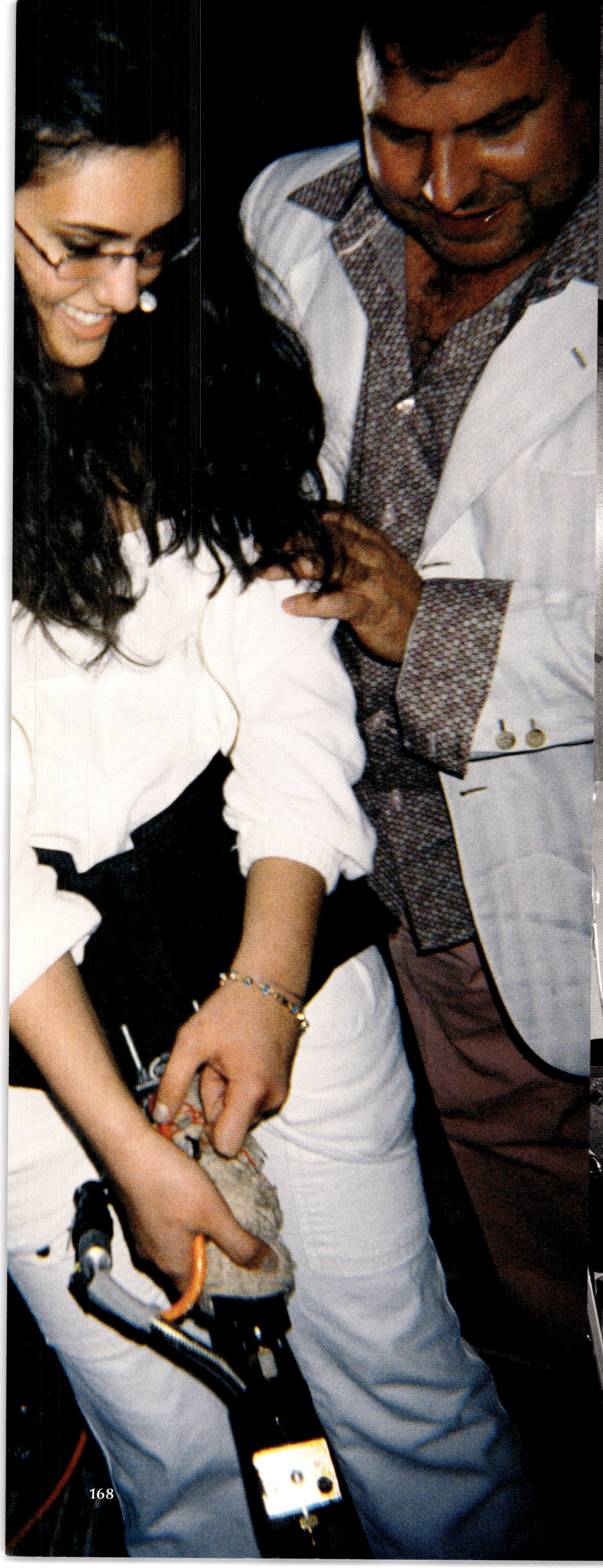

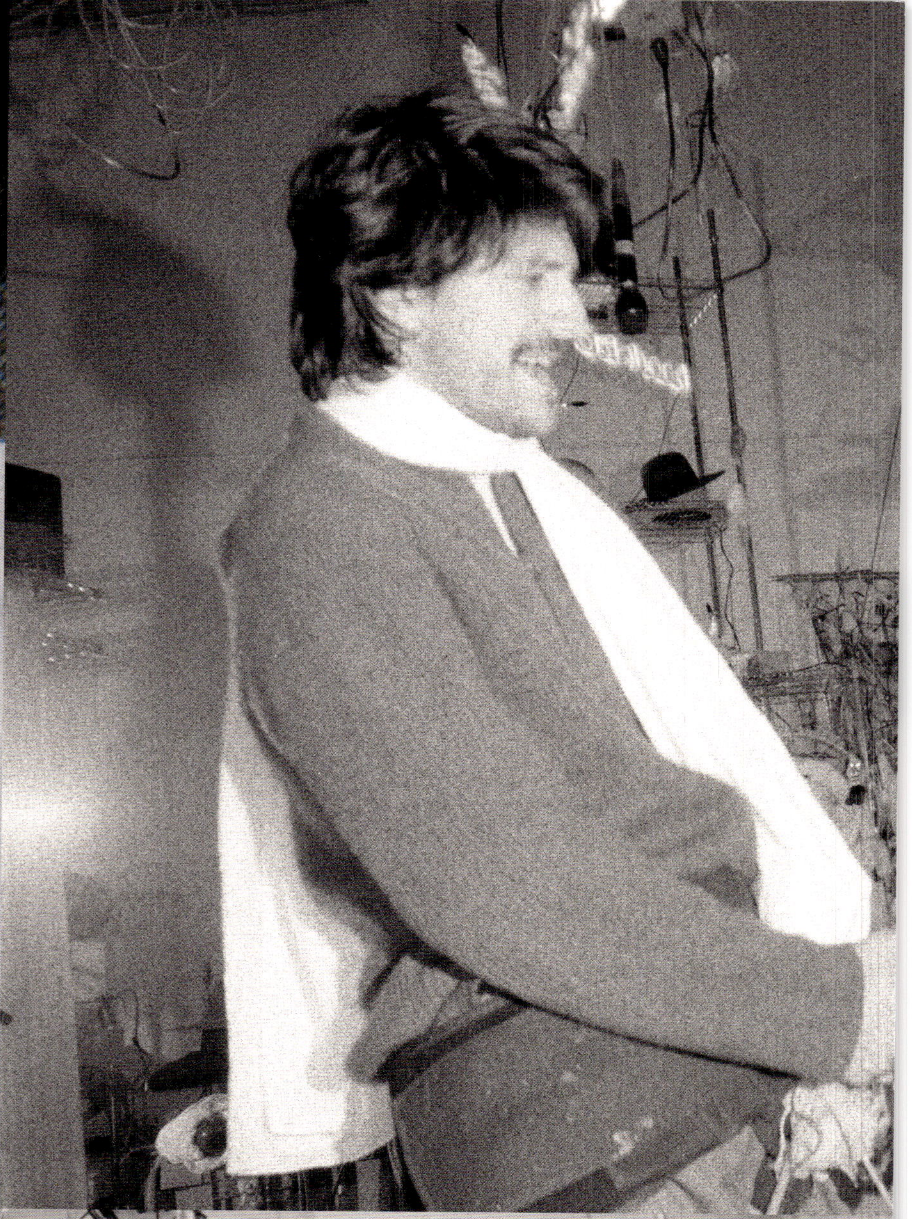

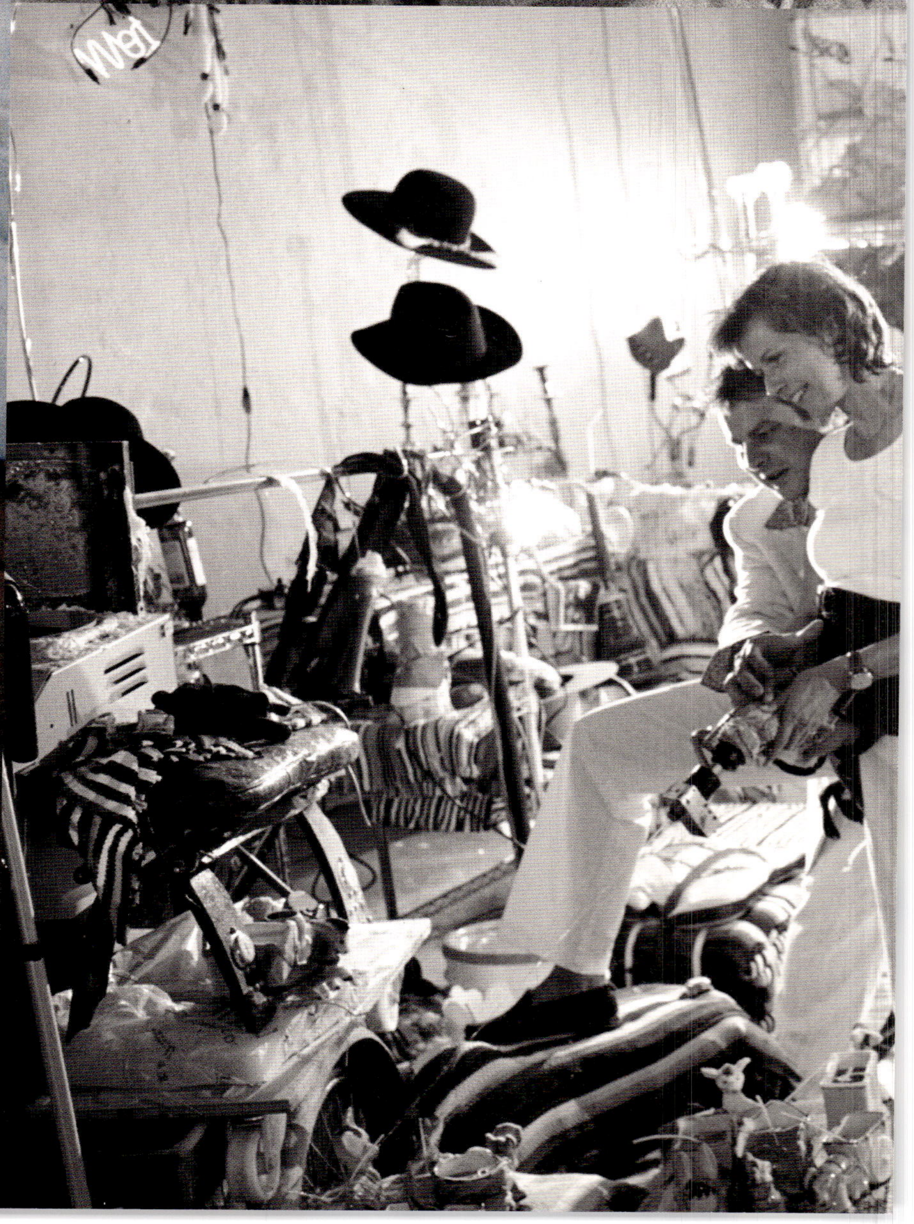

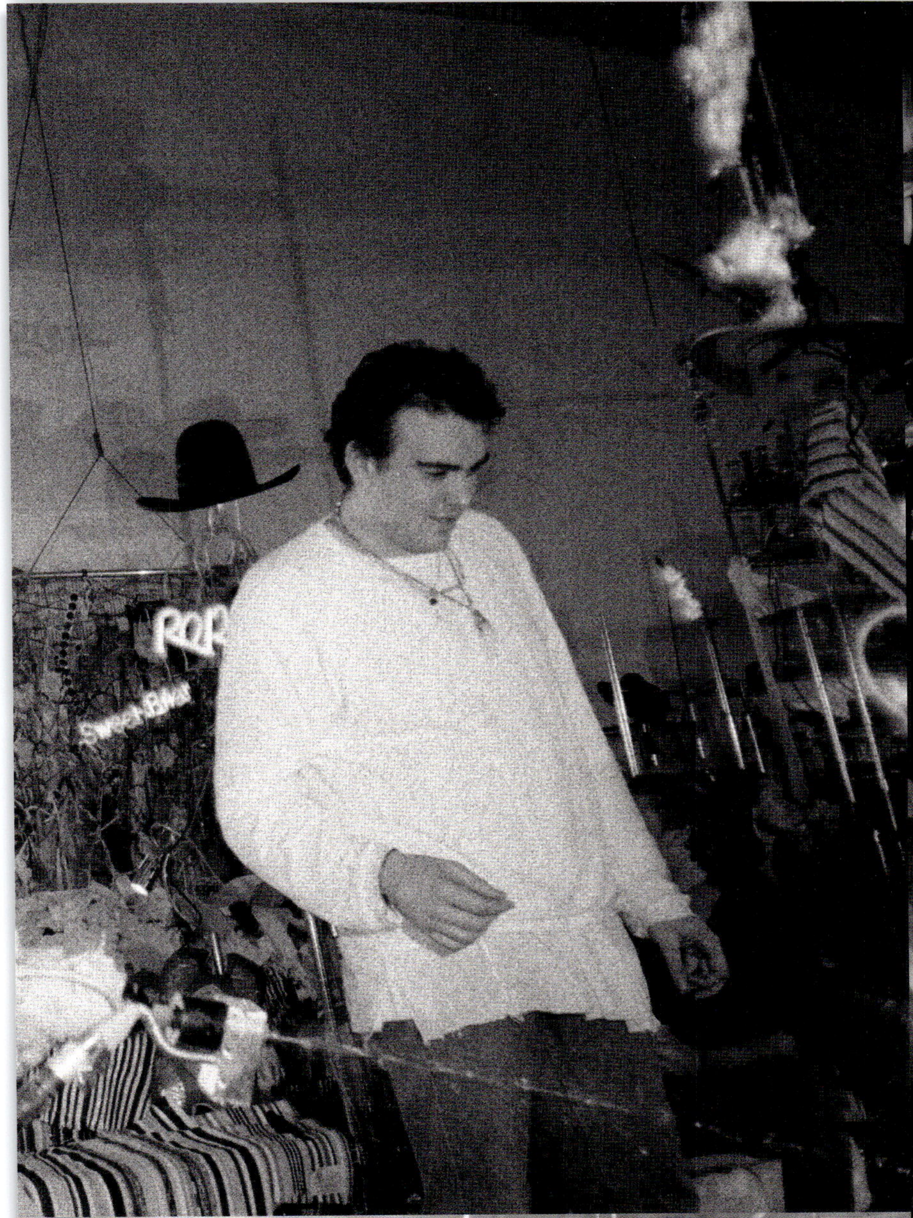

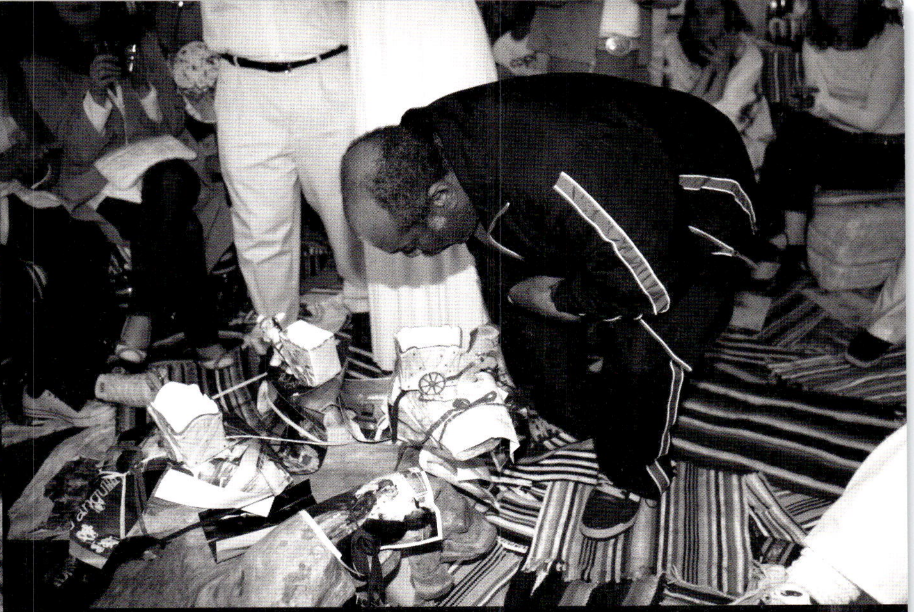

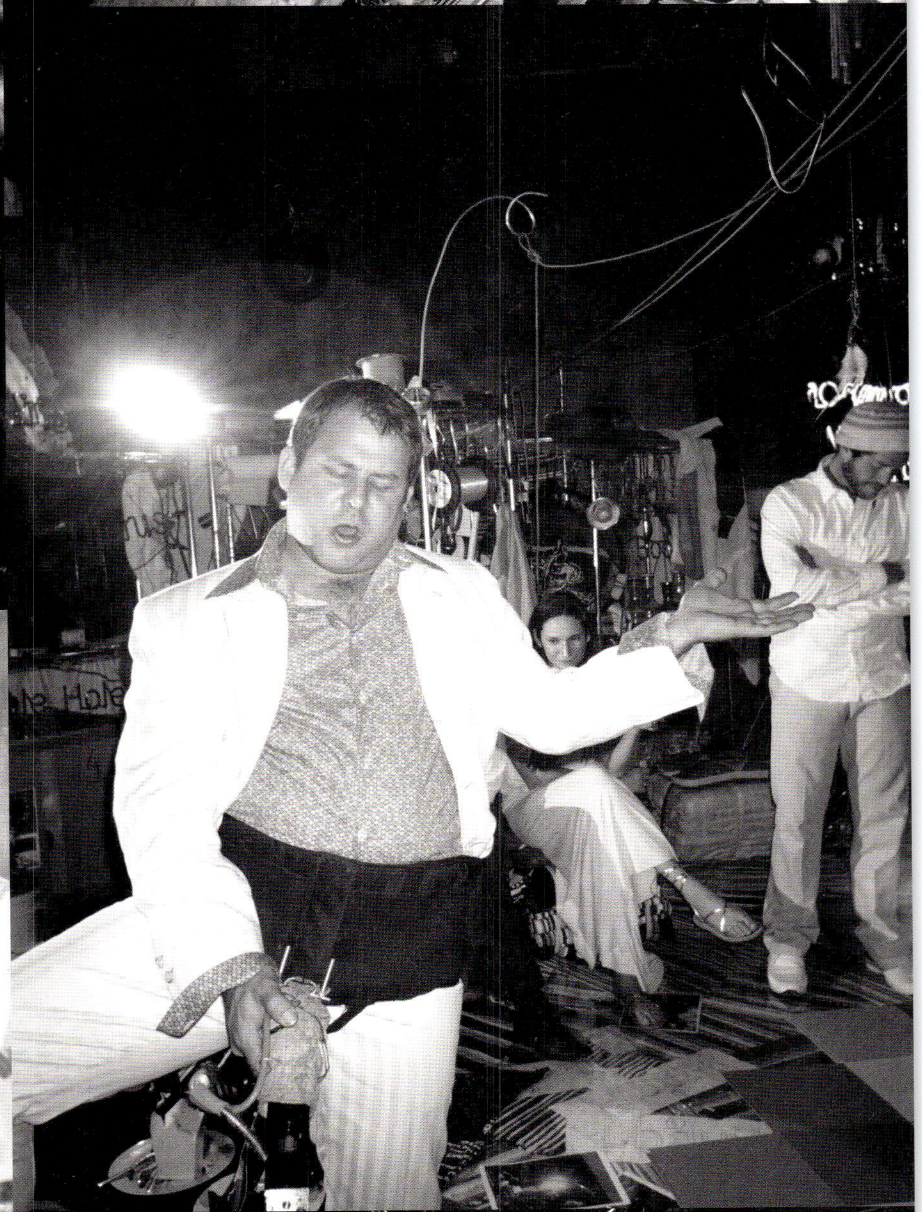

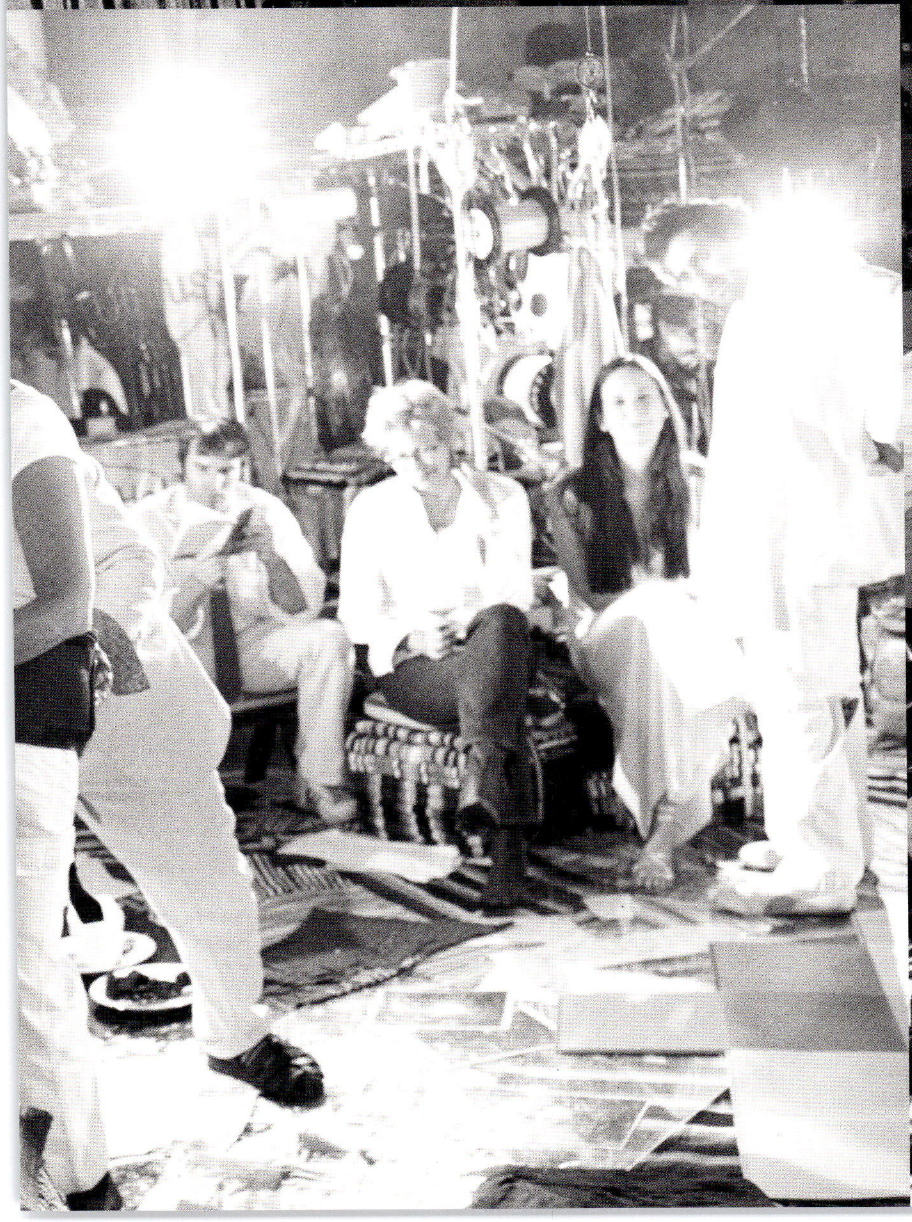

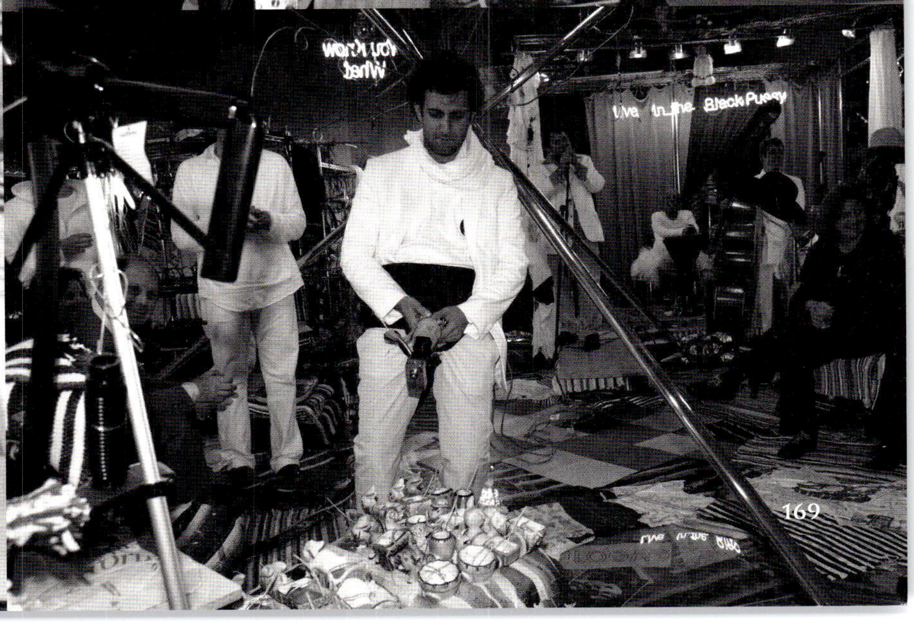

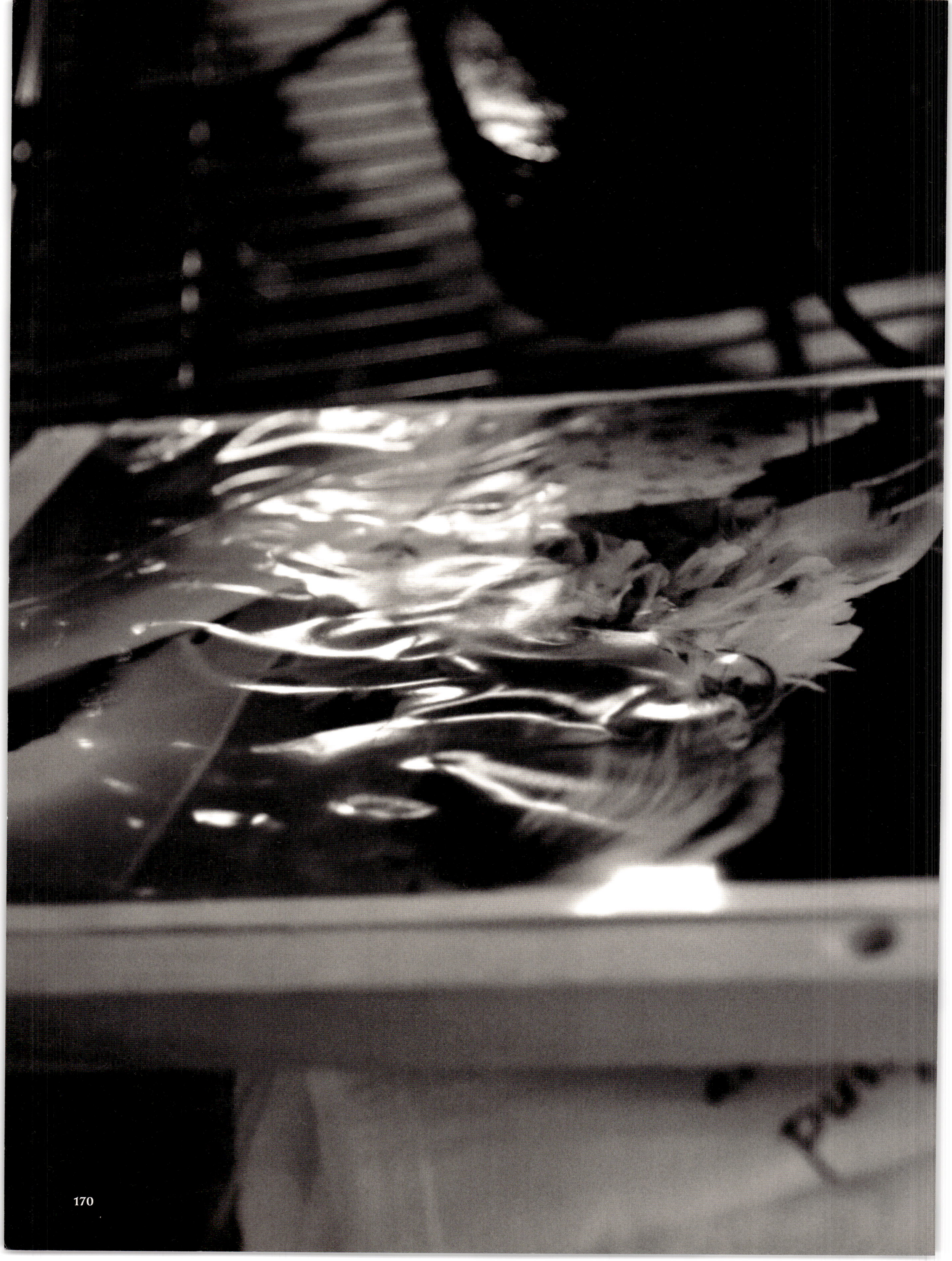

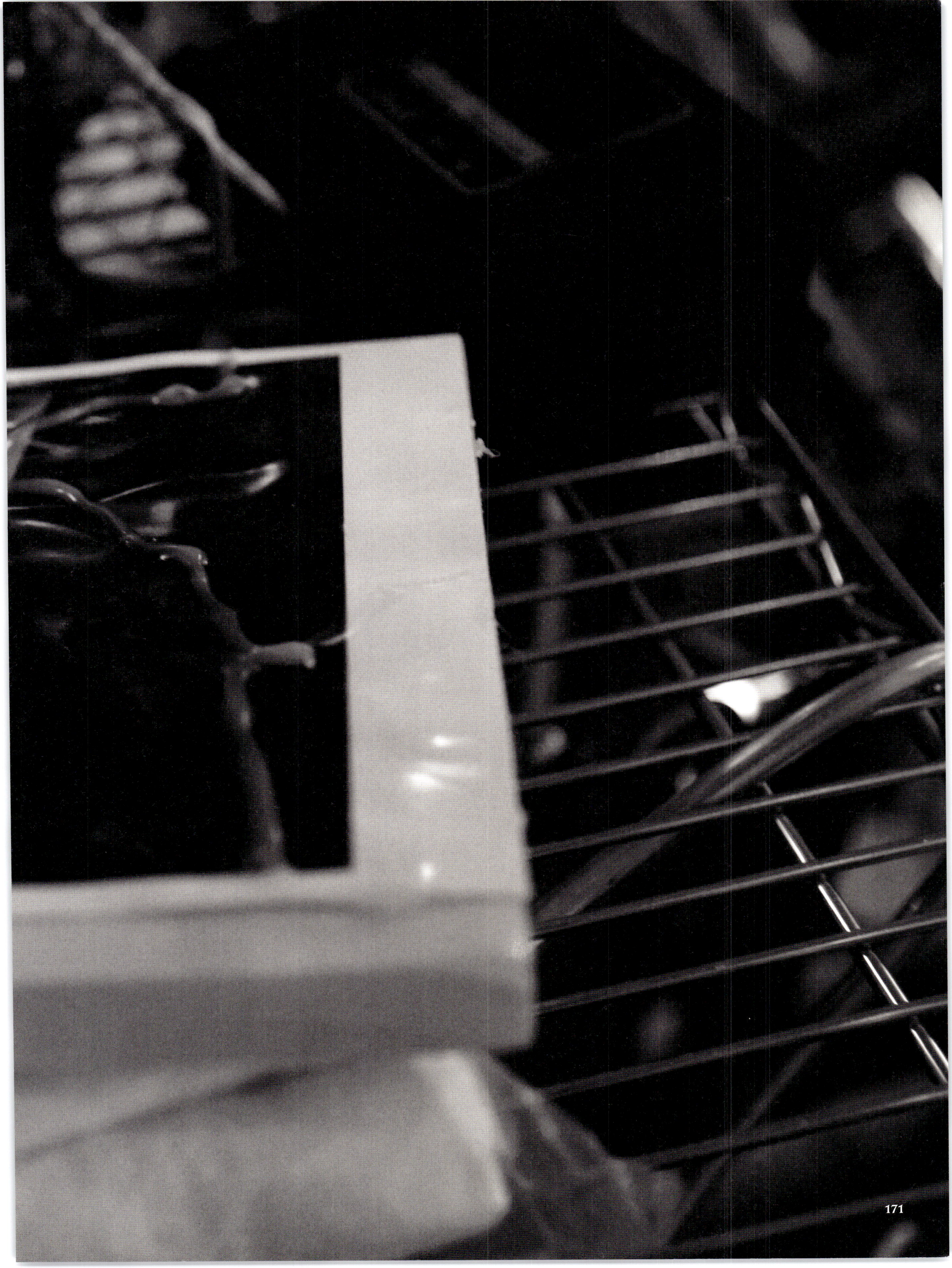

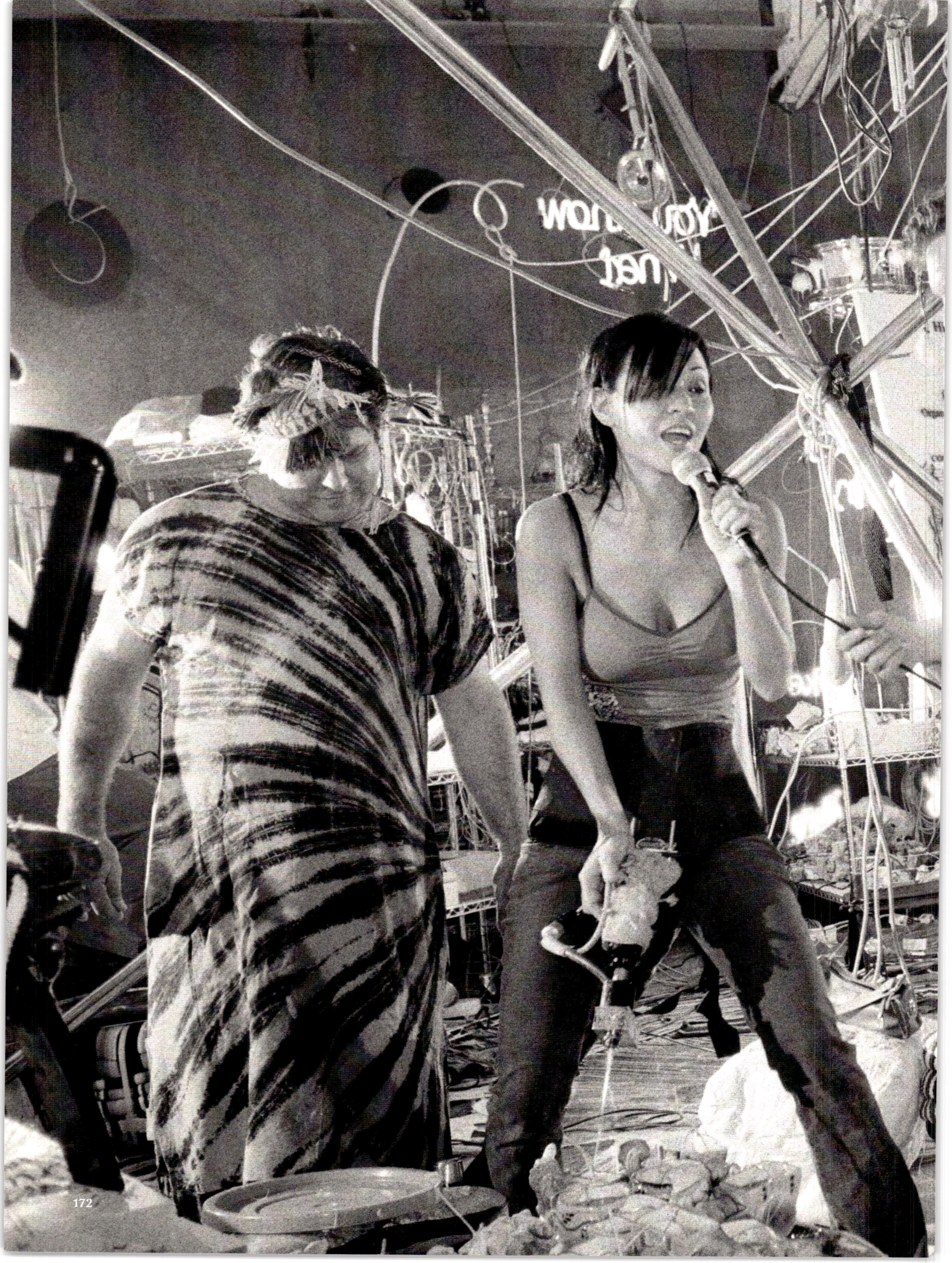

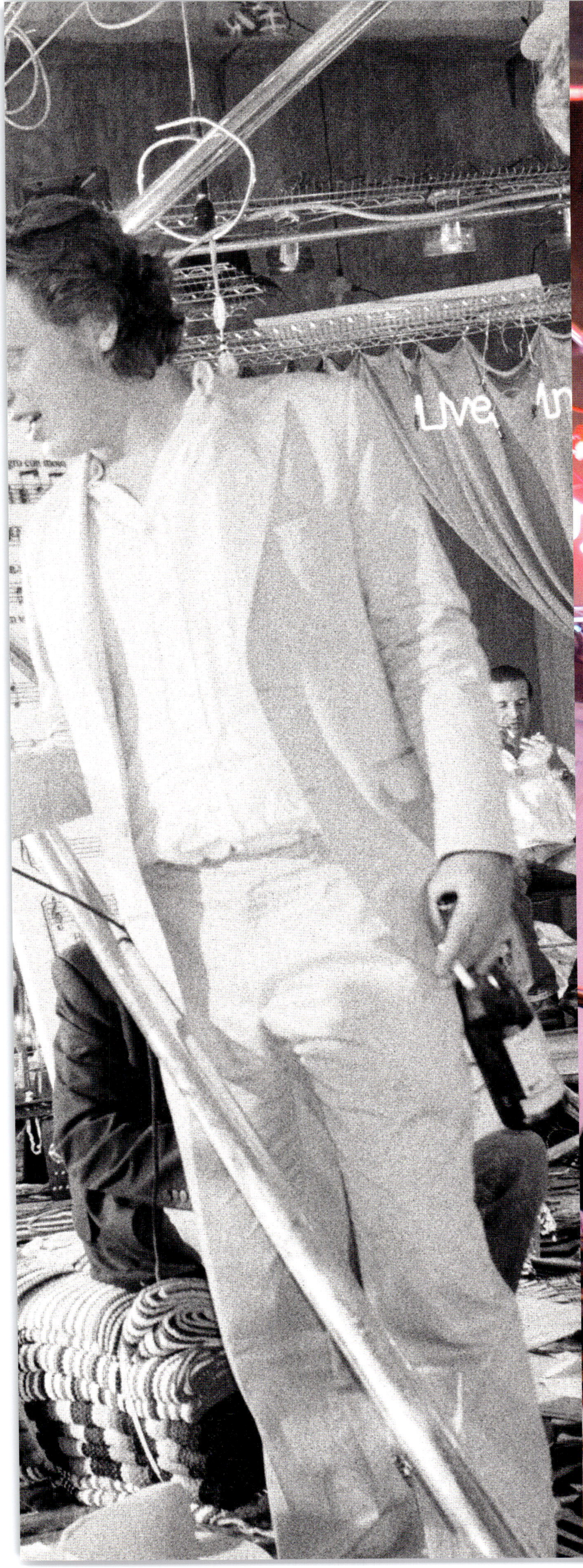
Live
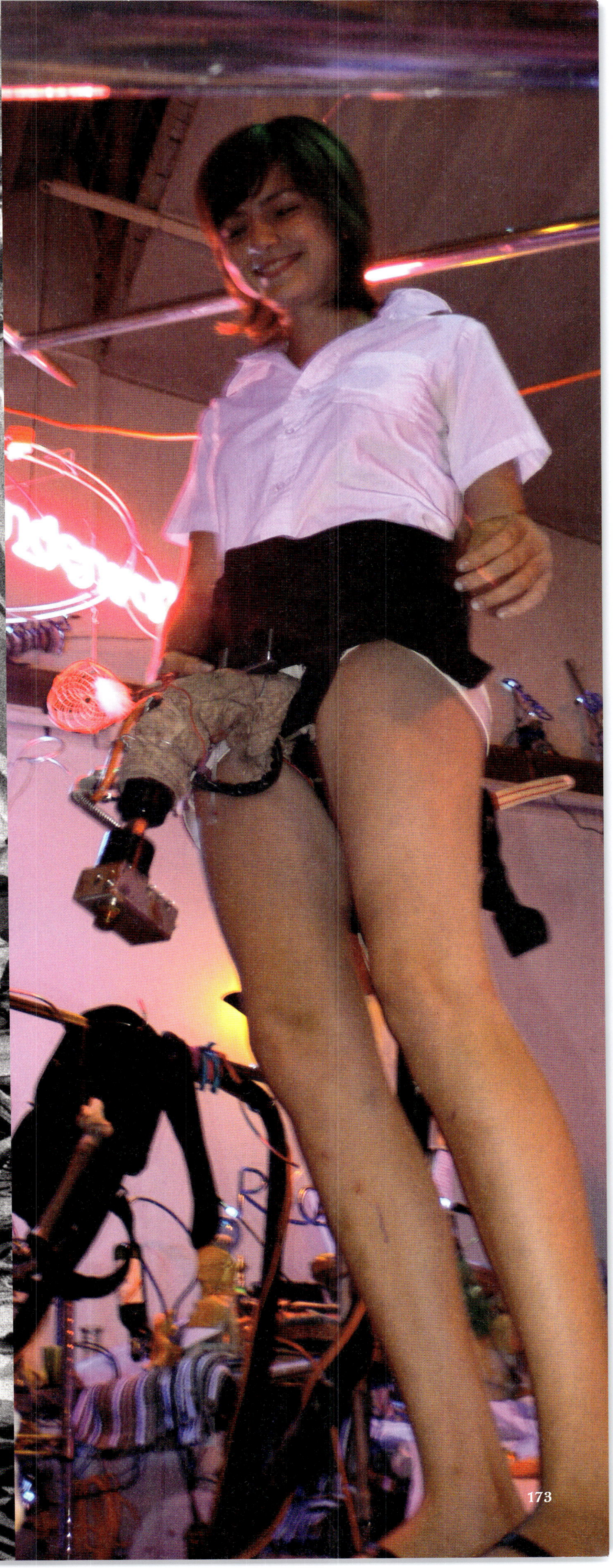

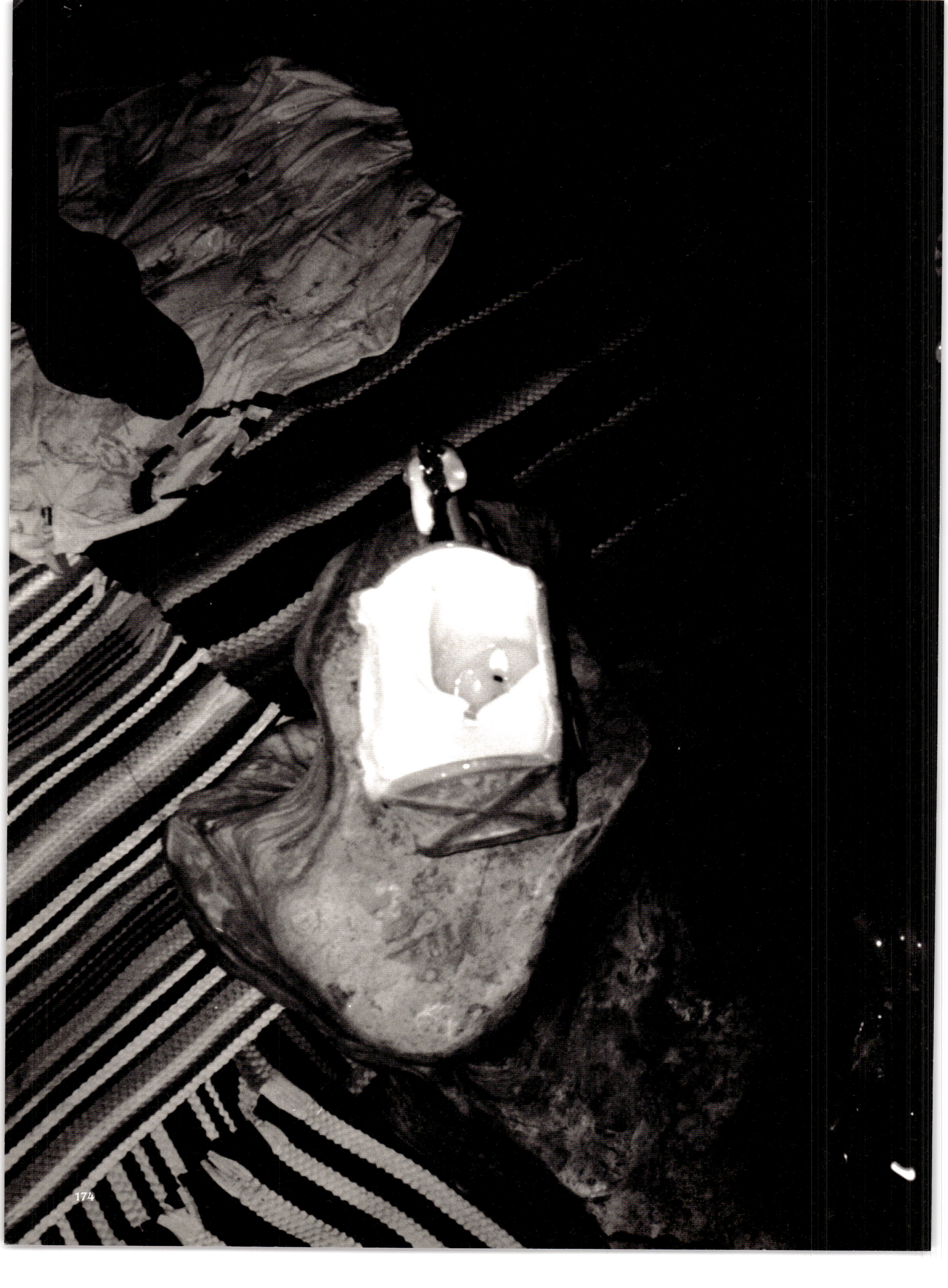

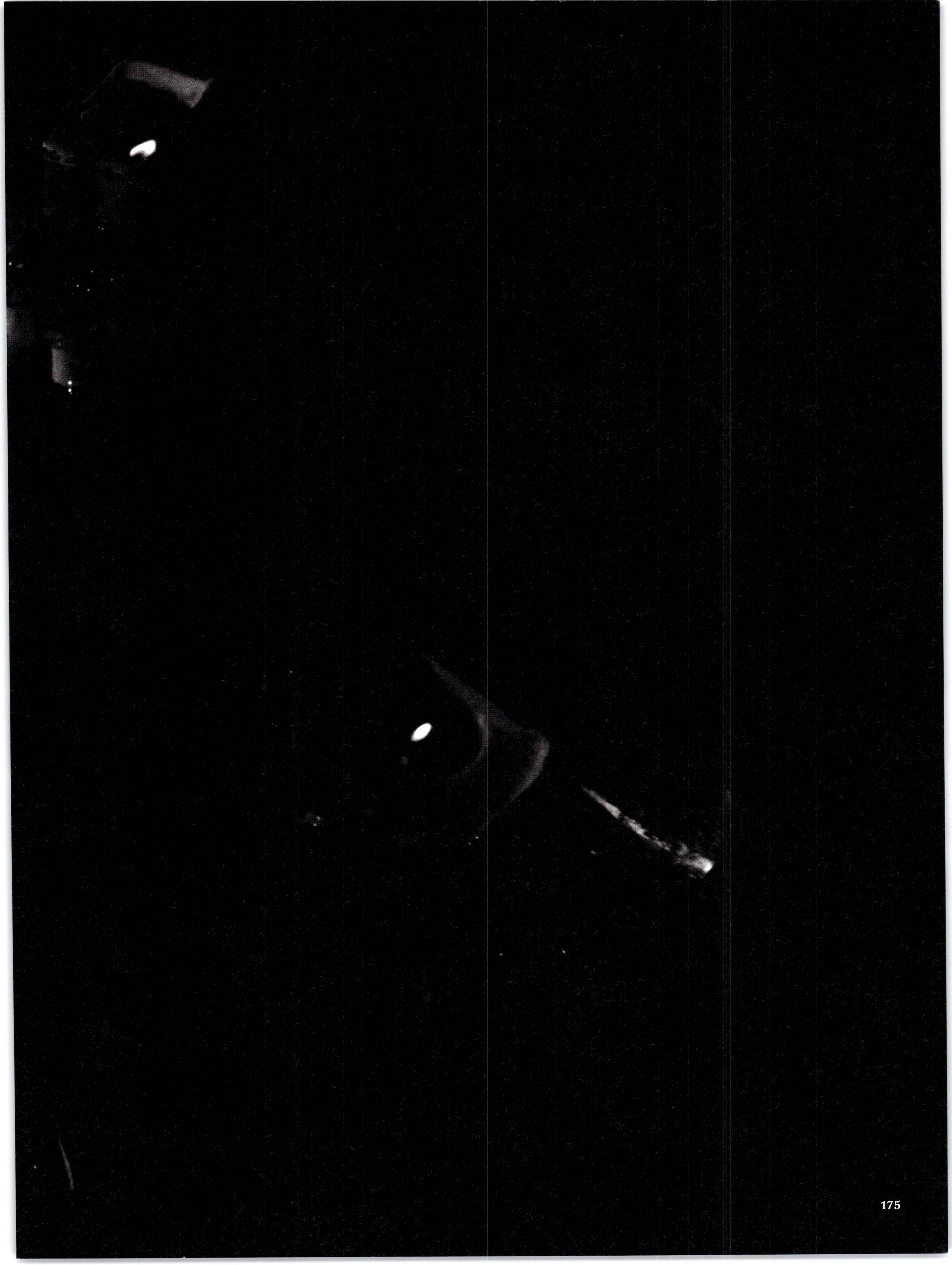

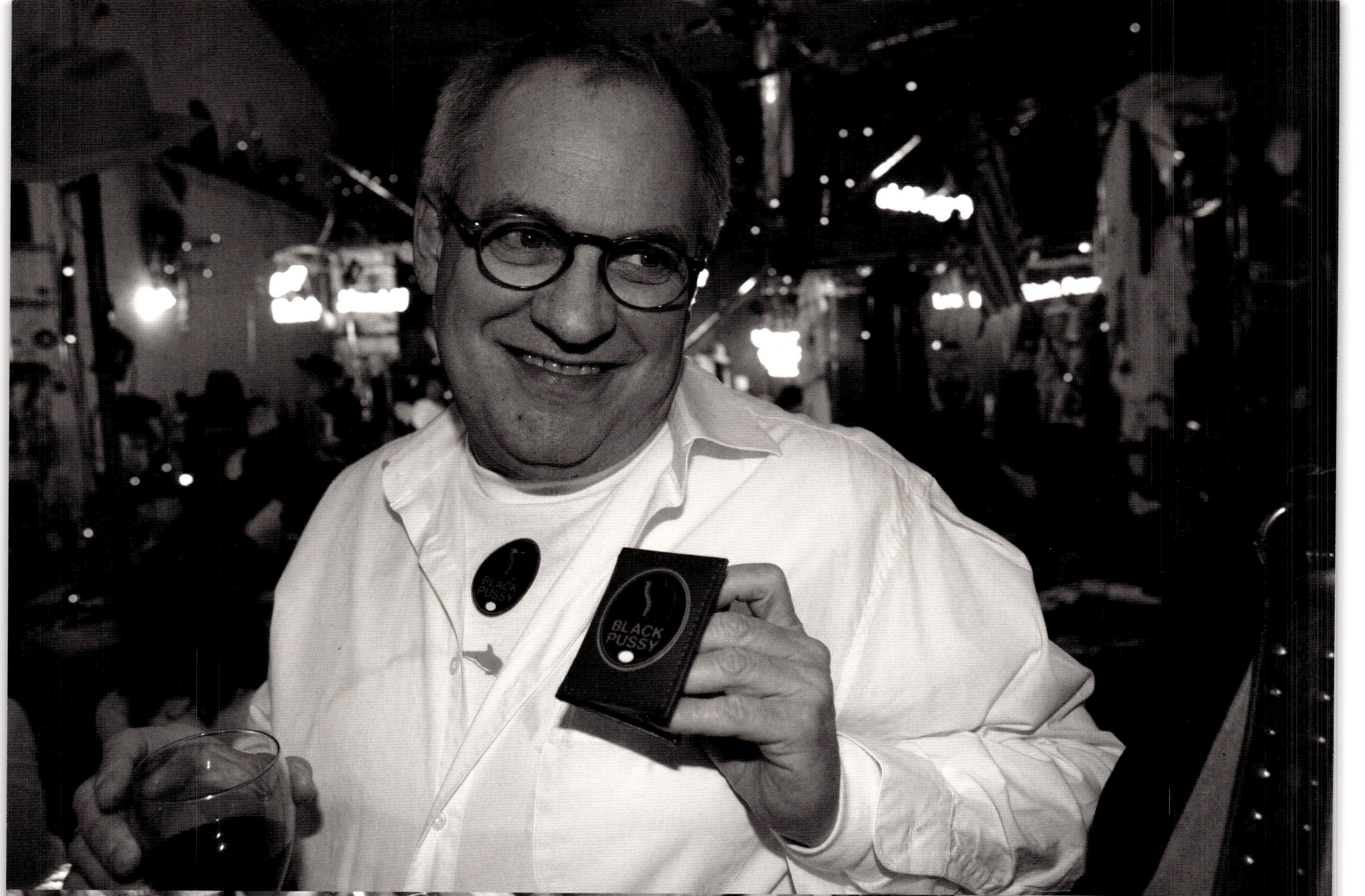
BLACK PUSSY
BLACK PUSSY

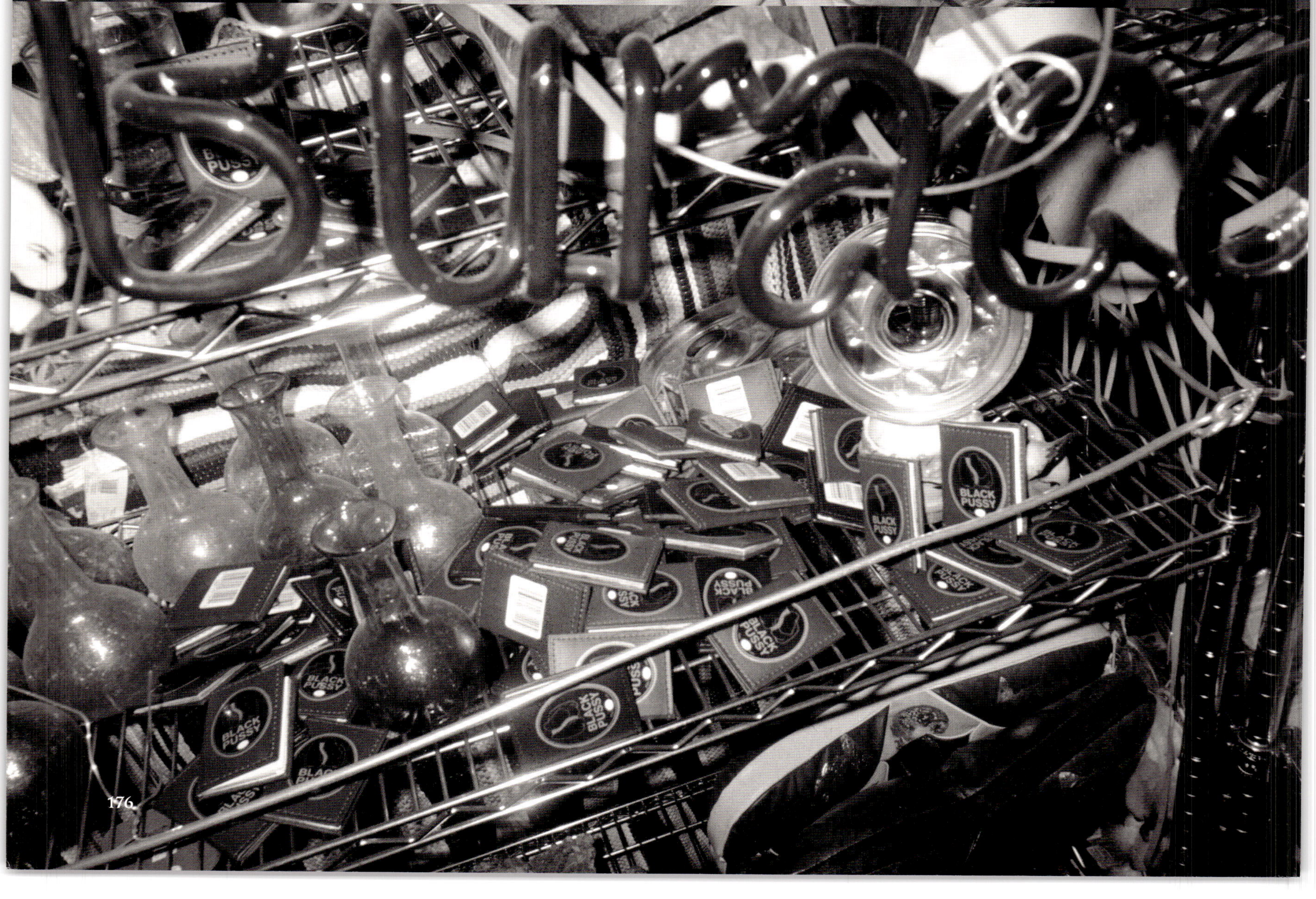
BLACK PUSSY
BLACK PUSSY
BLACK PUSSY

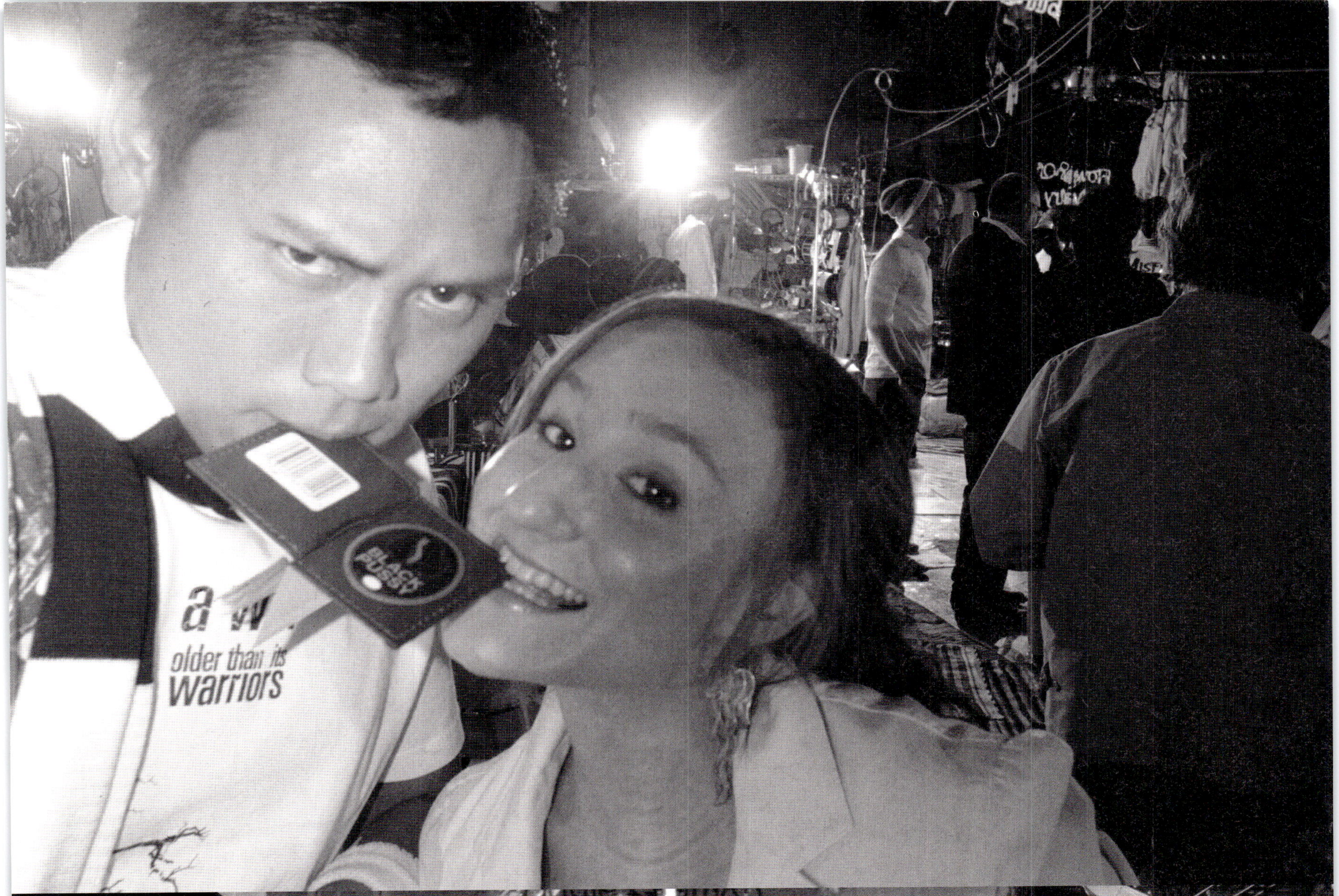
older than its
warriors

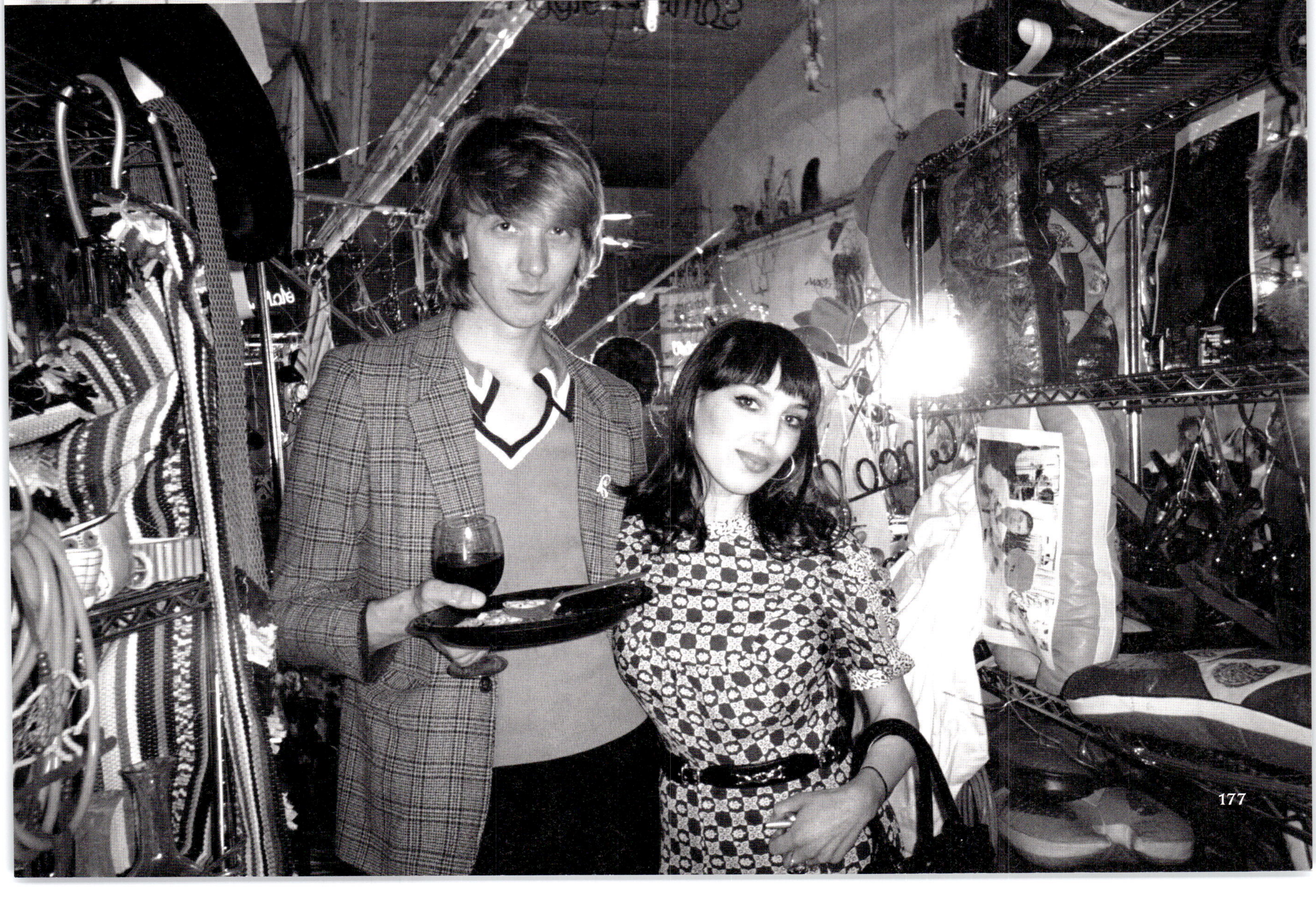

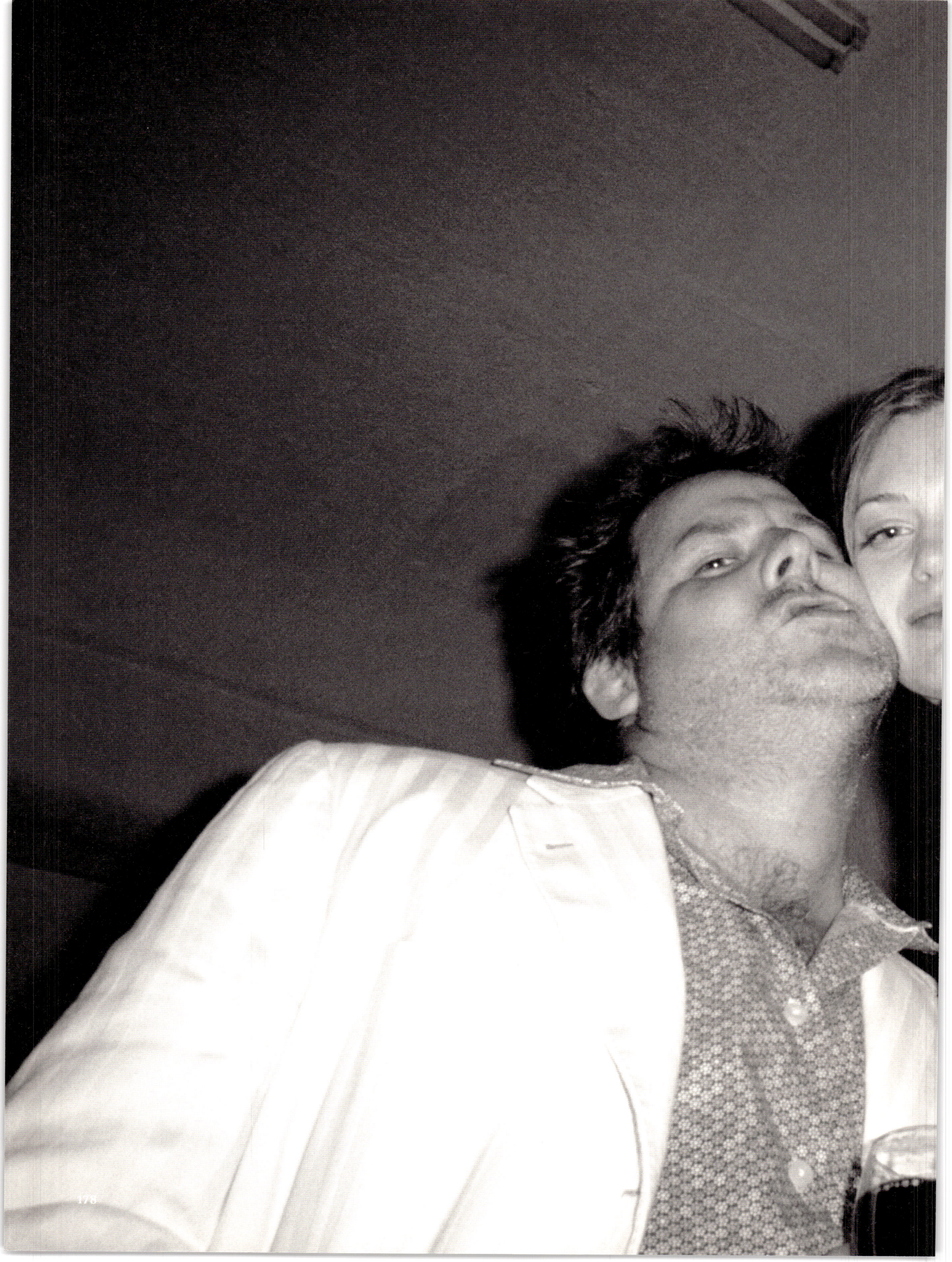

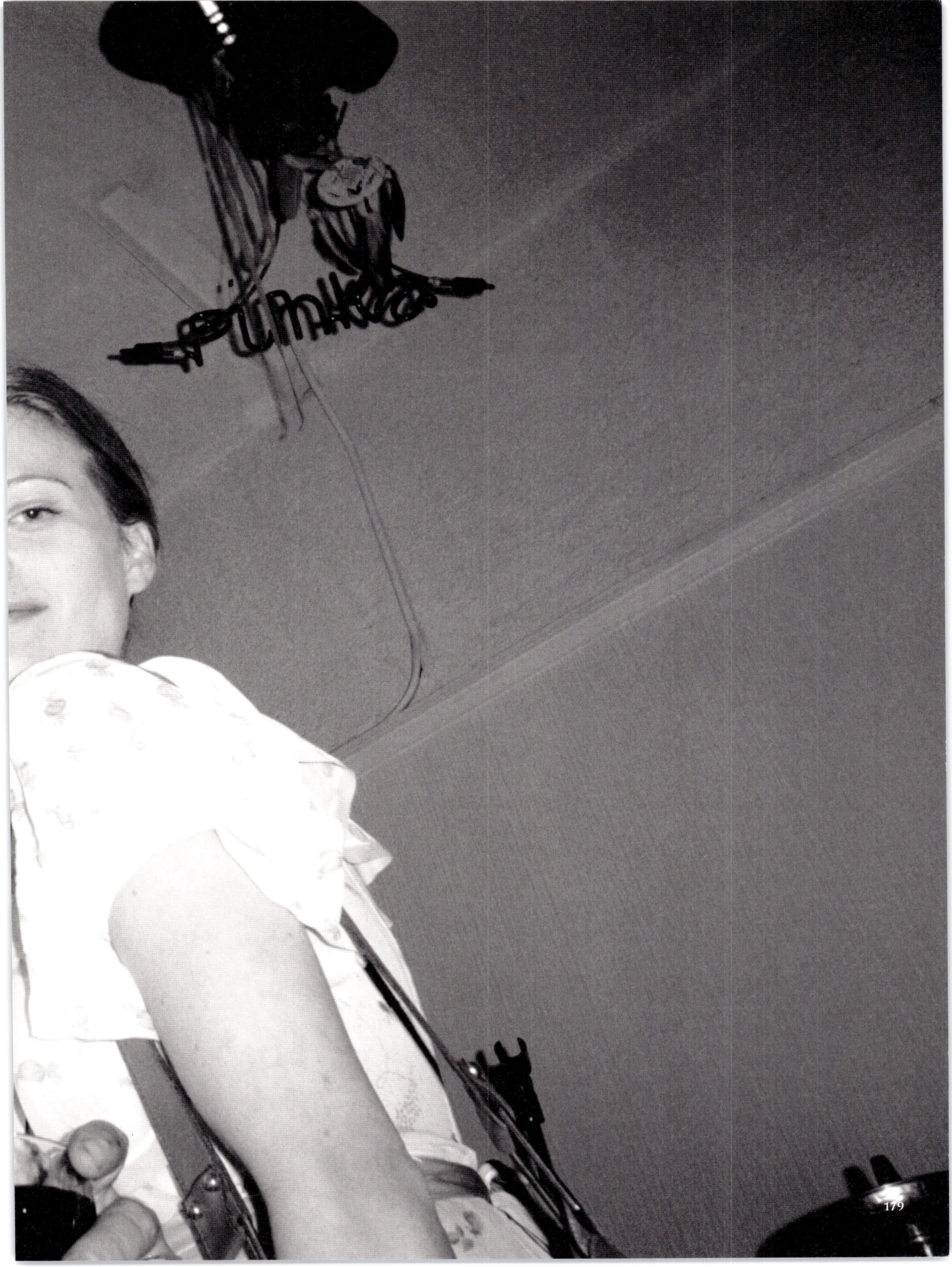

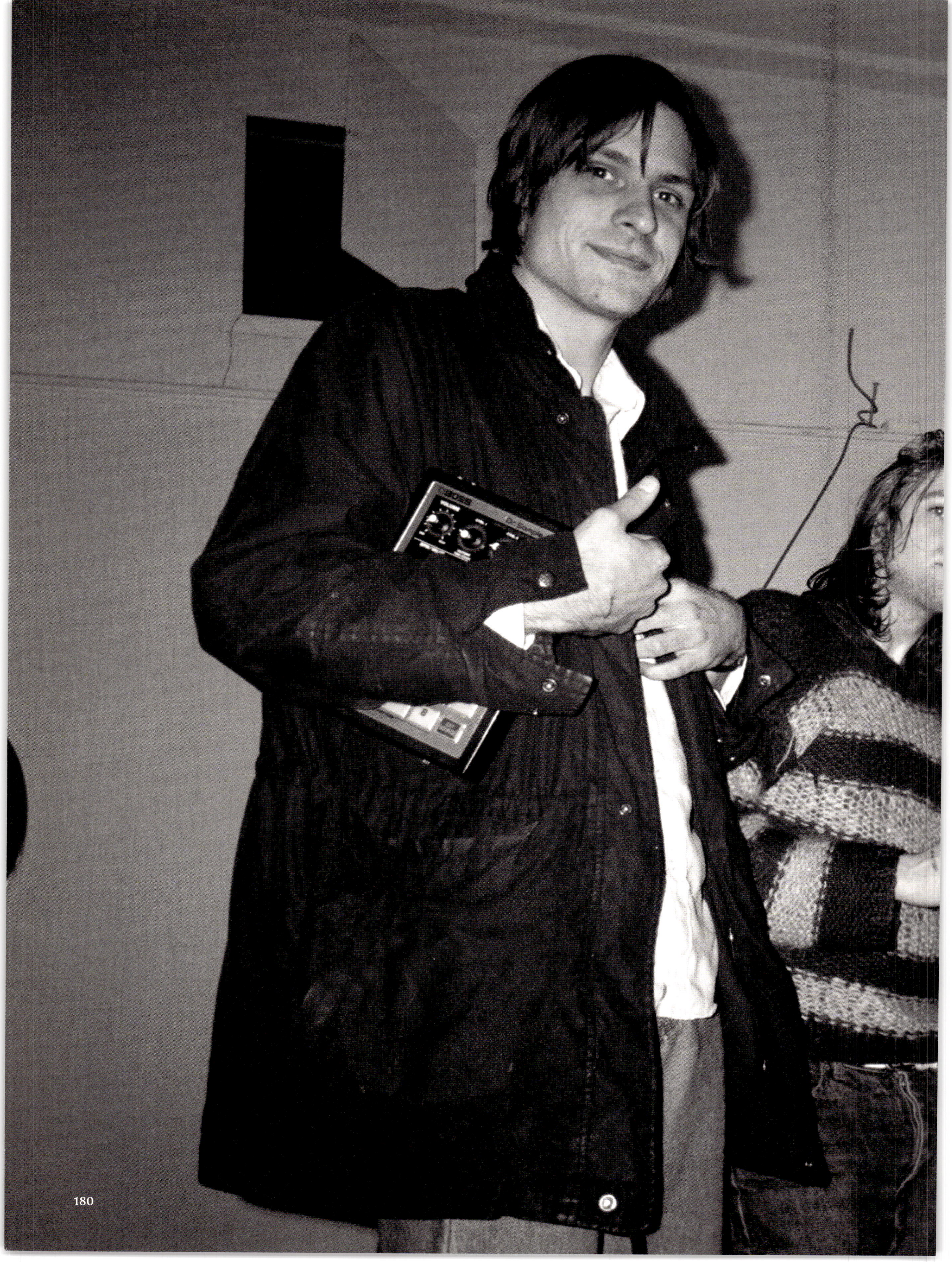

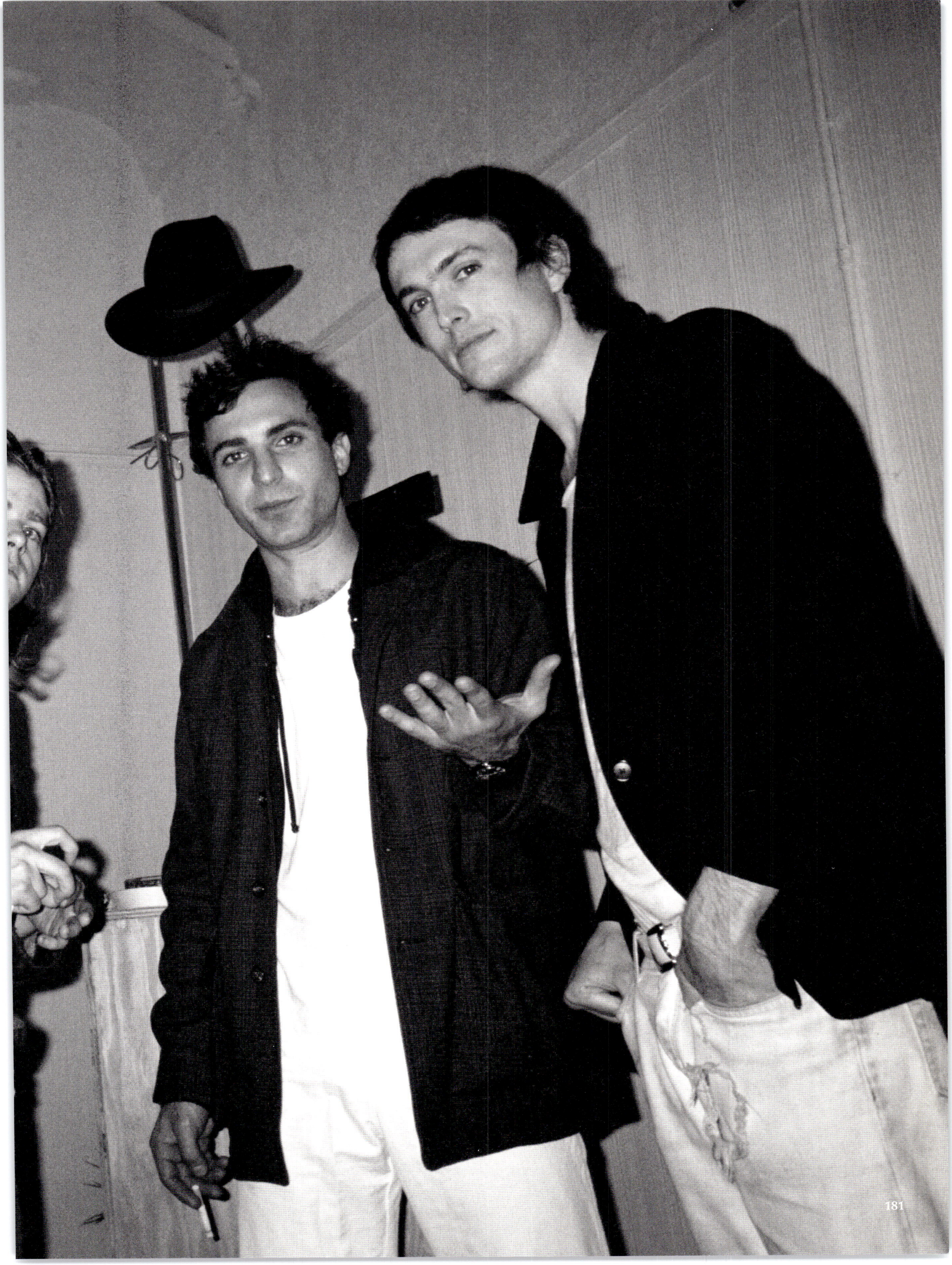

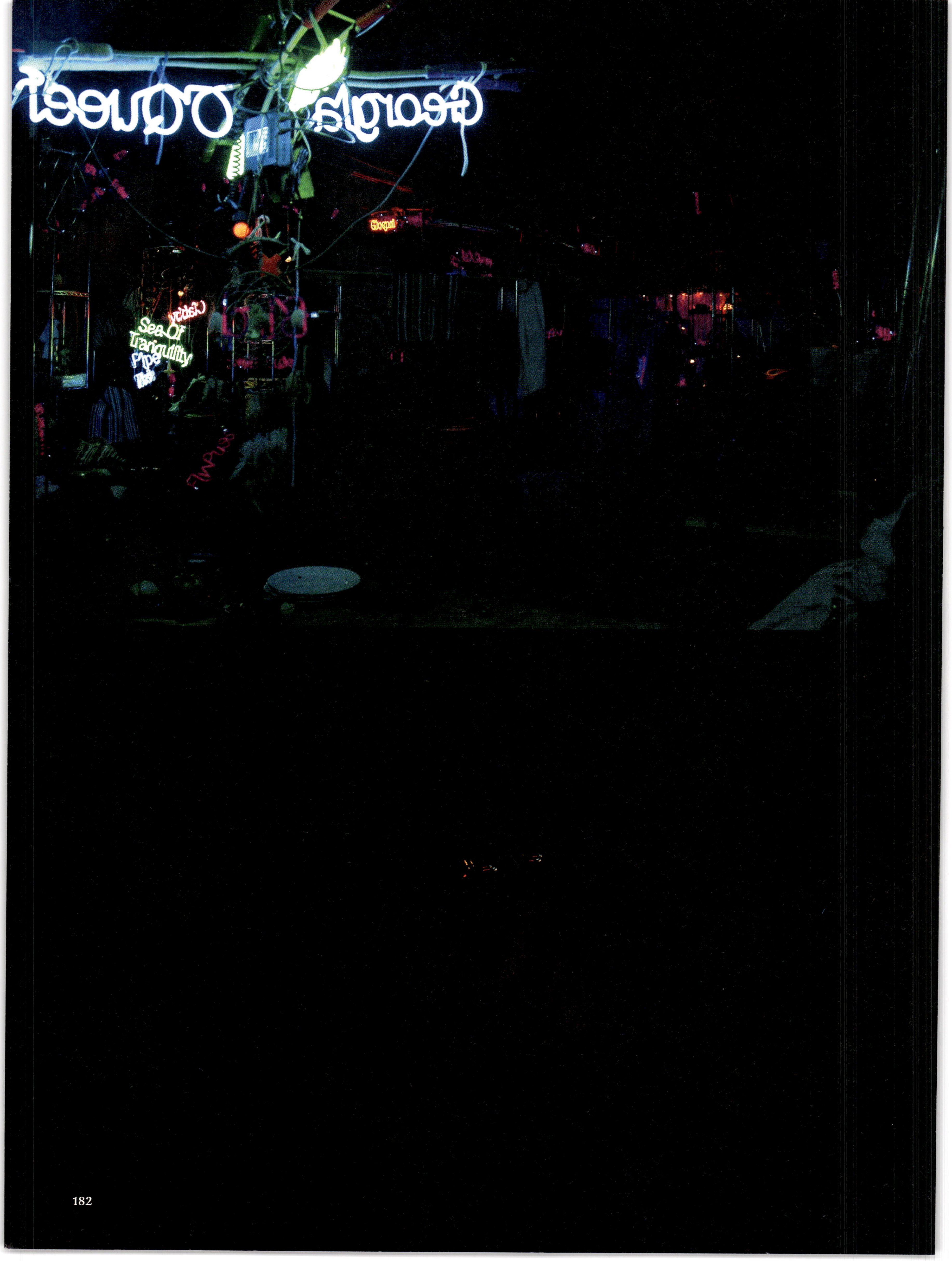
Sea Of
Tranquility
Pipe

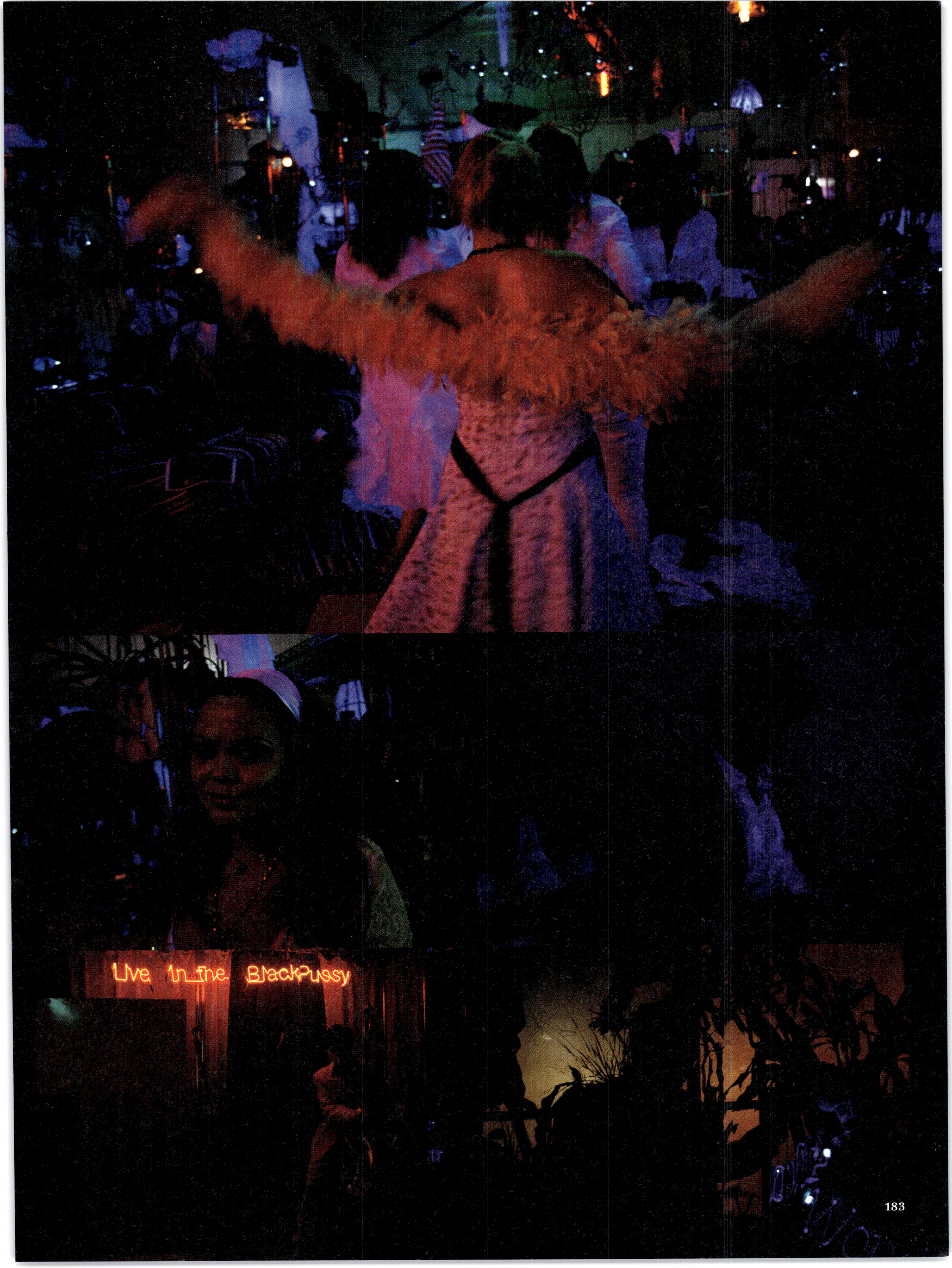
Live in the BlackPussy

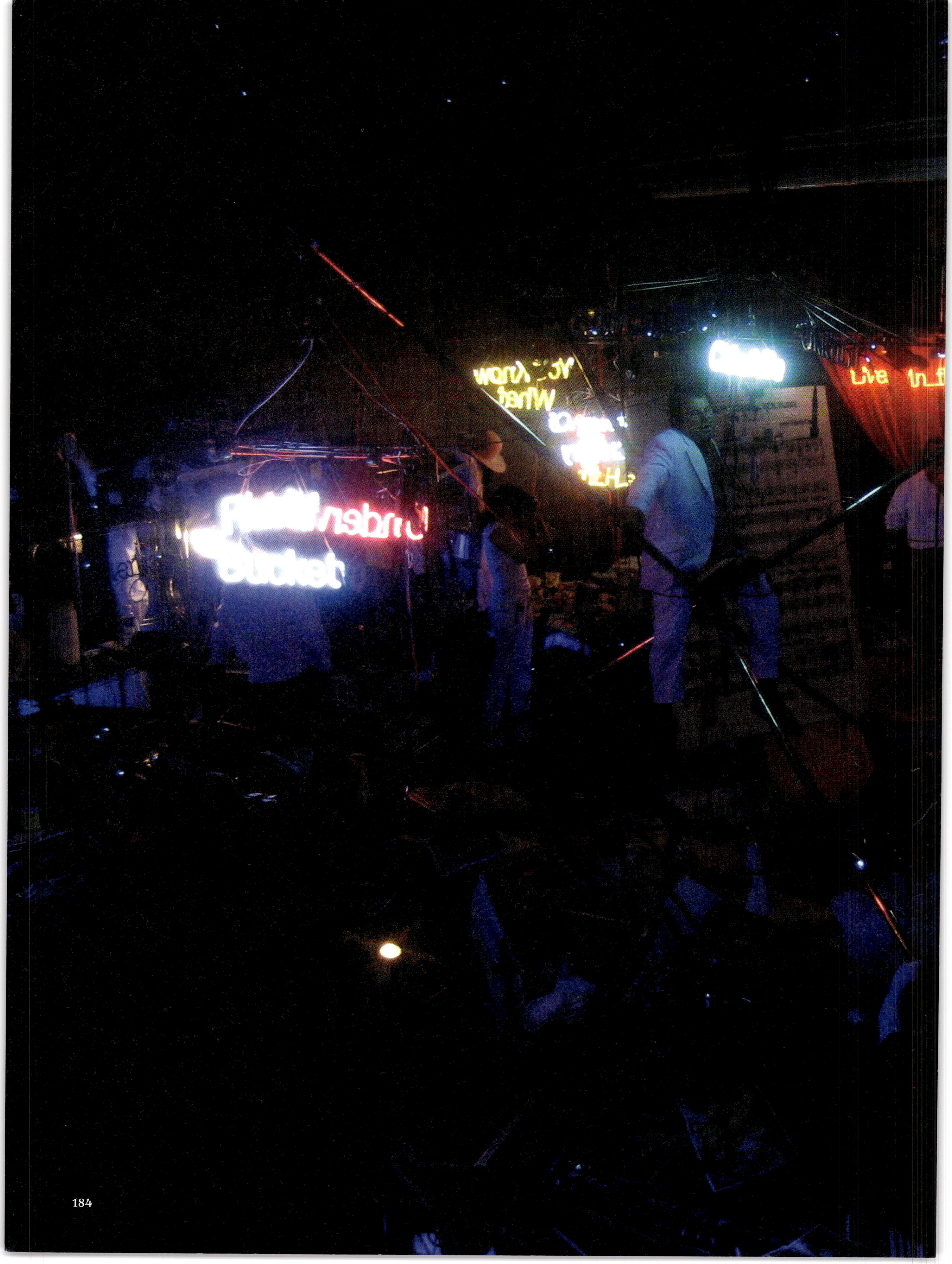

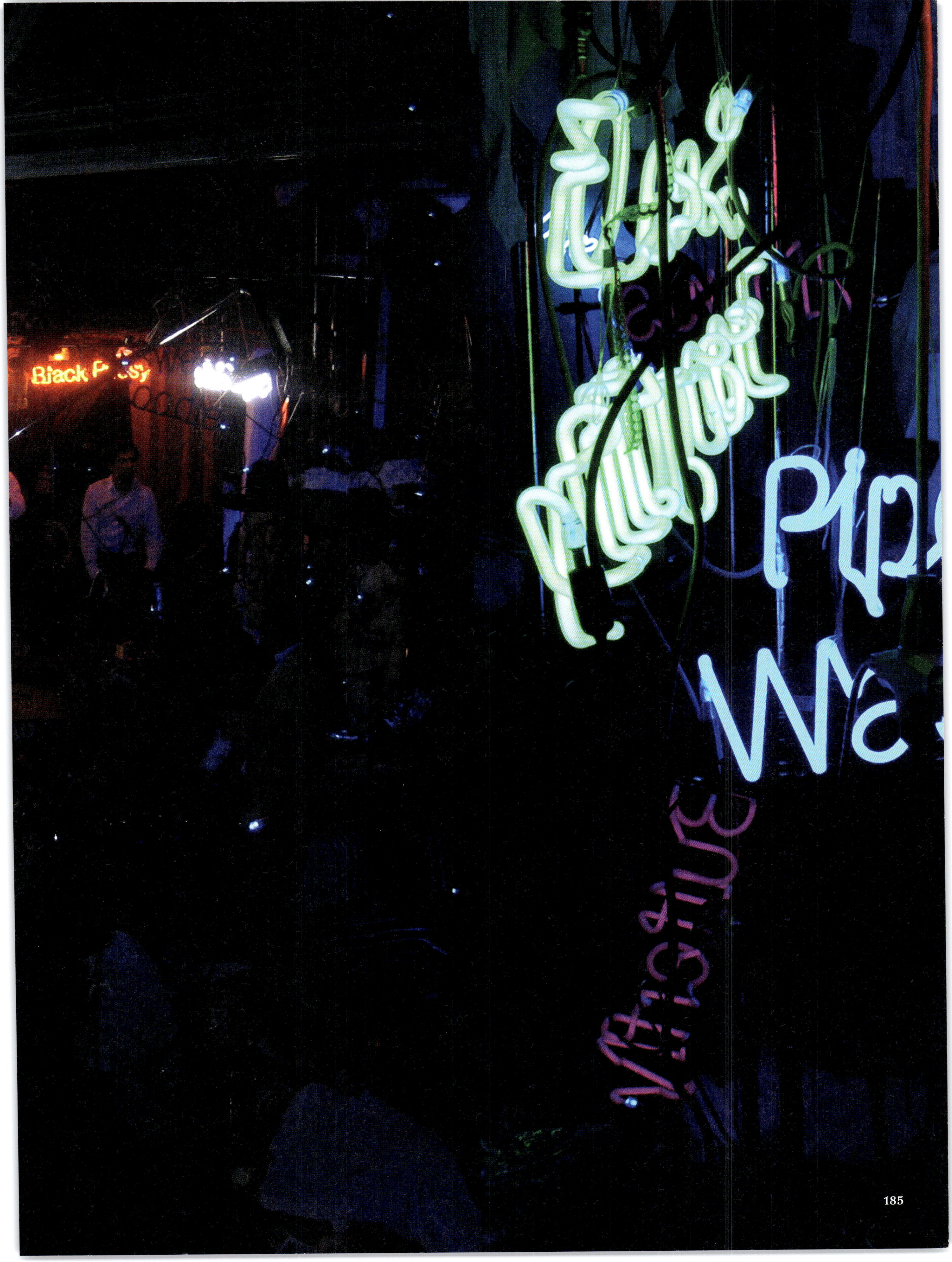
Black

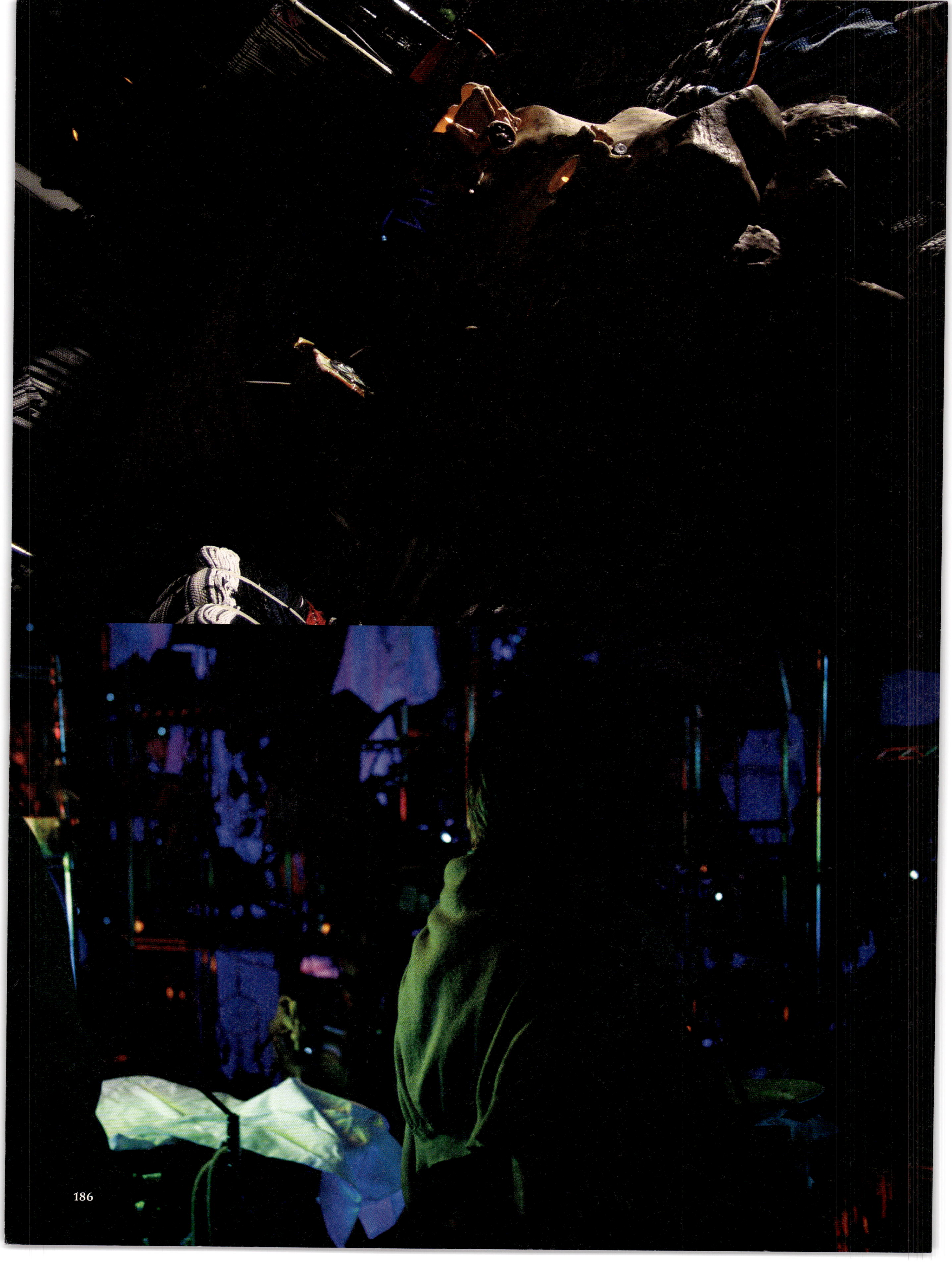

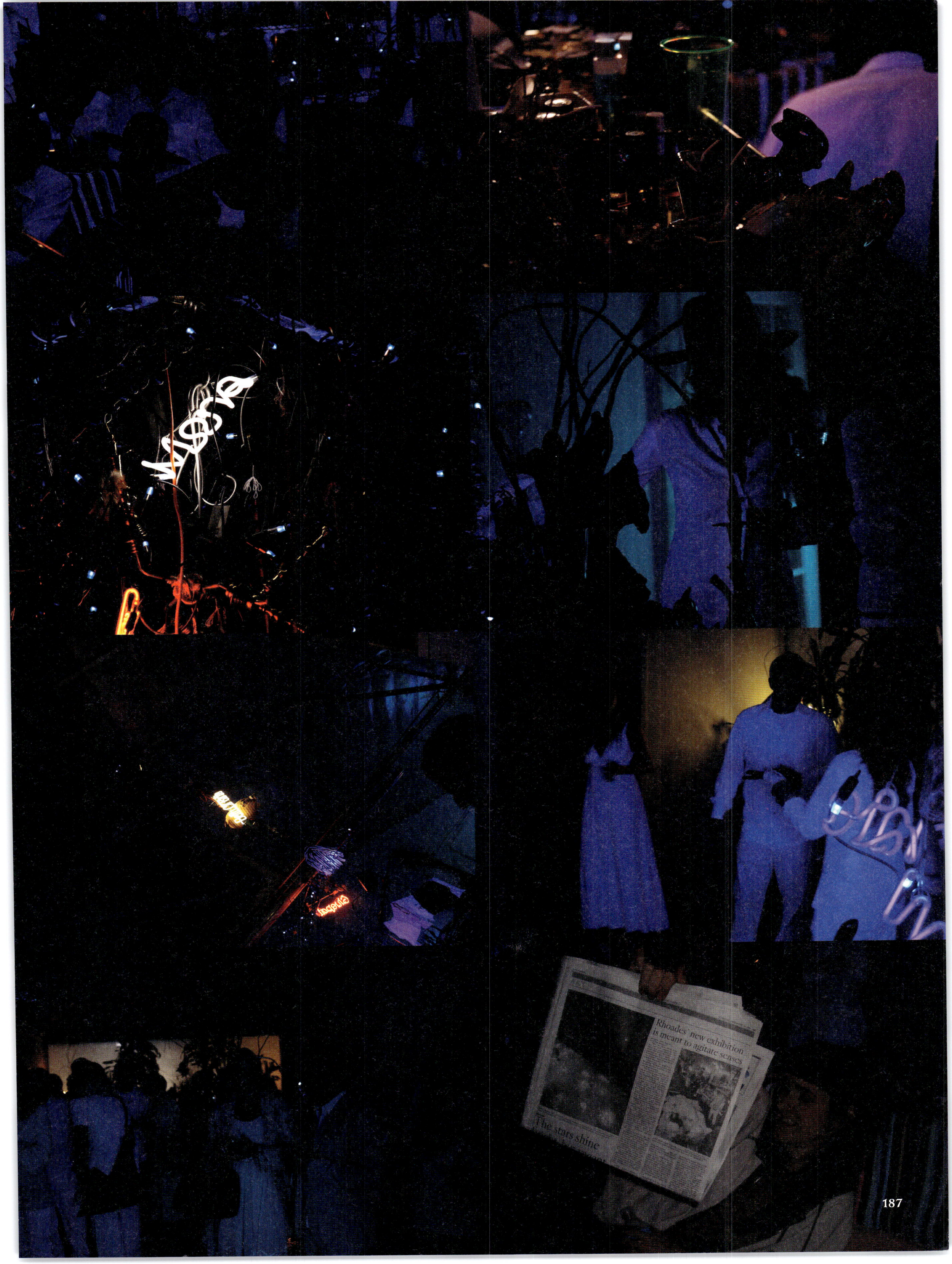
Rhoades' new exhibition
is meant to agitate senses
The stars shine

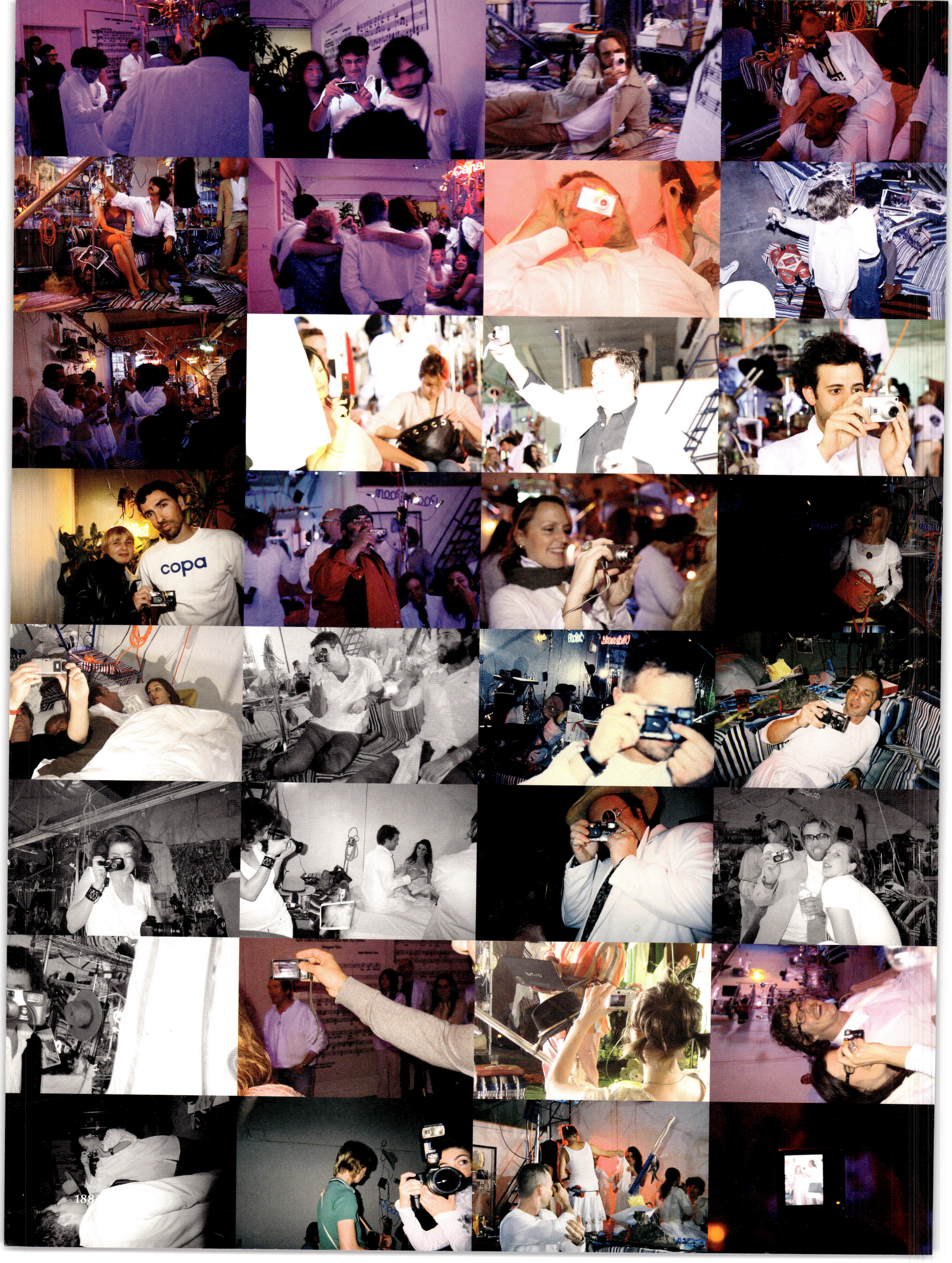
copa

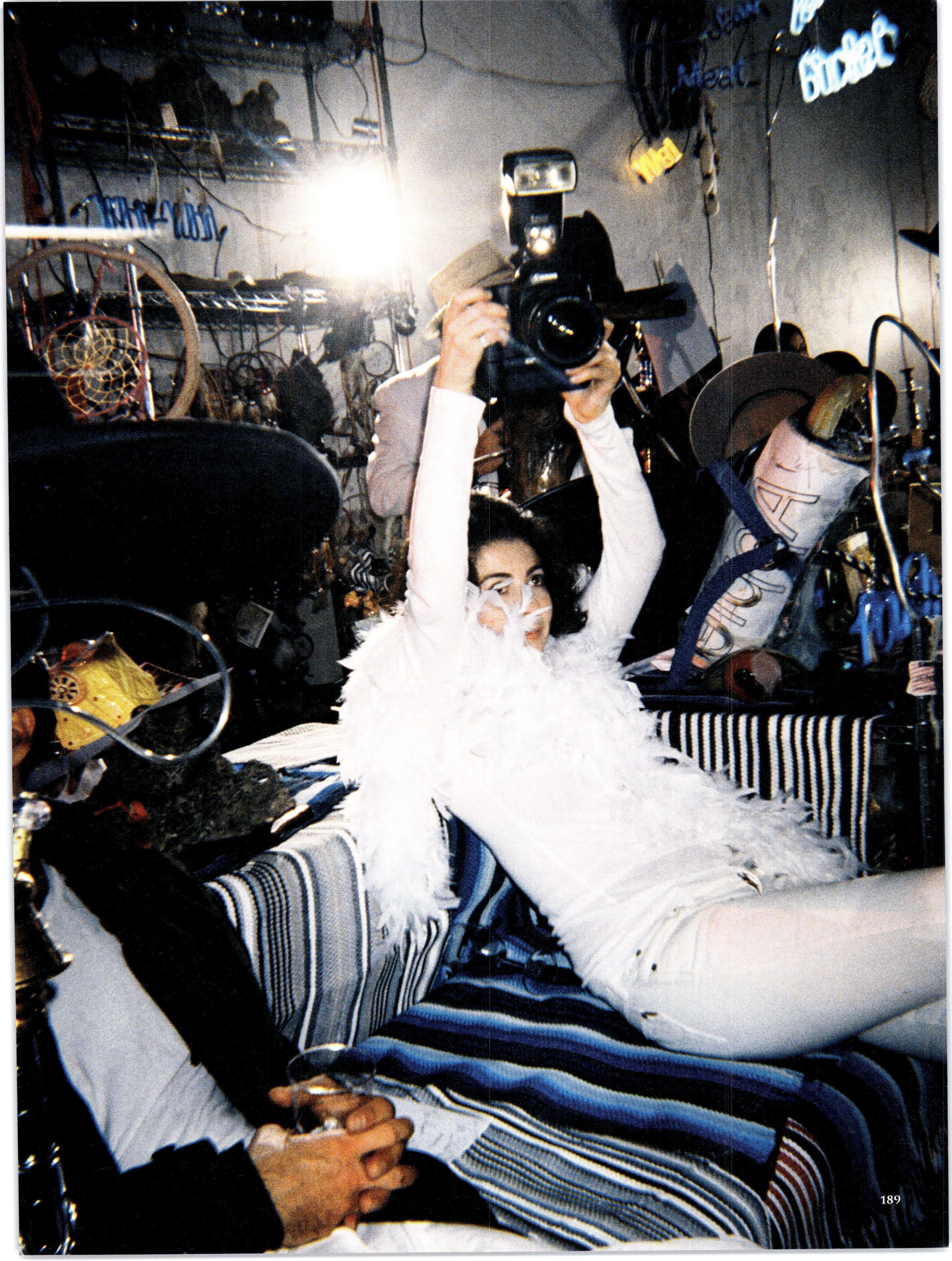

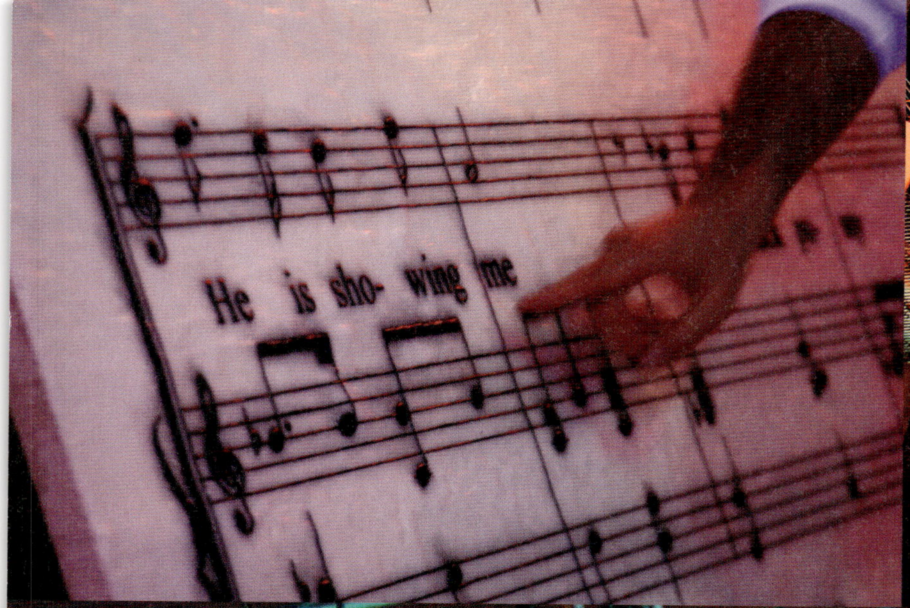
He is sho- wing me

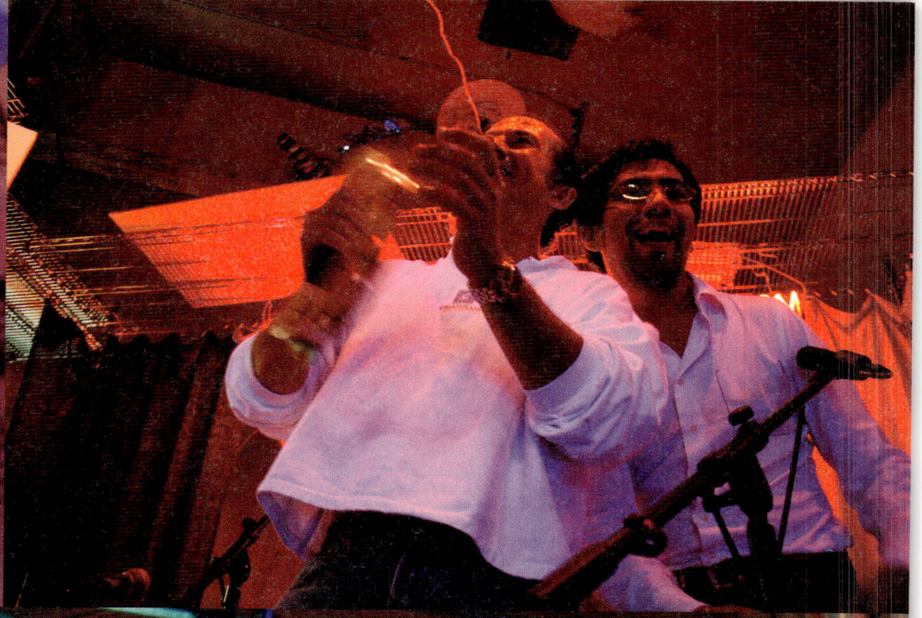

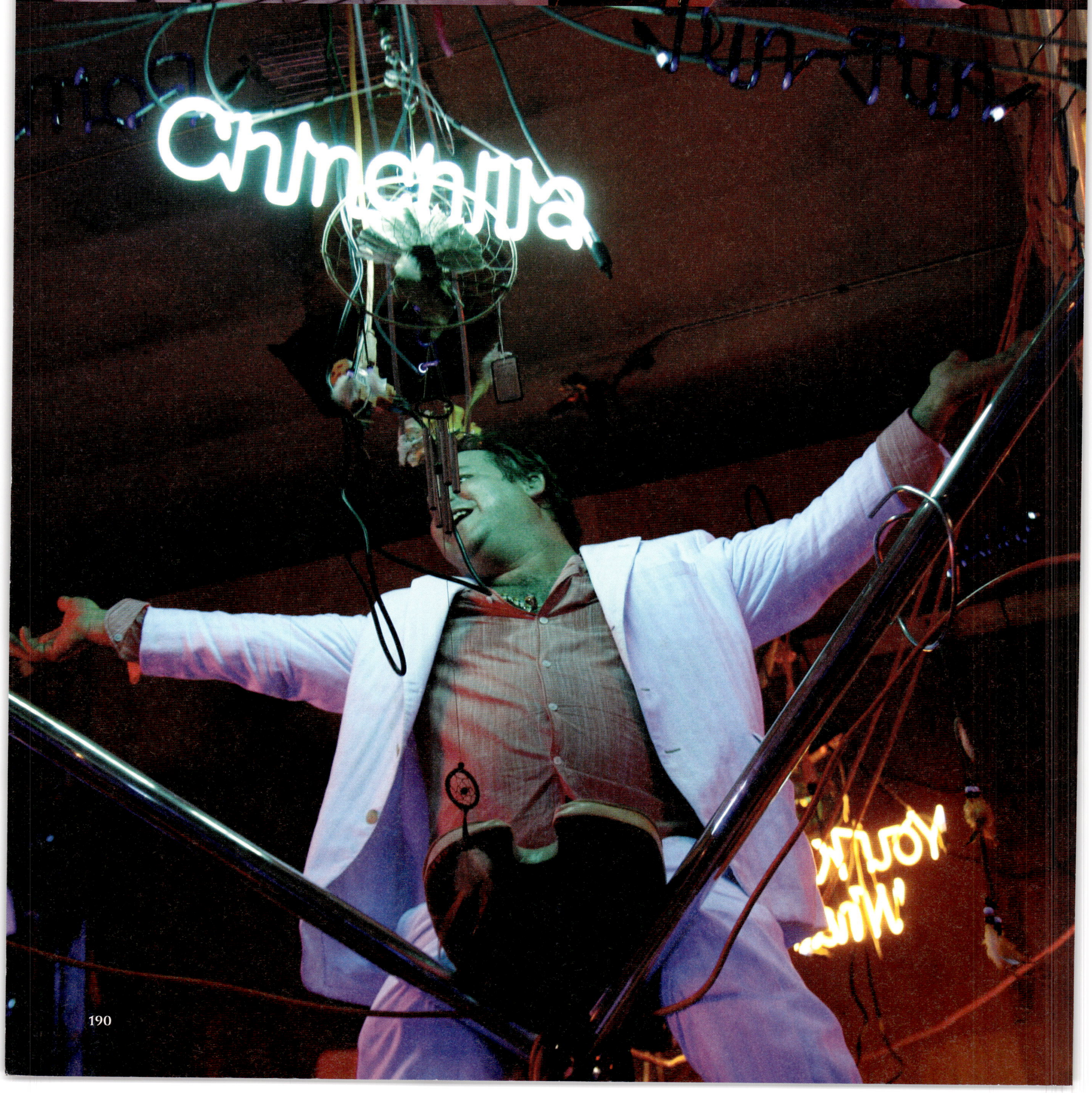

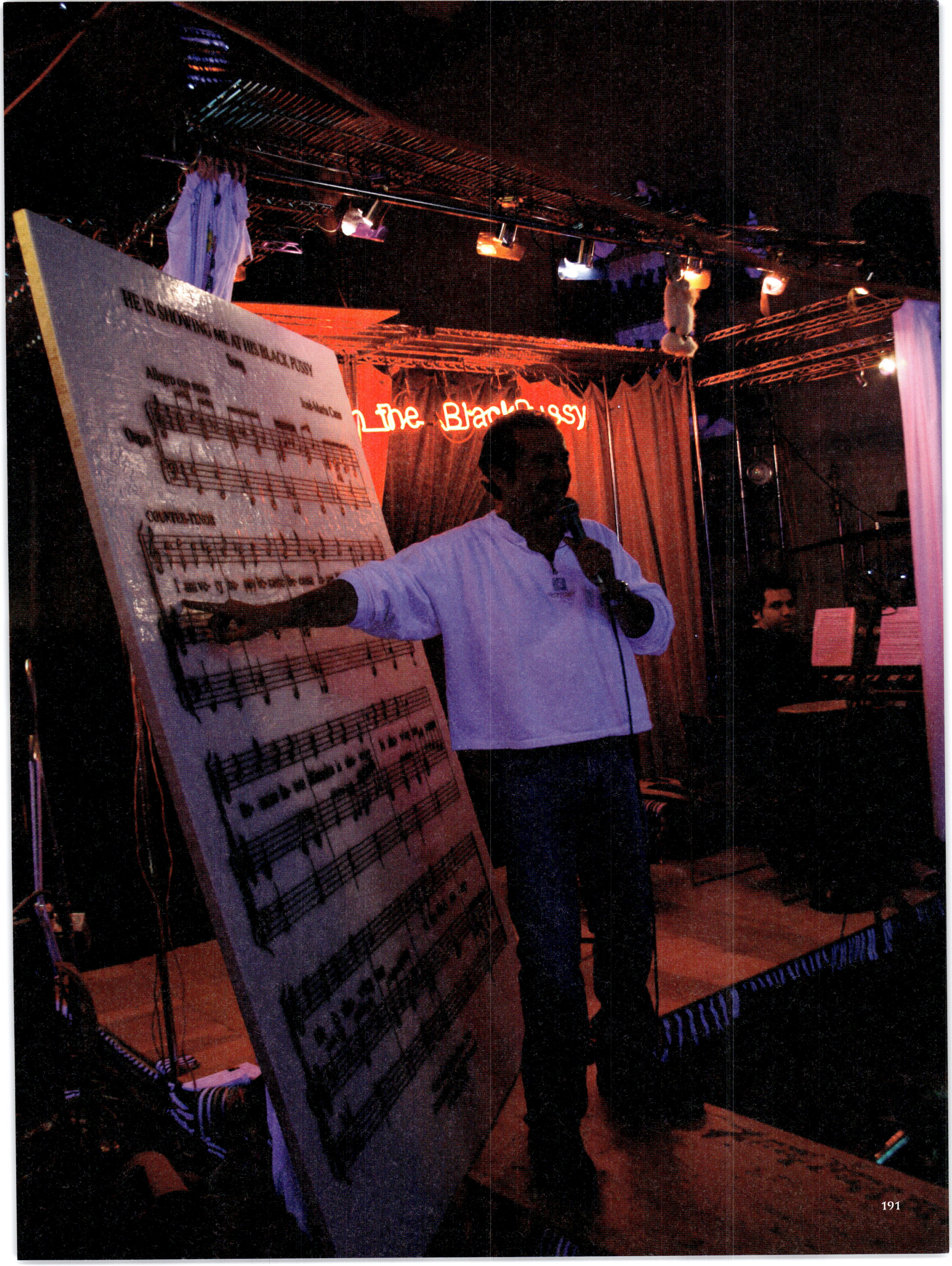
HE IS SHOWING ME AT HIS BLACK PUSSY
COUNTER-TENOR

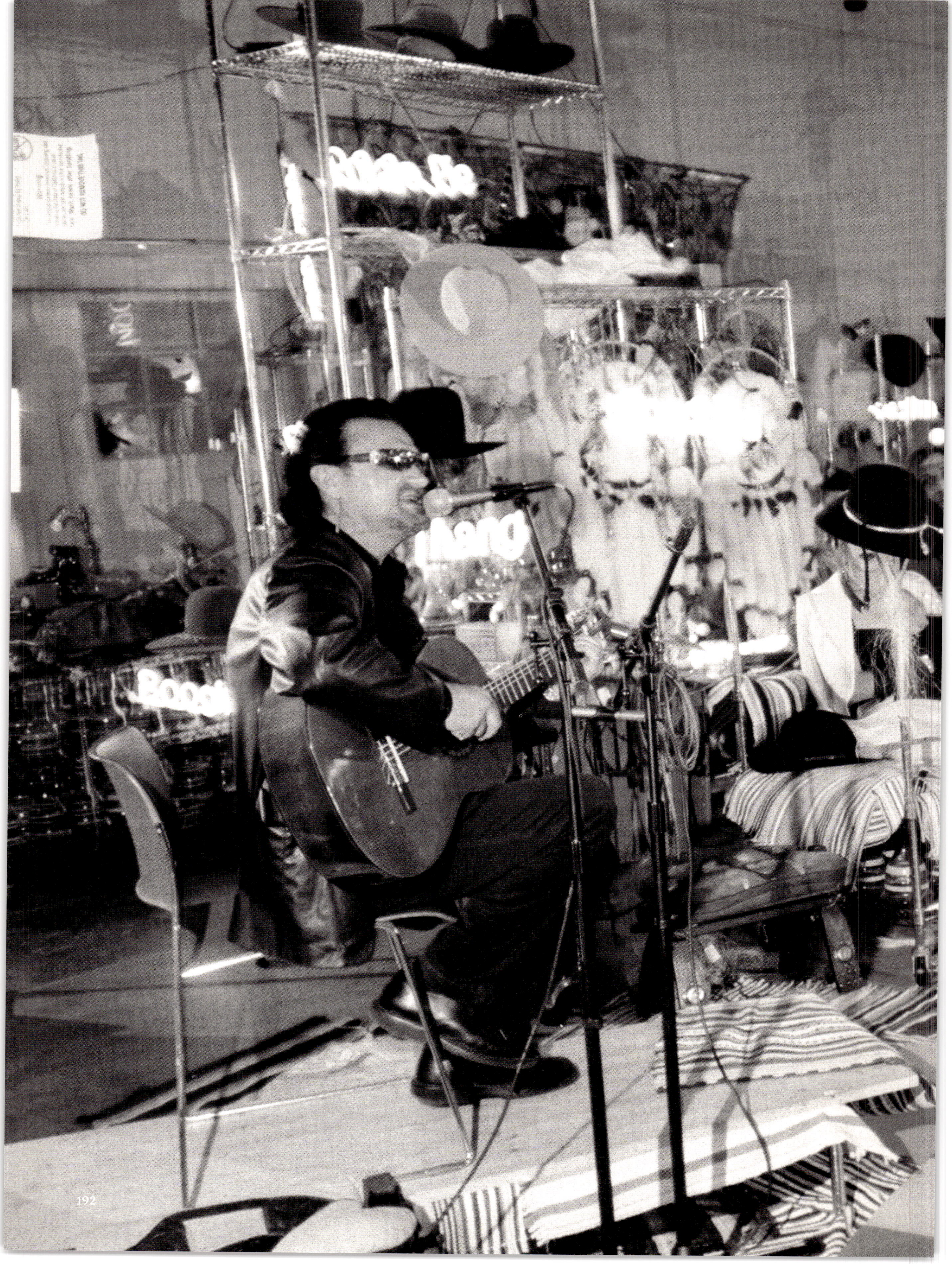

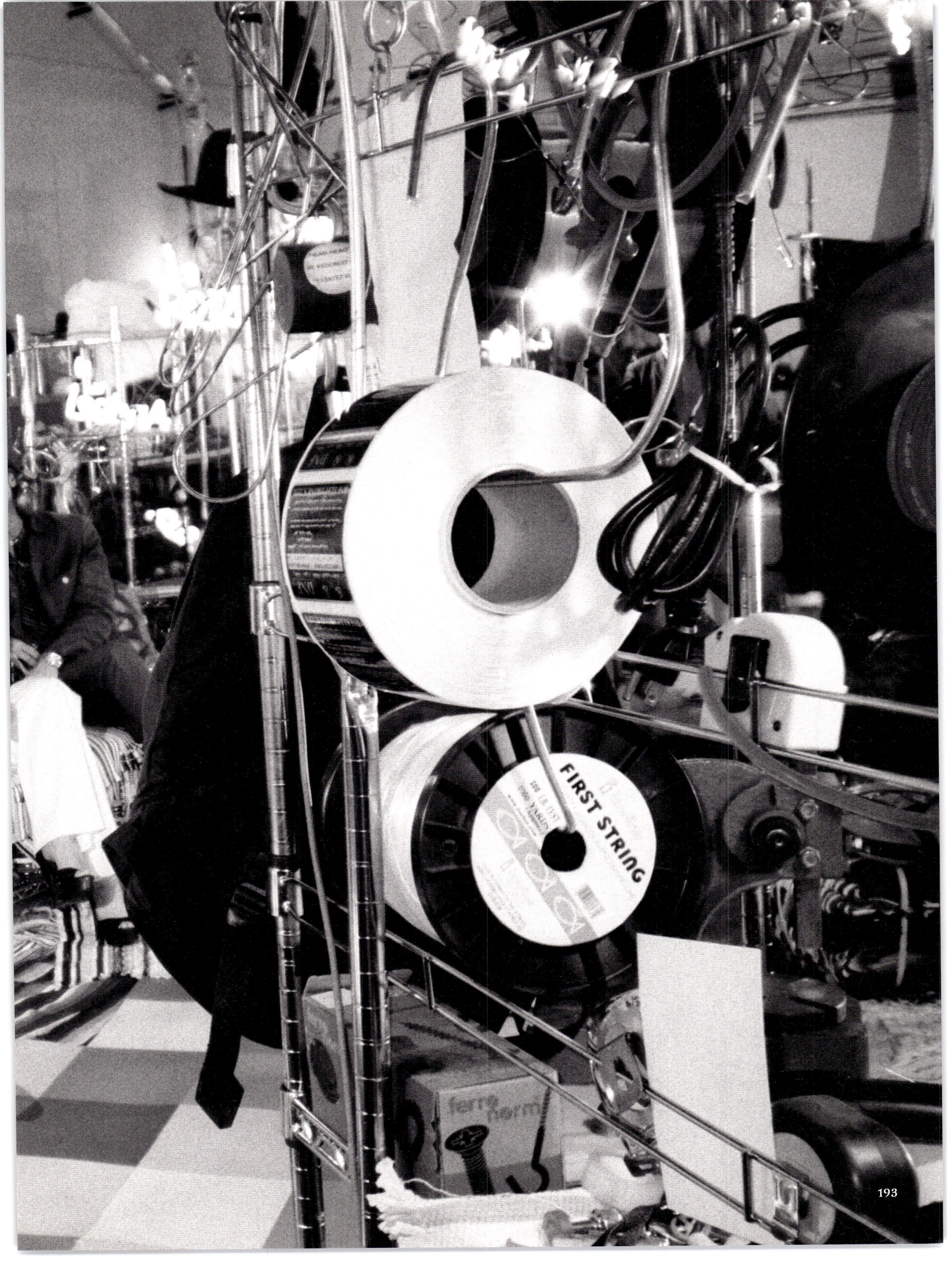
FIRST STRING

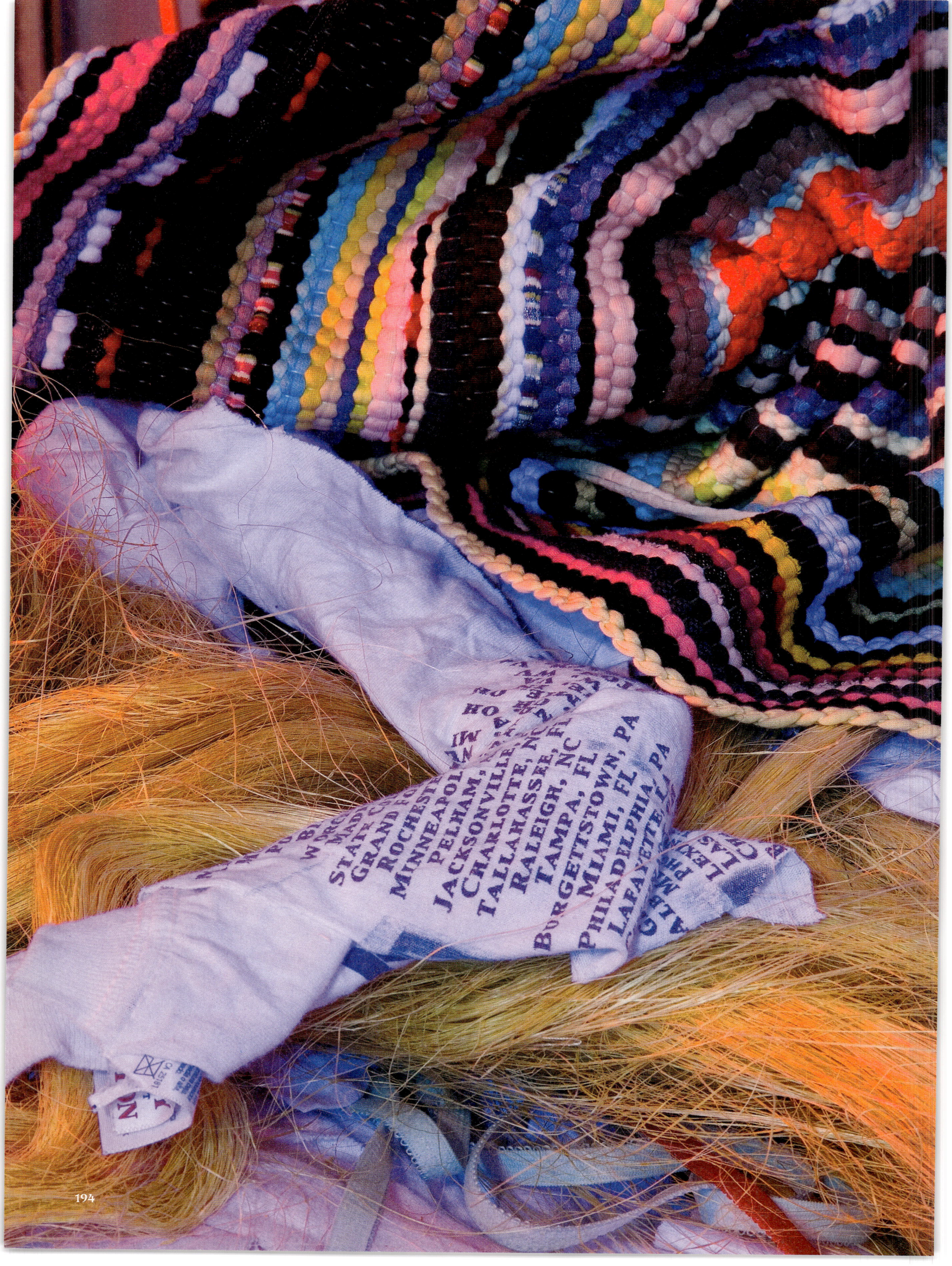
JACKSONVILLE, NC
TALLAHASSEE, FL
RALEIGH, NC
TAMPA, FL
BURGETTSTOWN, PA
MIAMI, FL
PHILADELPHIA, PA

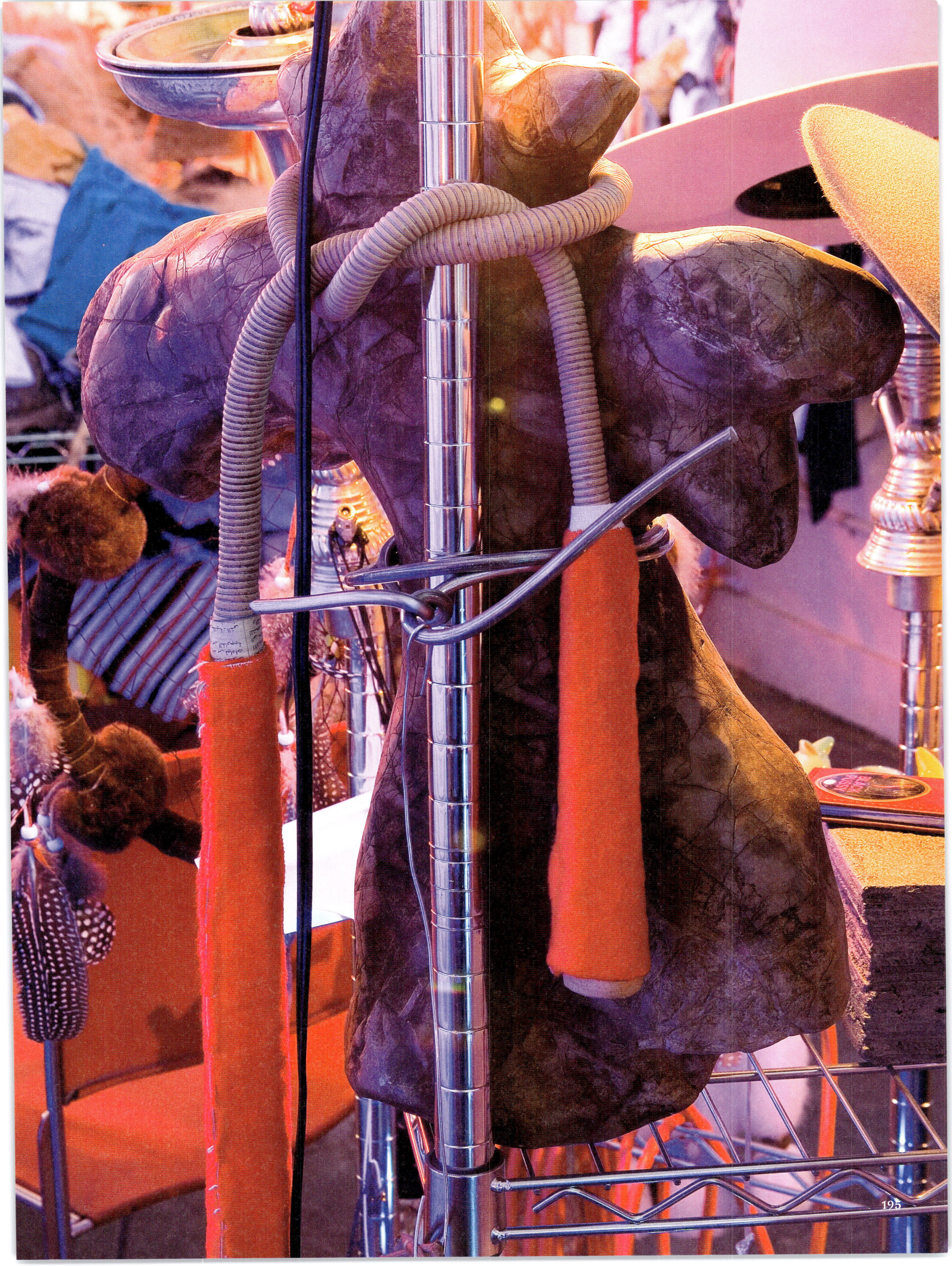

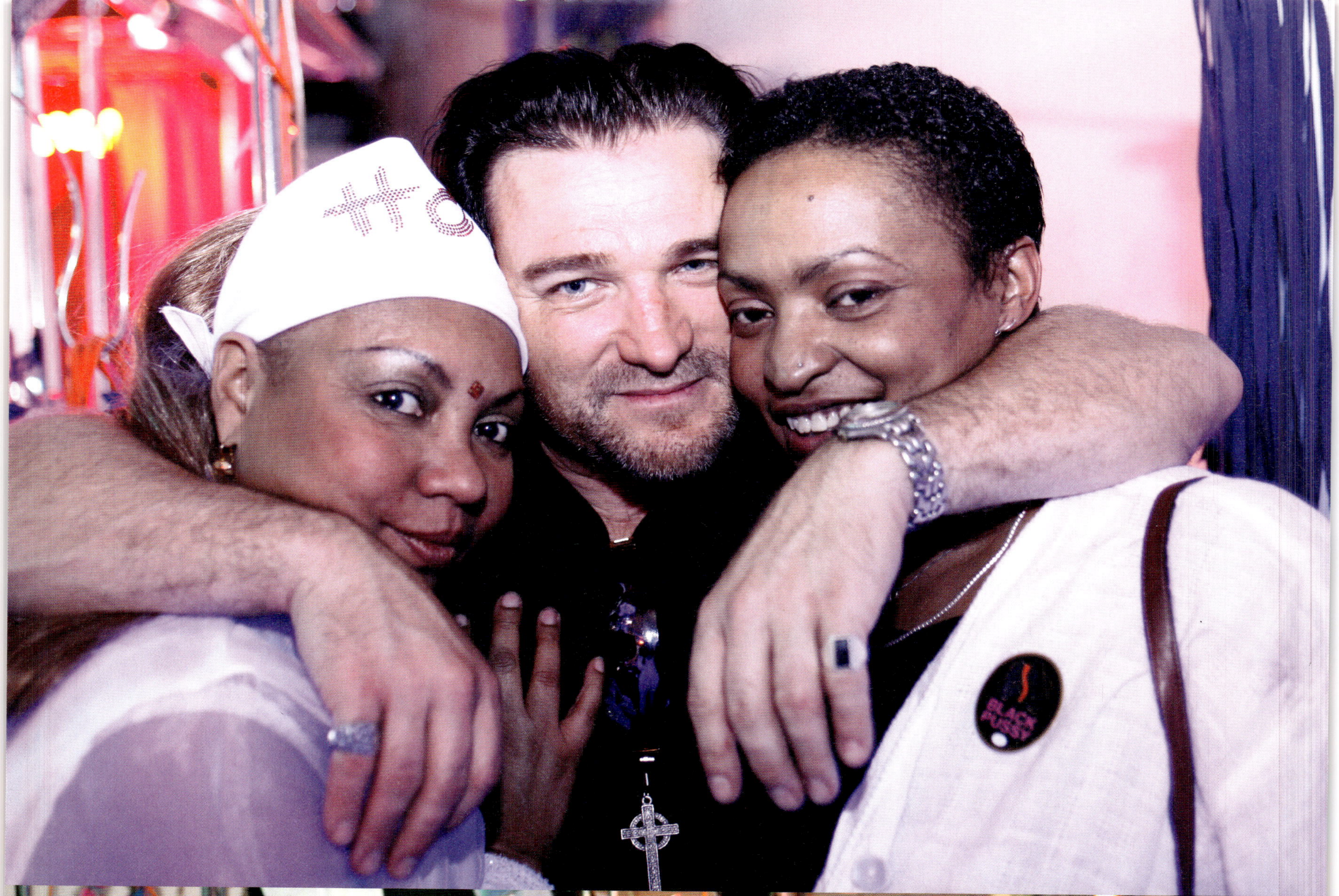
BLACK PUSSY

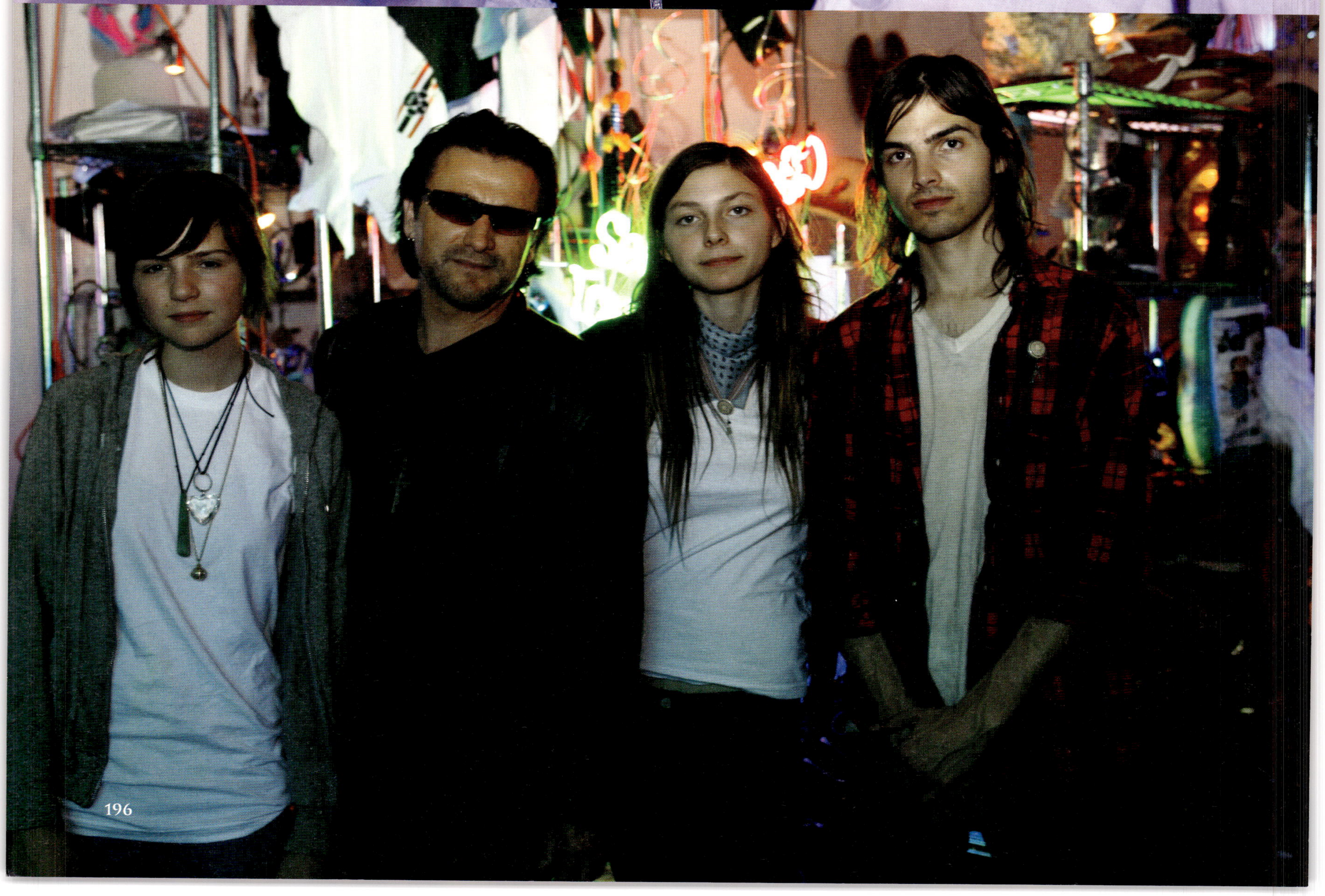

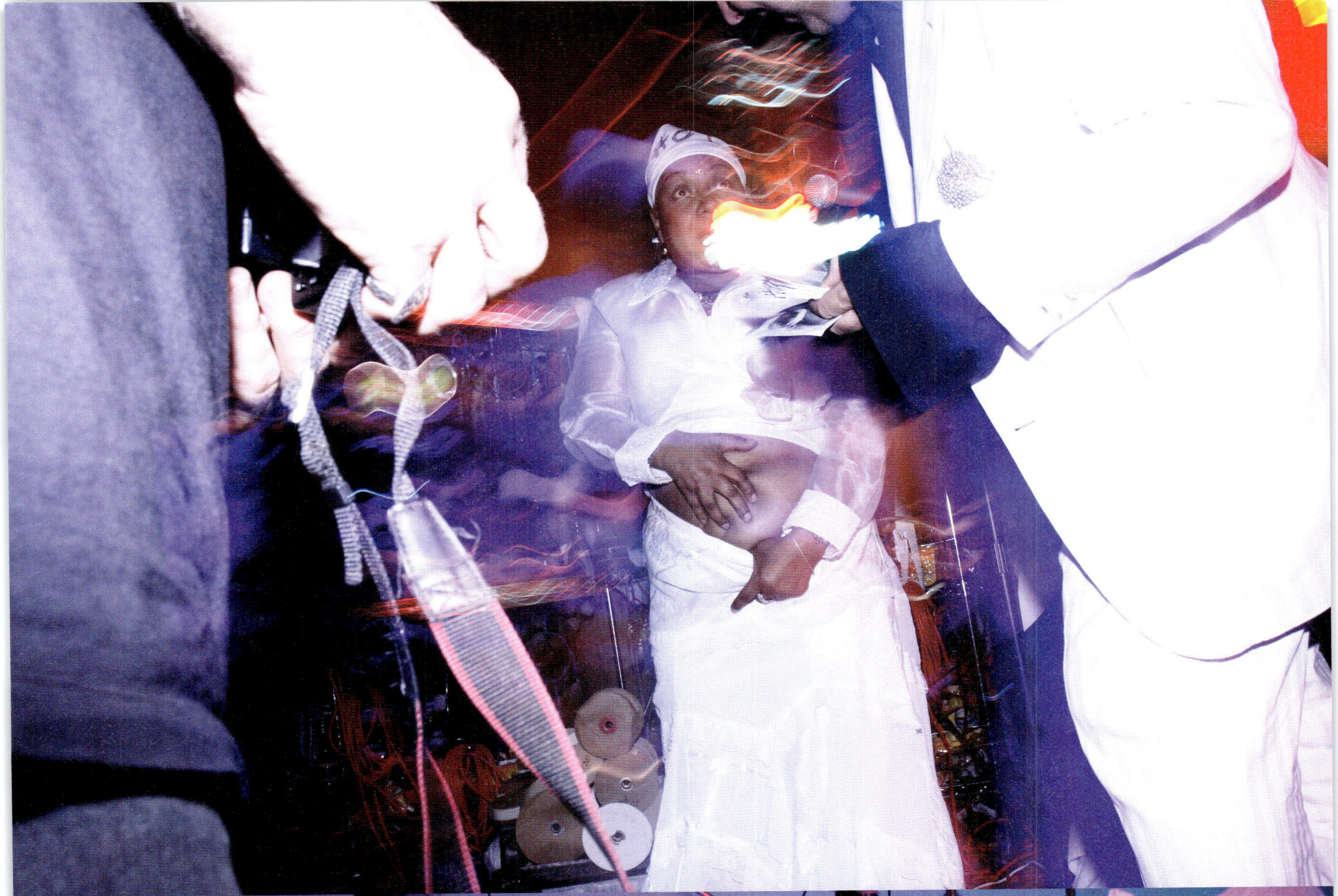

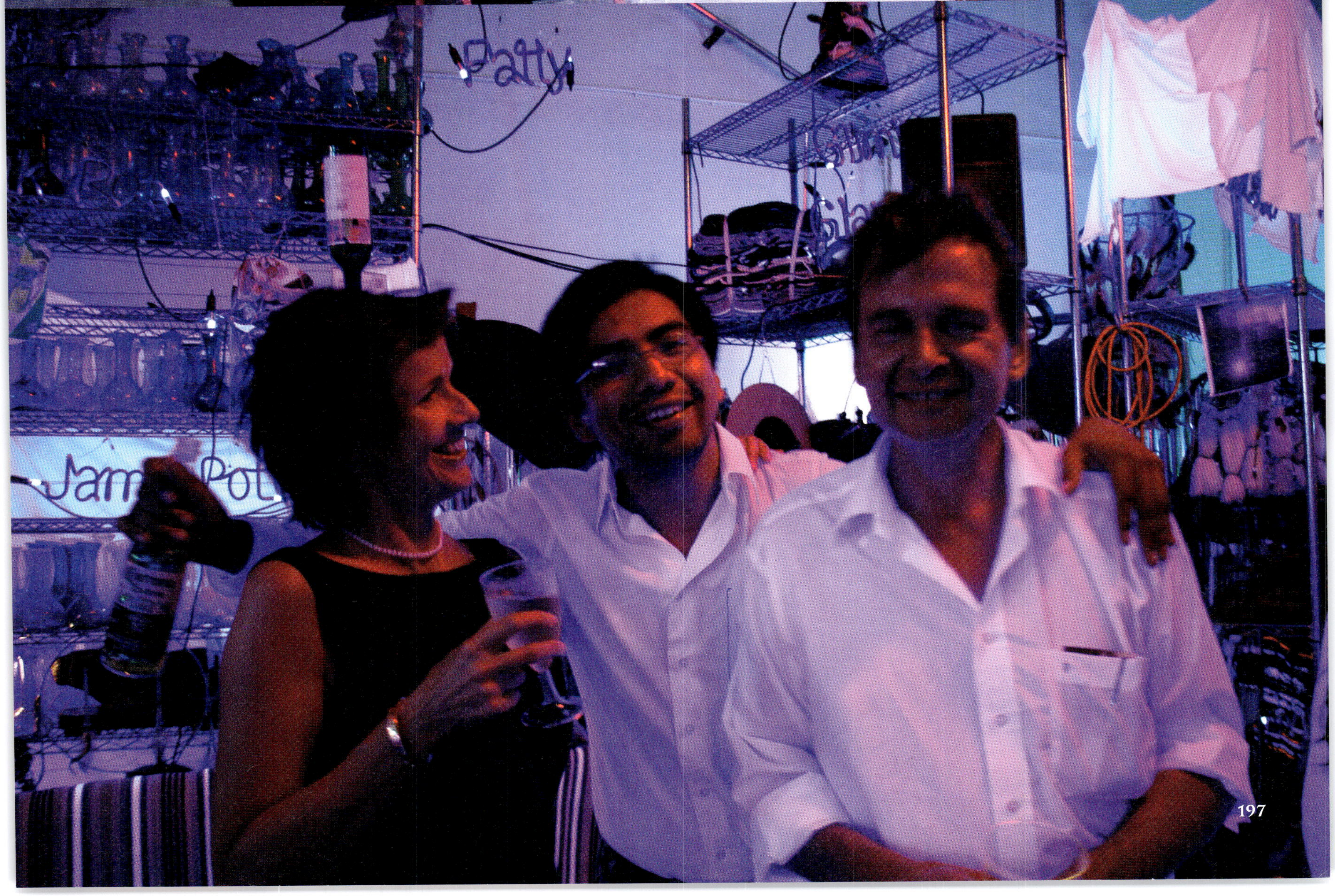
Party

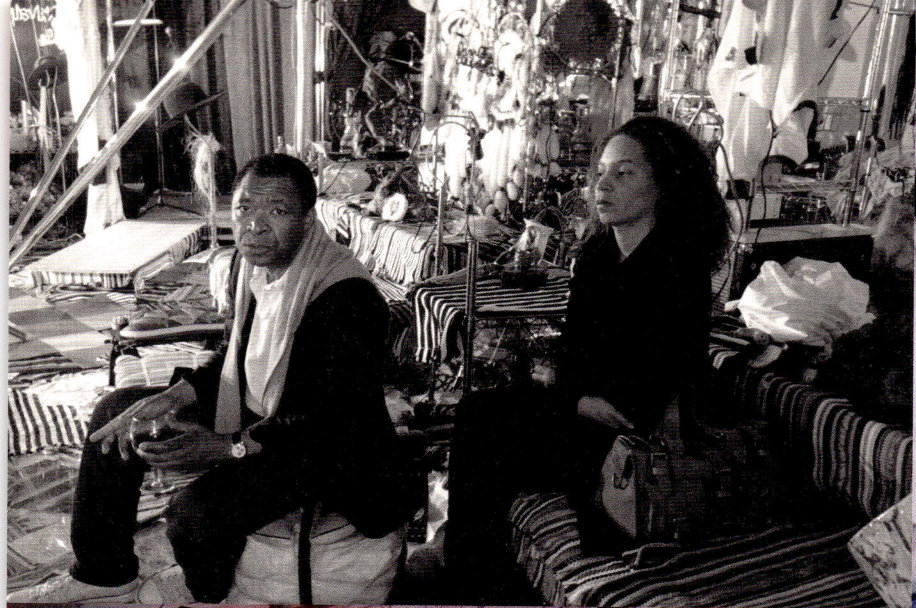

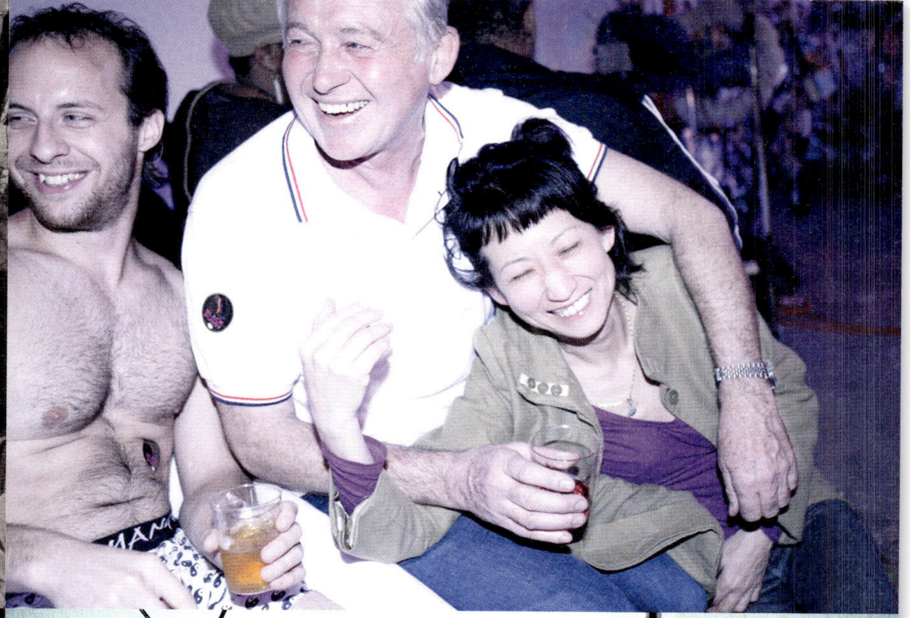

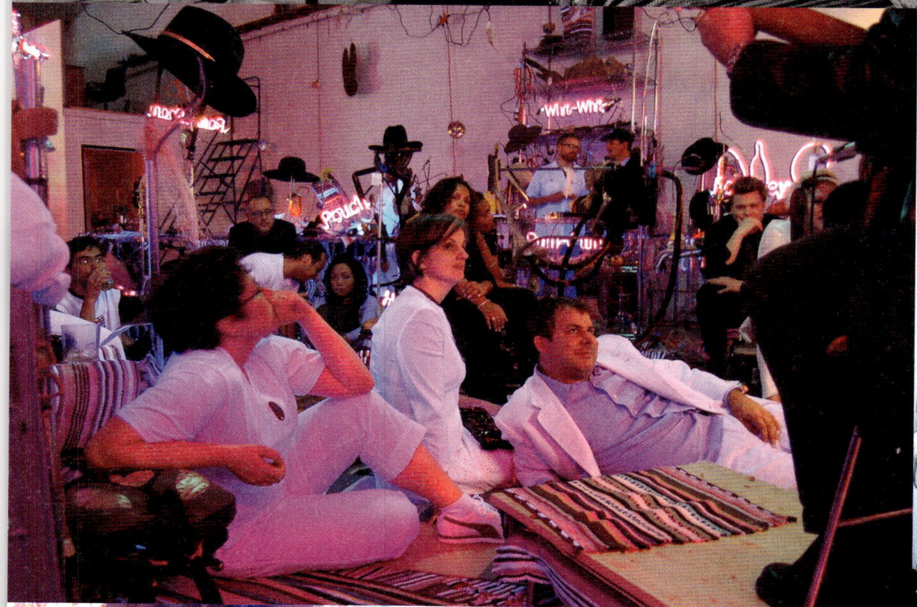

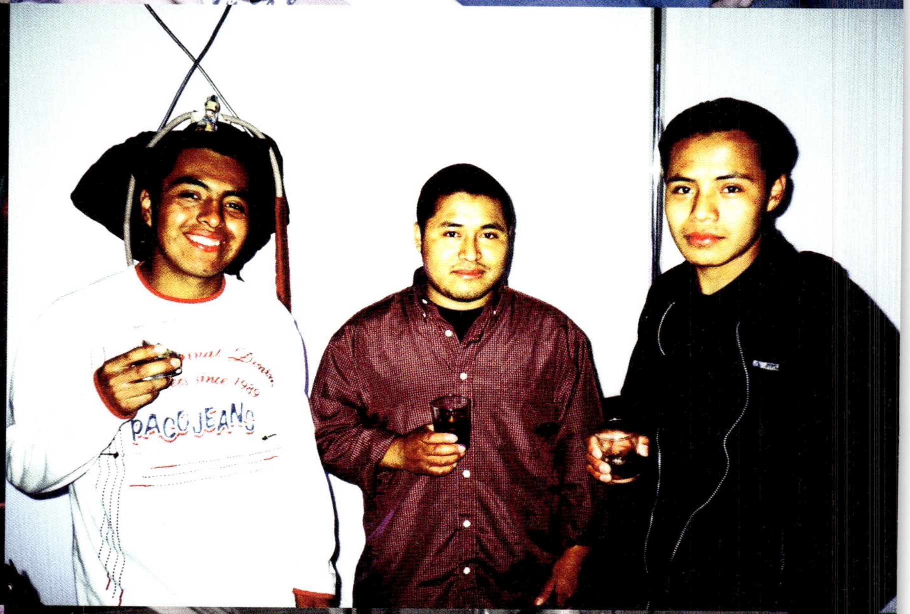
PACO JEANS

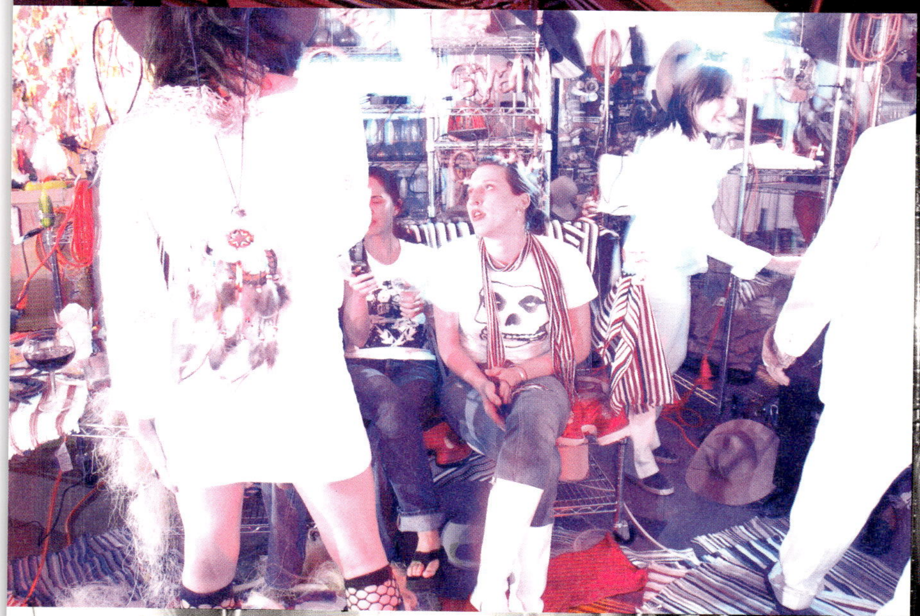

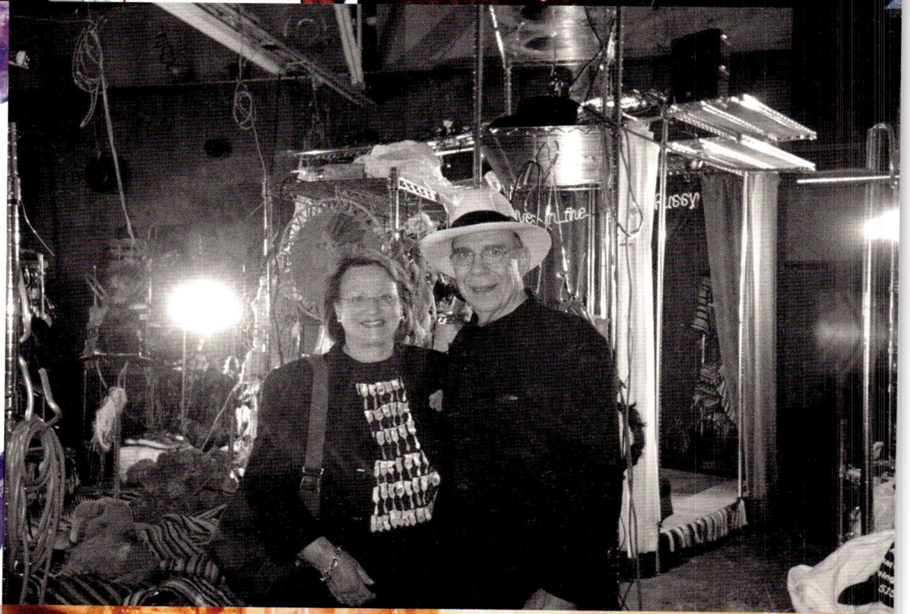

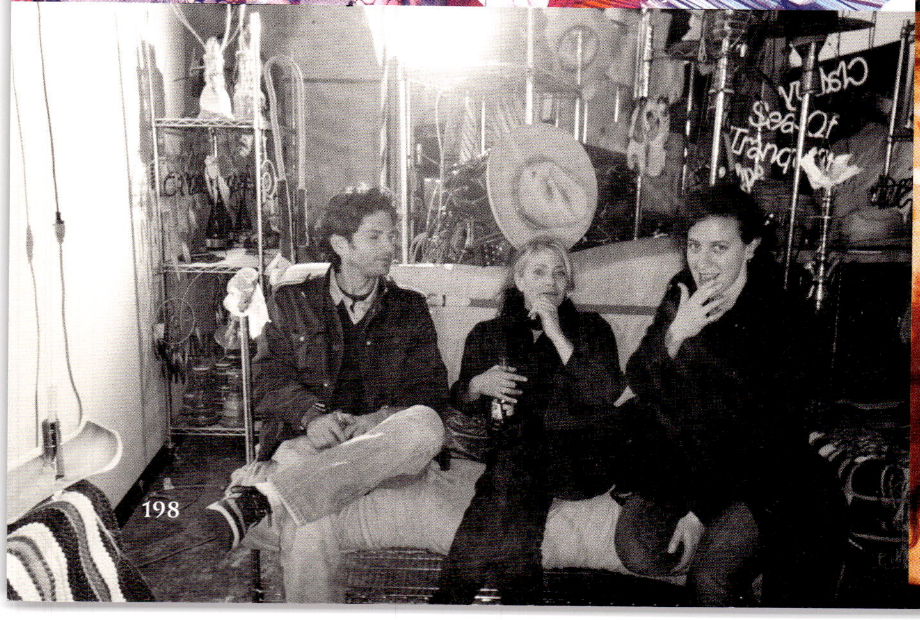

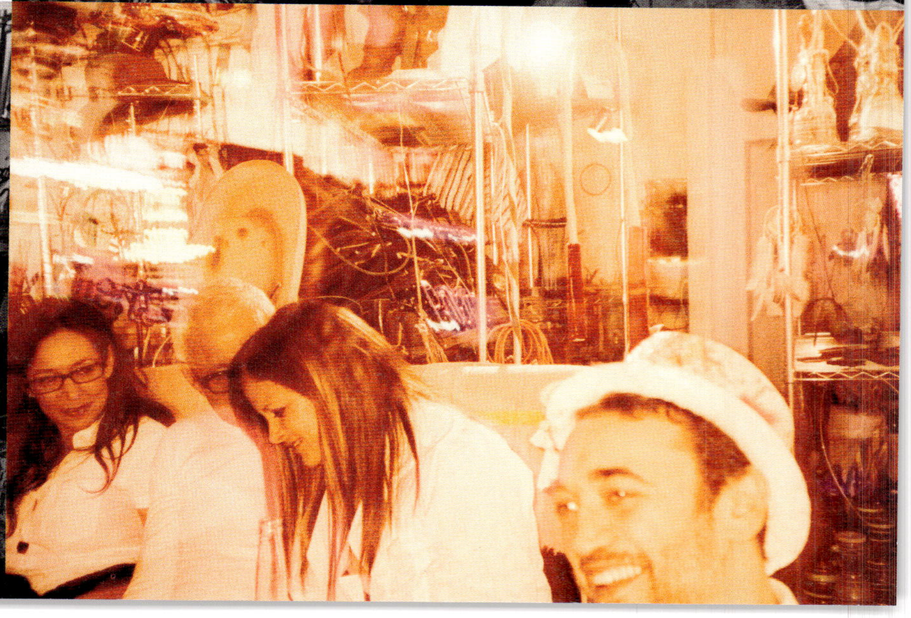

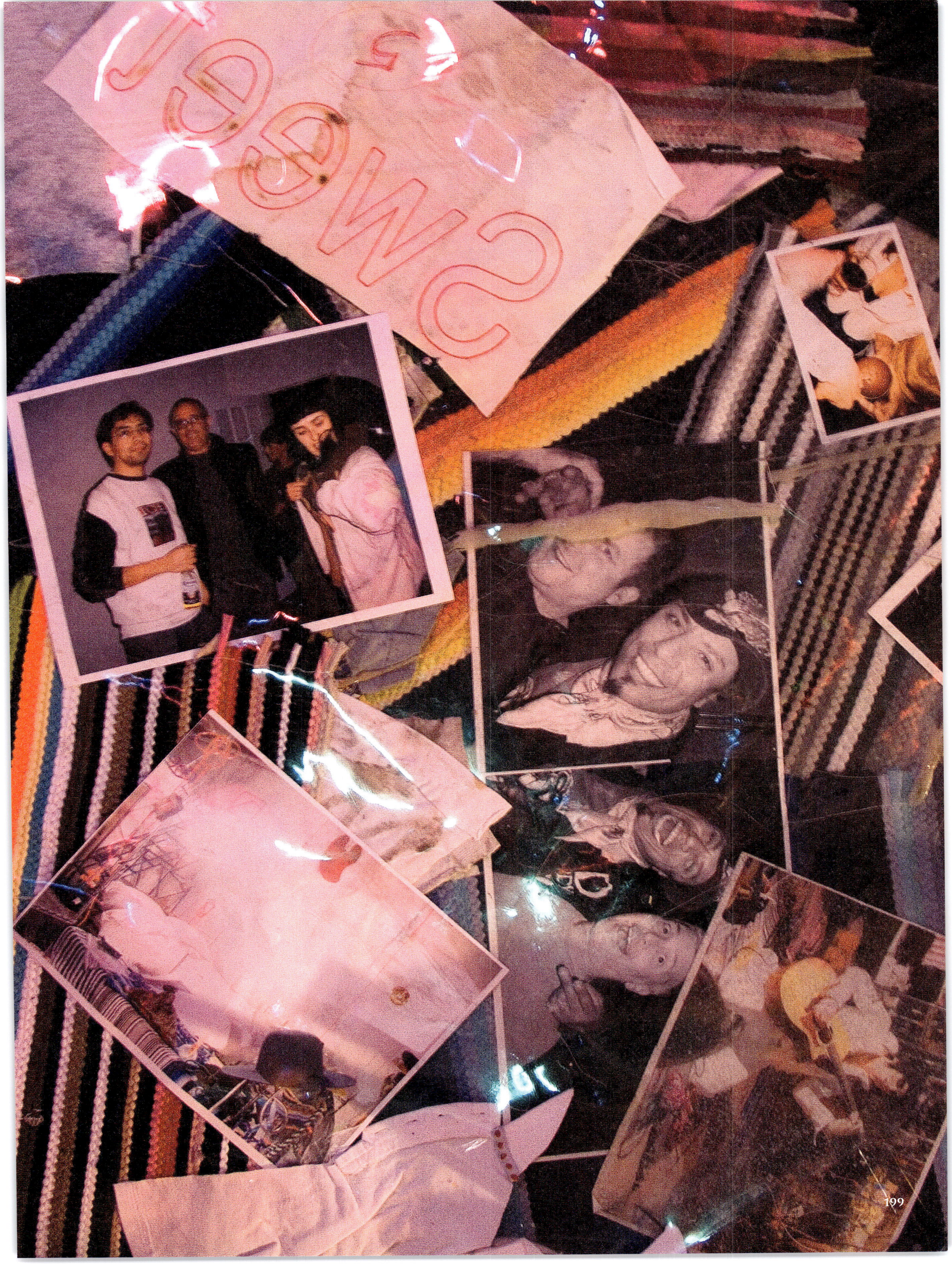
Sweet

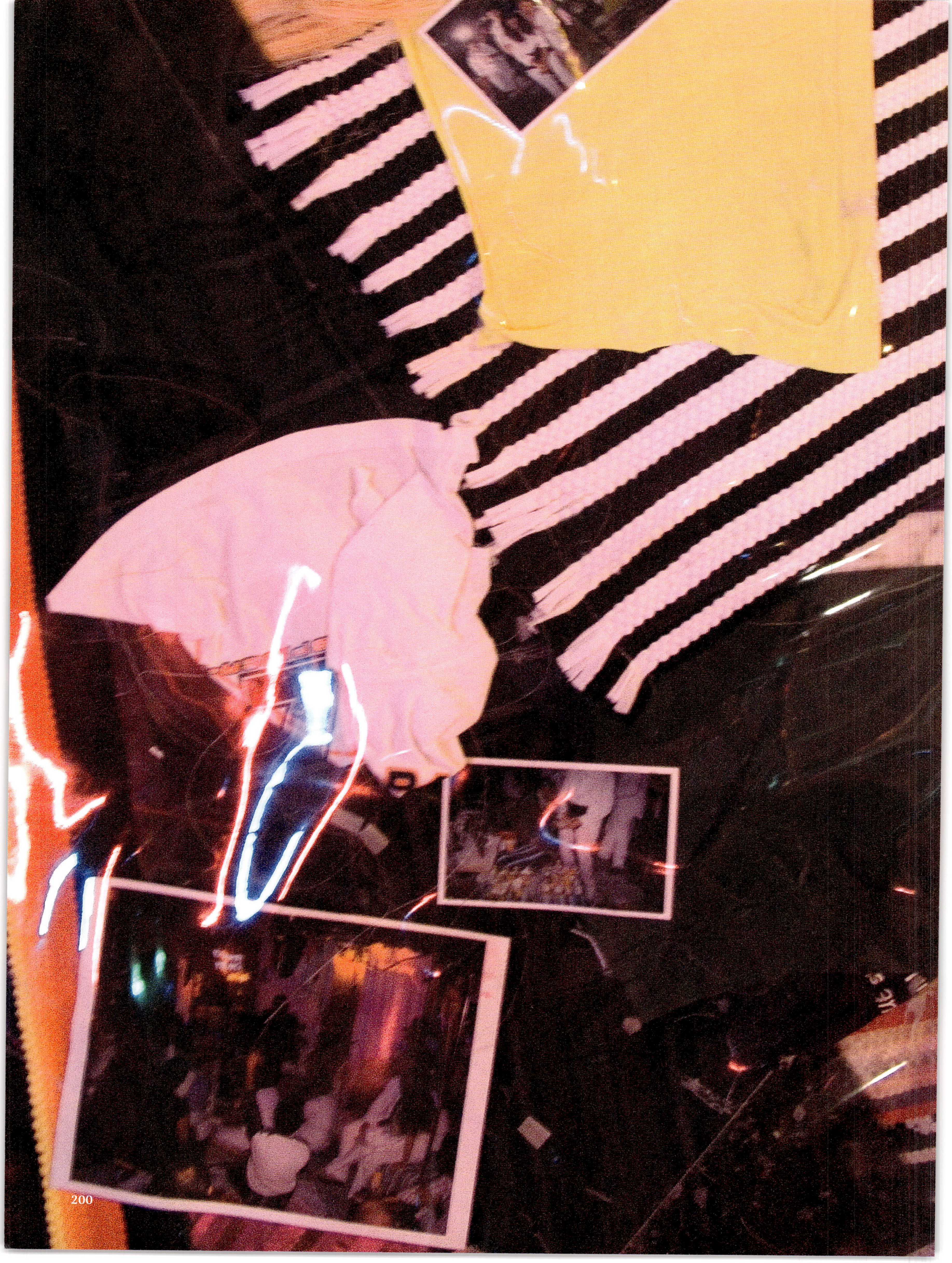

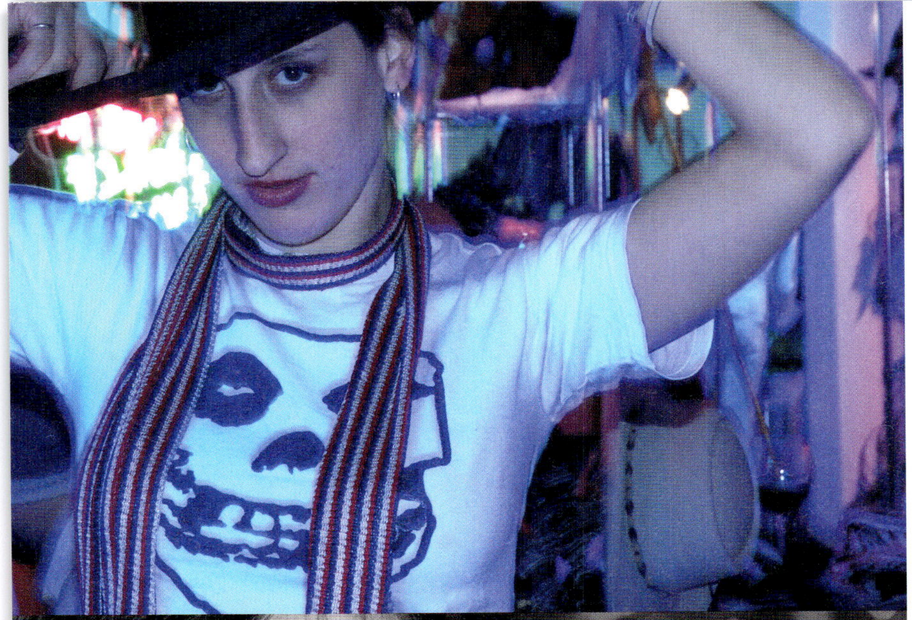

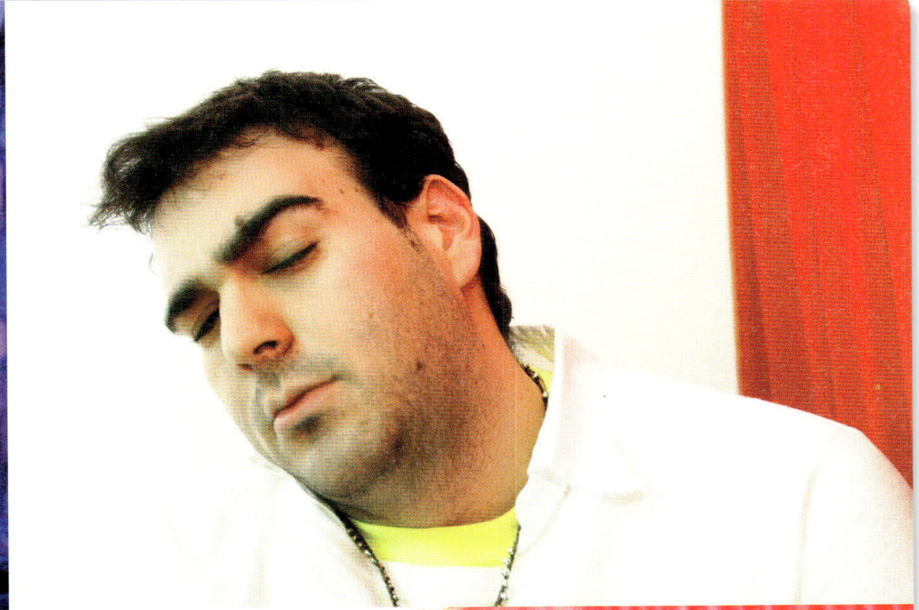

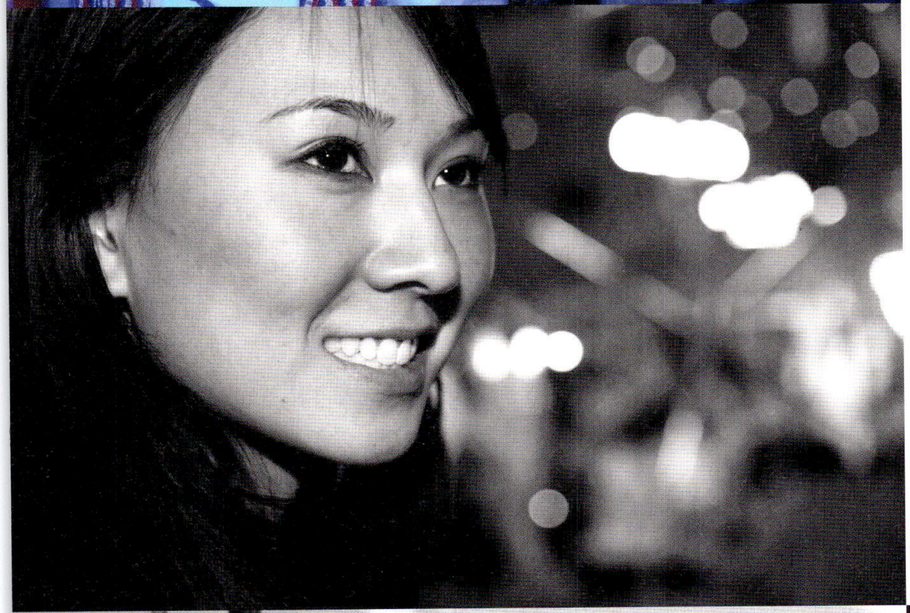

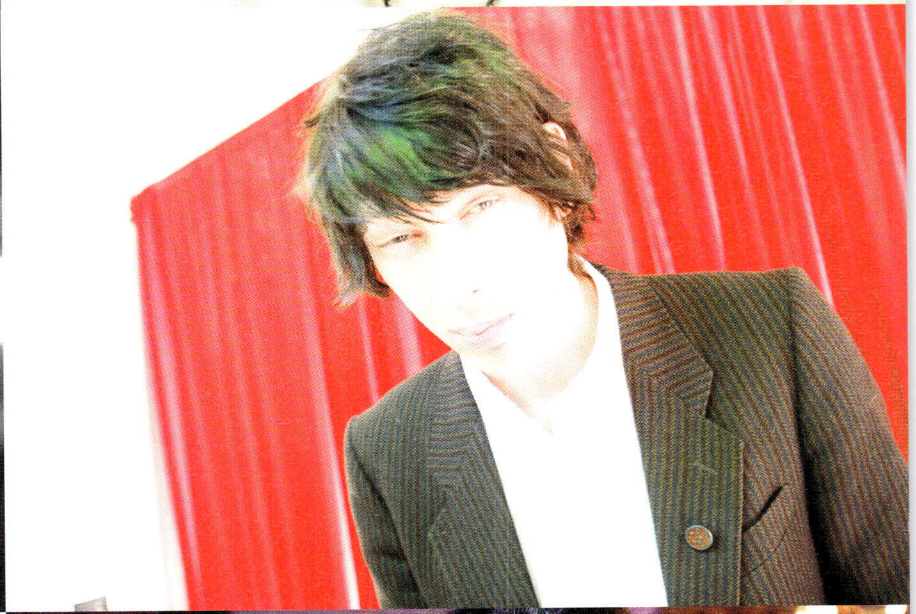

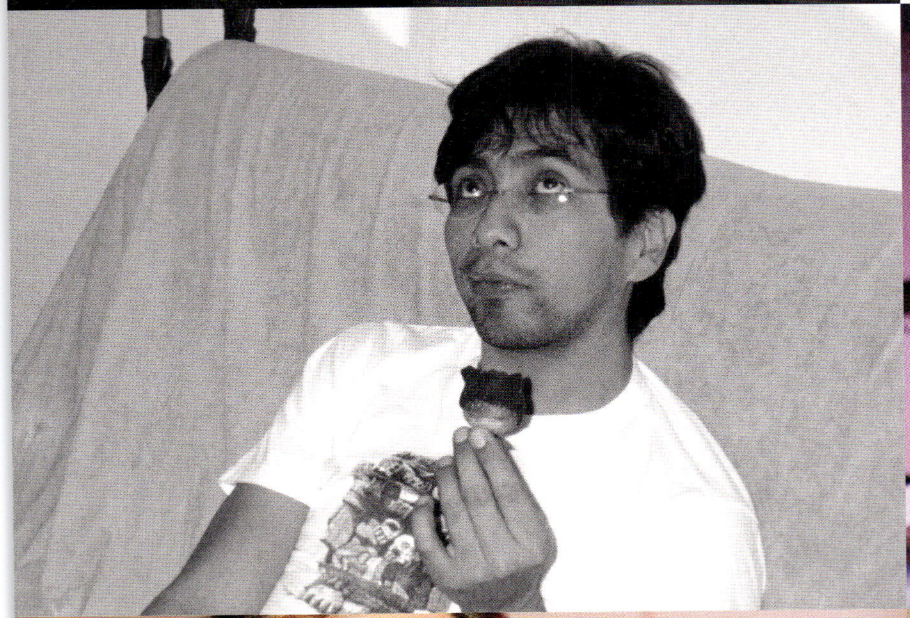

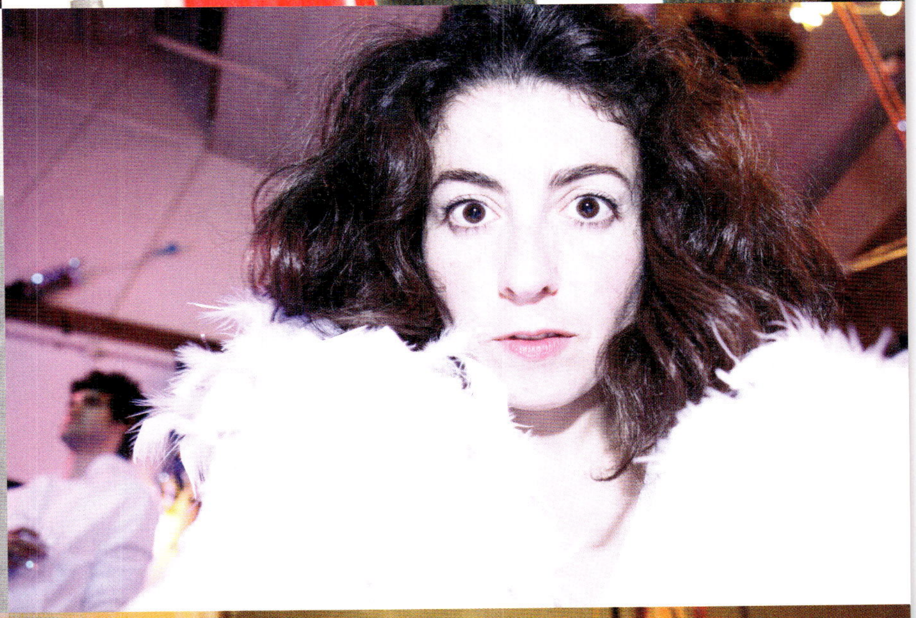

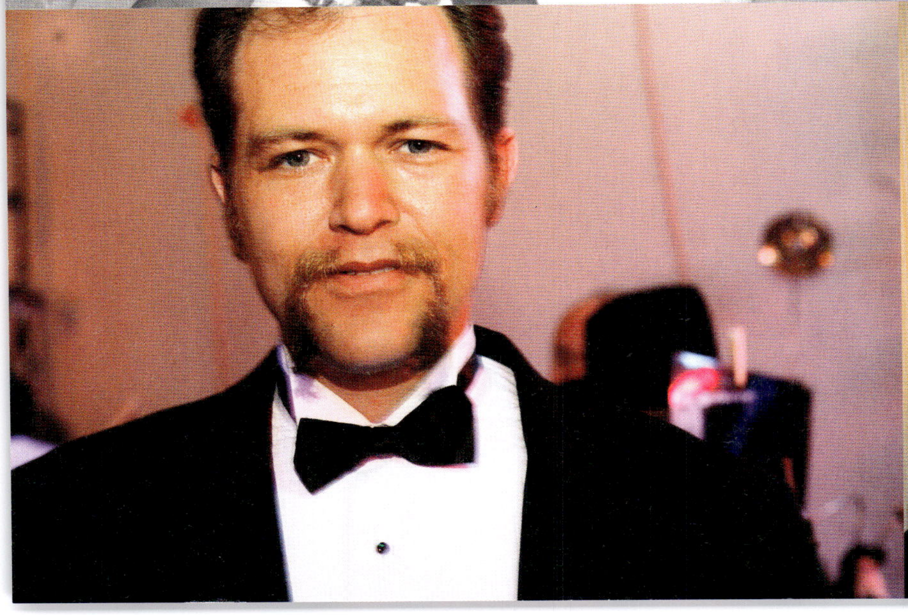

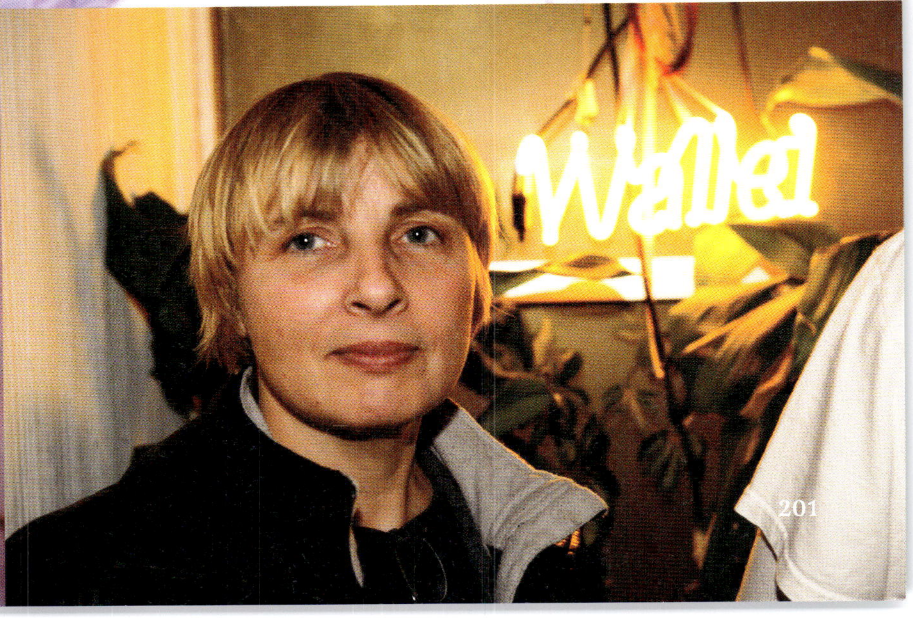

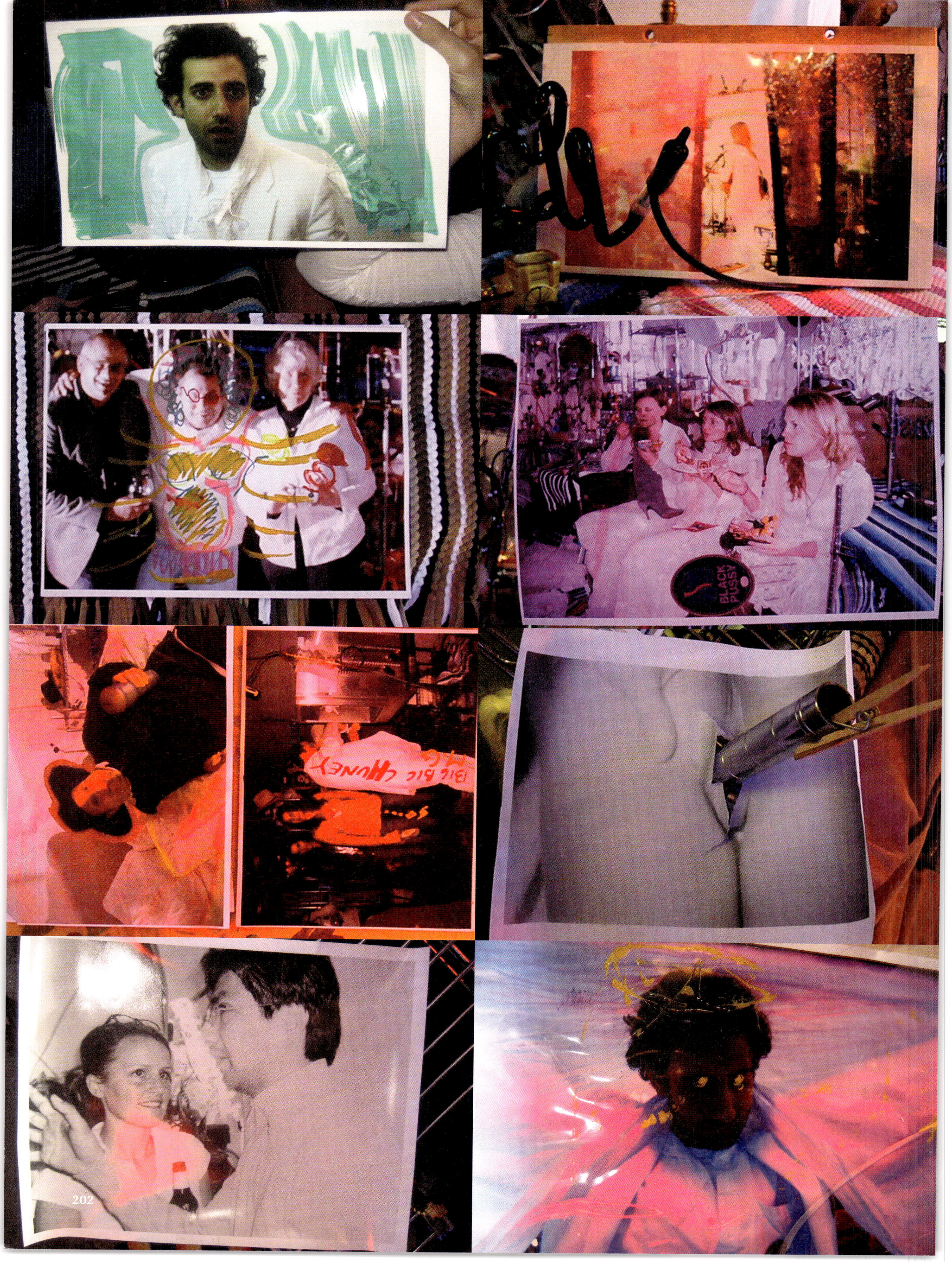
BLACK PUSSY

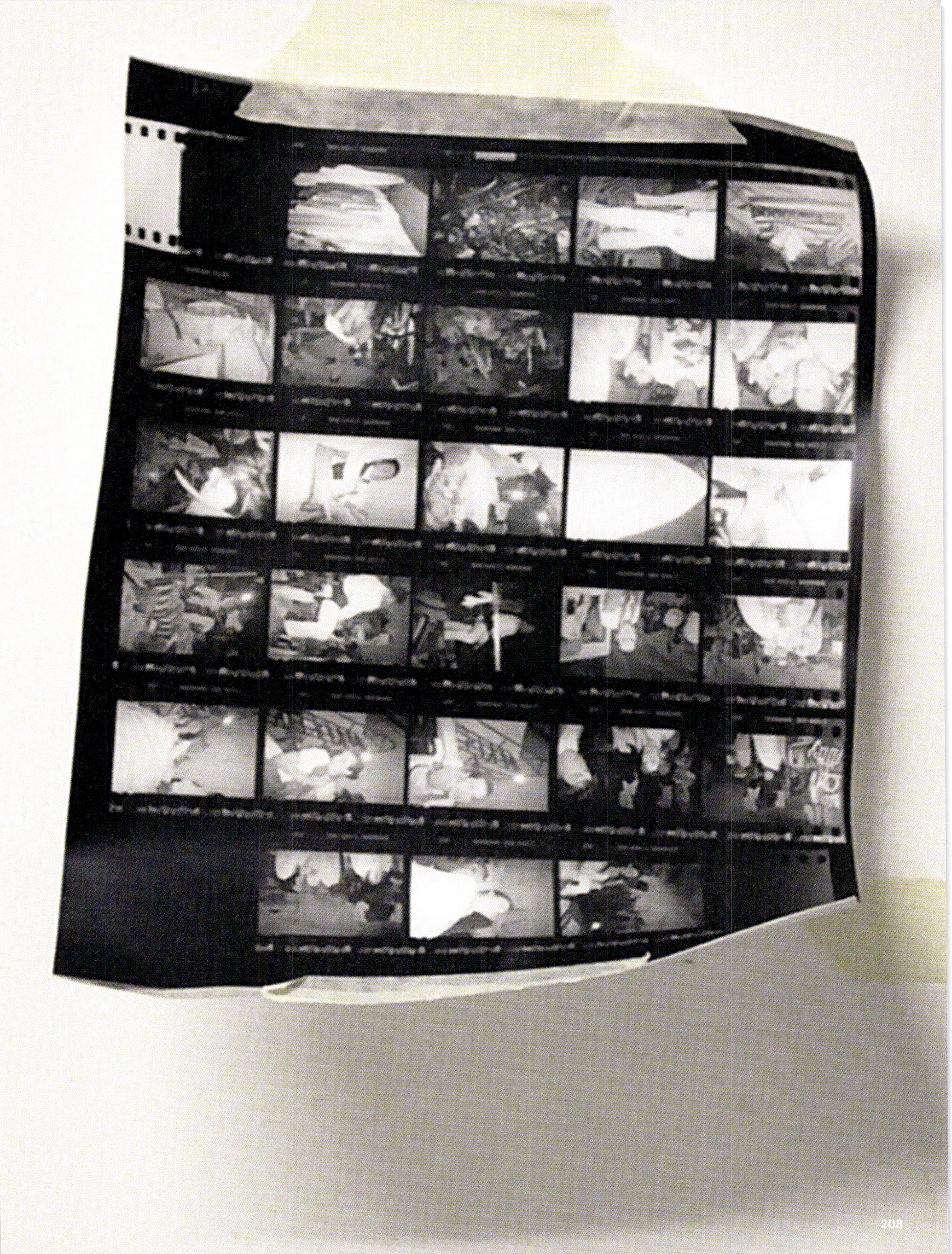

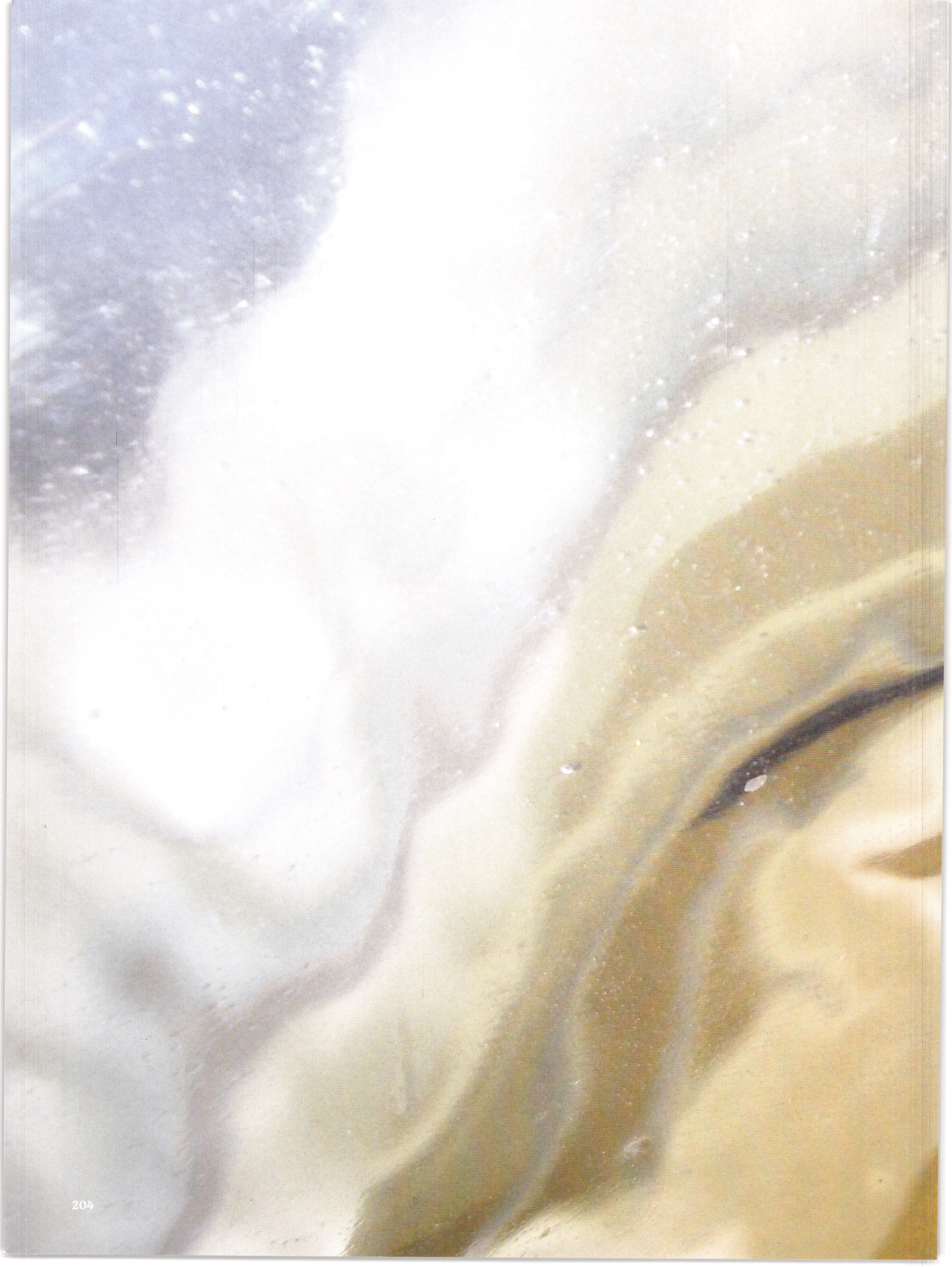

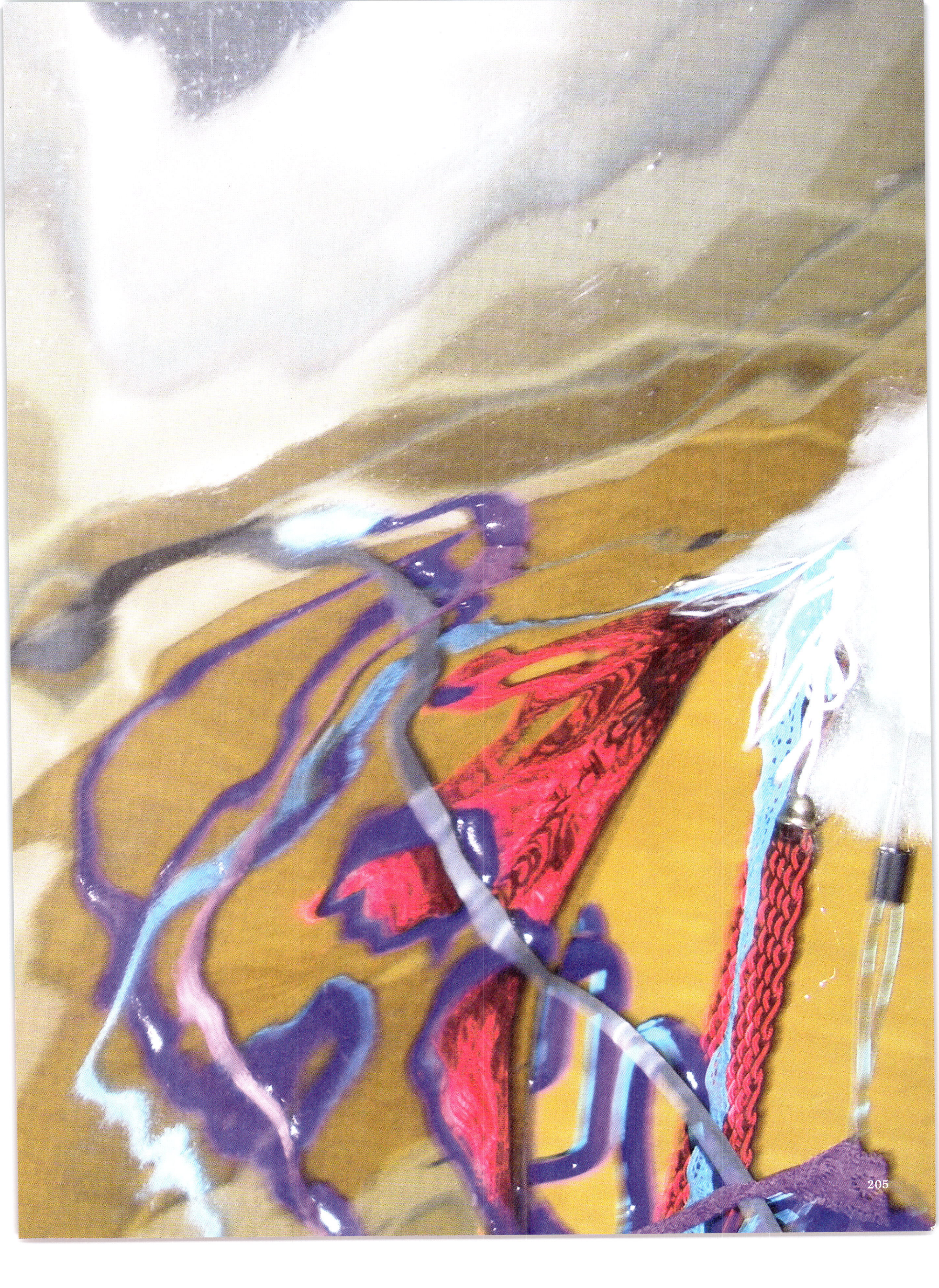

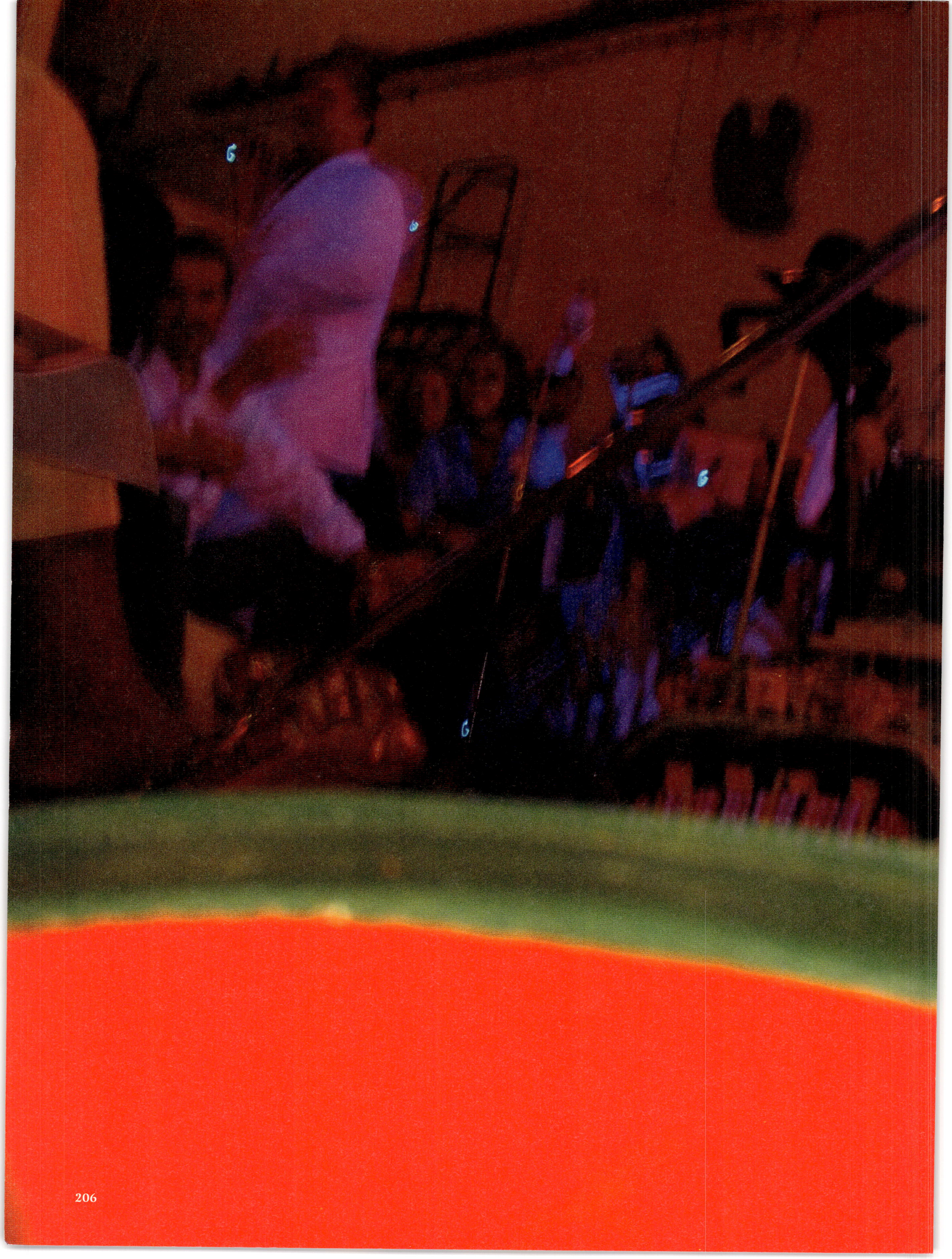

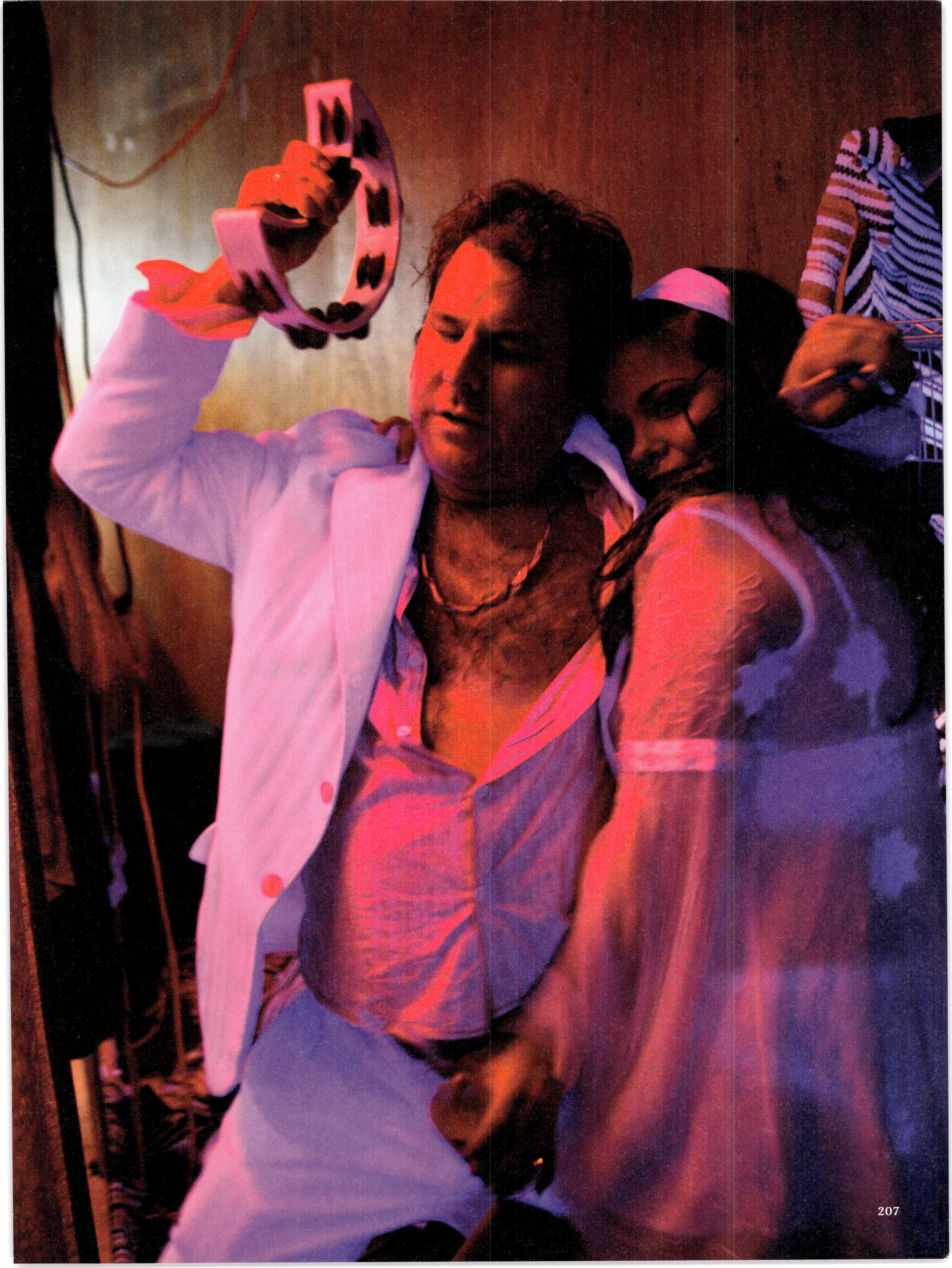

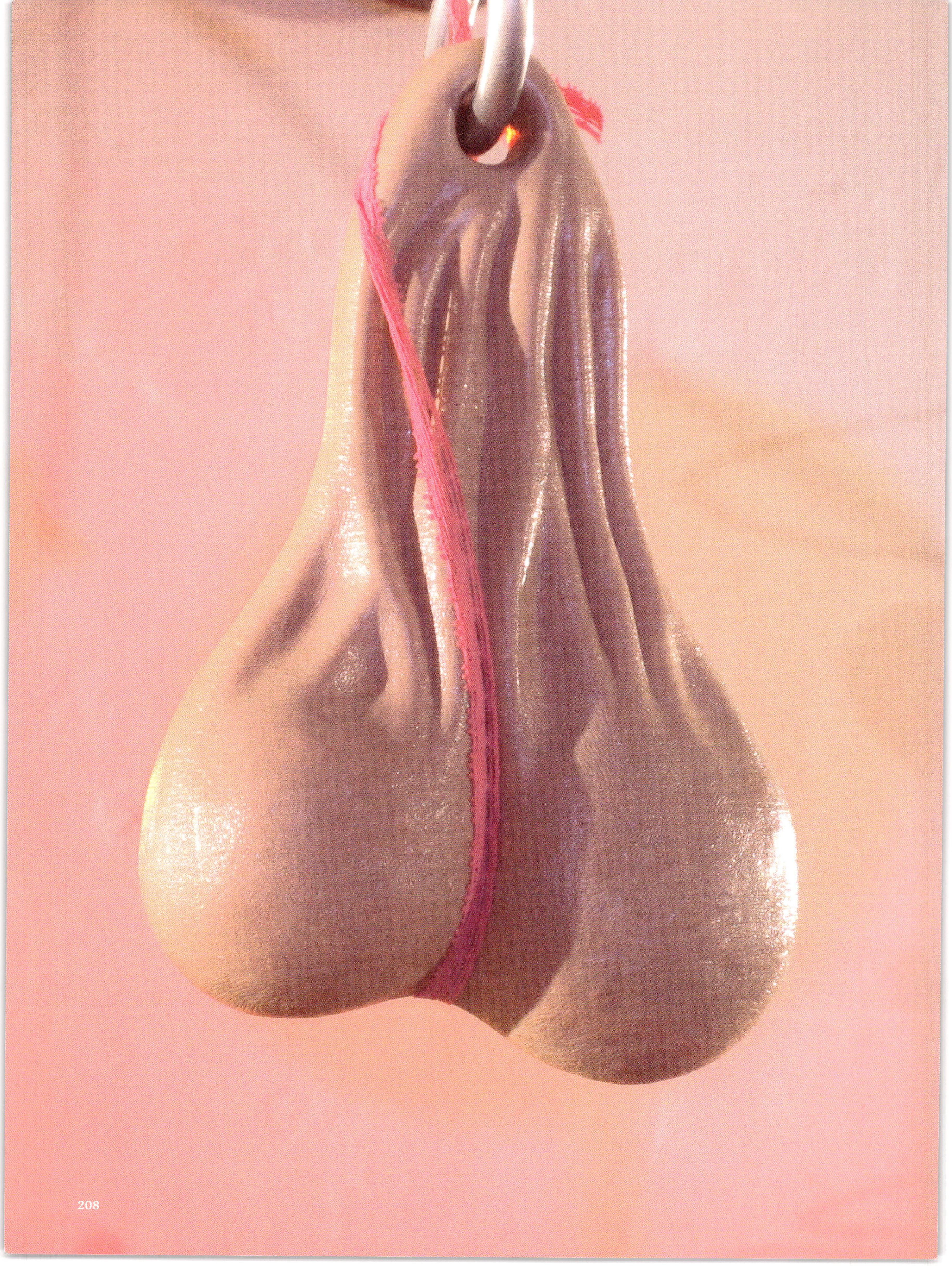

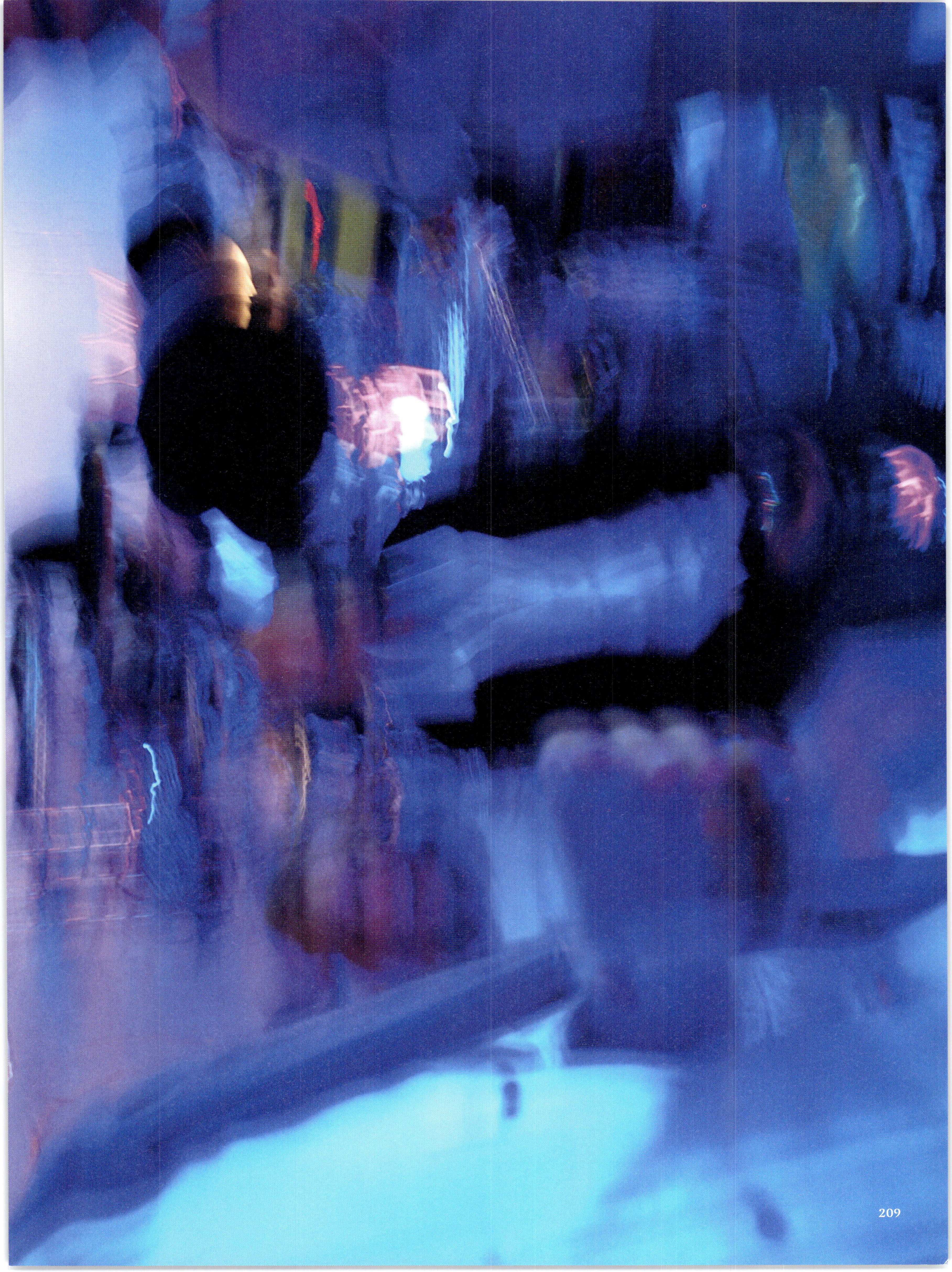

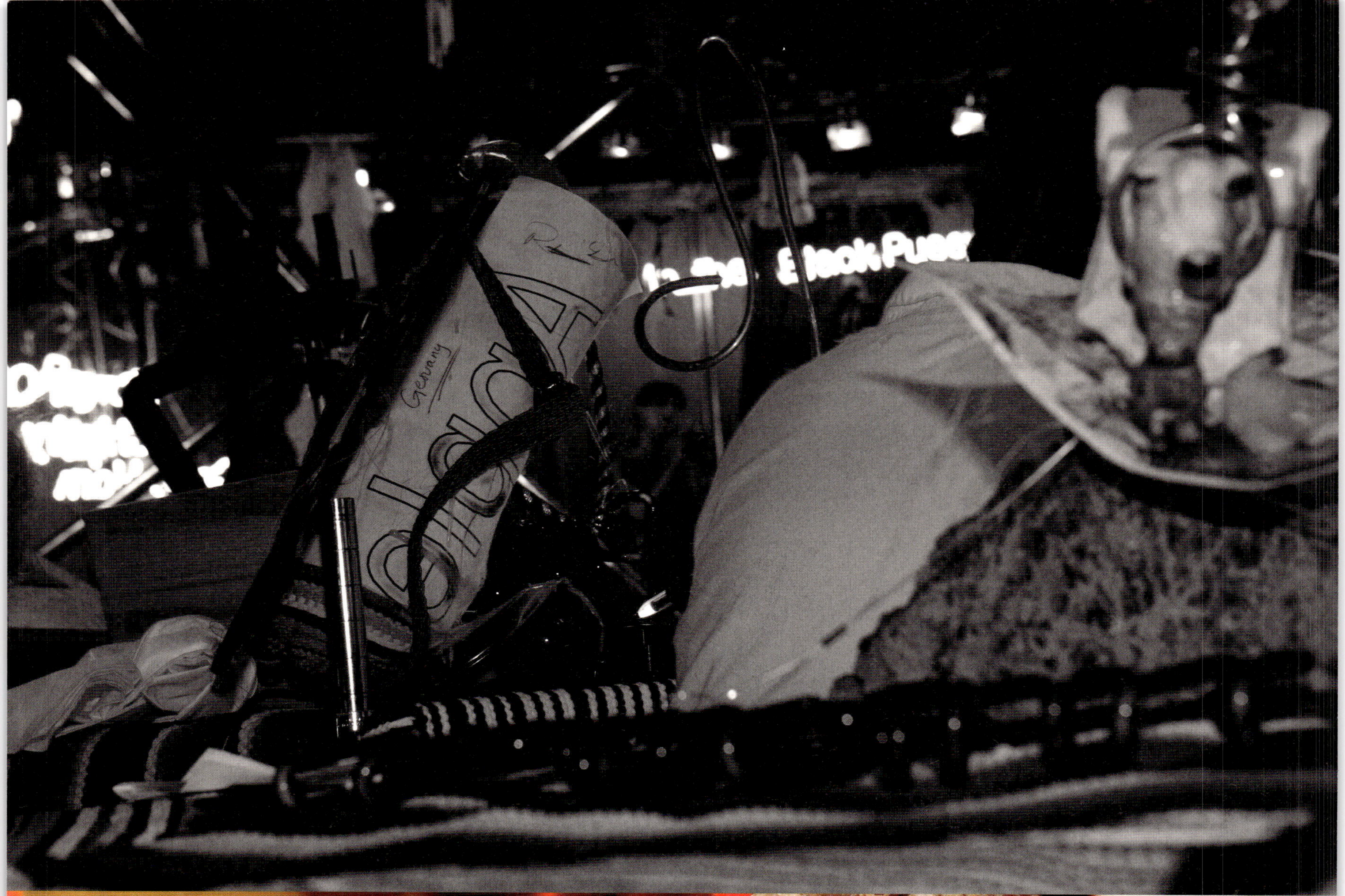

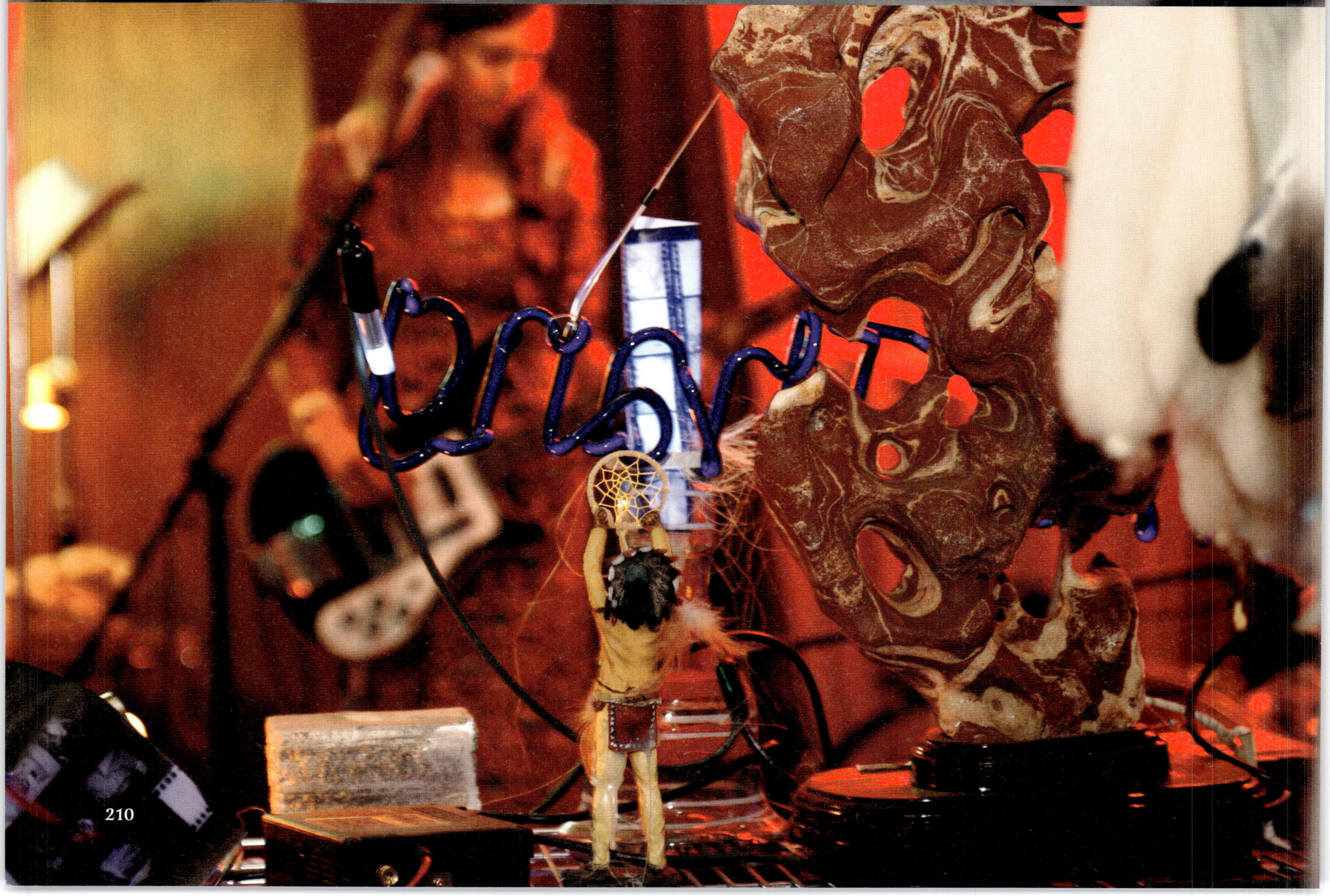

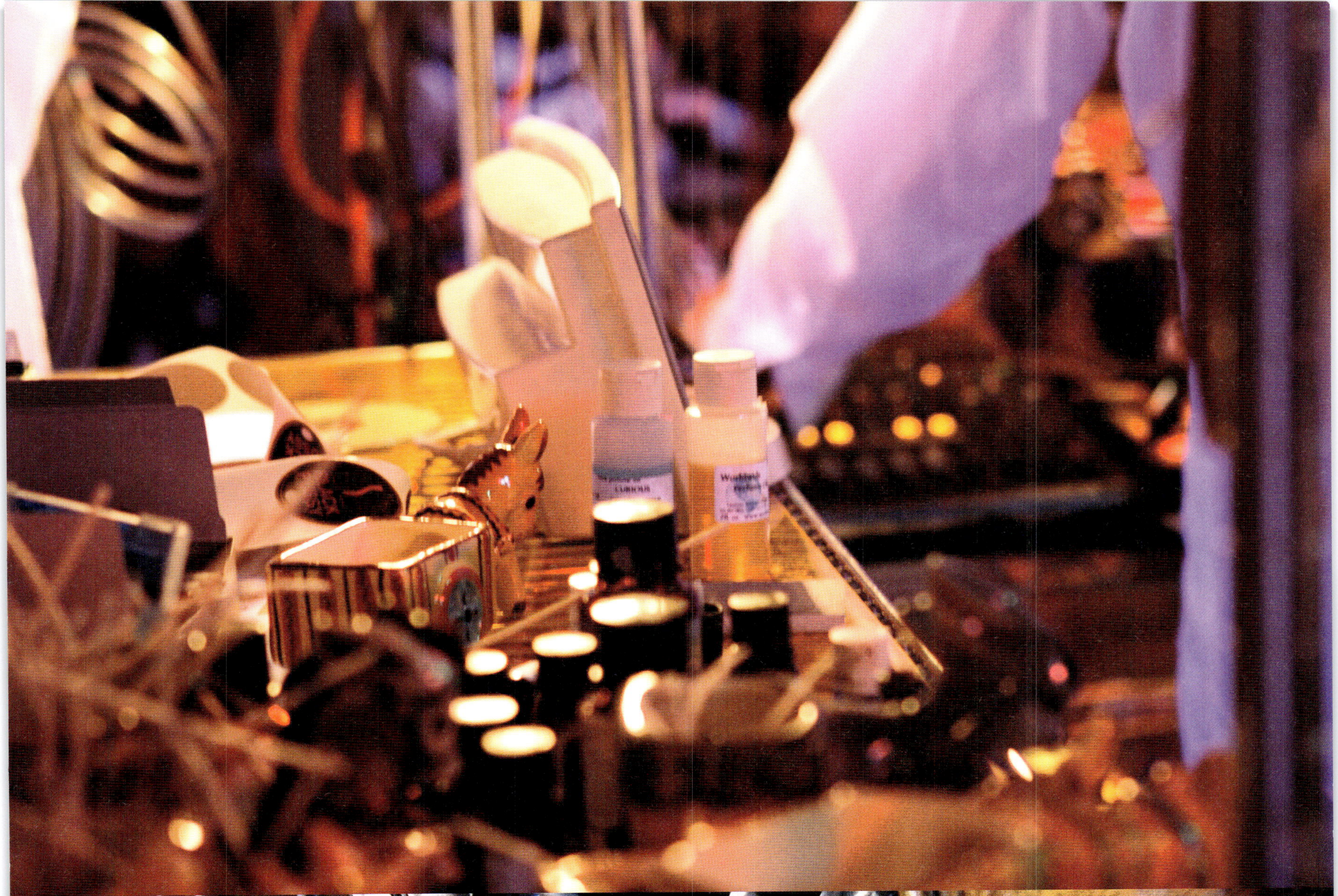

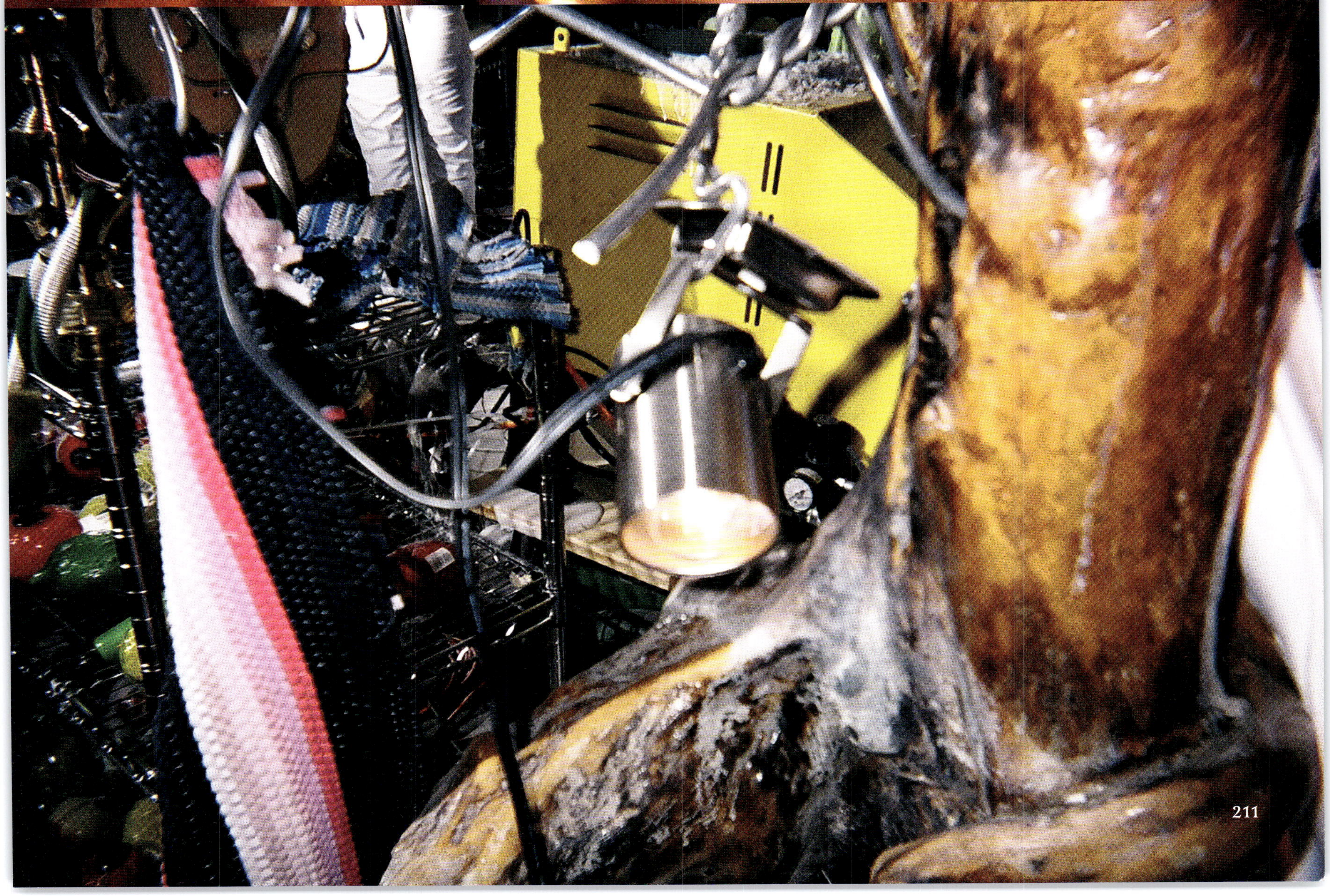

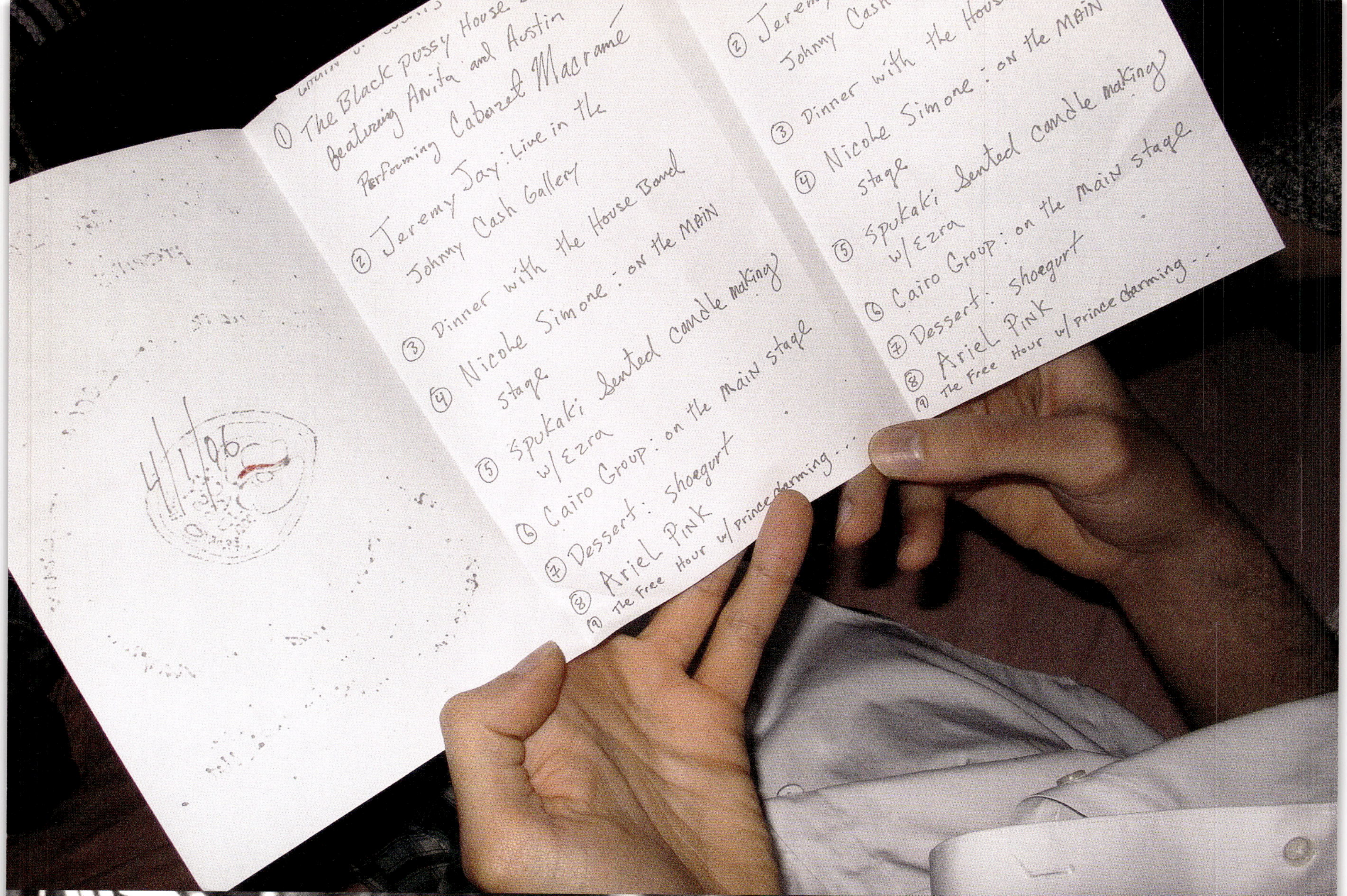
4/1/06
① The Black pussy House featuring Anita and Austin Performing Cabaret Macramé
② Jeremy Jay: Live in the Johnny Cash Gallery
③ Dinner with the House Band
④ Nicole Simone: on the MAIN stage
⑤ Spukaki Sented candle making w/Ezra
⑥ Cairo Group: on the main stage
⑦ Dessert: shoegurt
⑧ Ariel Pink
⑨ The Free Hour w/ Prince charming...

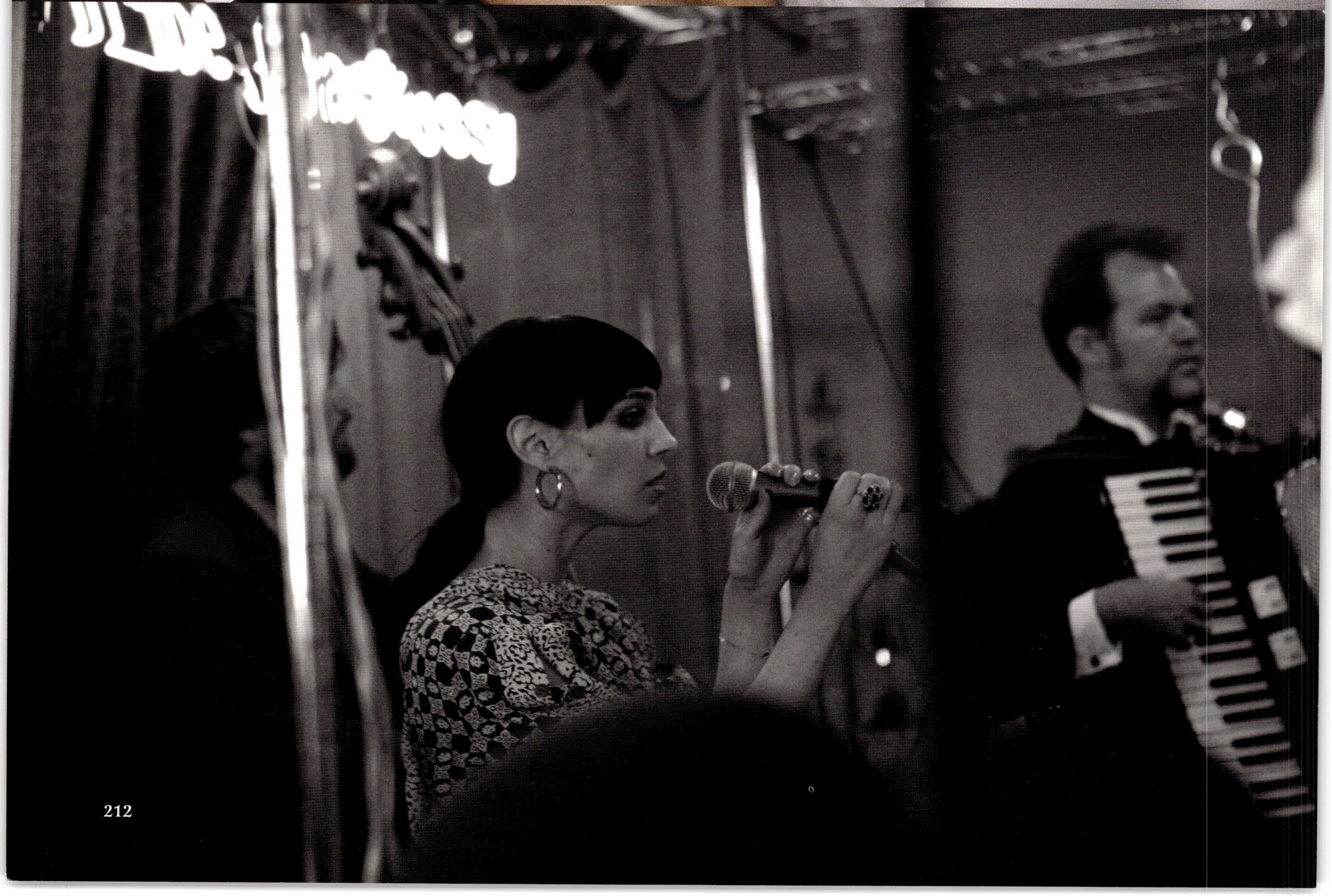

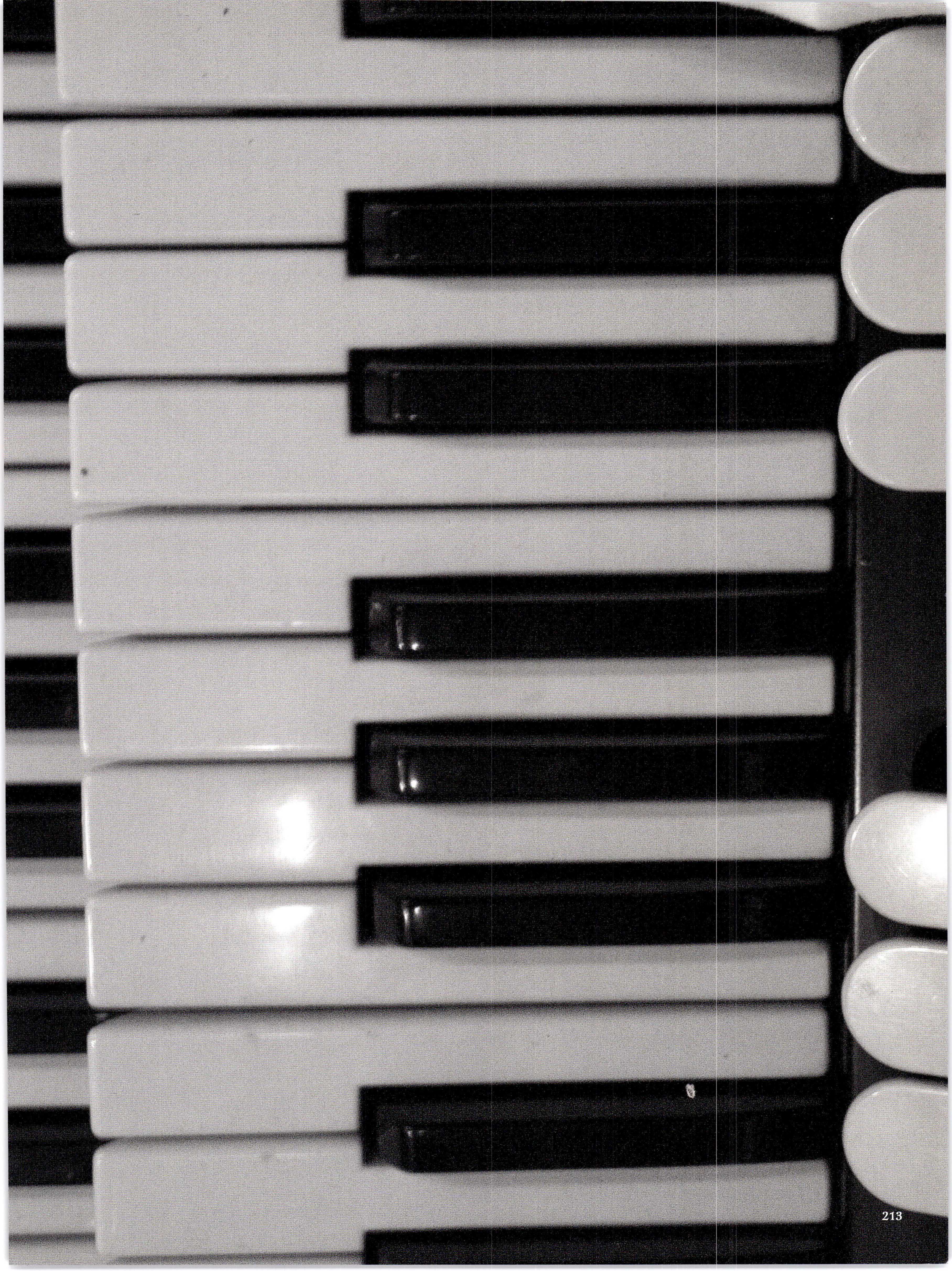

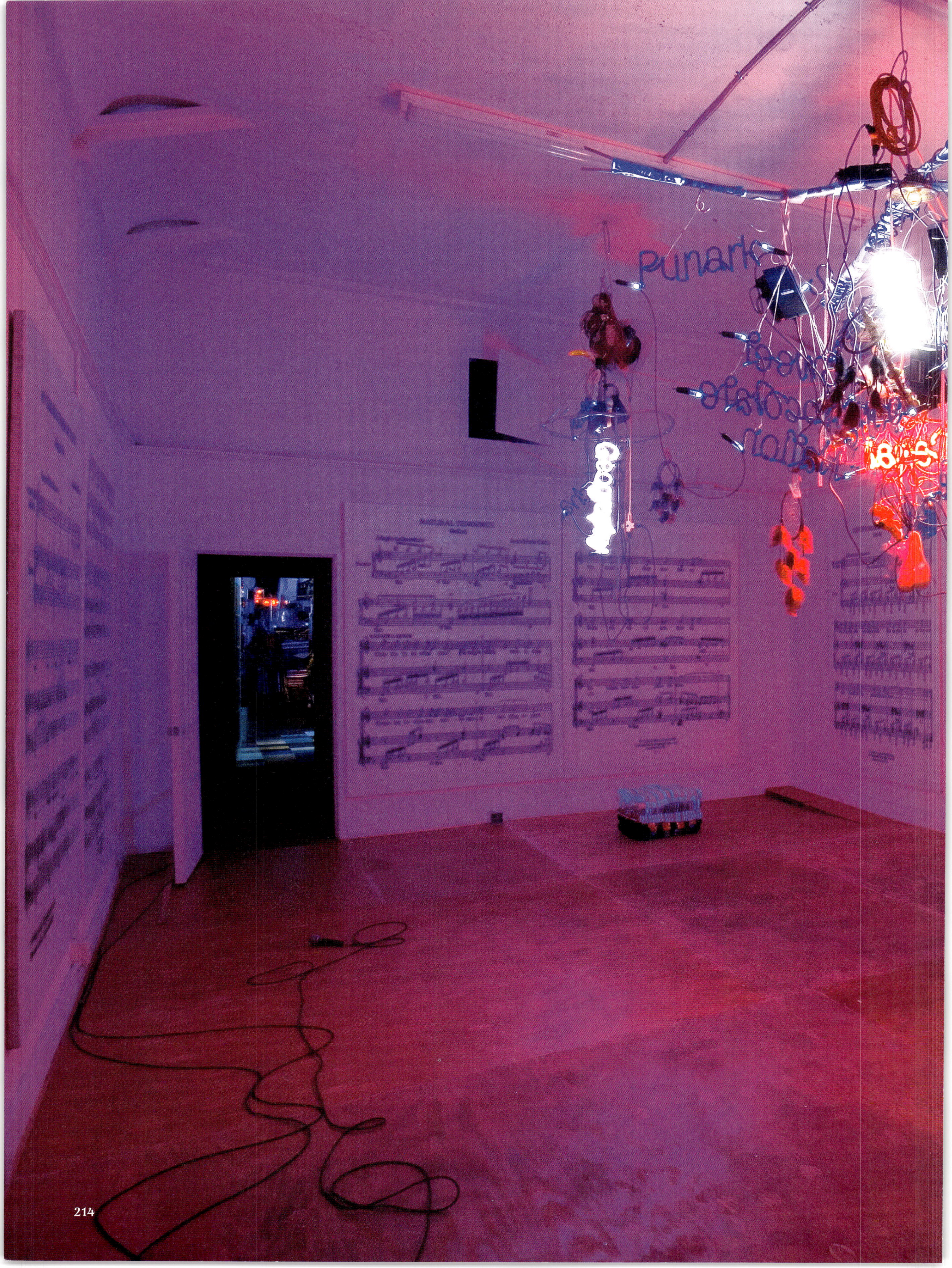
Punark

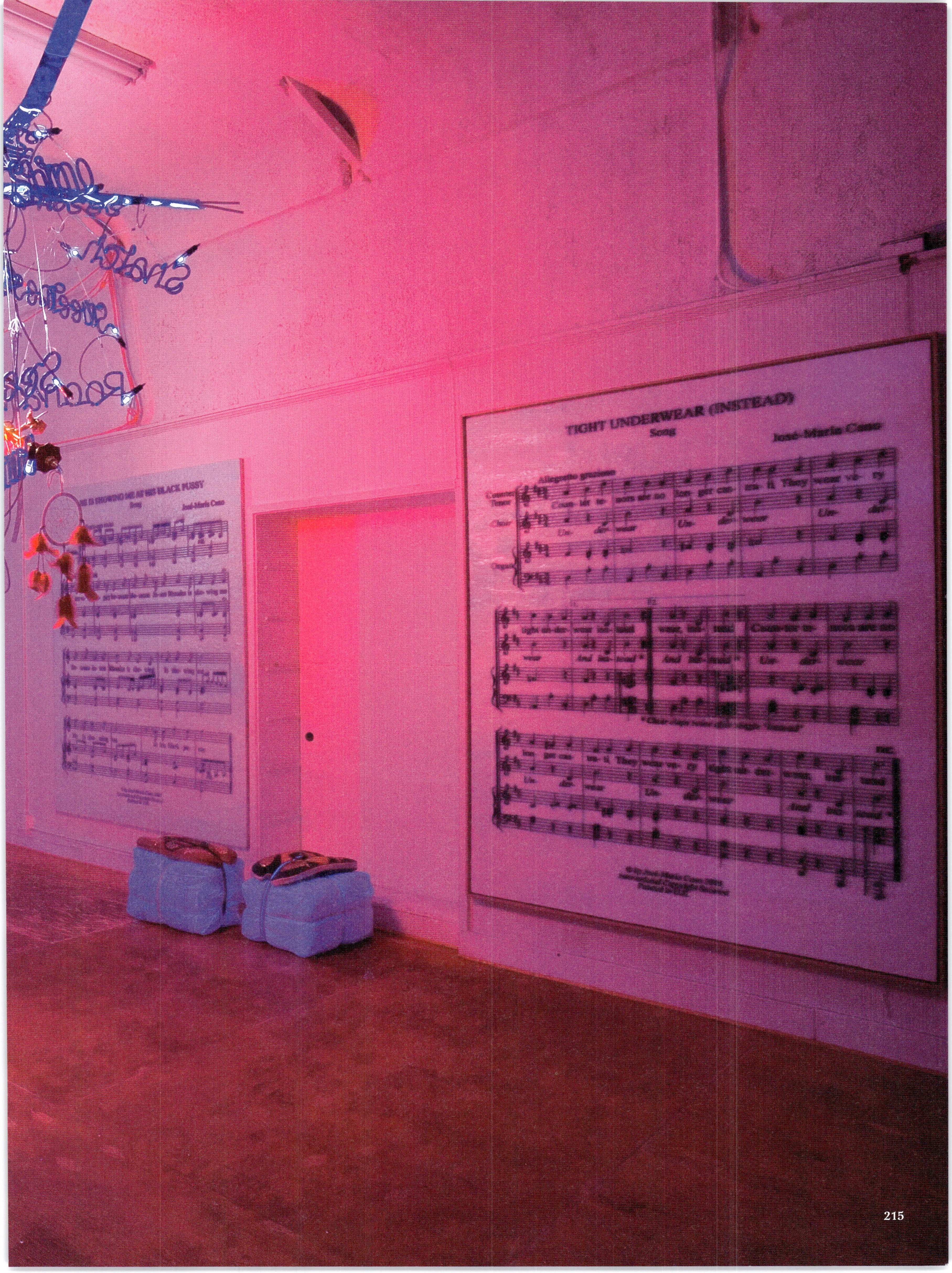
TIGHT UNDERWEAR (INSTEAD)
Song
José-Maria Cano

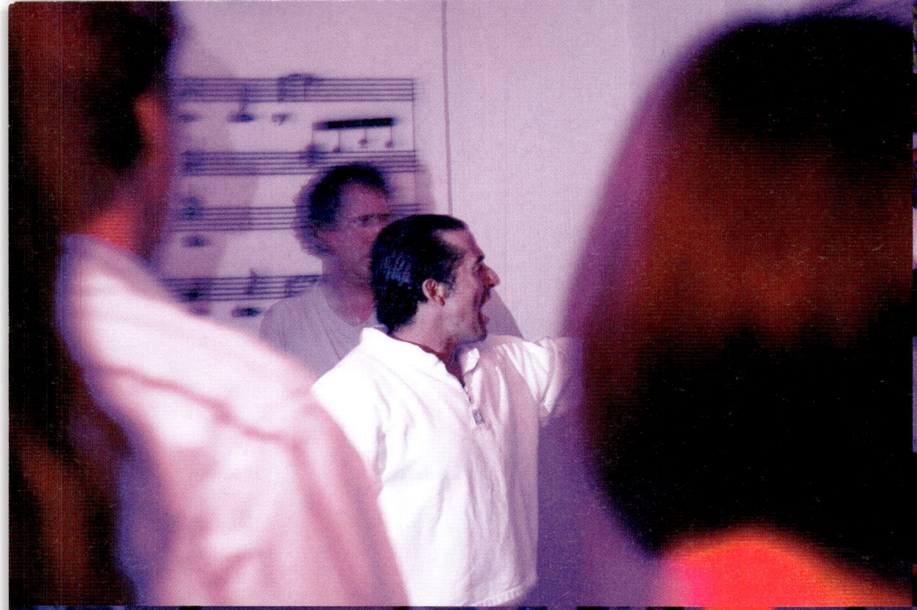
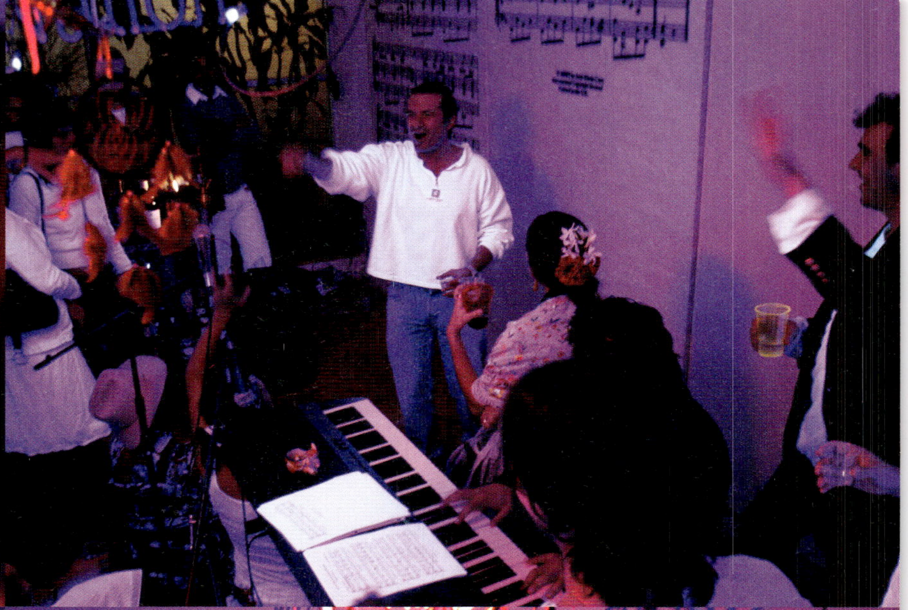
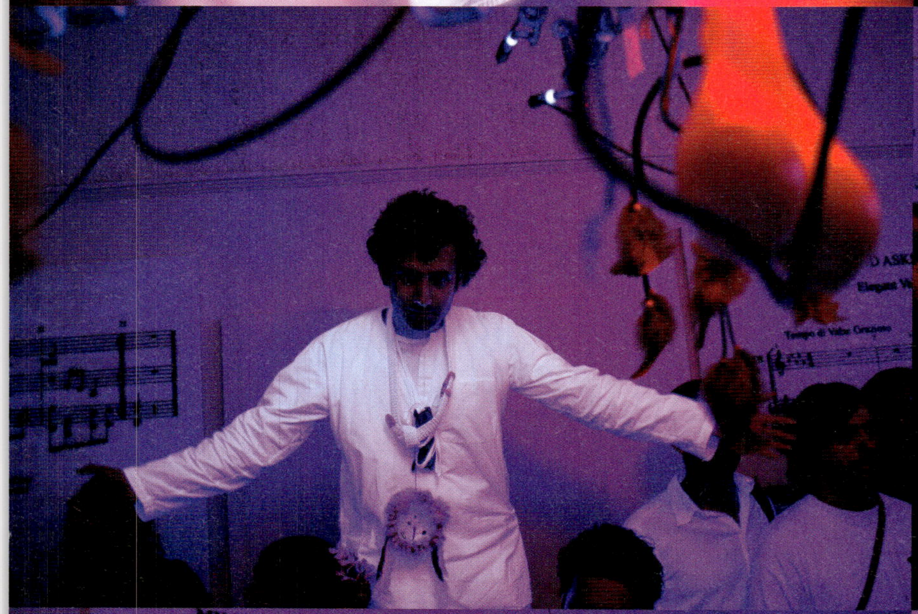
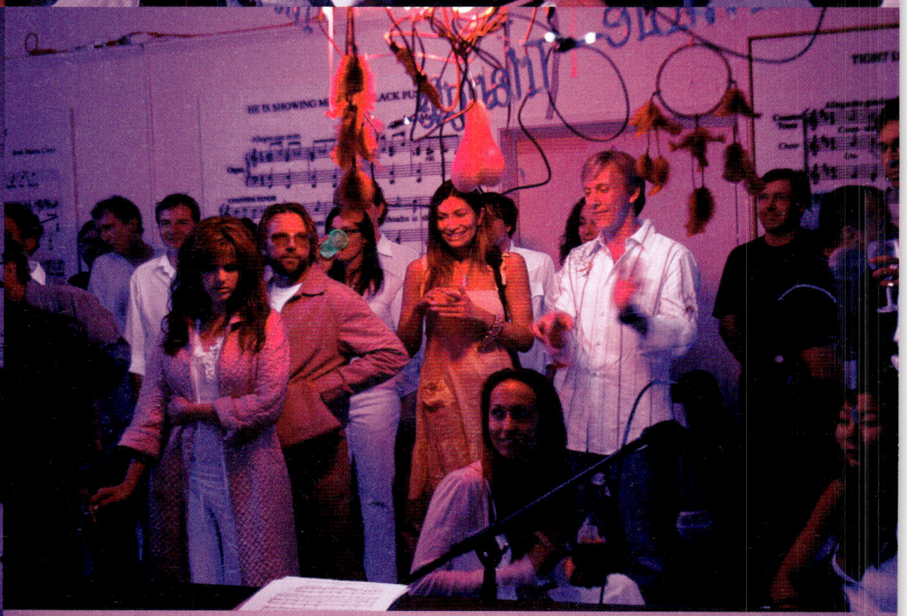
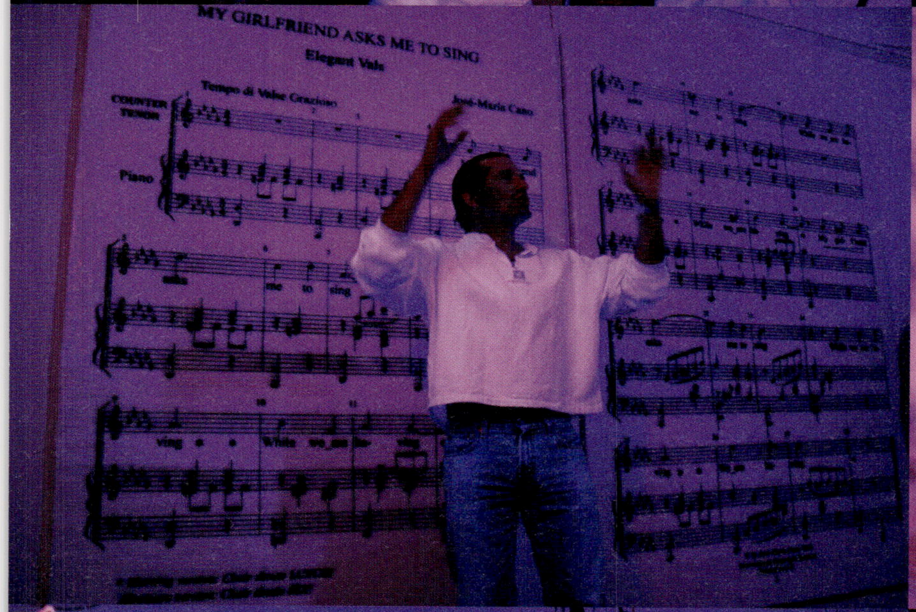
MY GIRLFRIEND ASKS ME TO SING
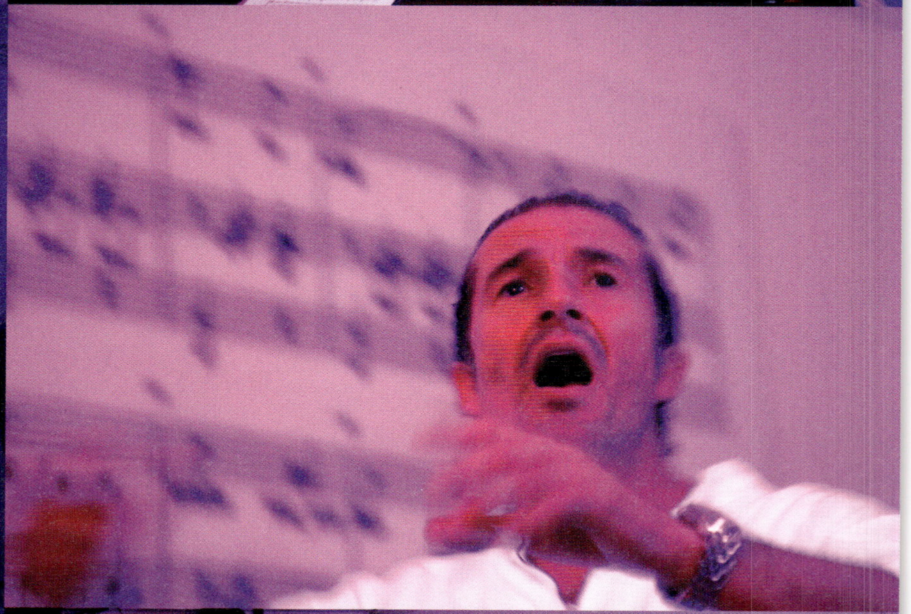
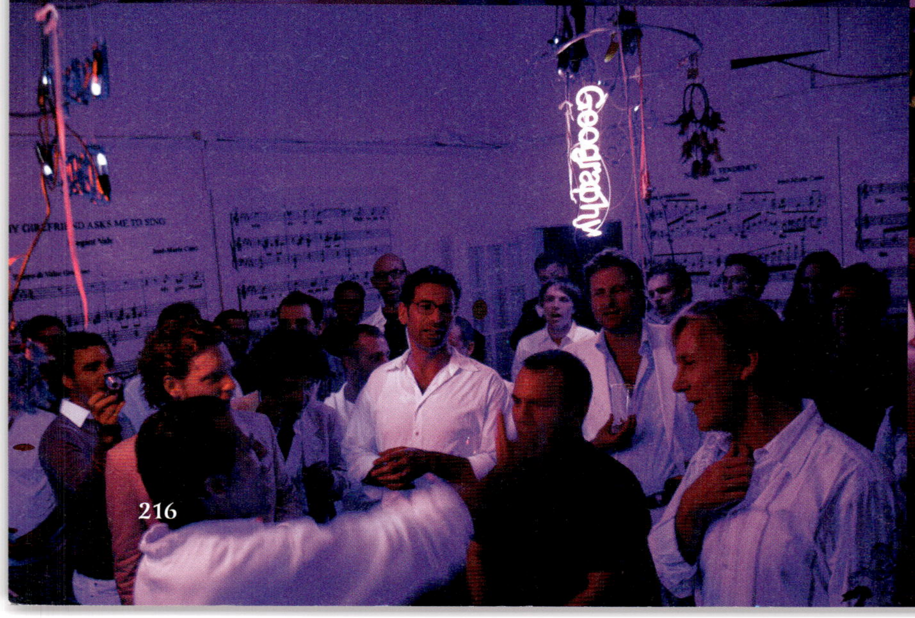
Geography
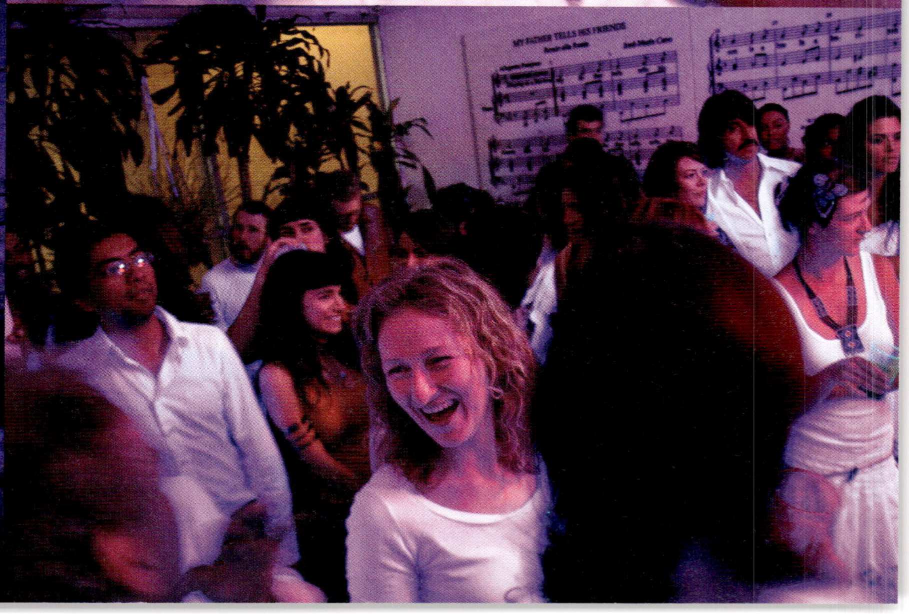

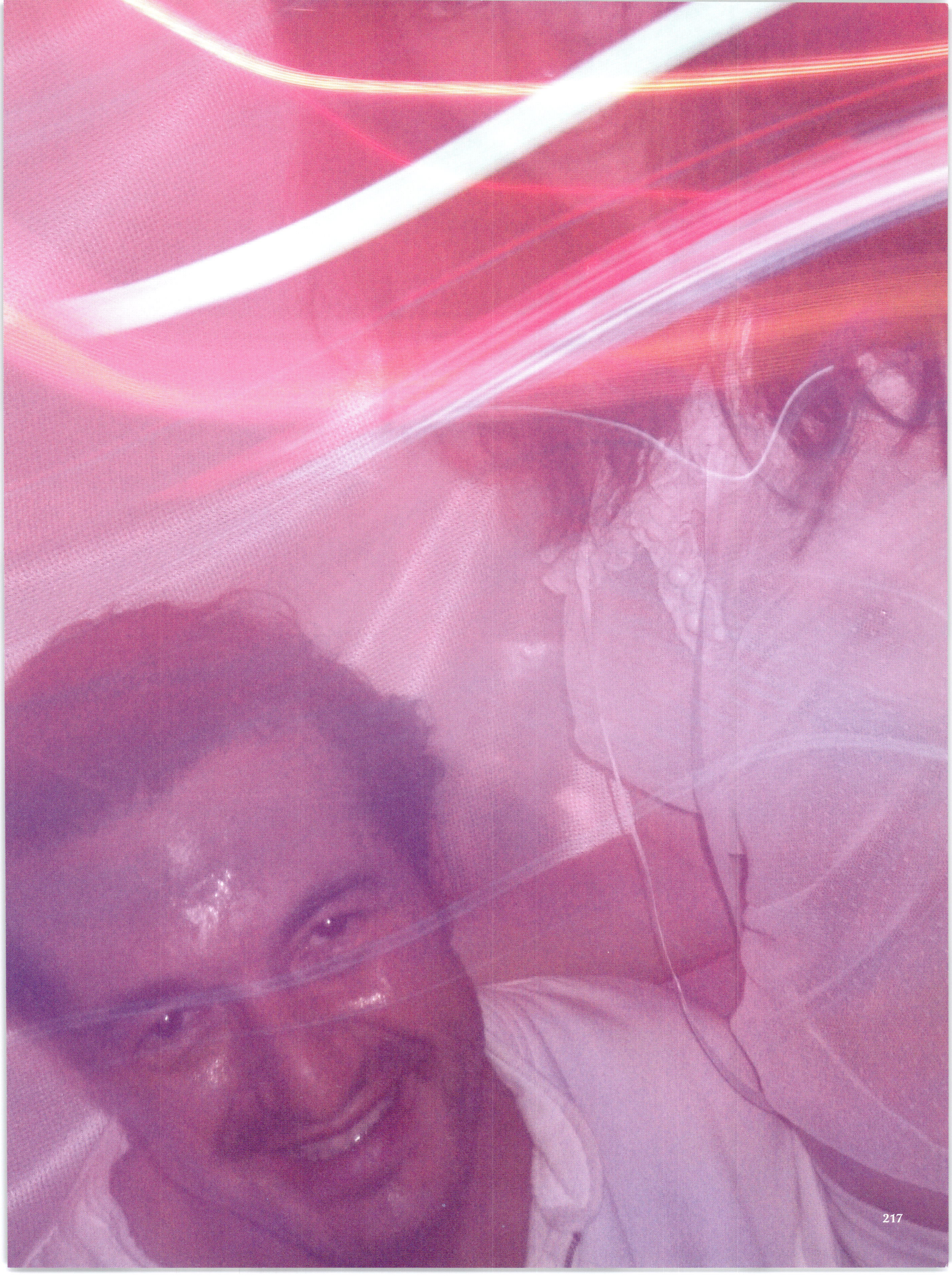

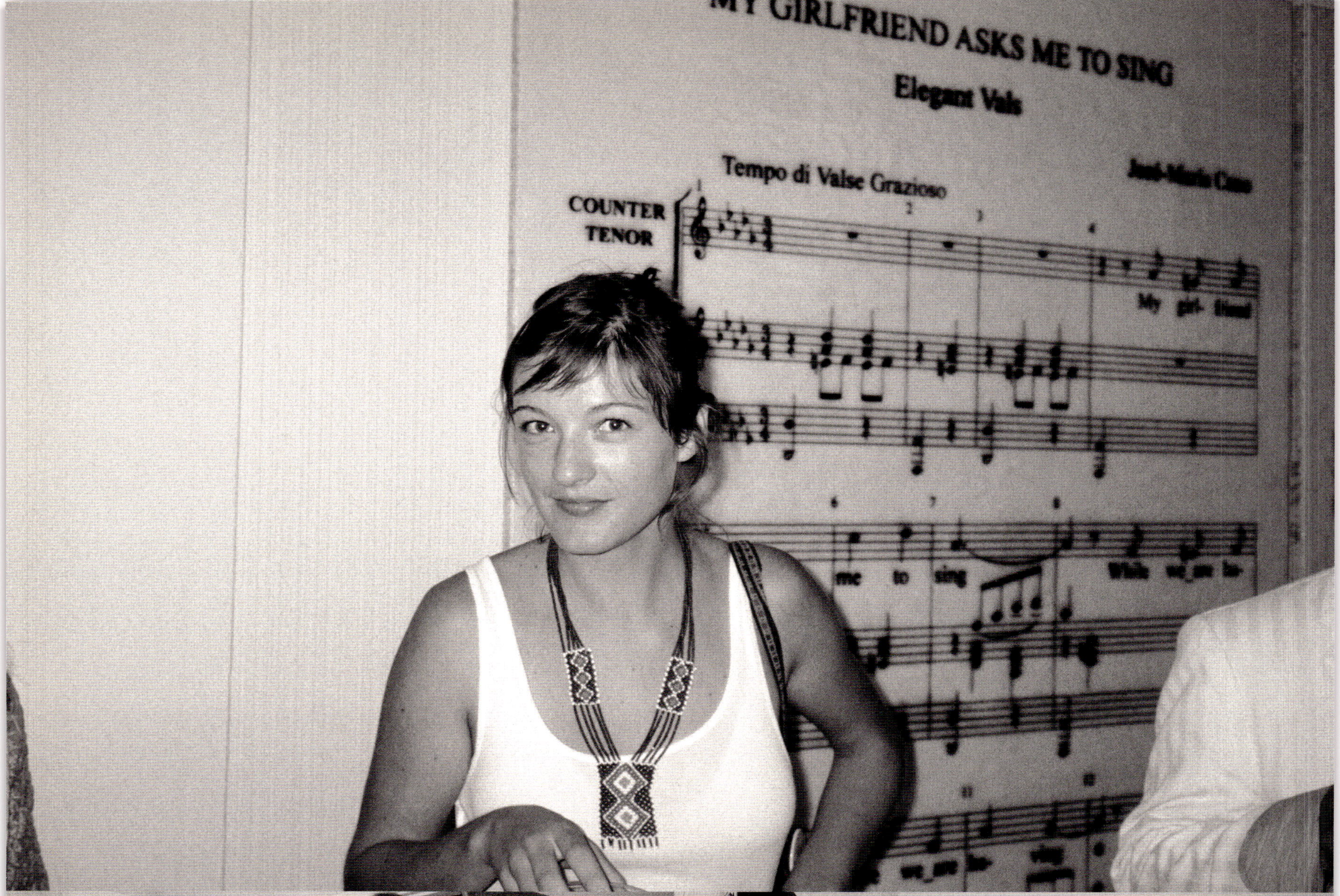
MY GIRLFRIEND ASKS ME TO SING
Elegant Vals
Tempo di Valse Grazioso
COUNTER TENOR
me to sing

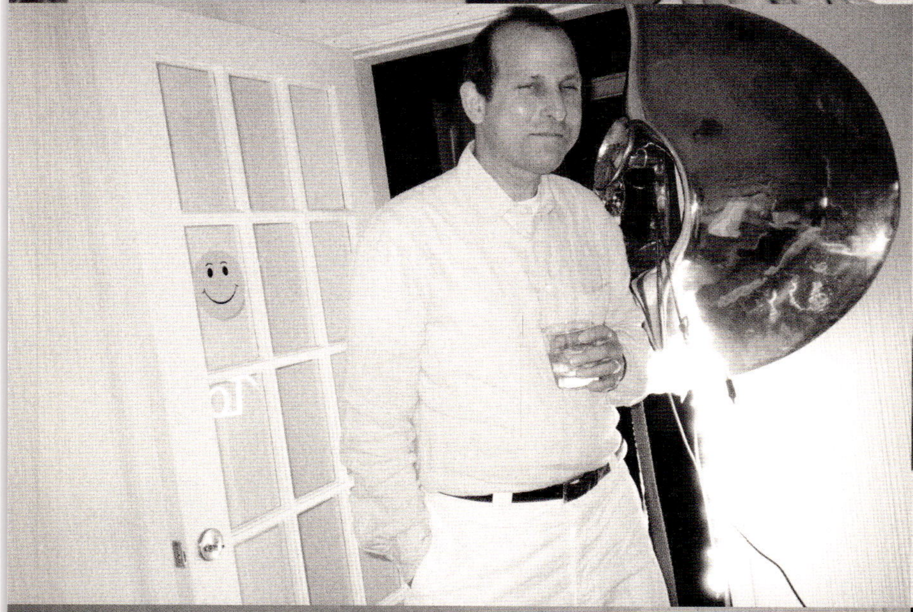

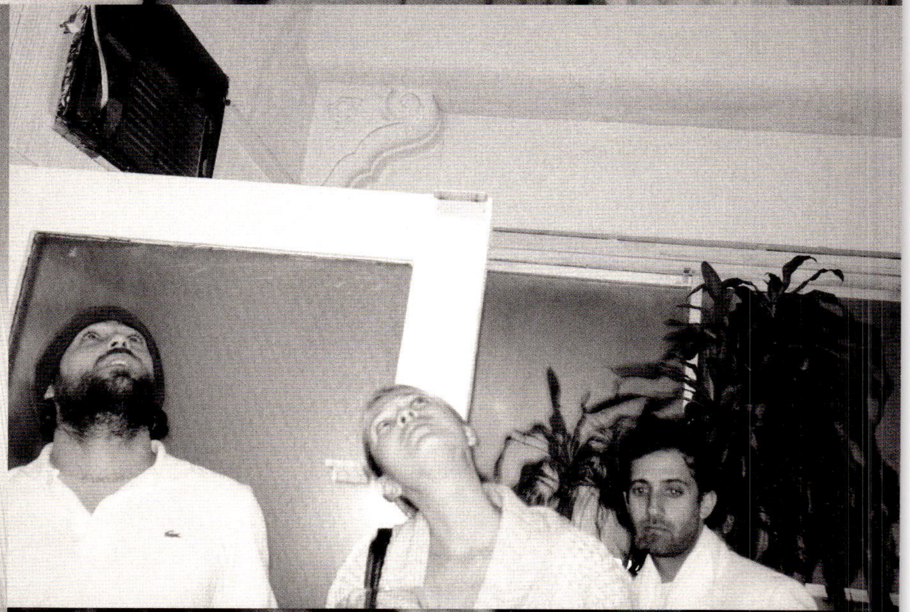

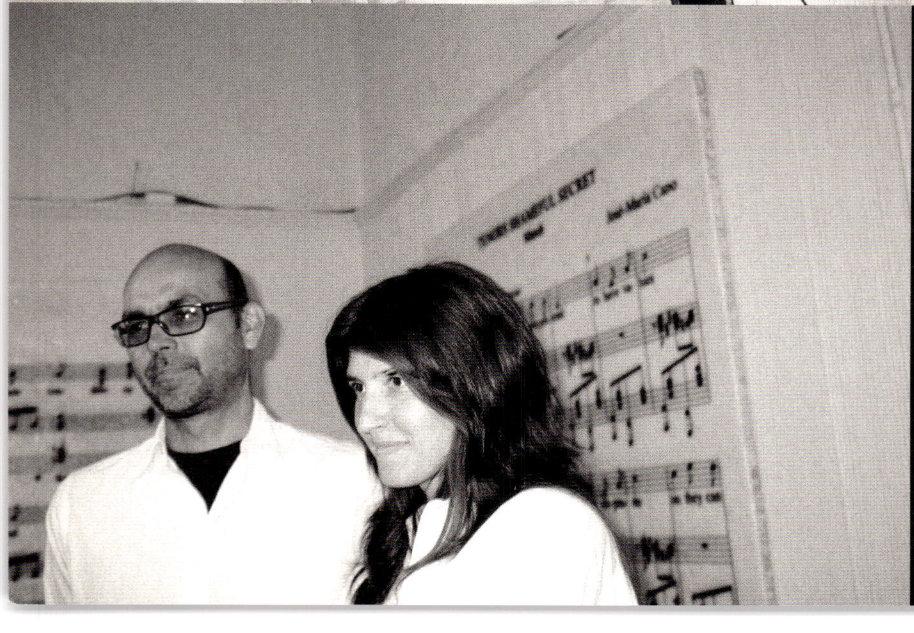

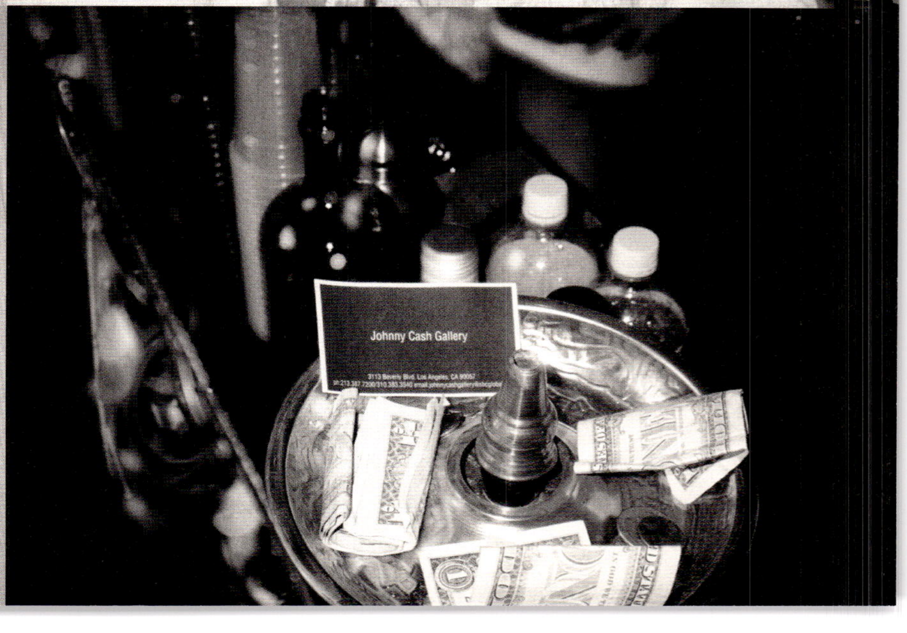
Johnny Cash Gallery

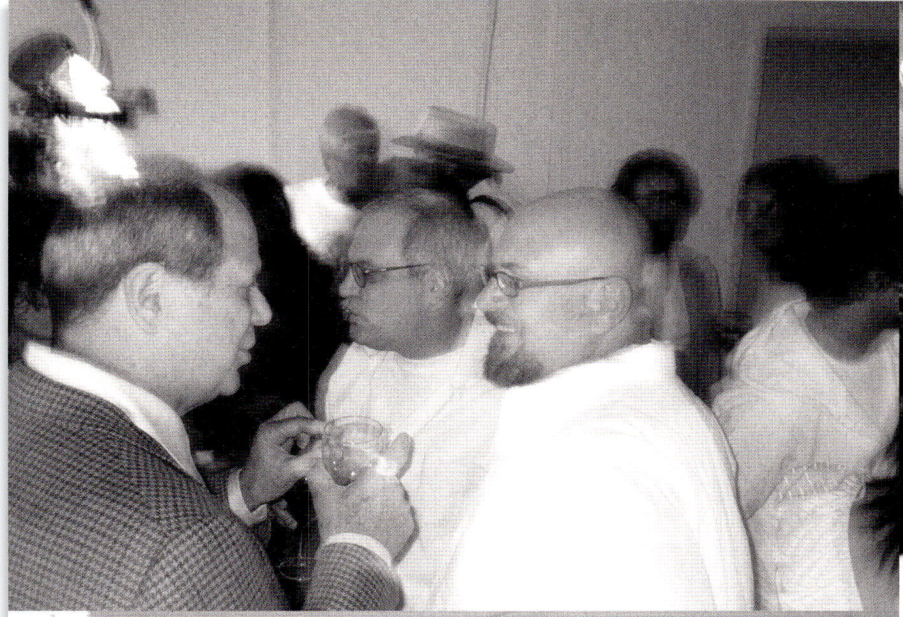
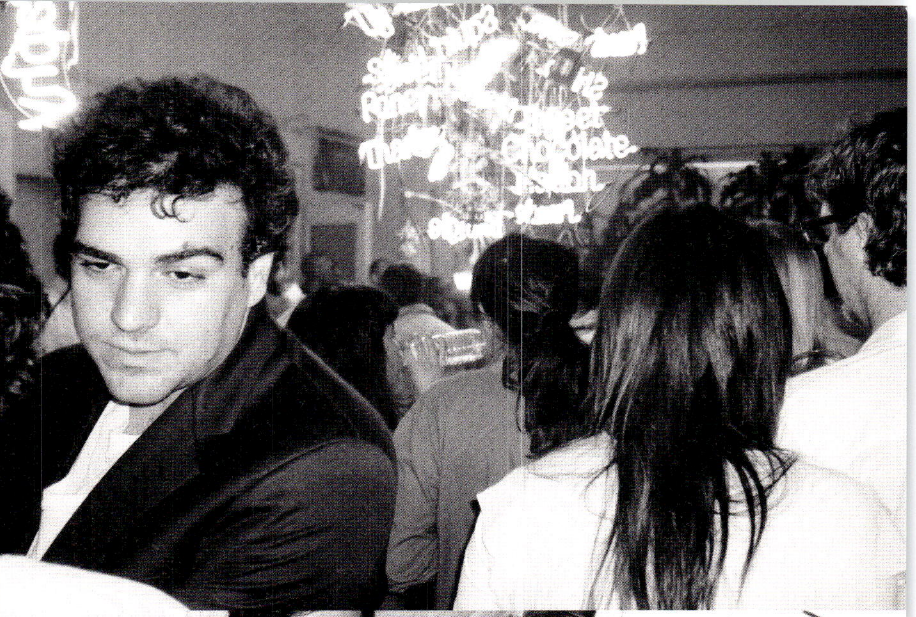
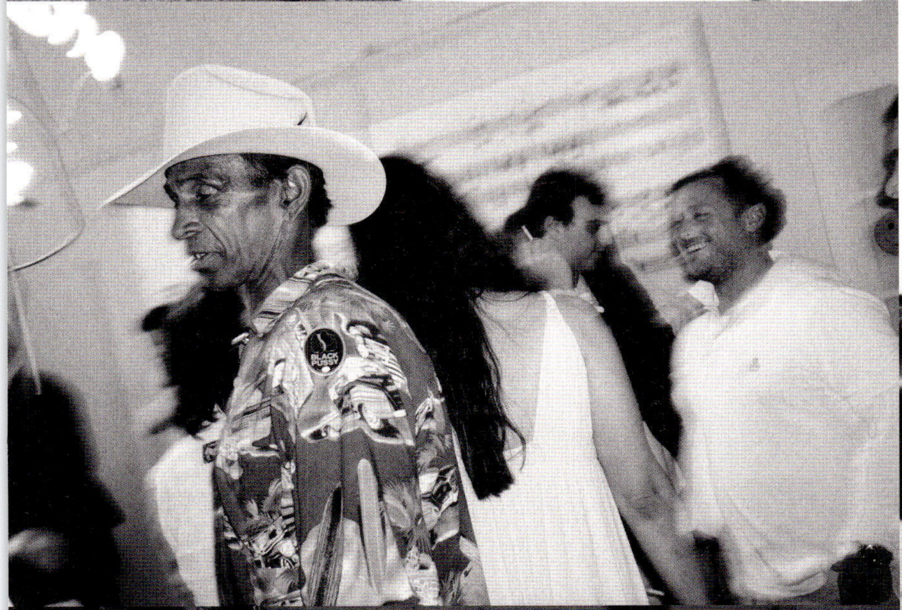
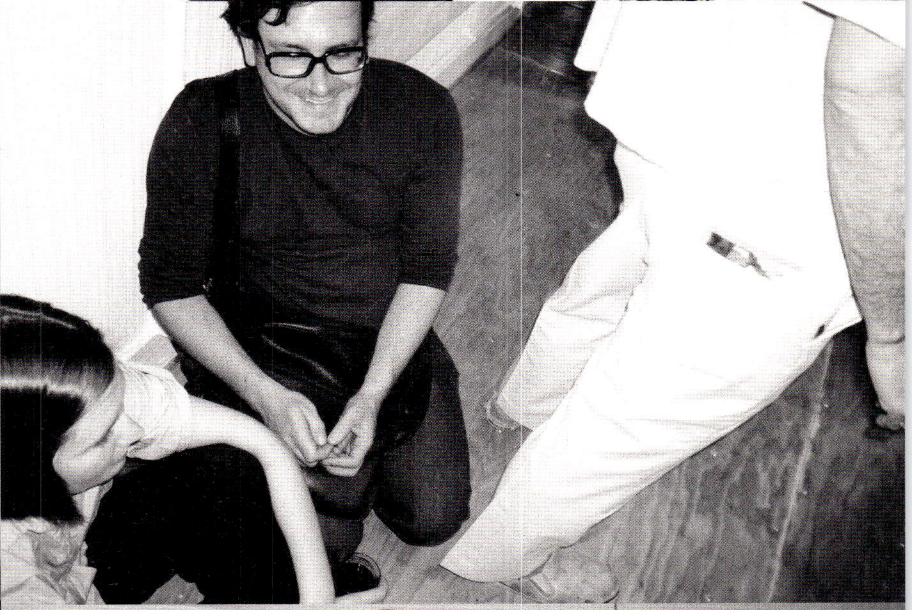
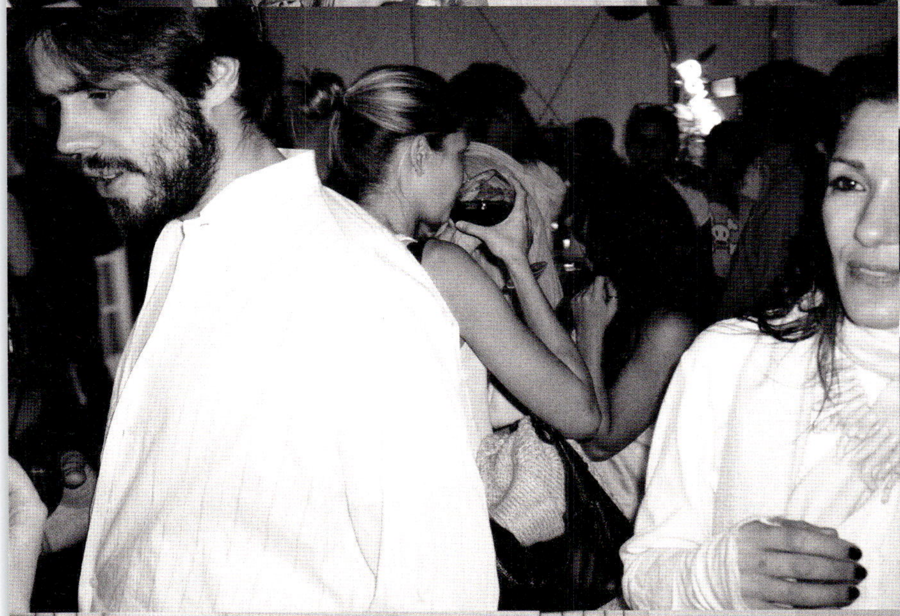
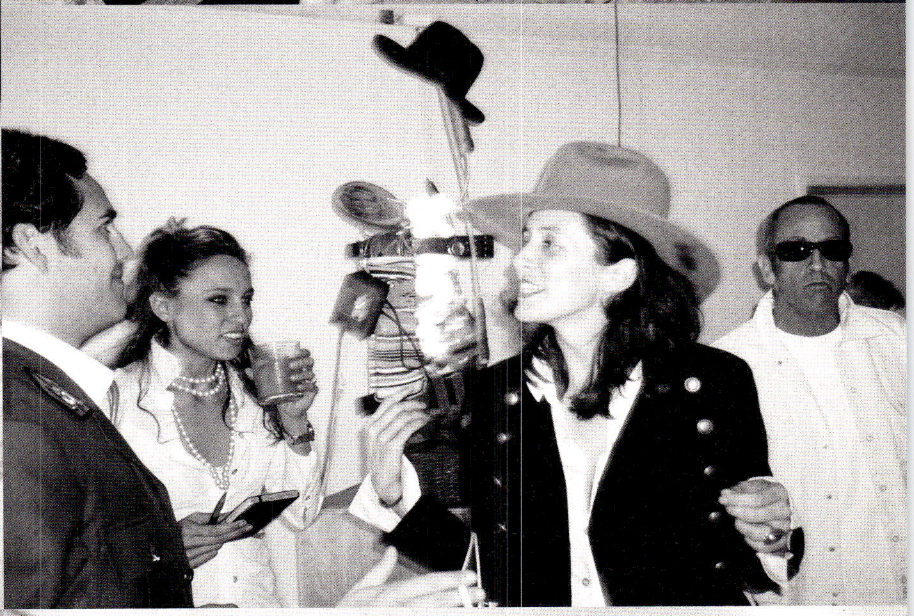
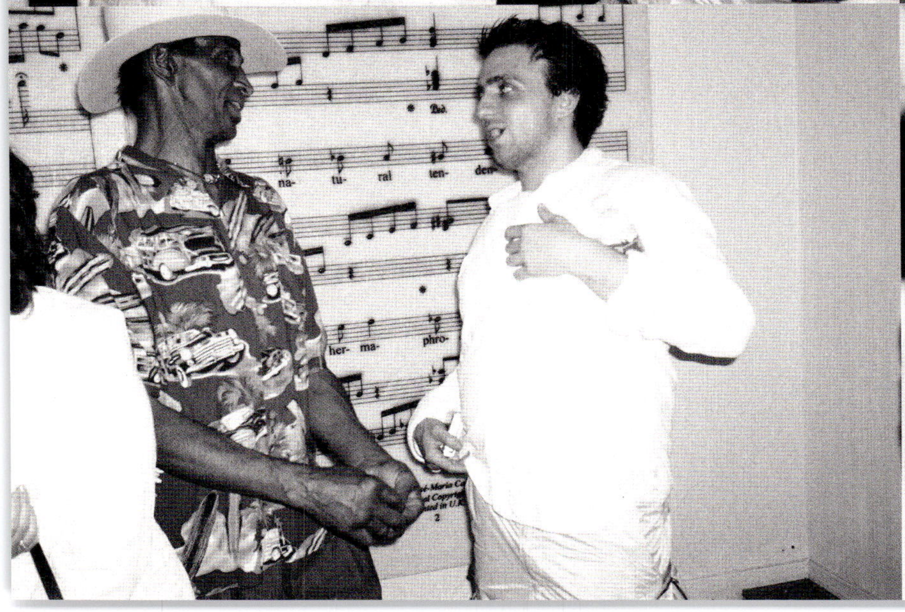
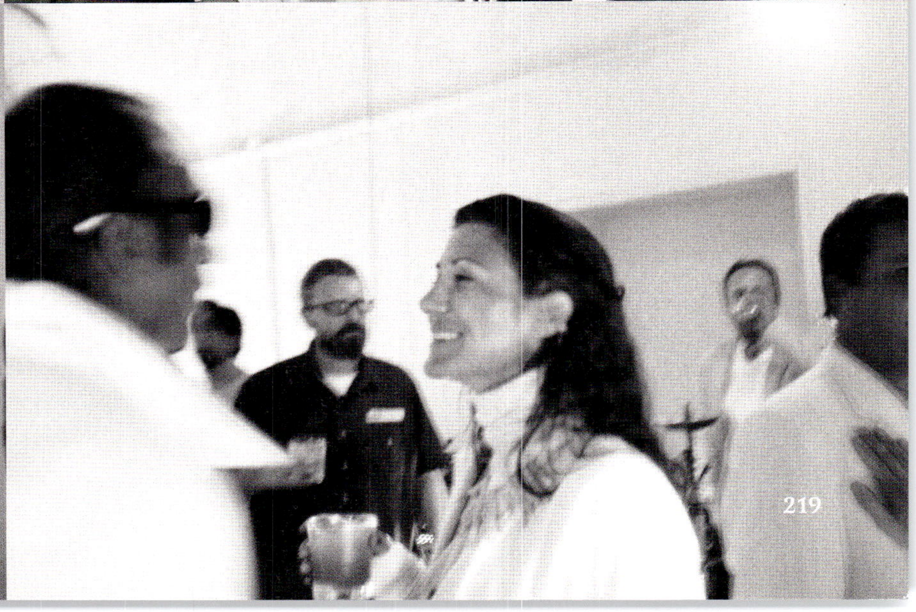

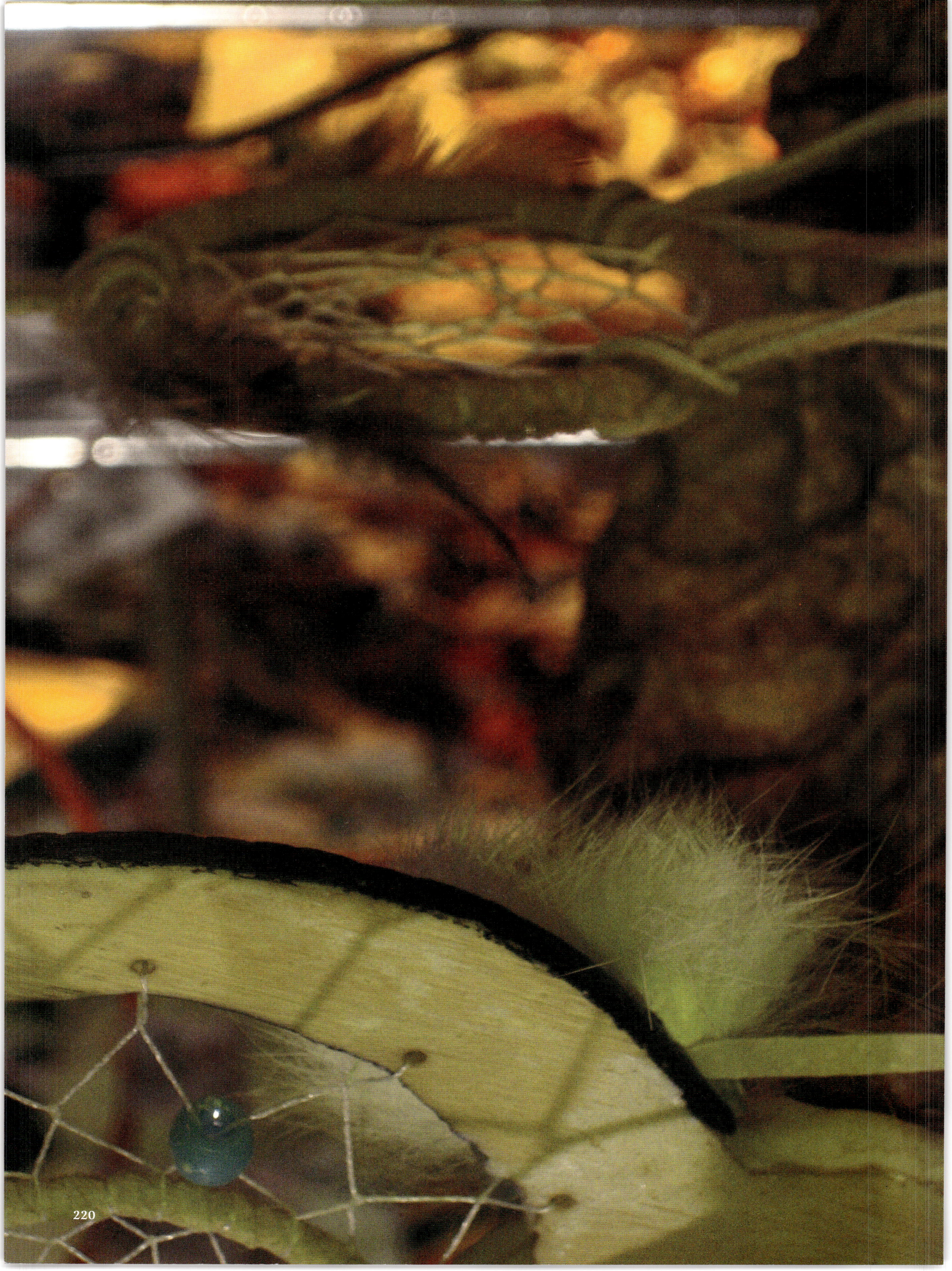

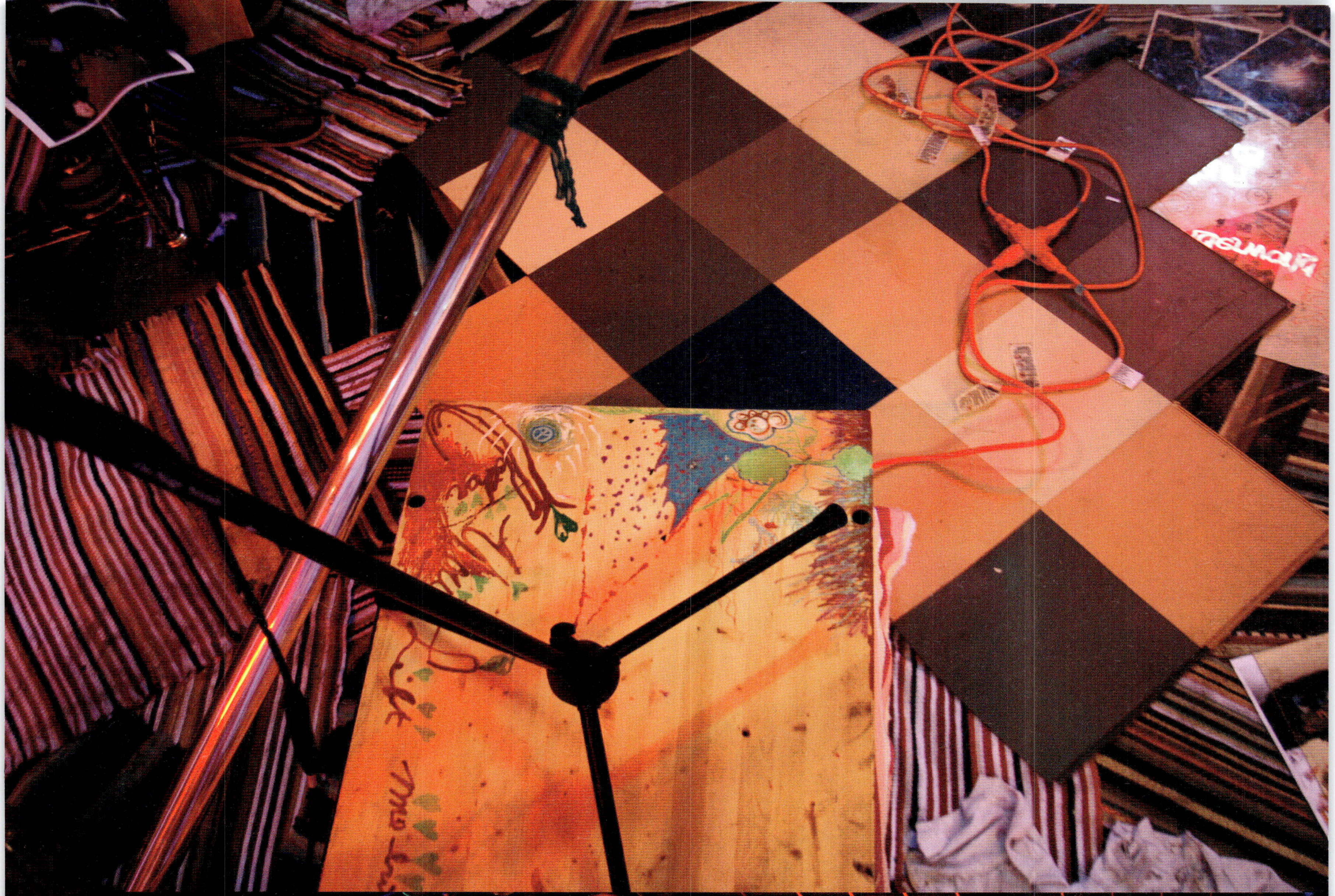

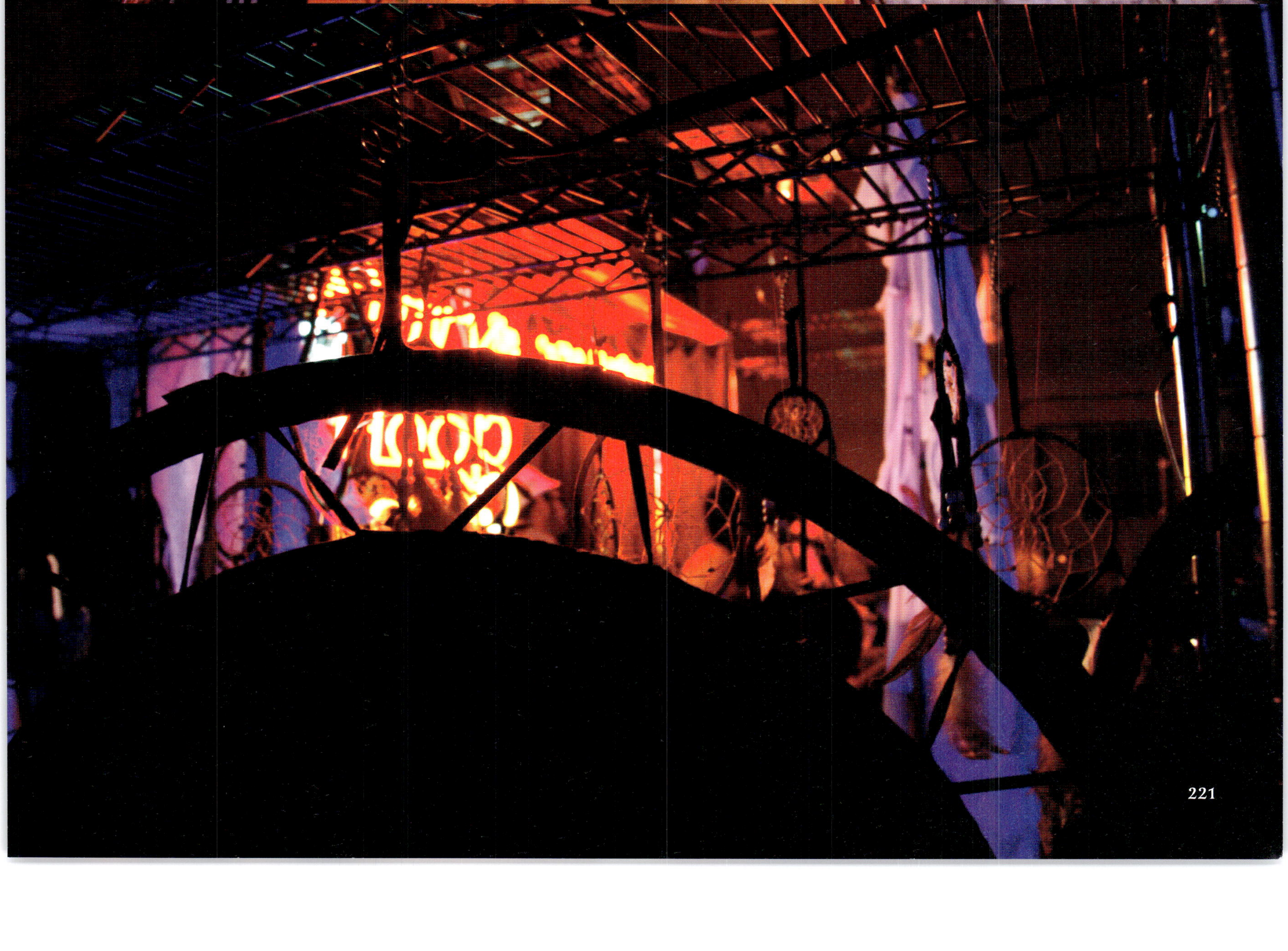

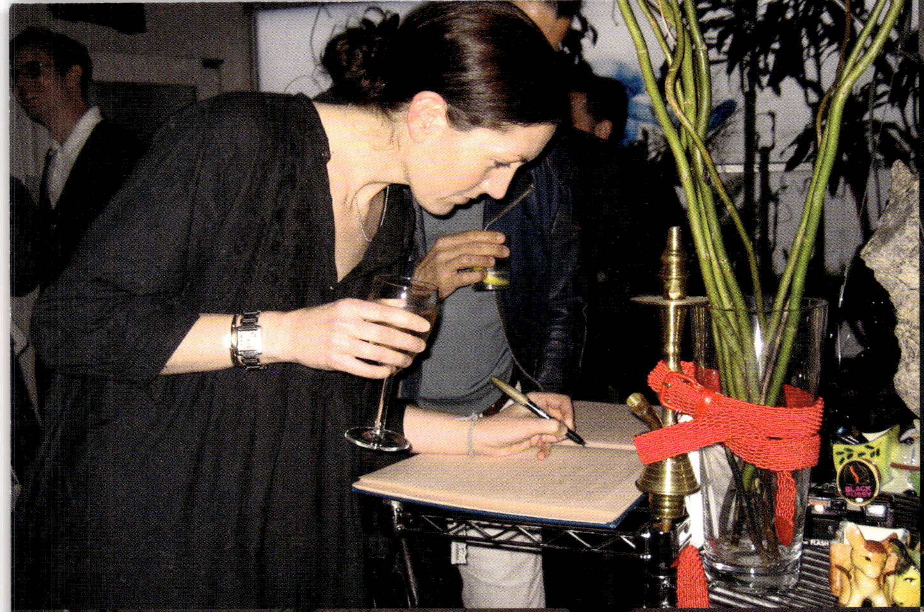

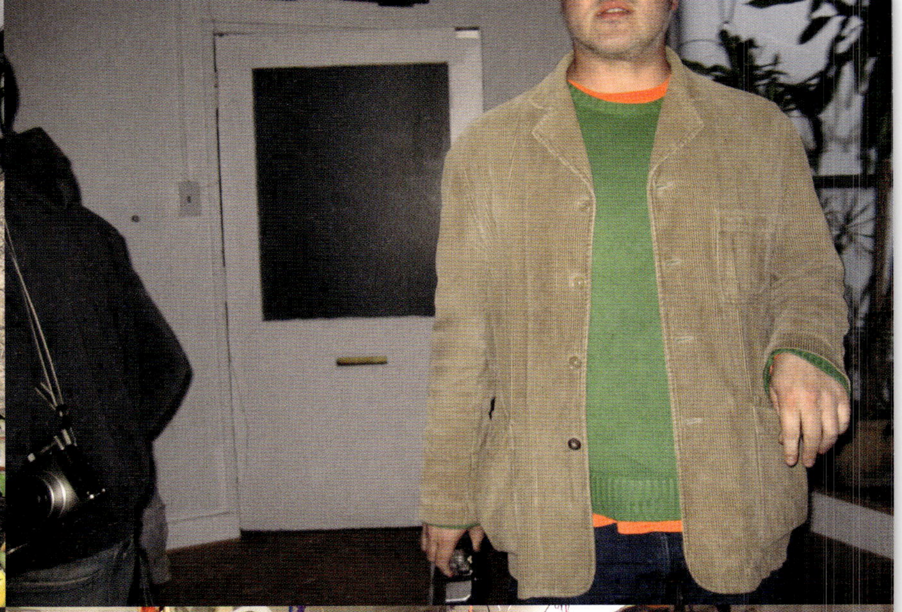

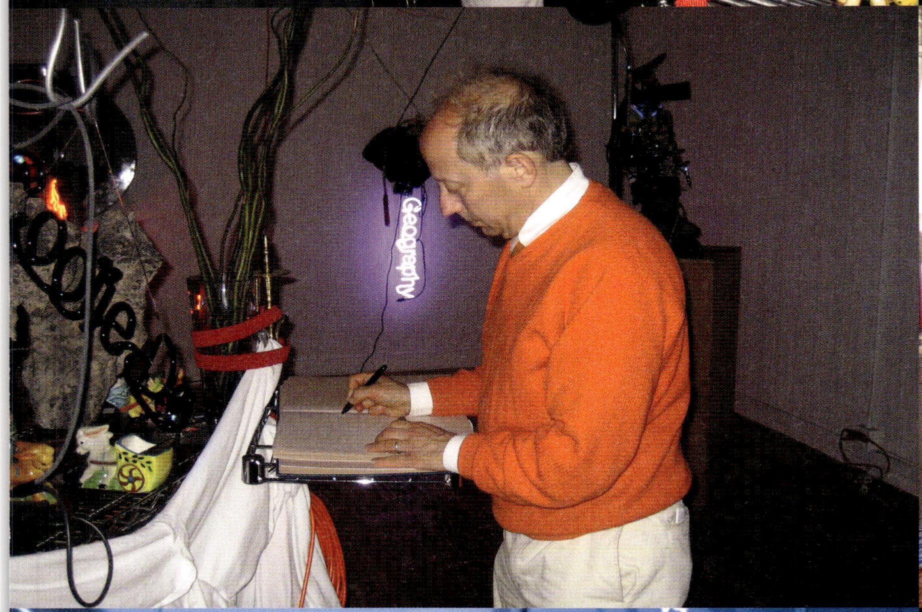
Geography

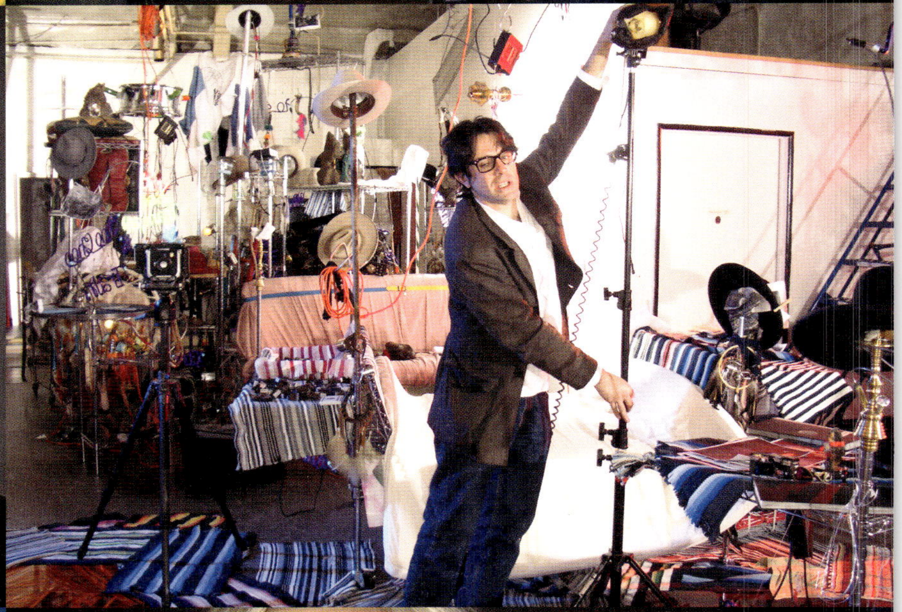

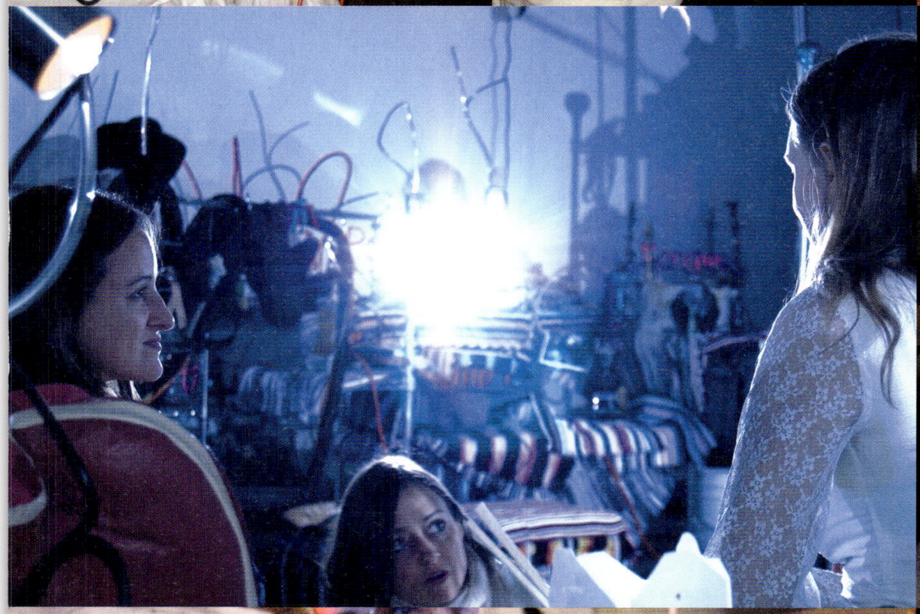

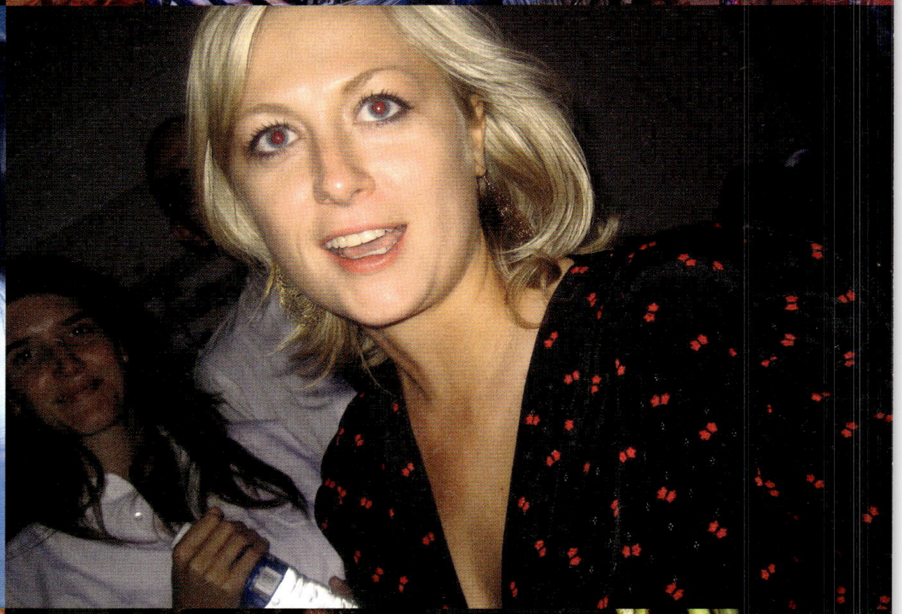

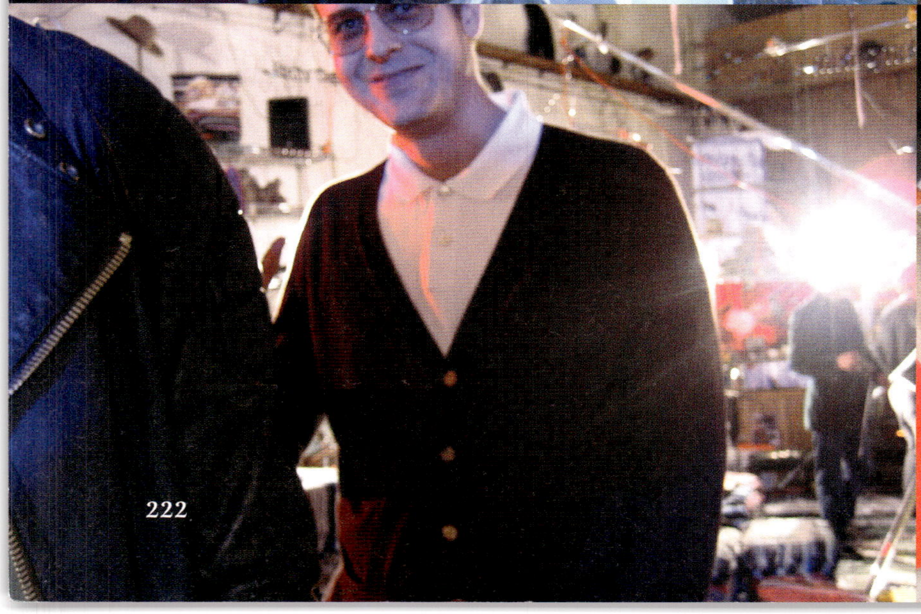

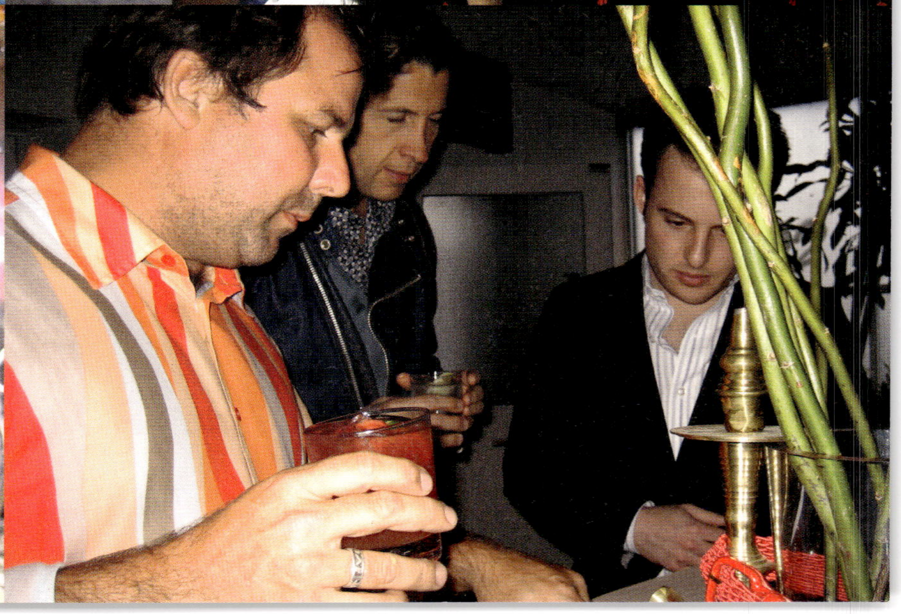

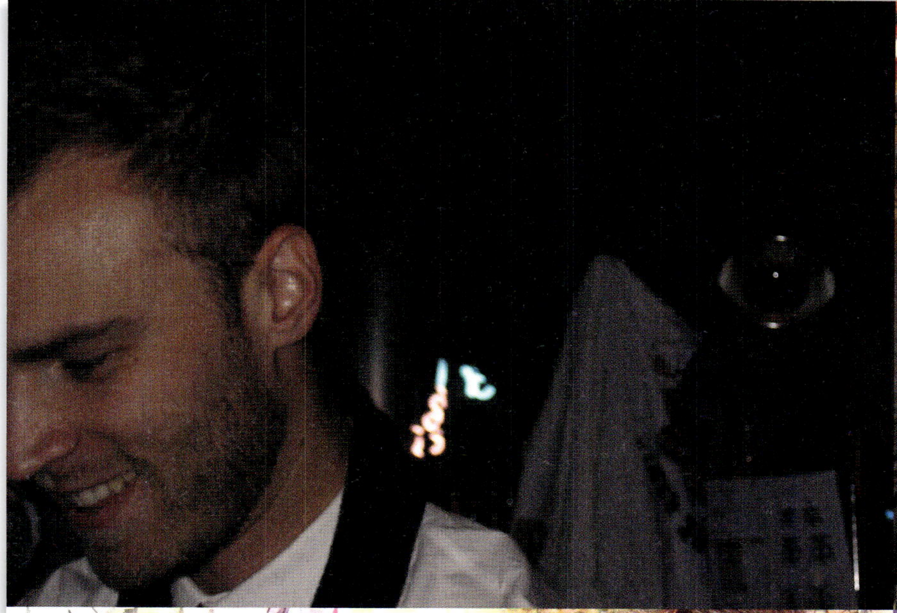
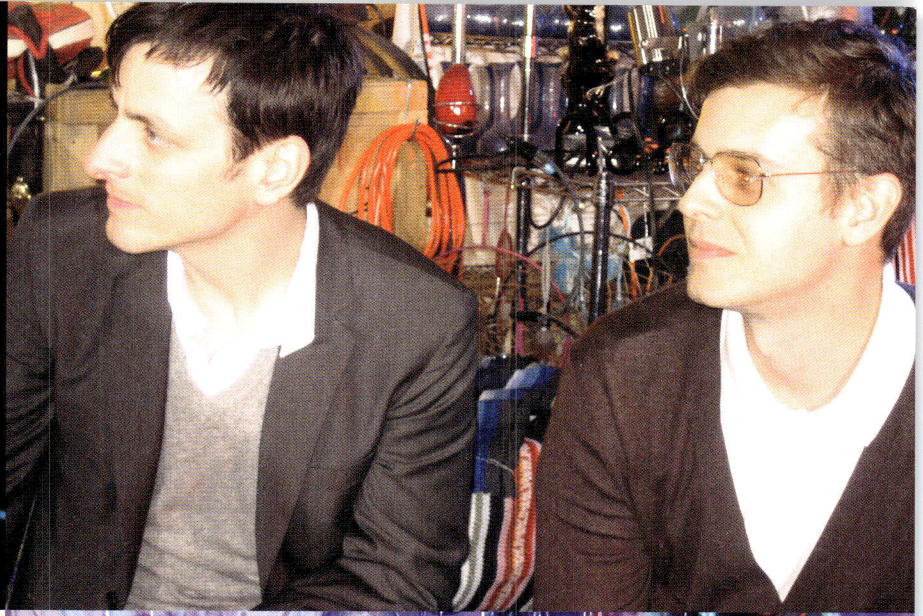
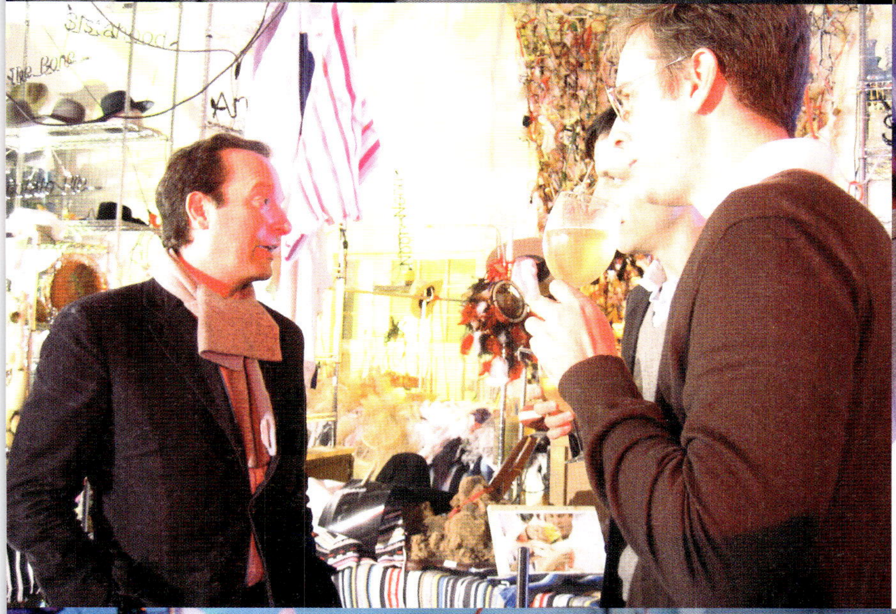
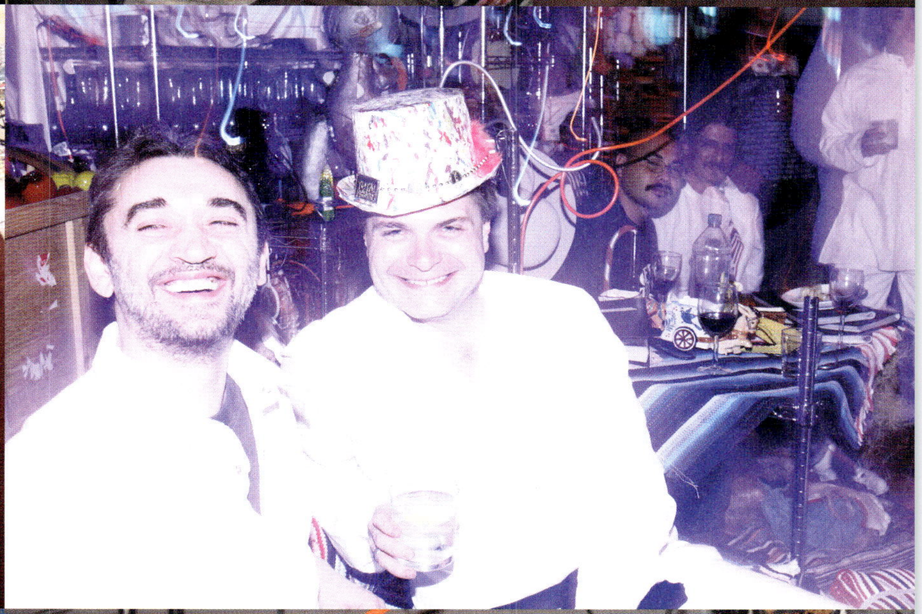
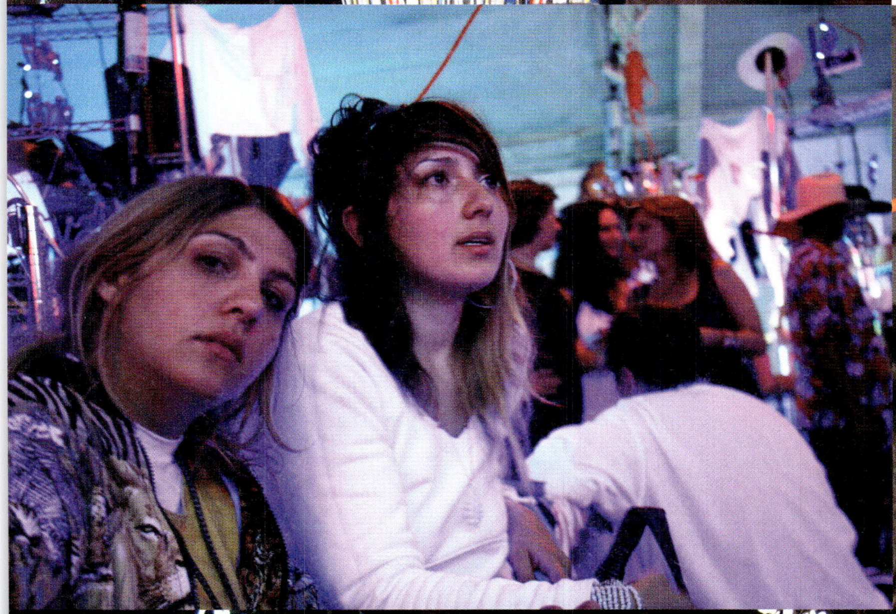
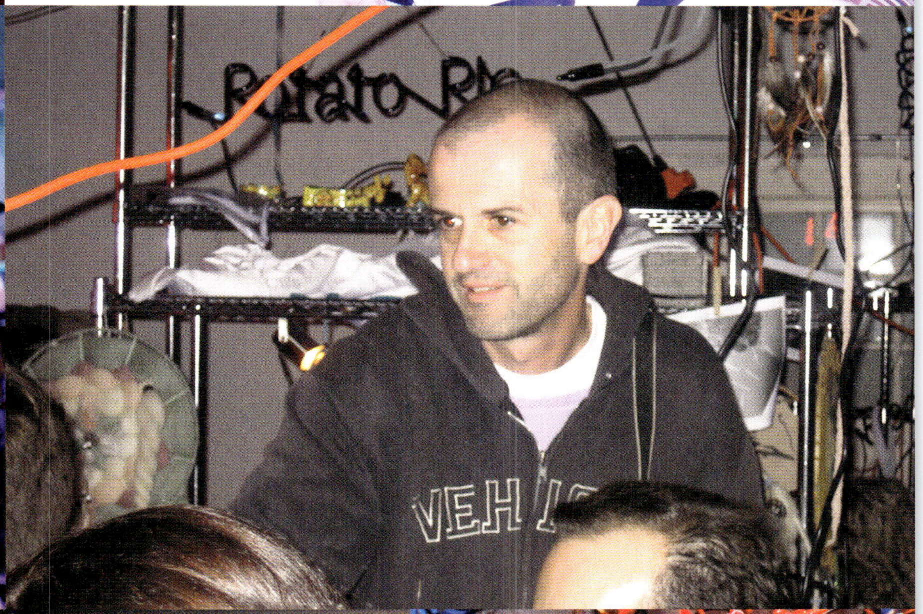
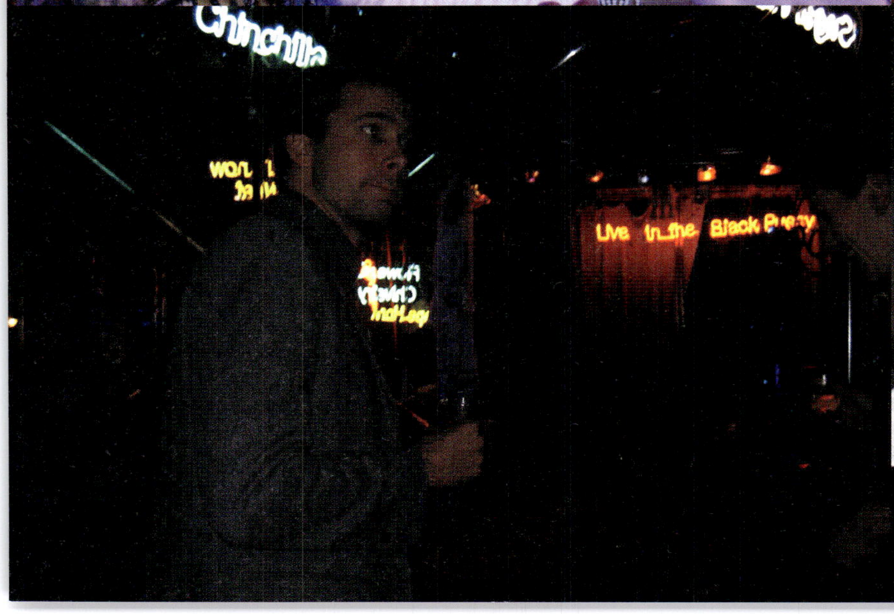
Chinchilla
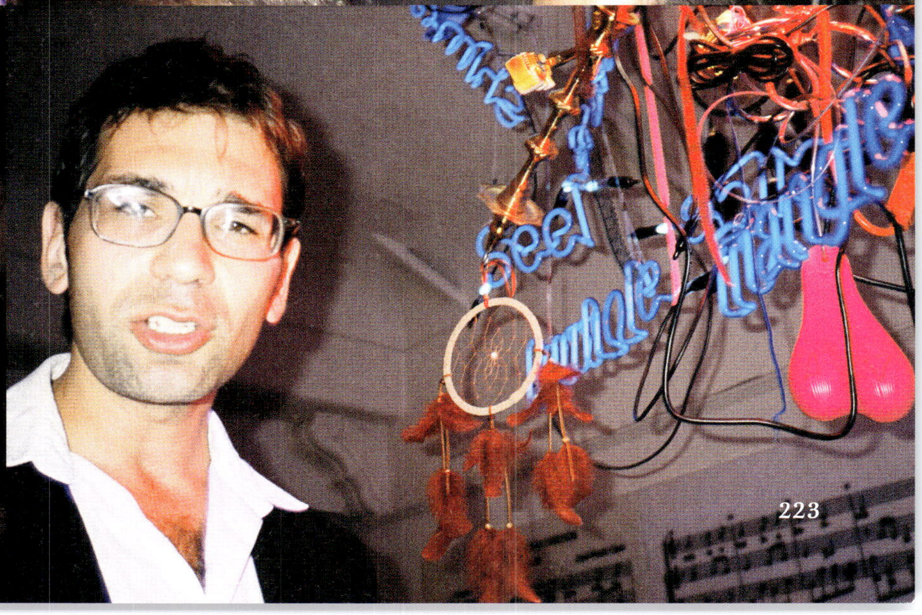

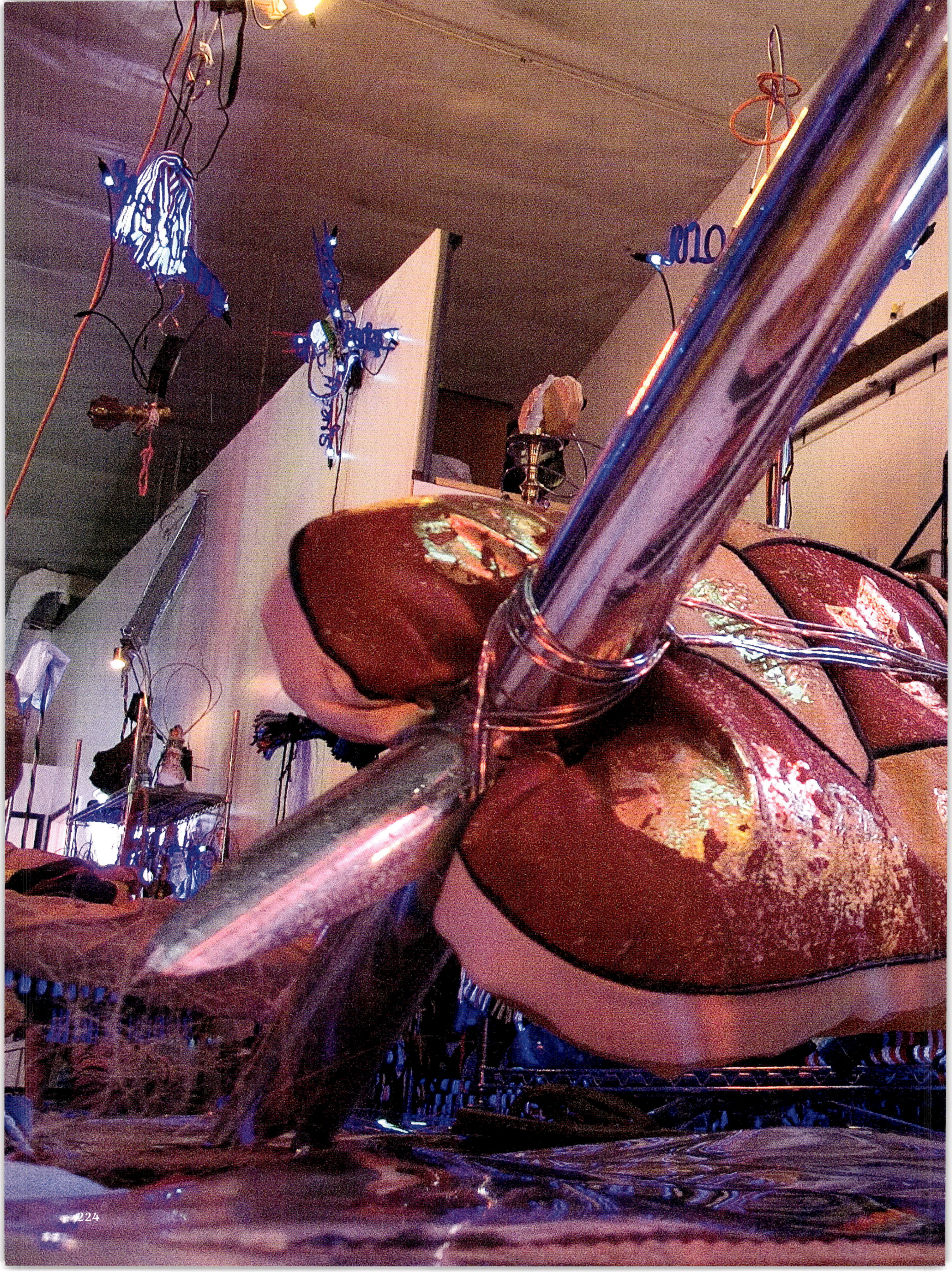

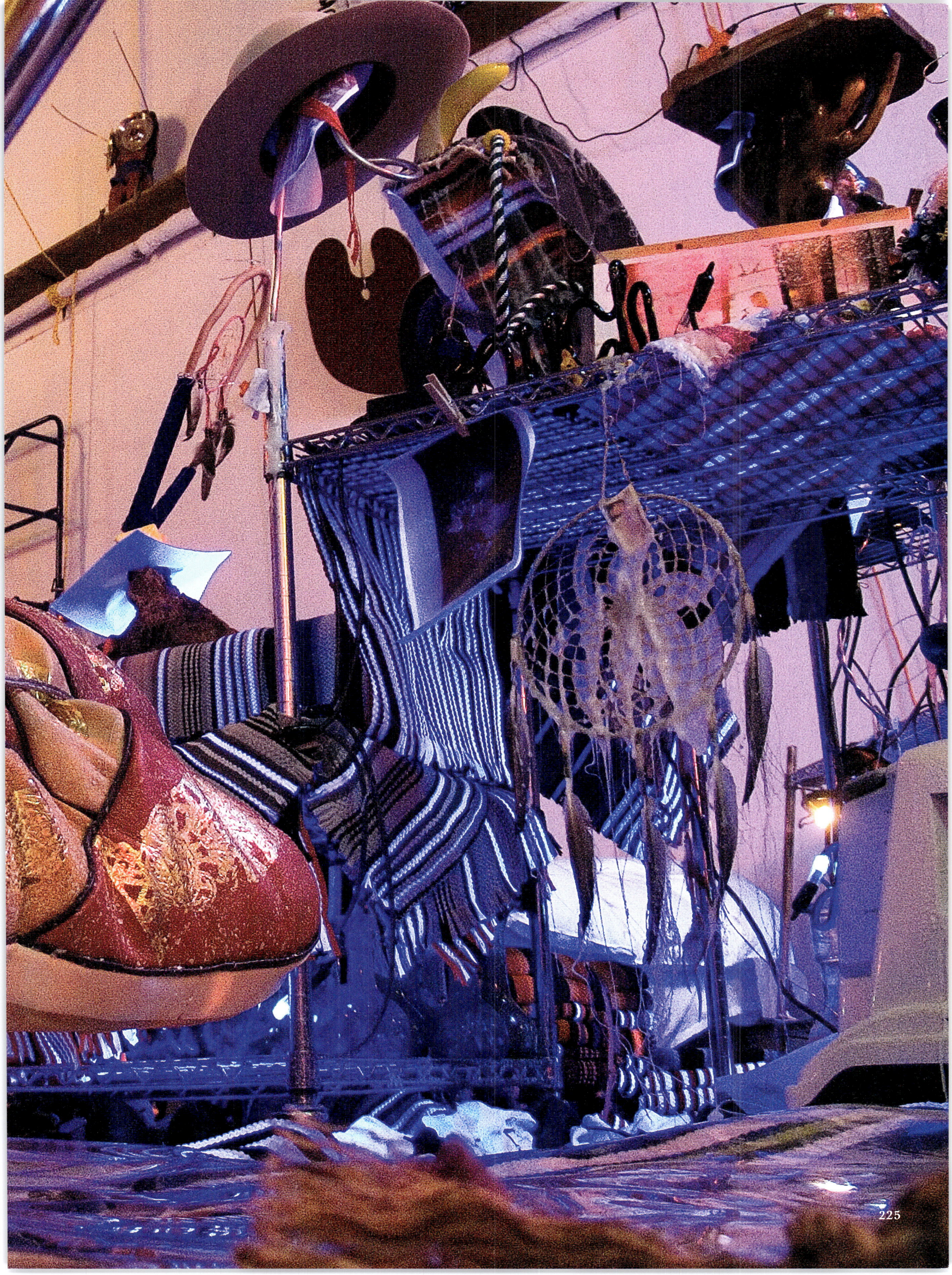

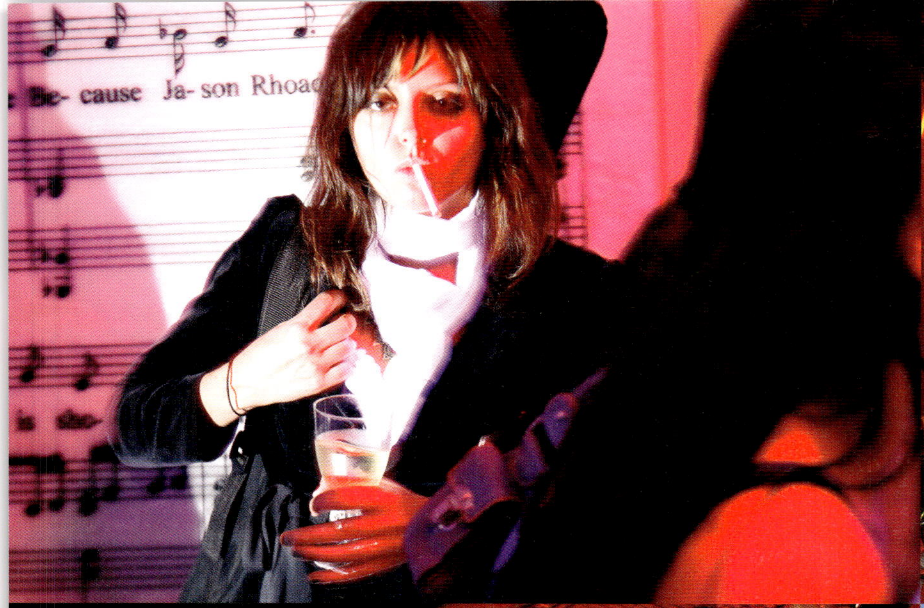
Be- cause Ja- son Rhoad

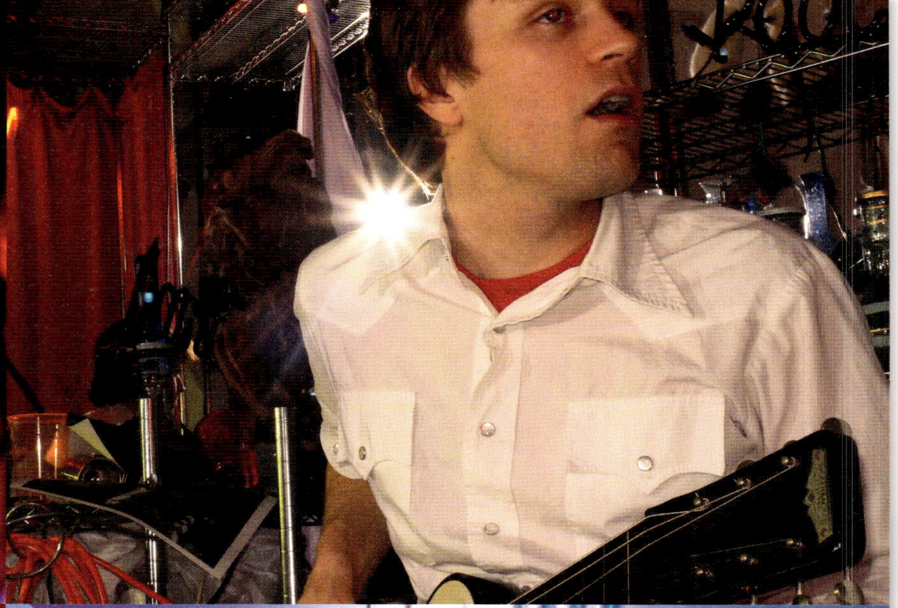

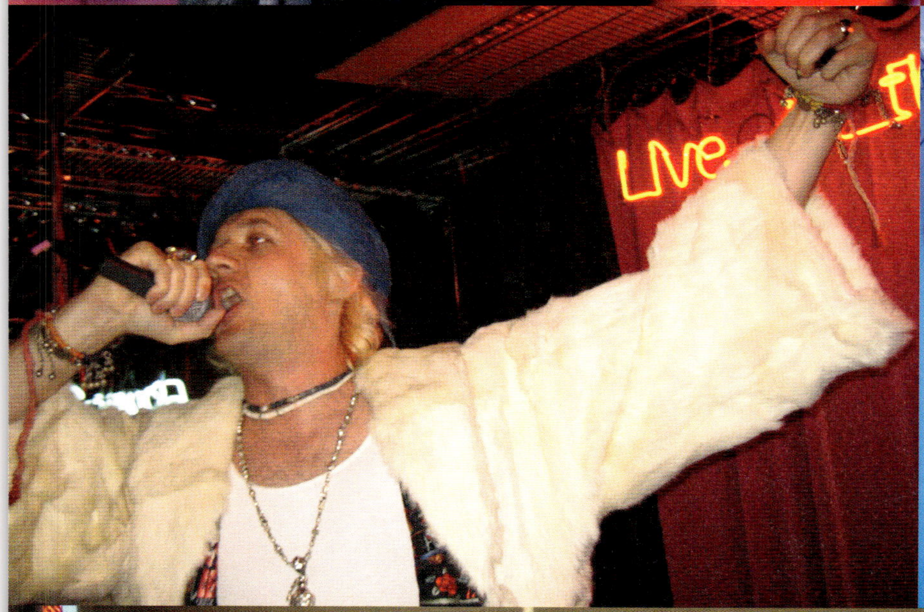
Live

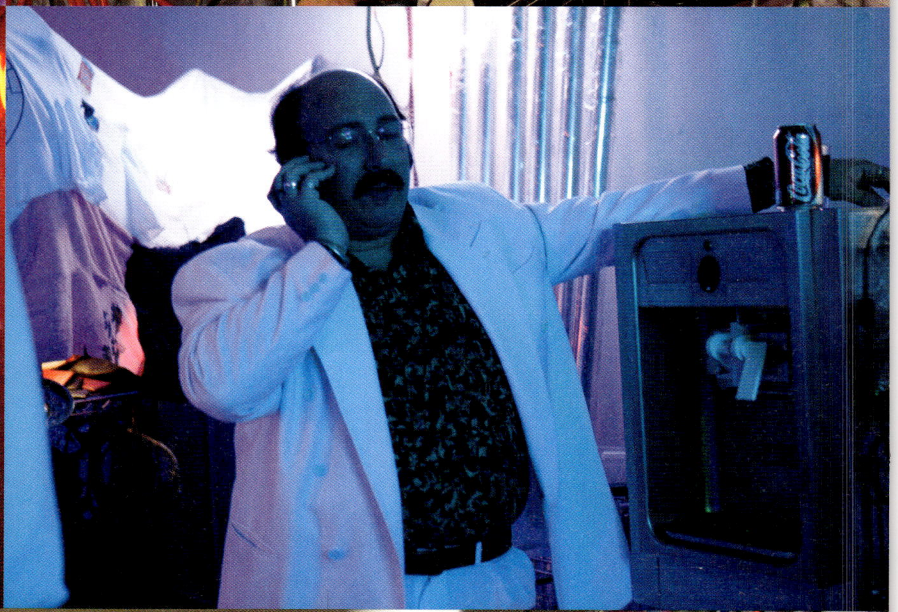

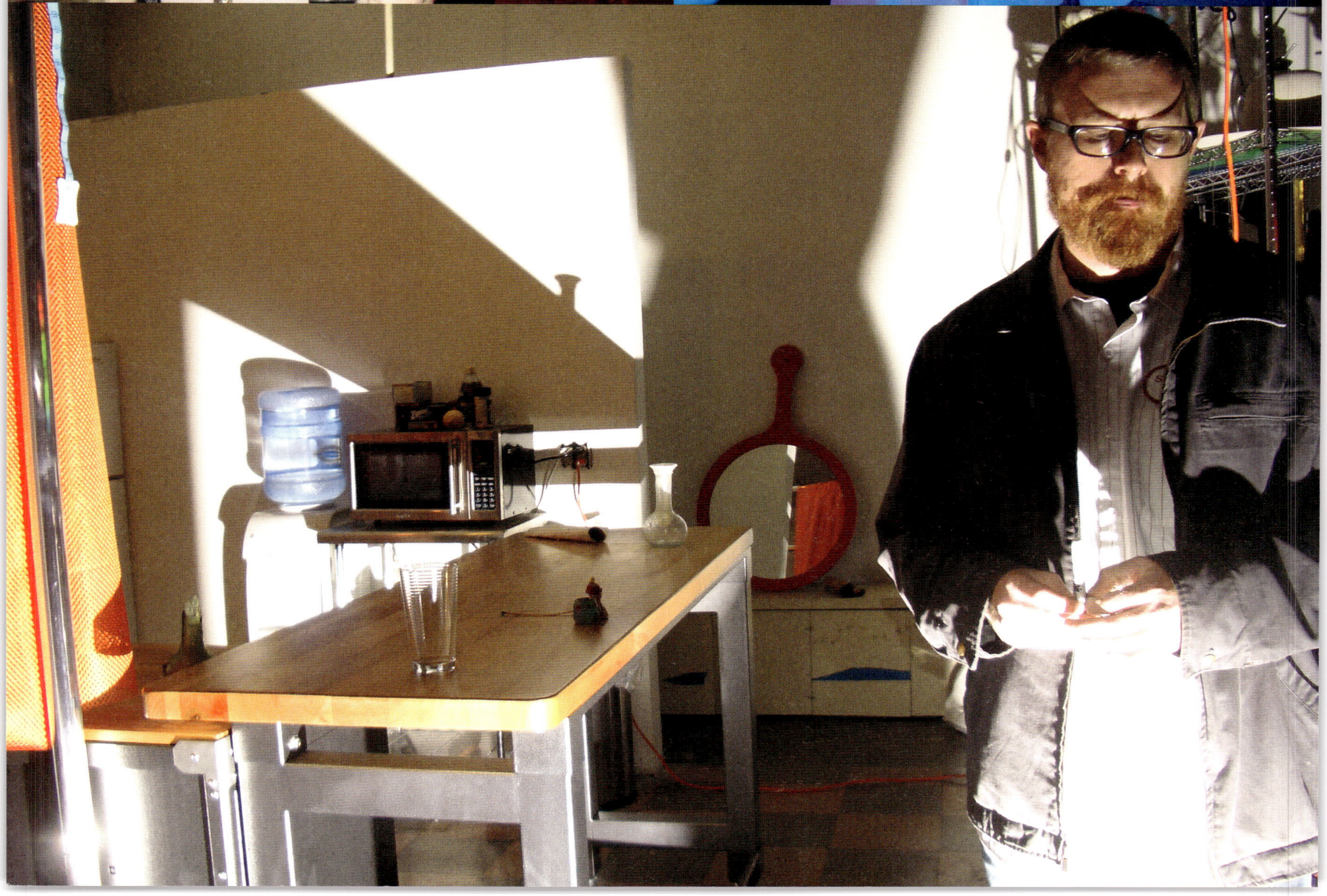

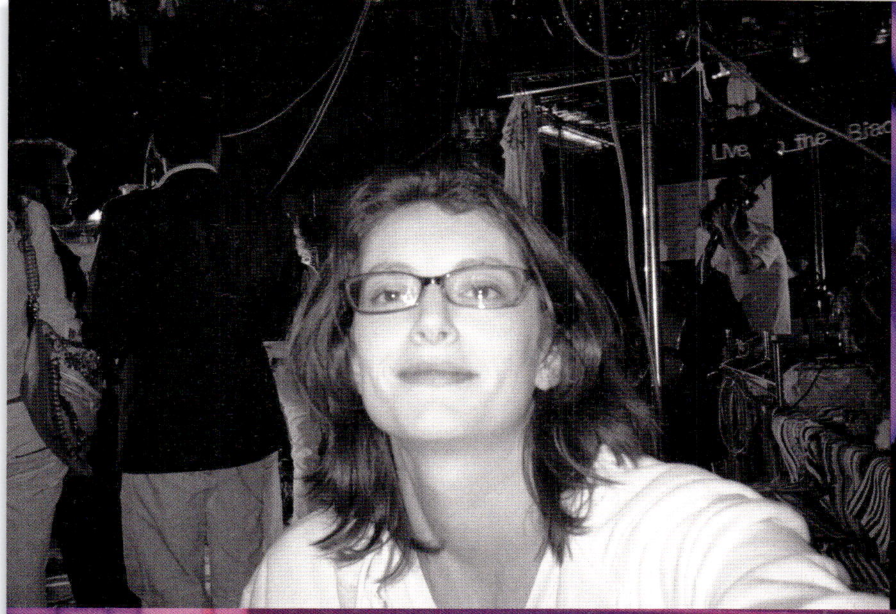

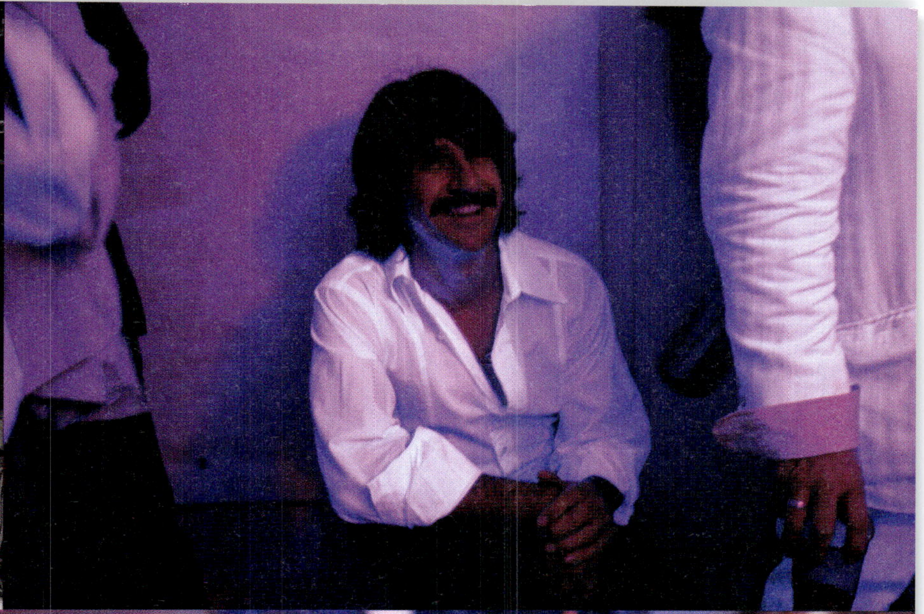

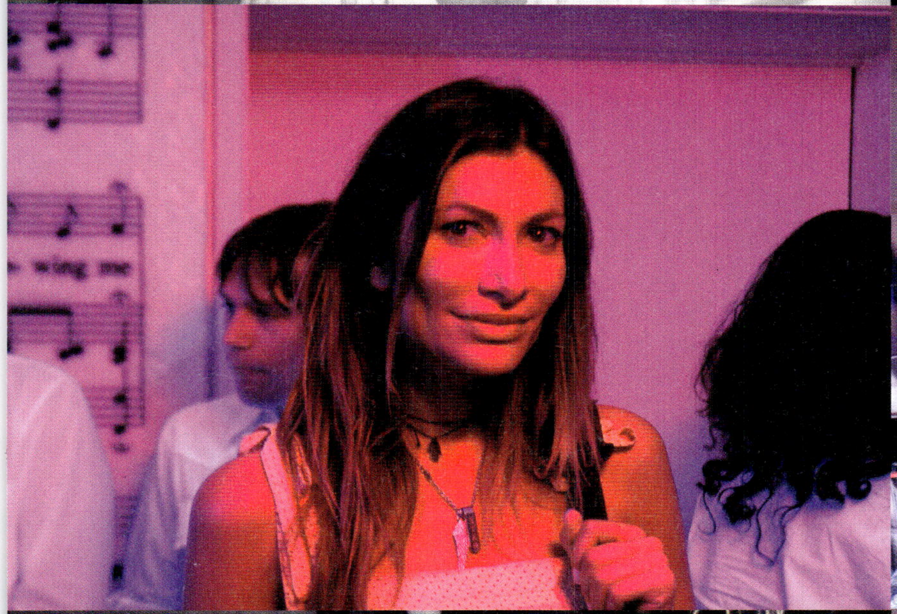

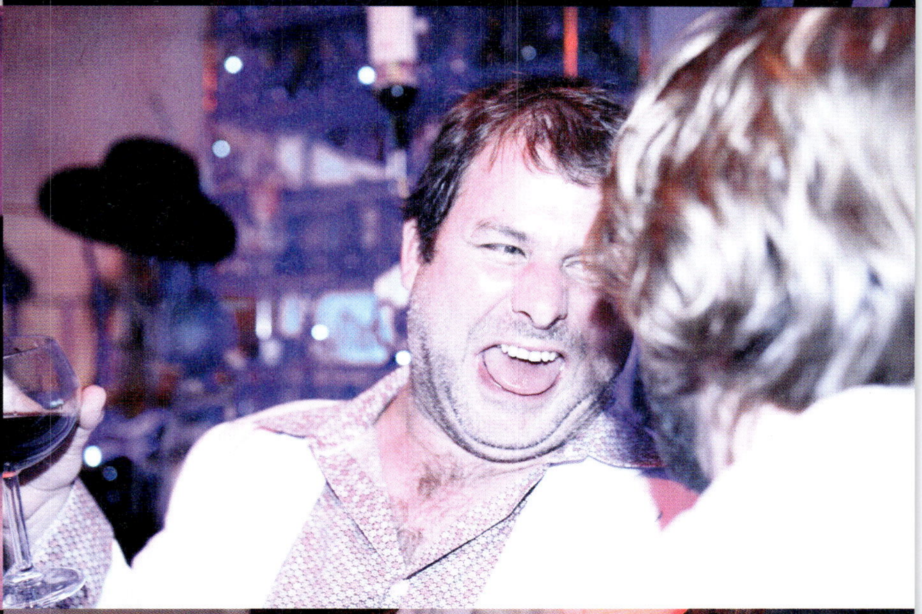

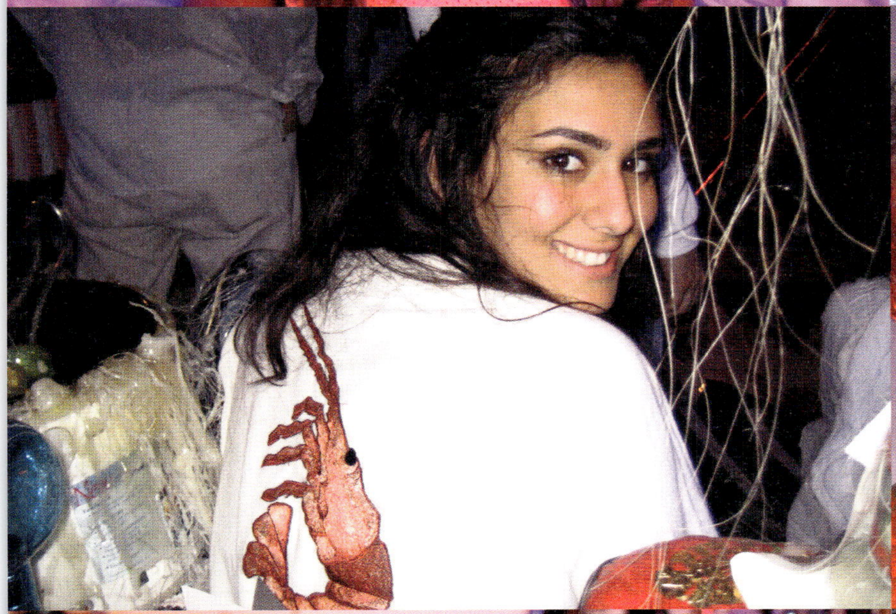

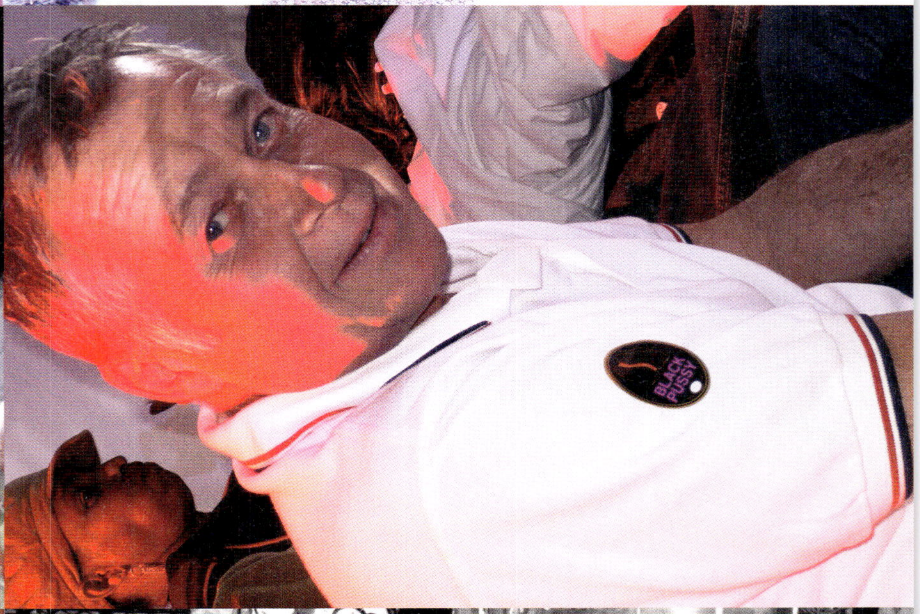

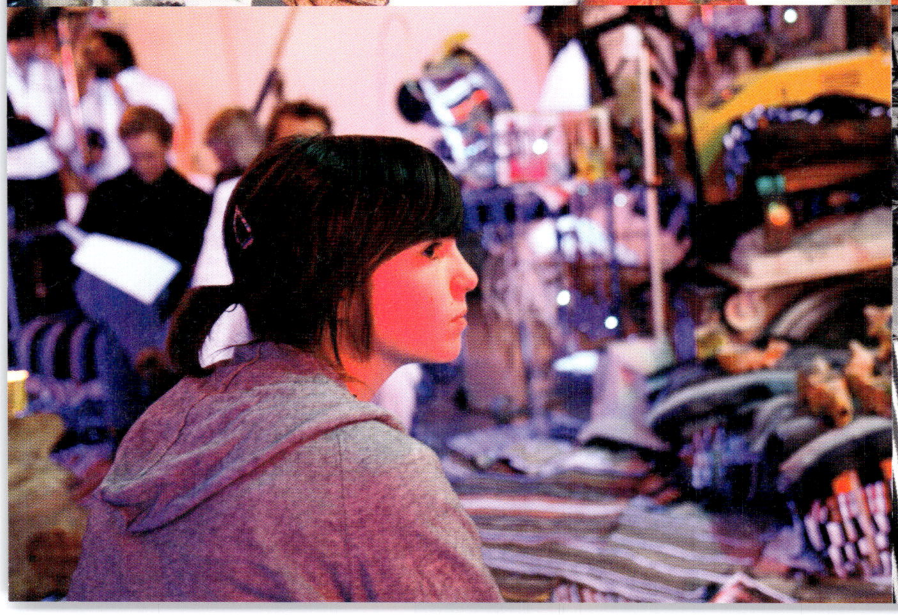

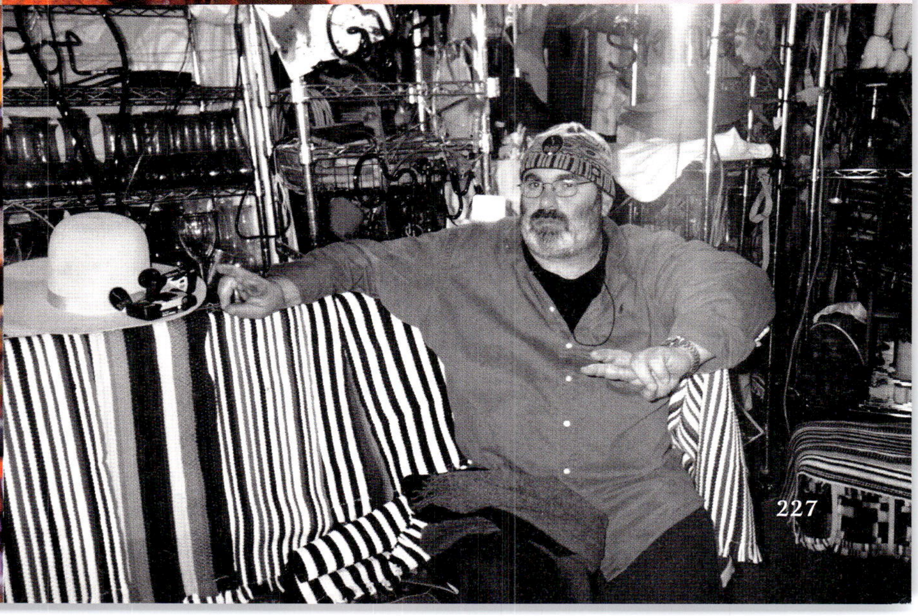

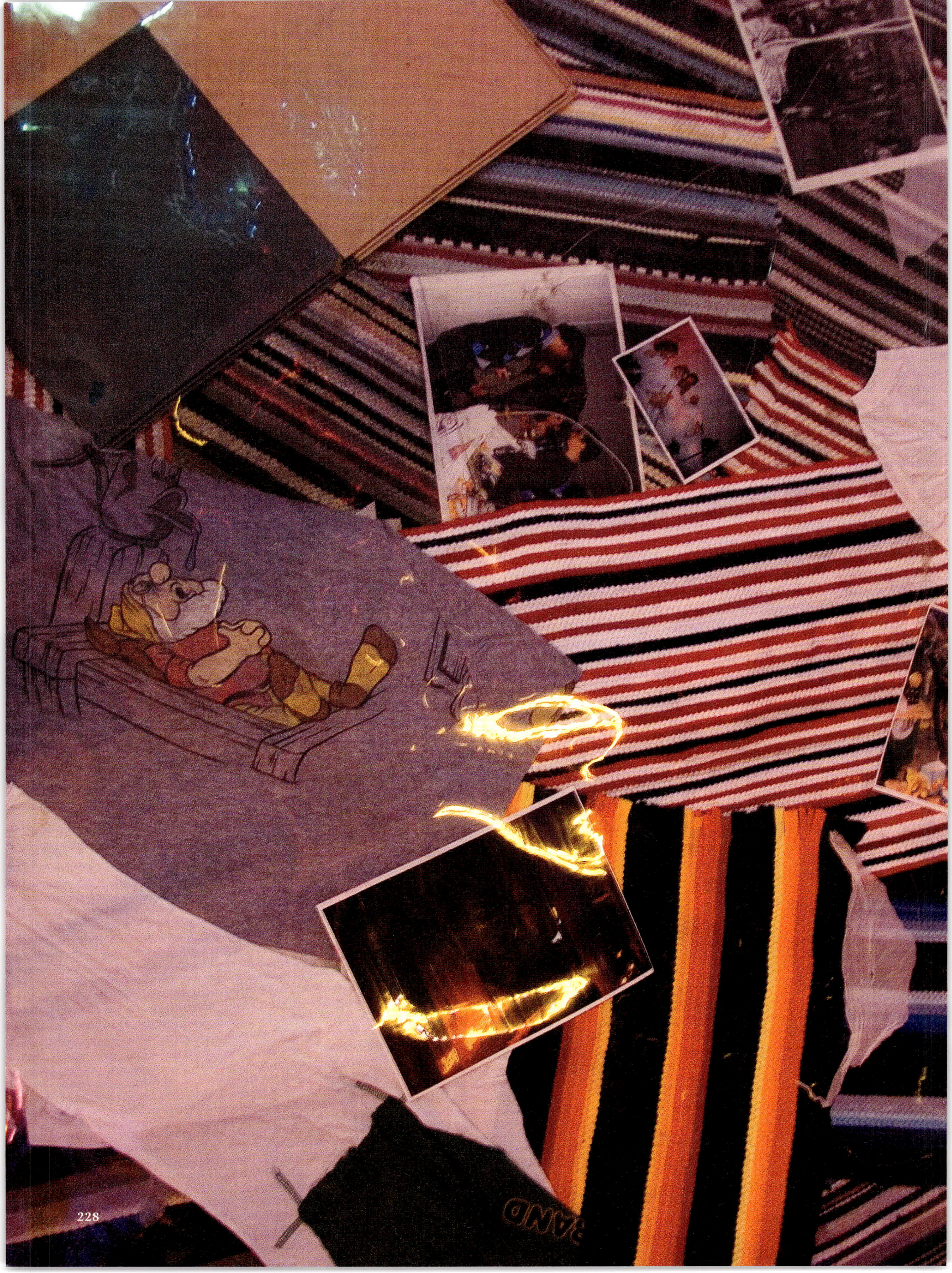

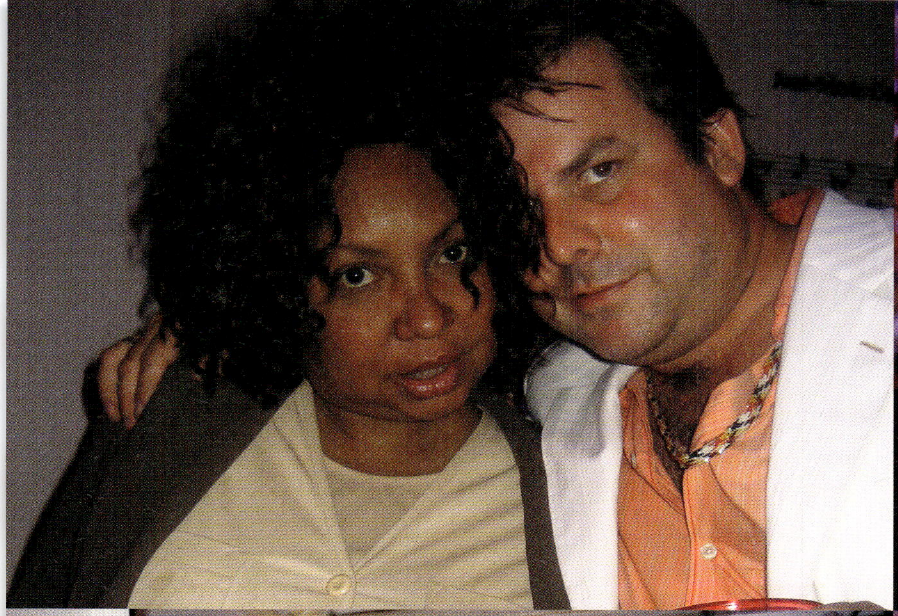
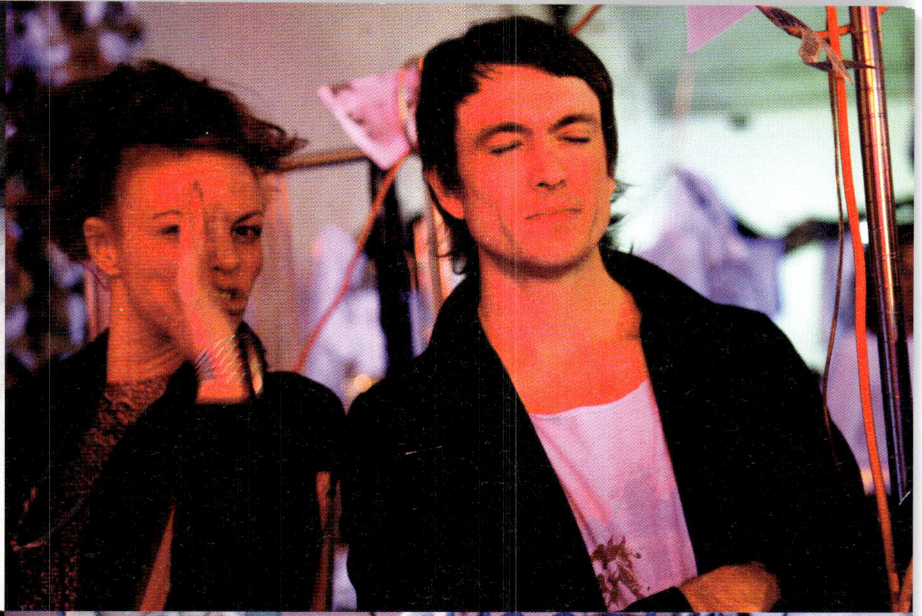
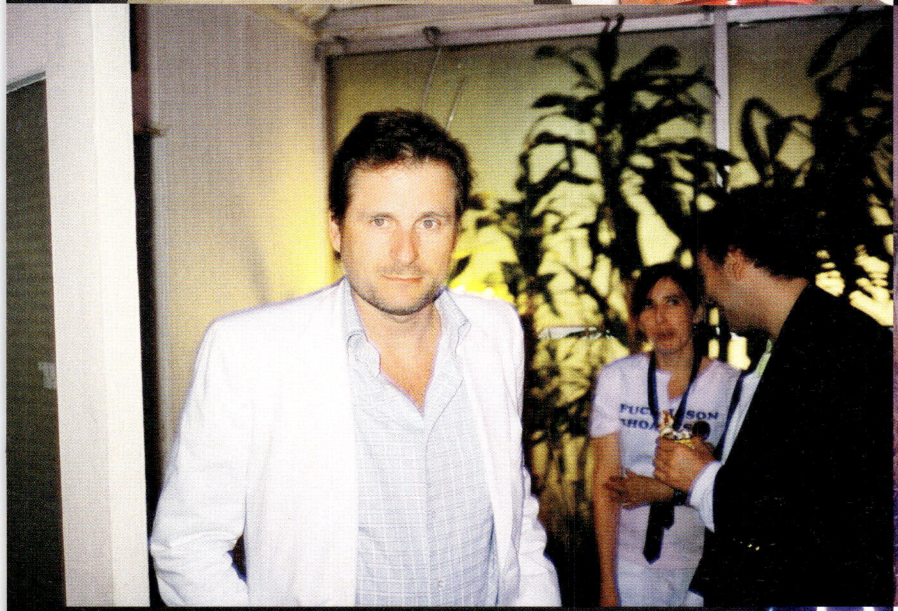
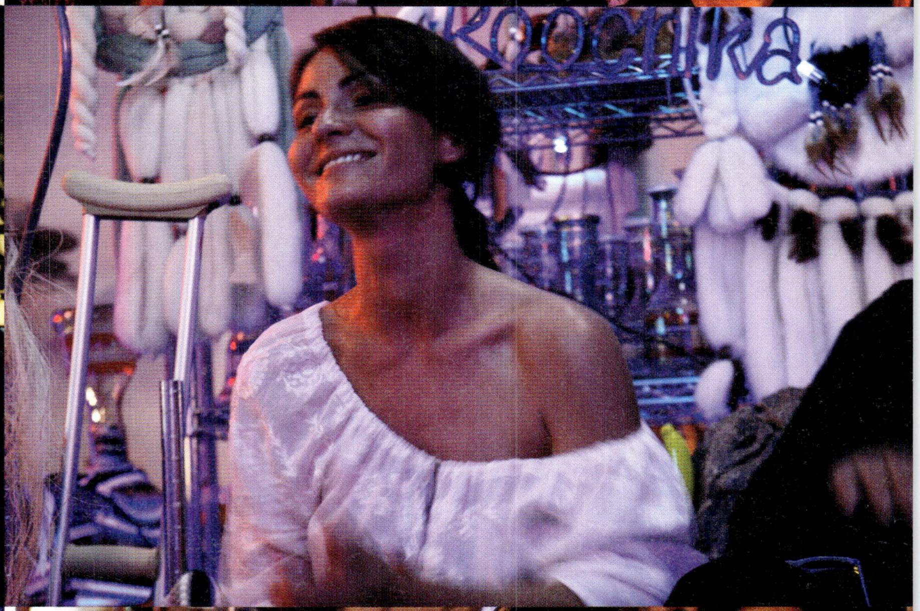
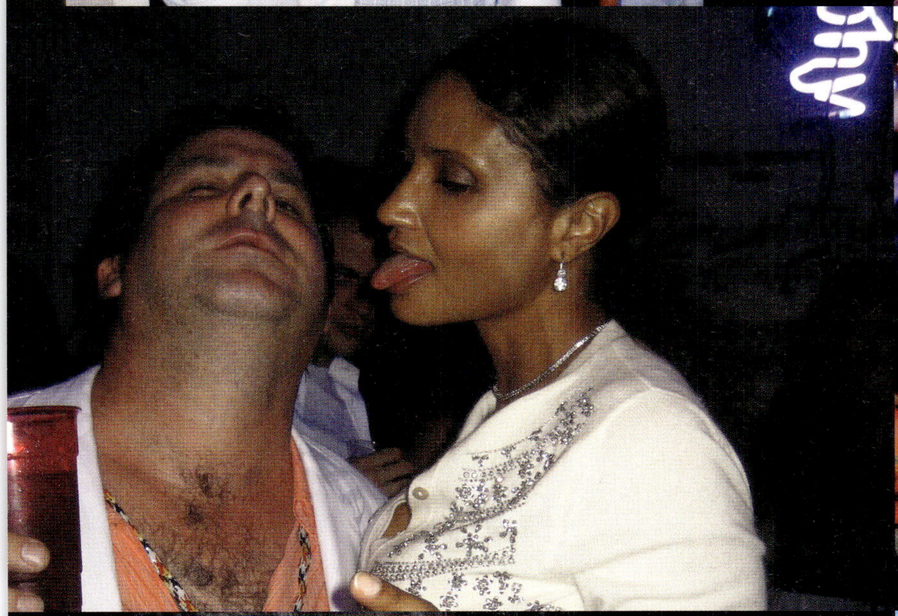
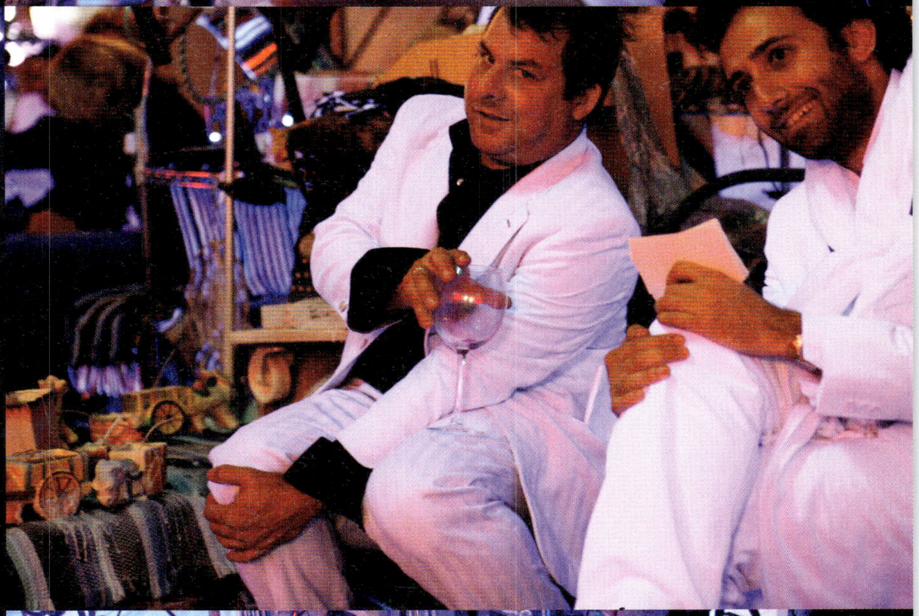
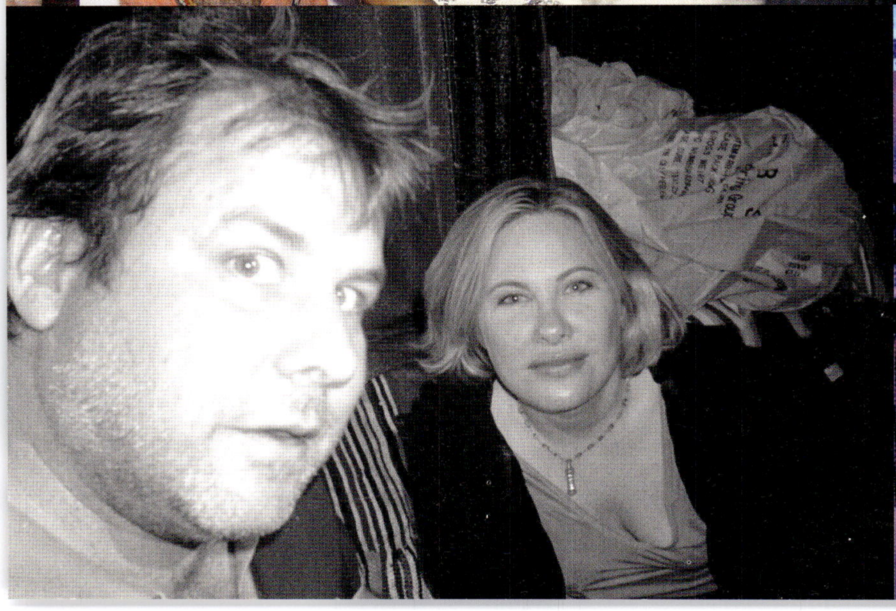
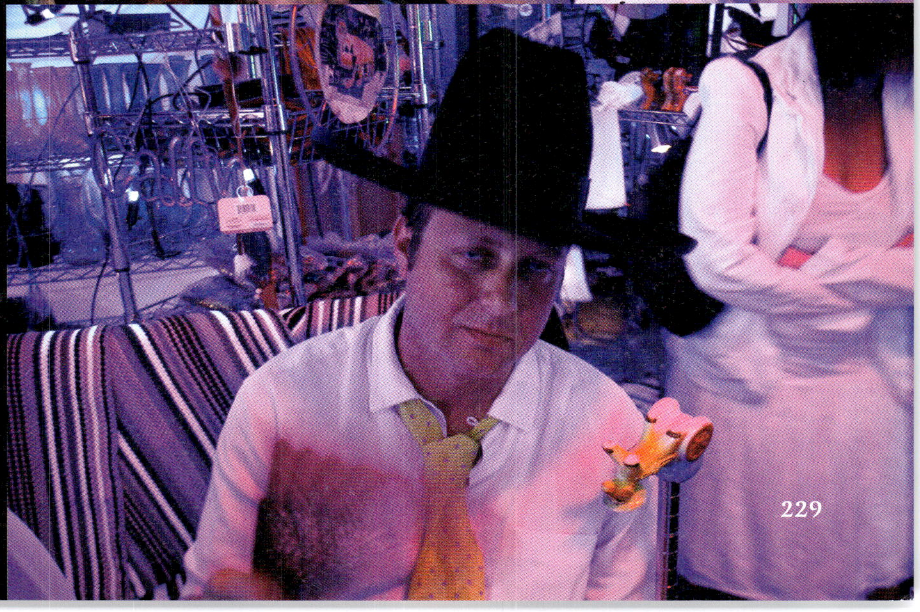

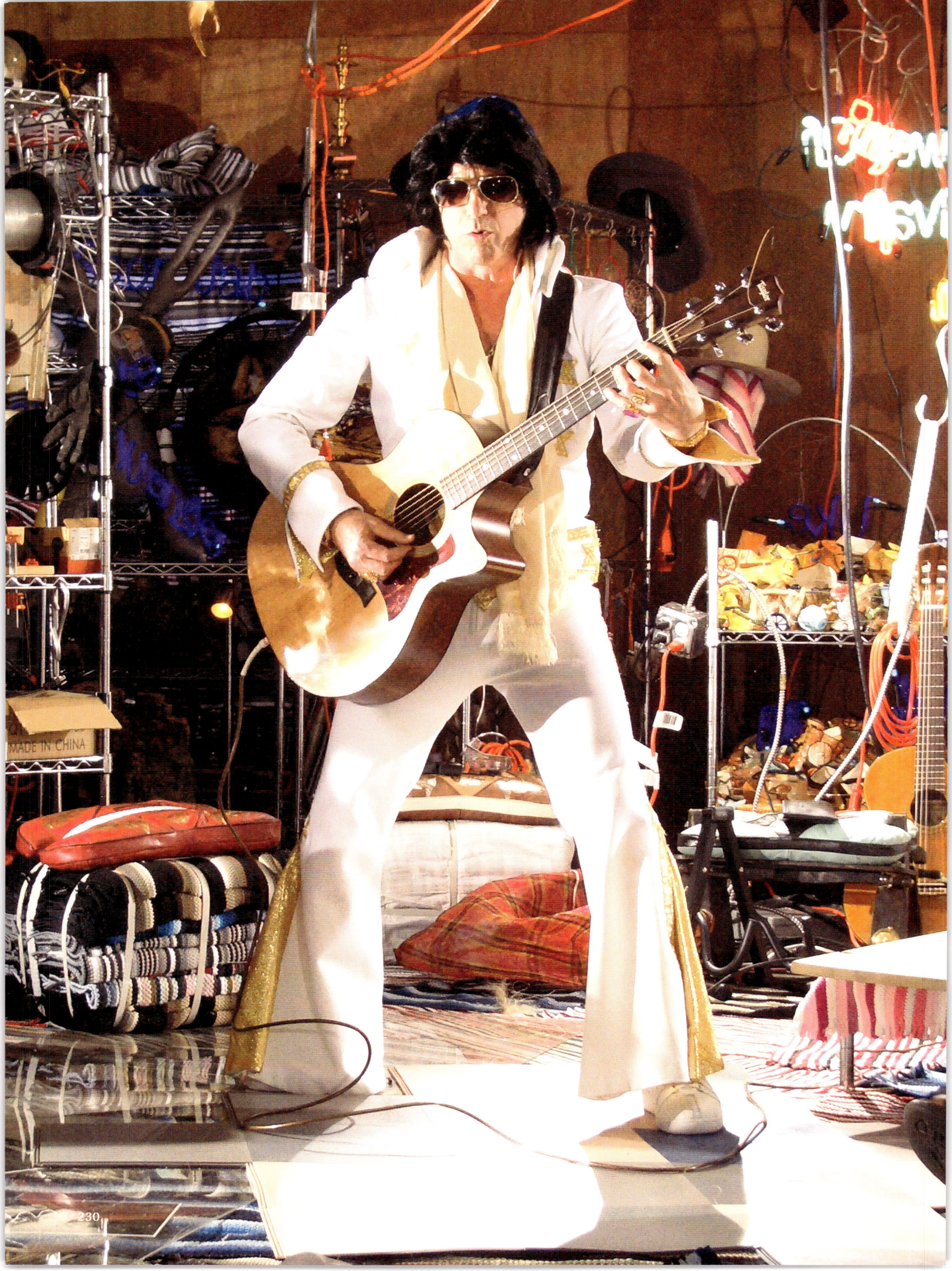
MADE IN CHINA

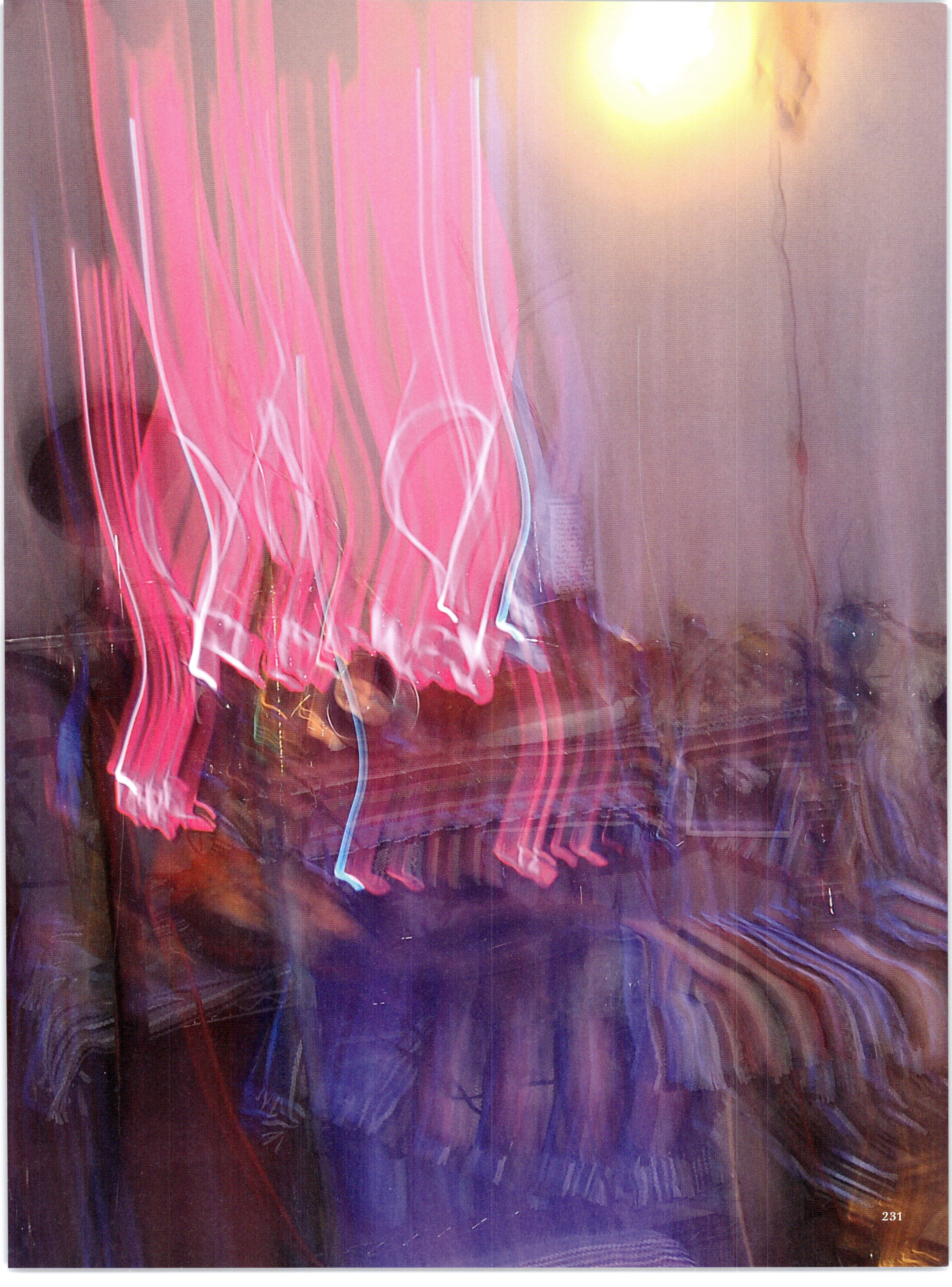

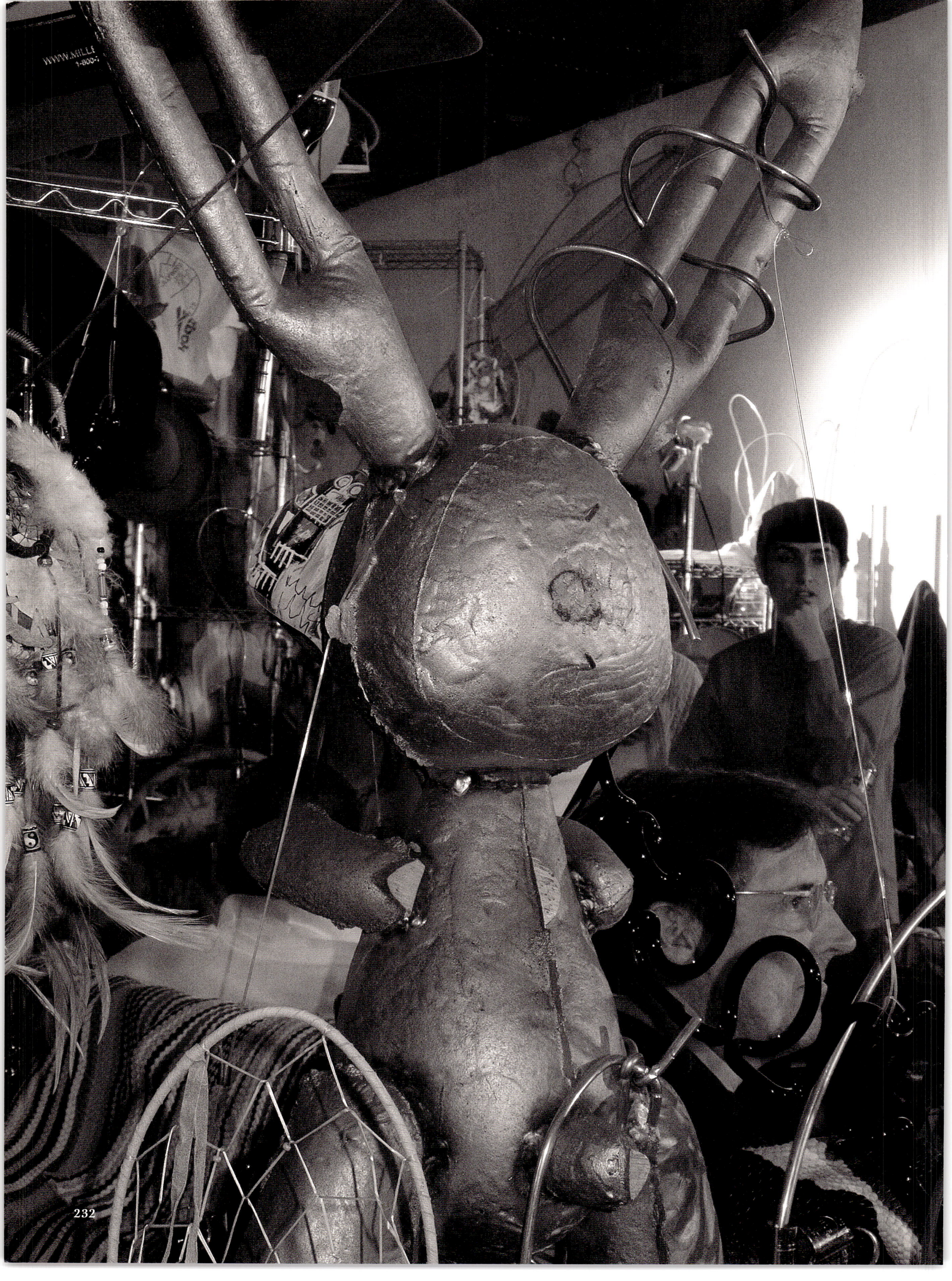

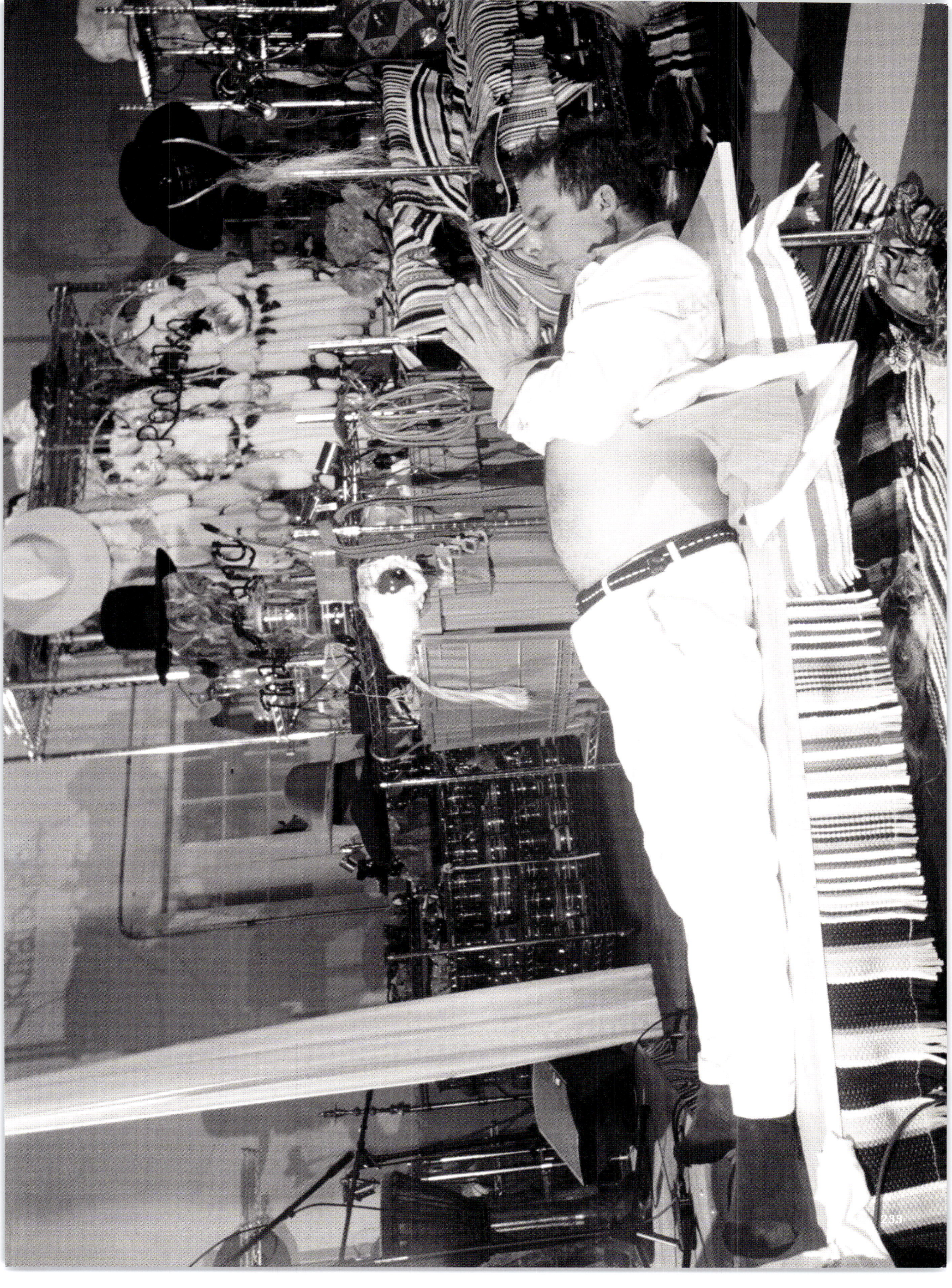

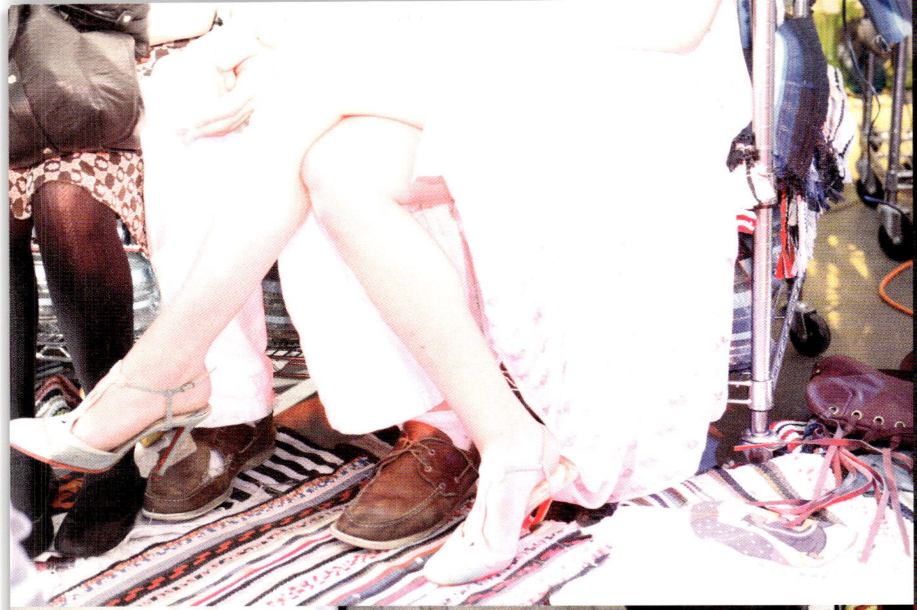

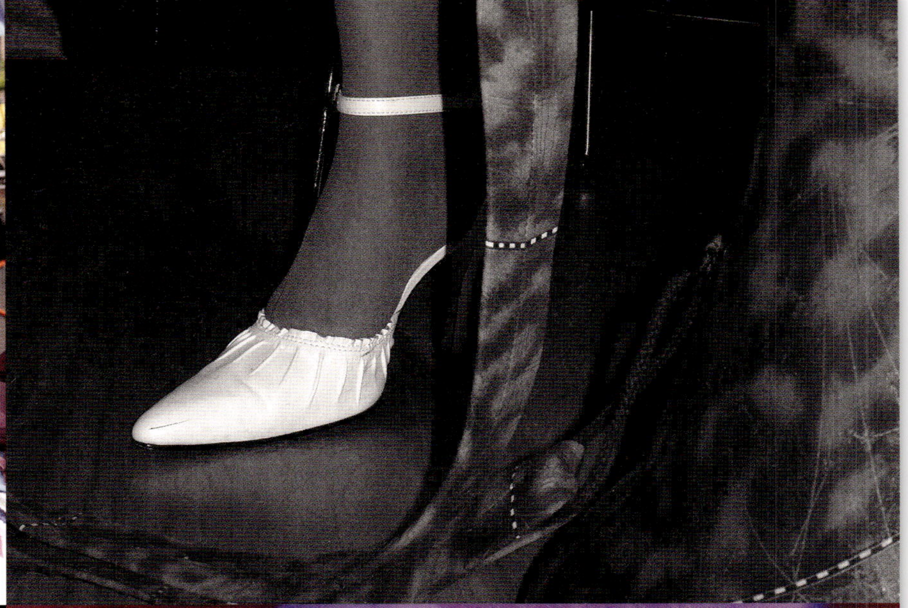

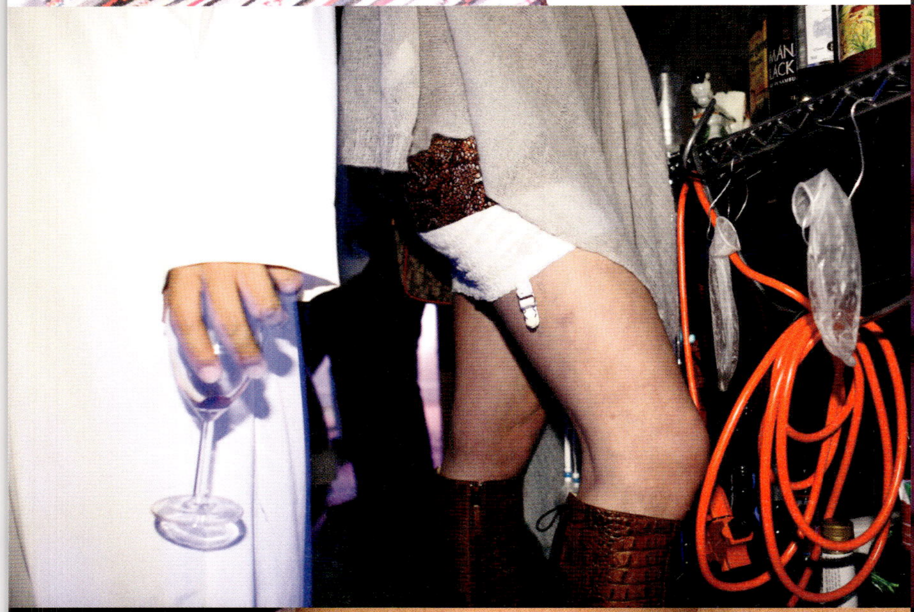

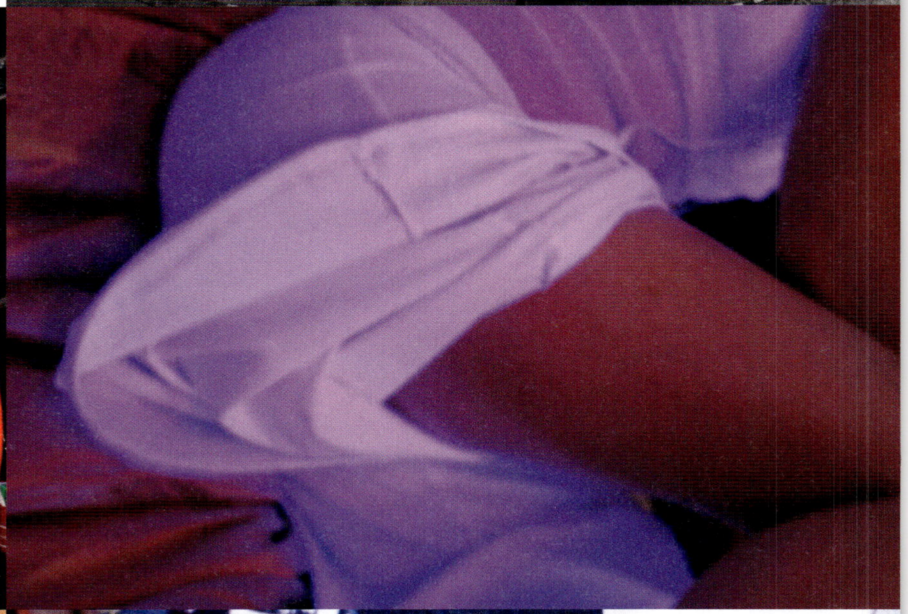

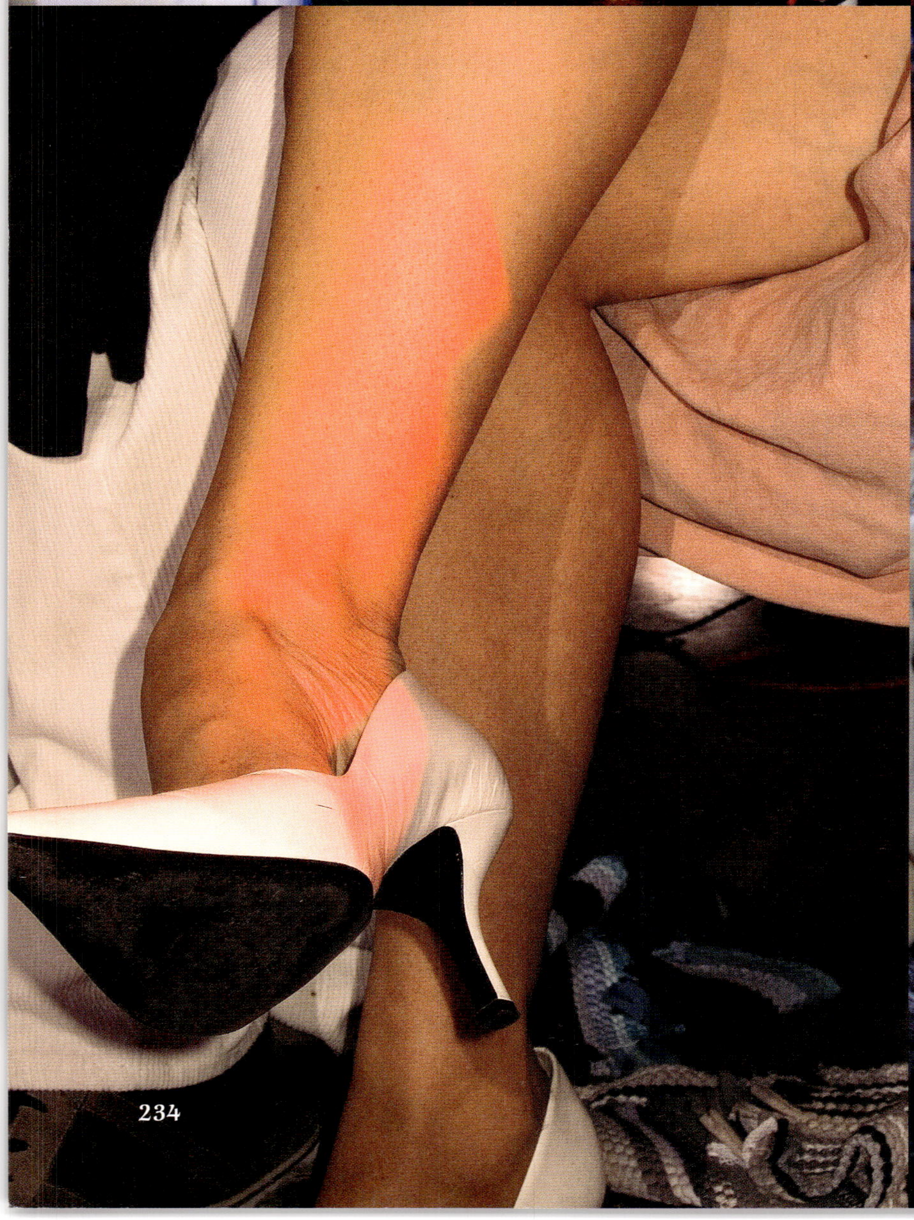

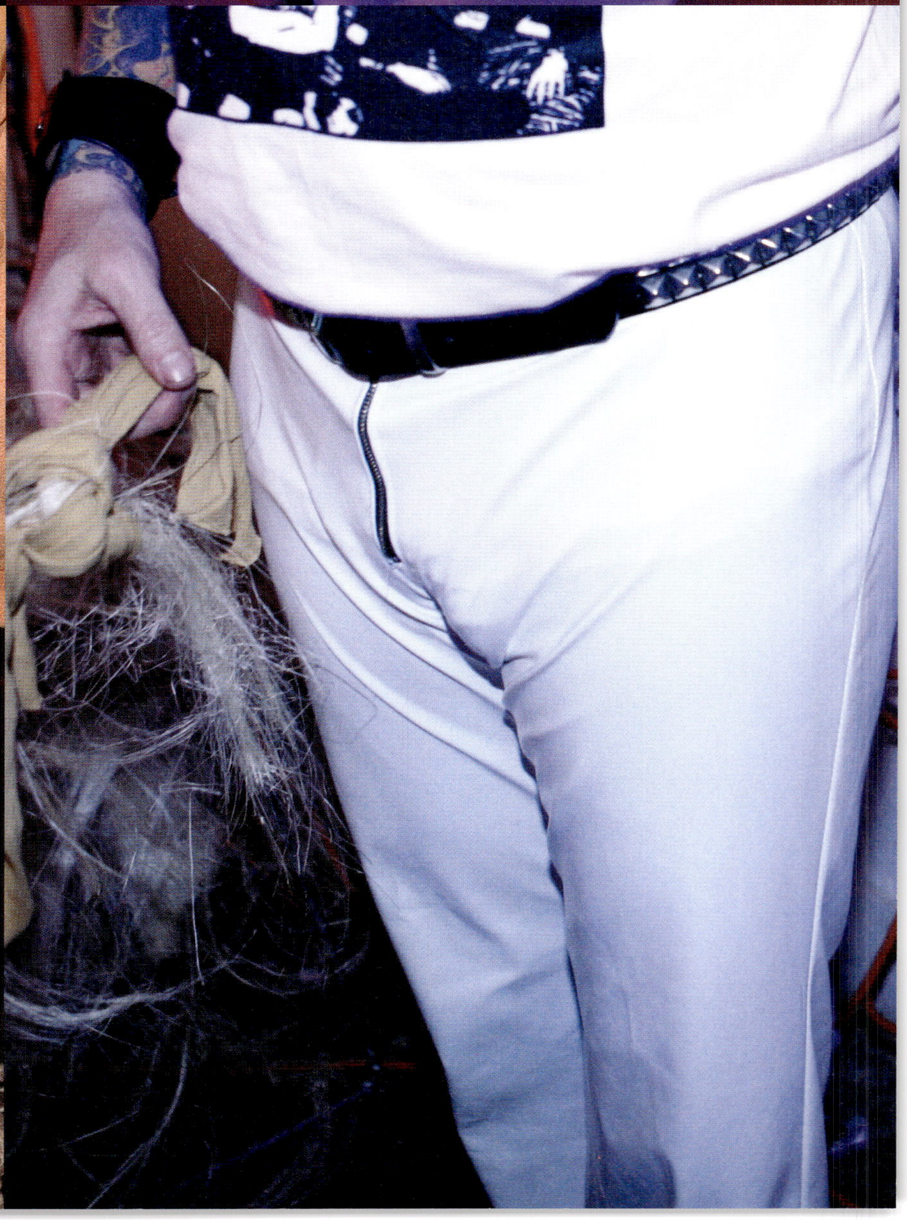

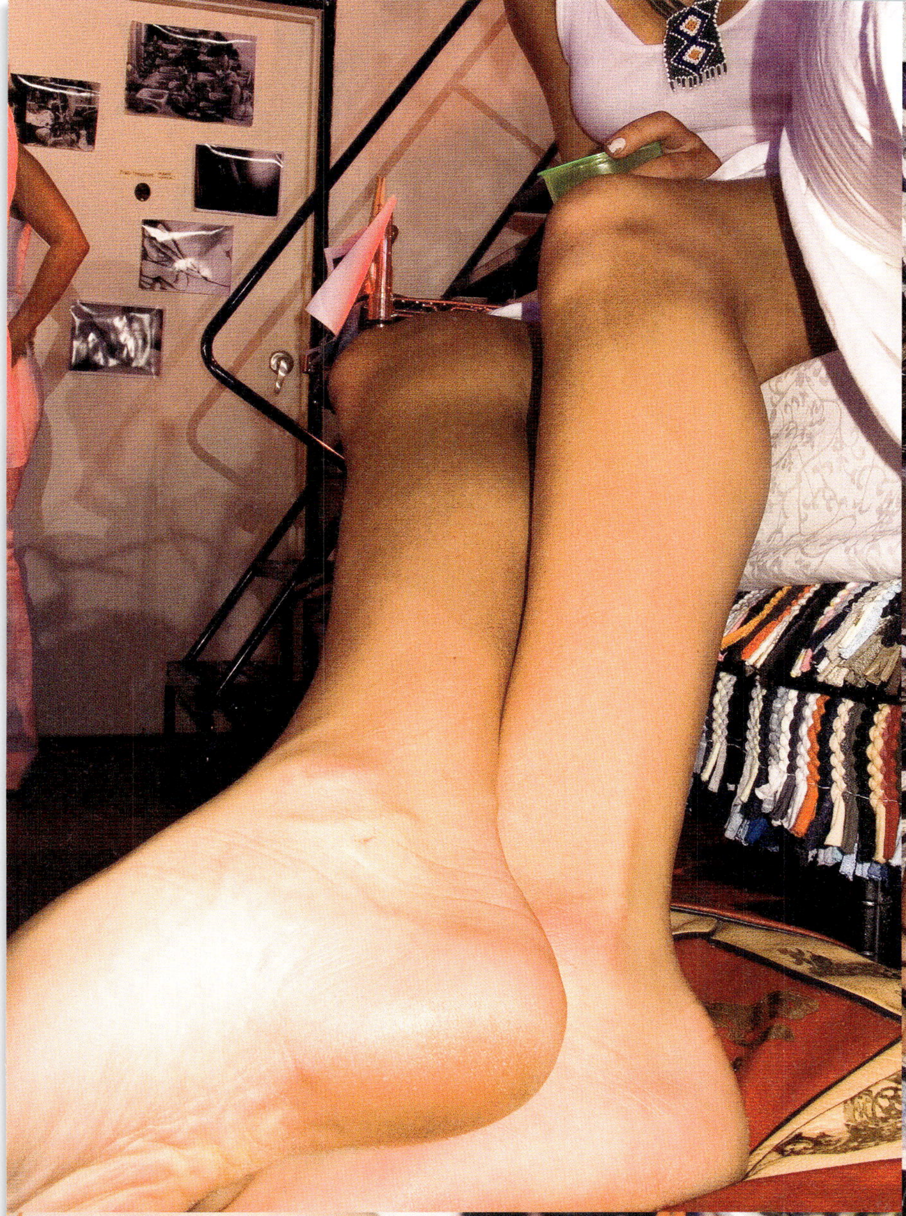
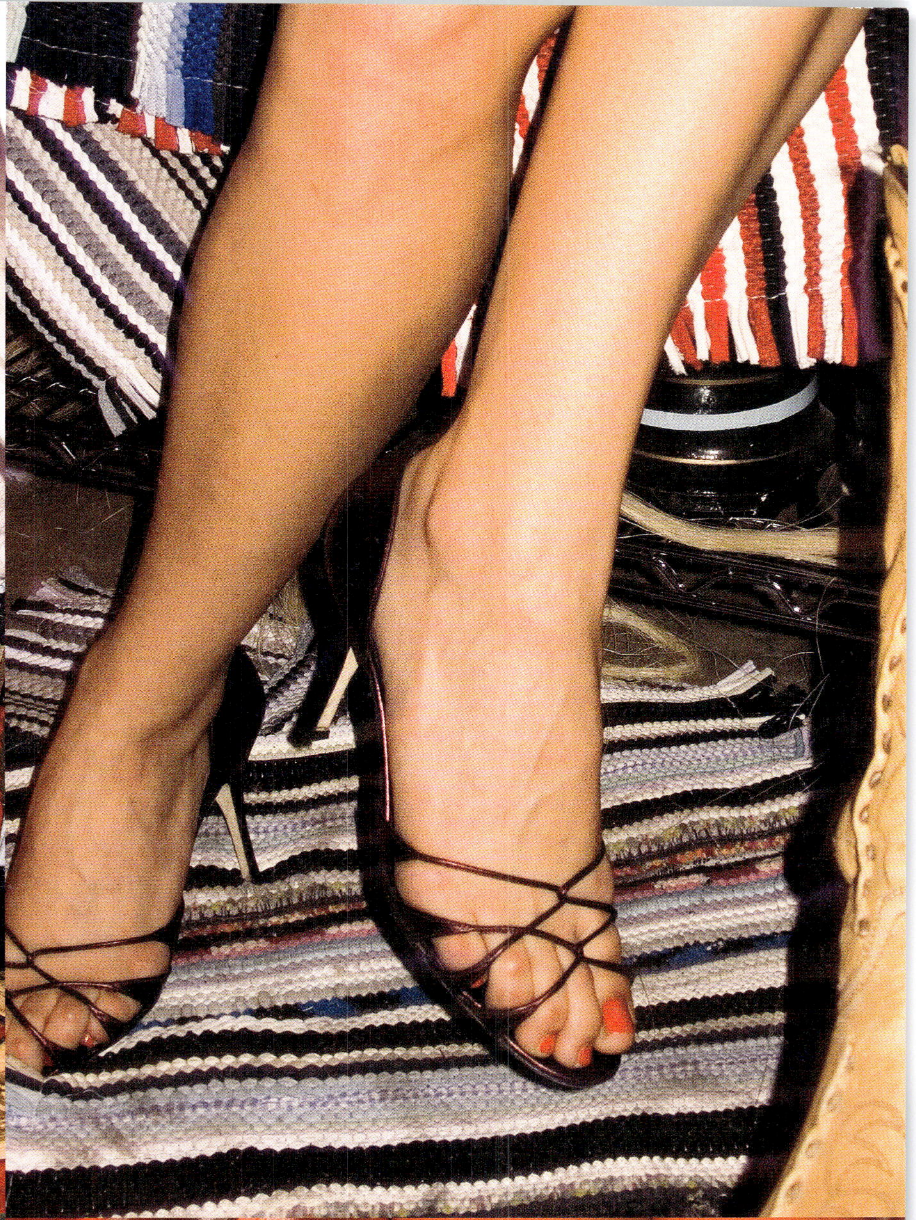
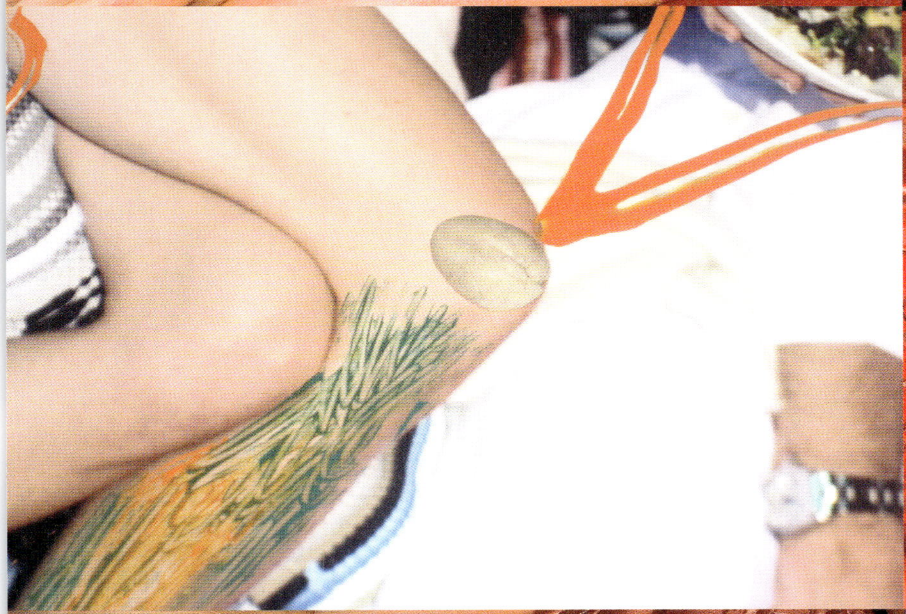
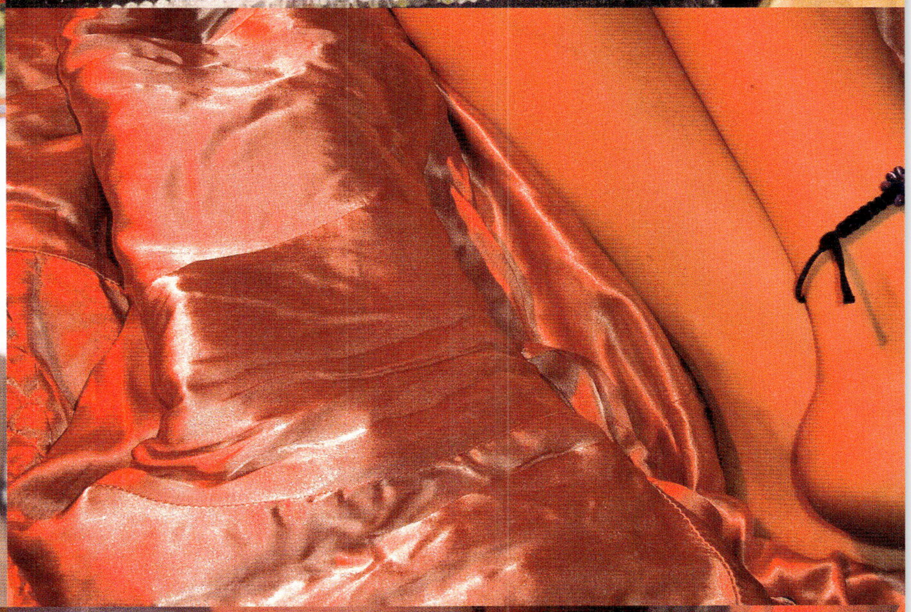
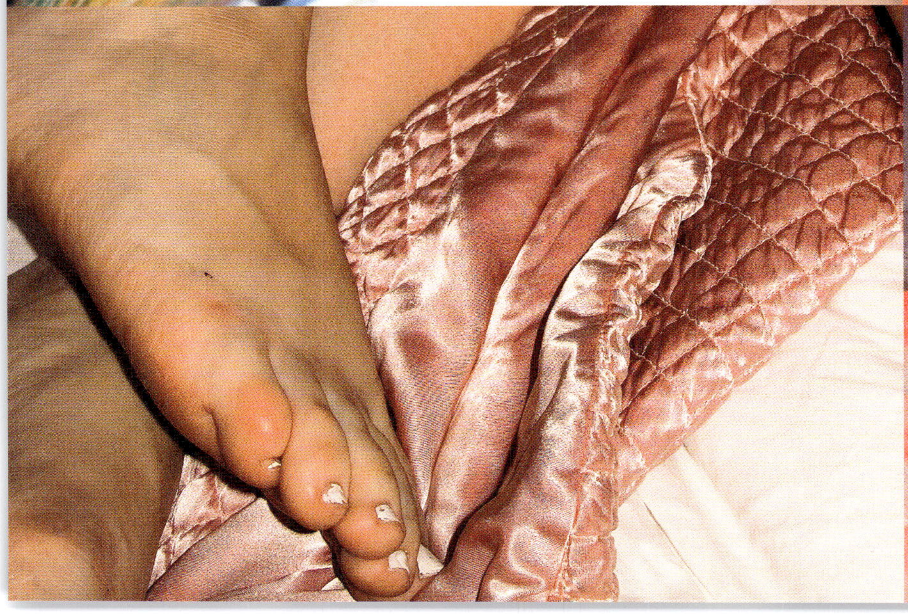
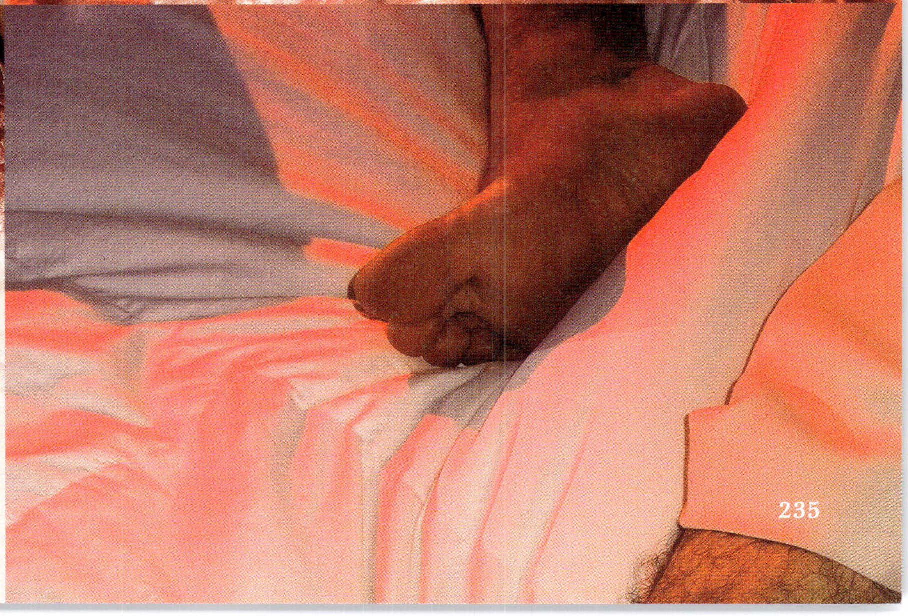

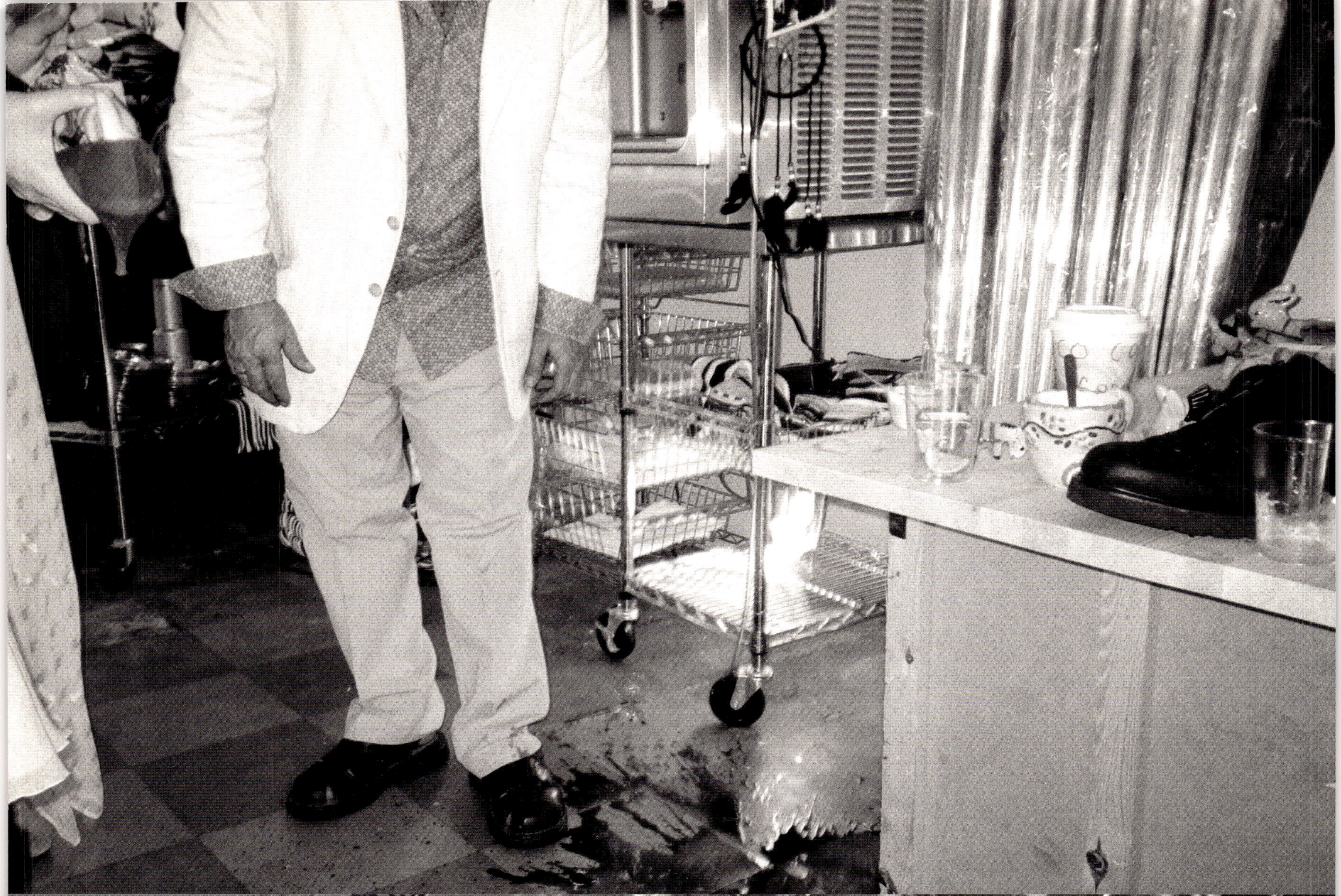

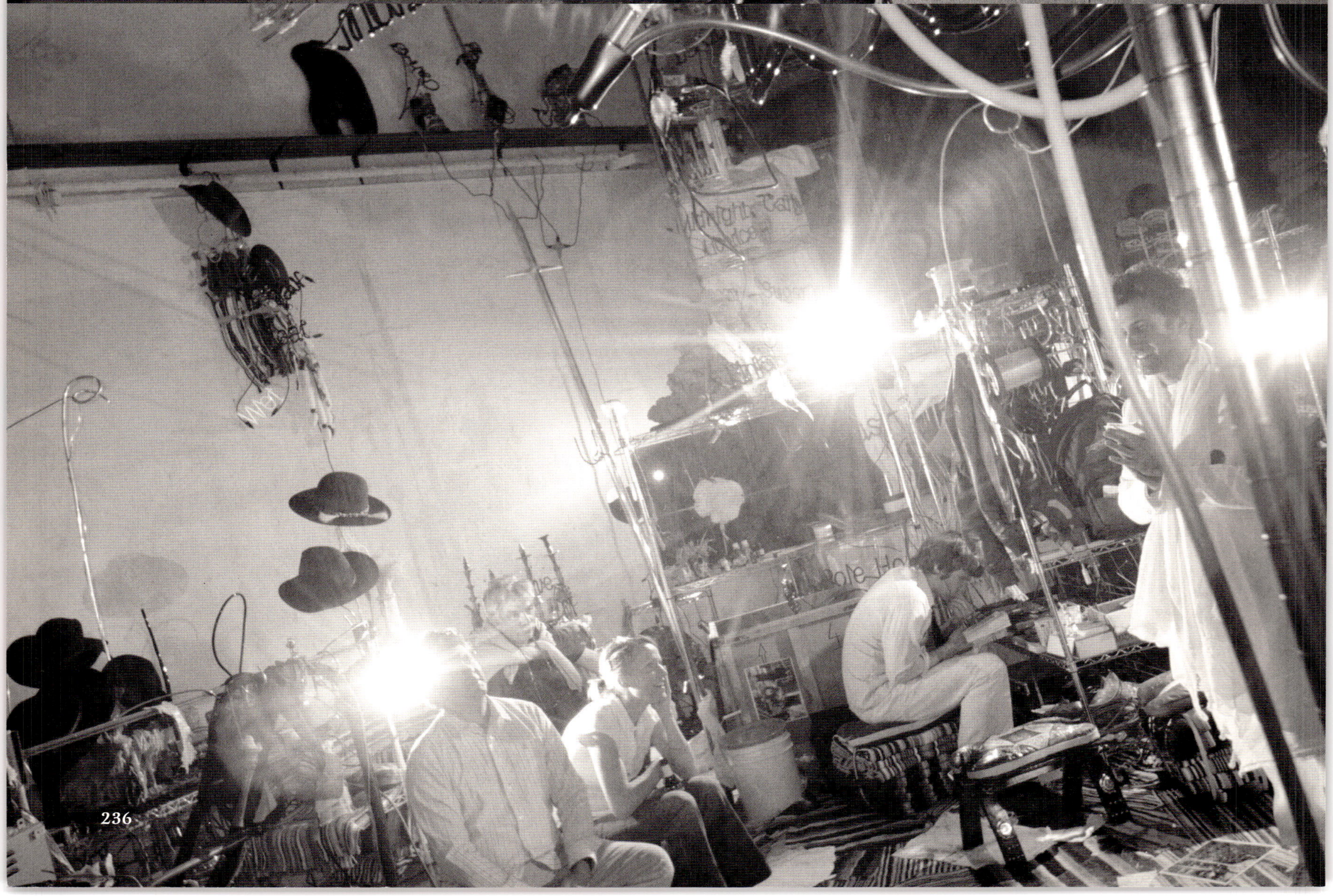

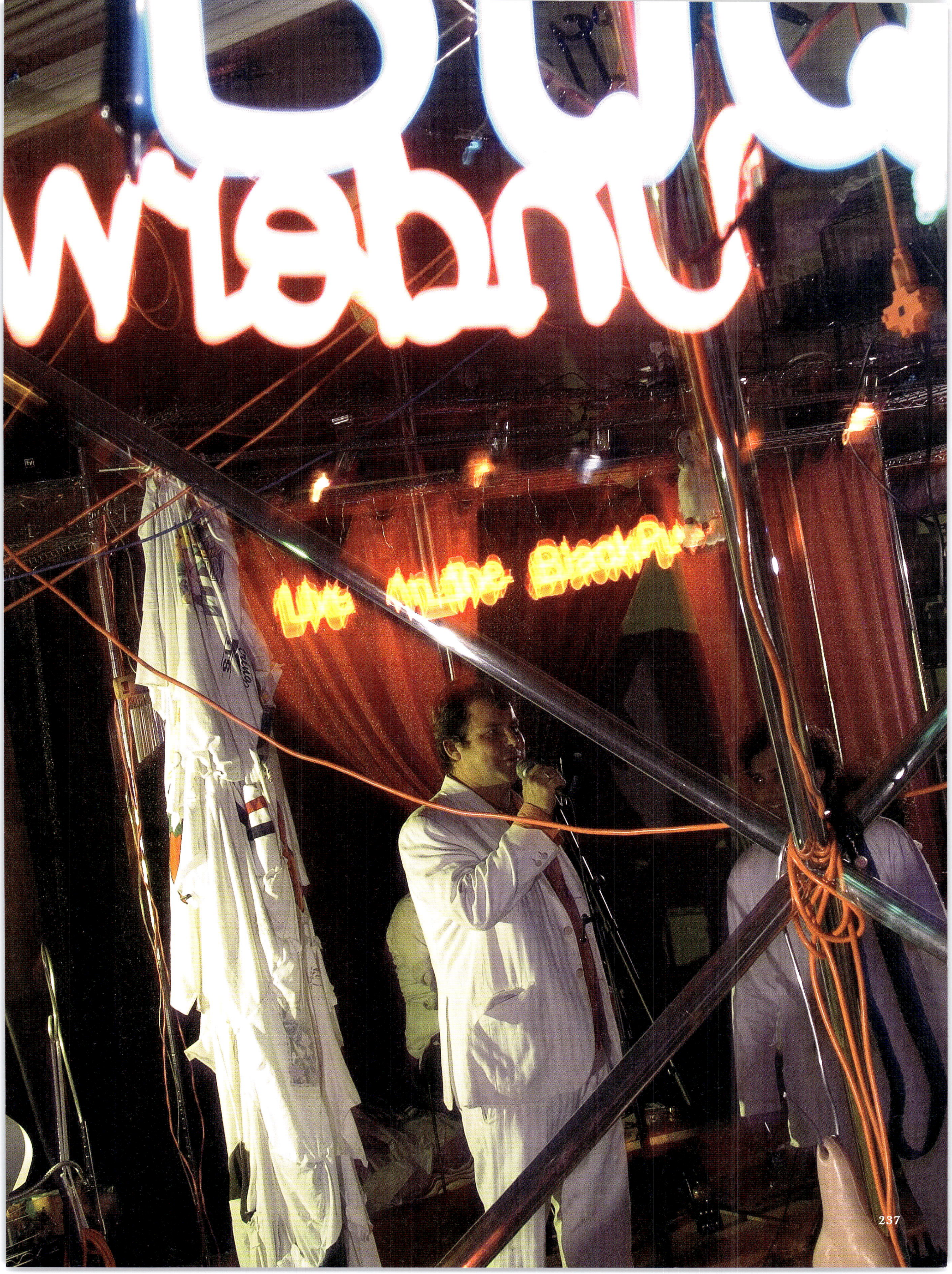

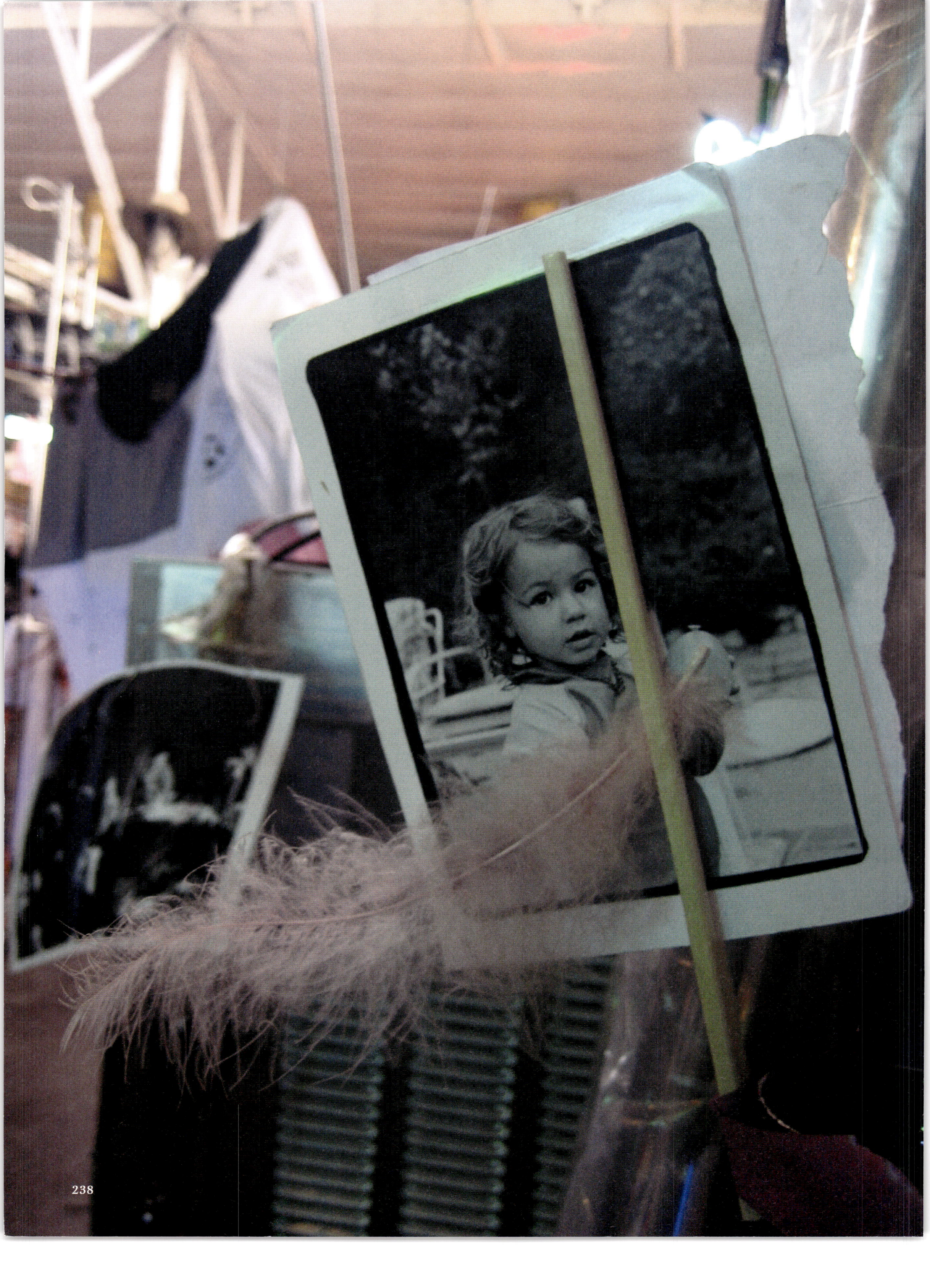

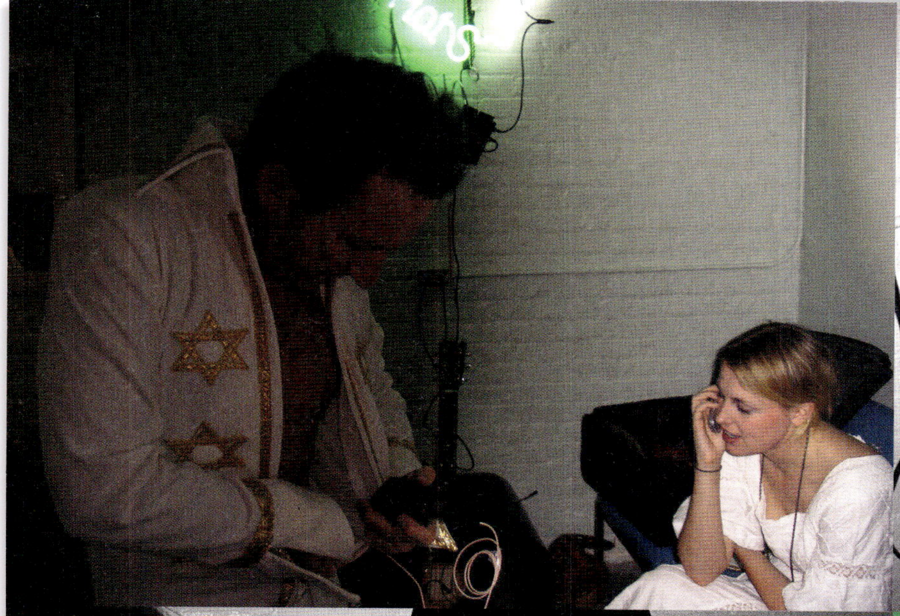
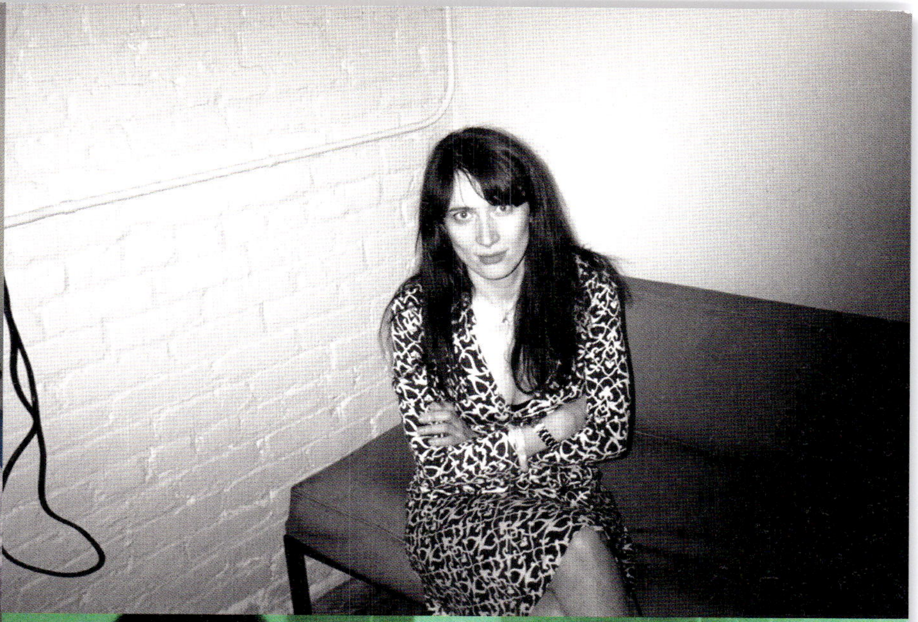
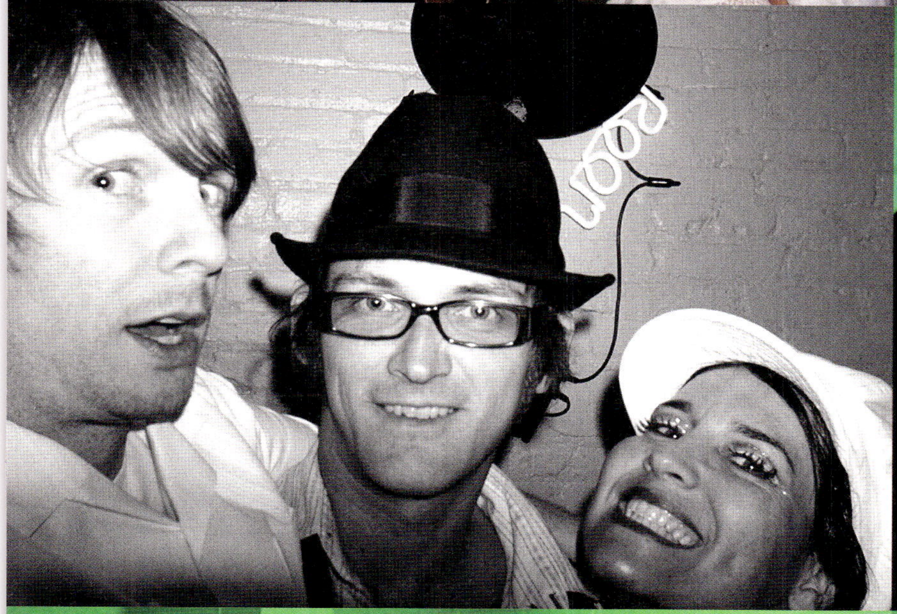
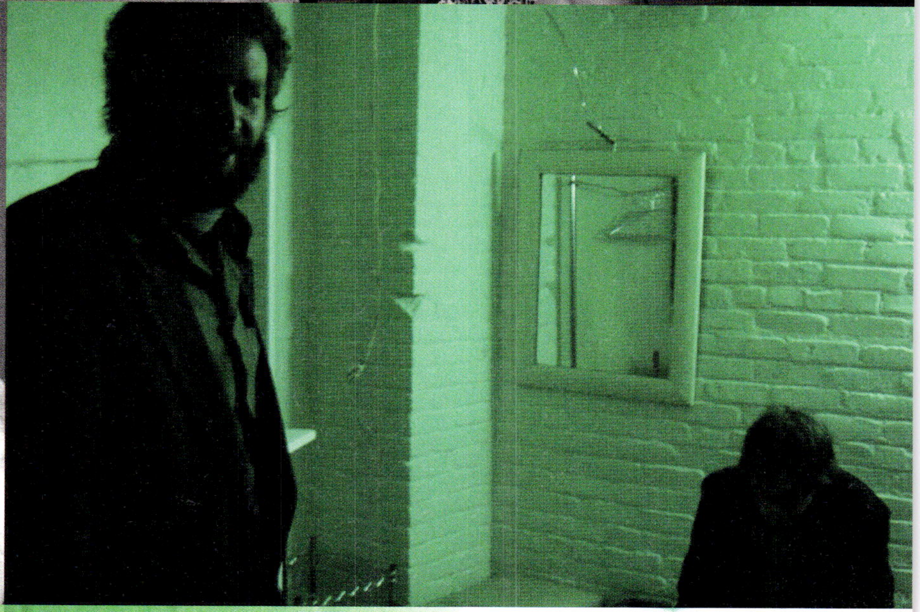
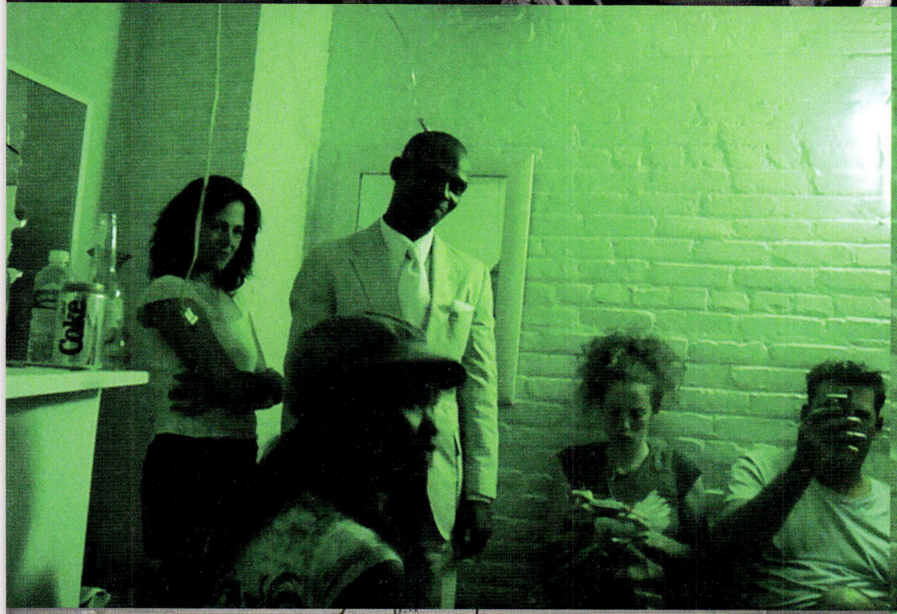
Coke
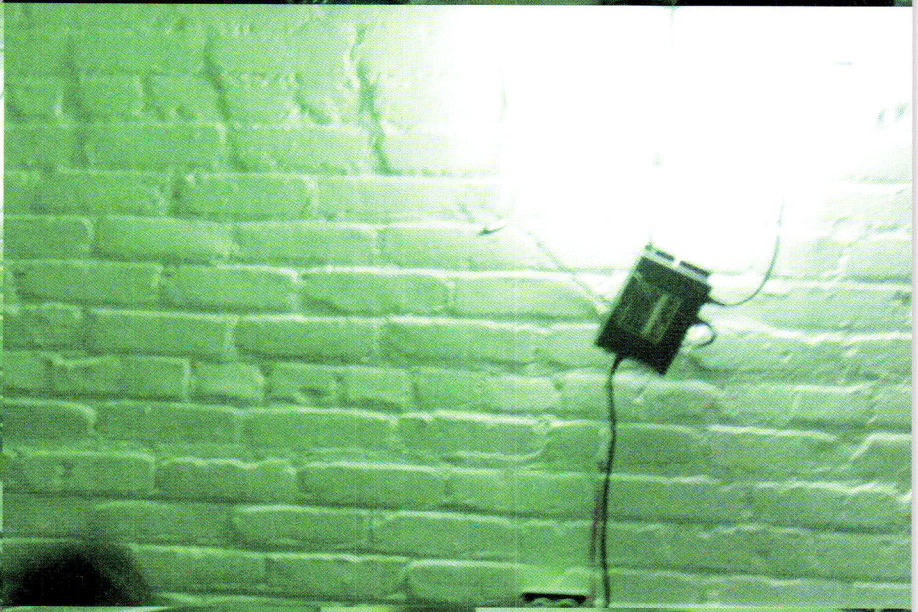
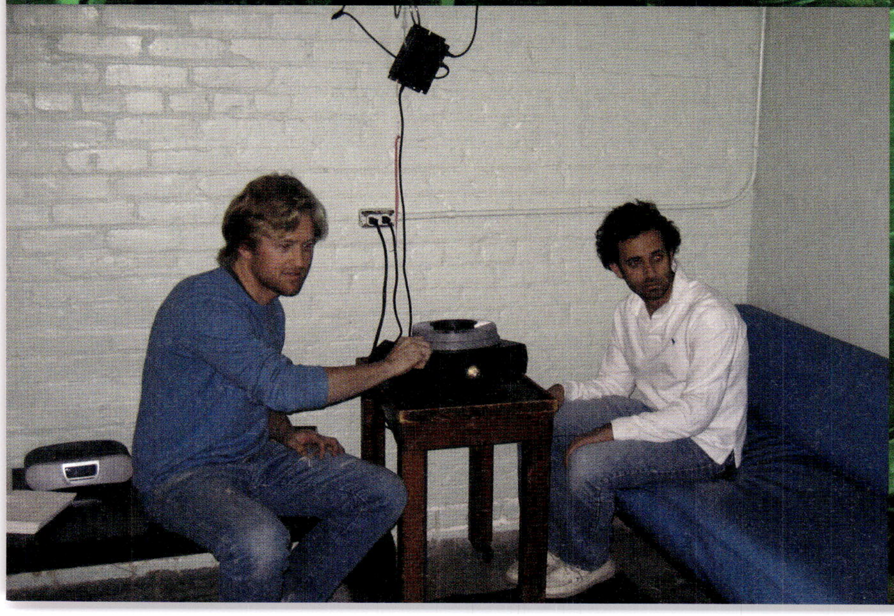
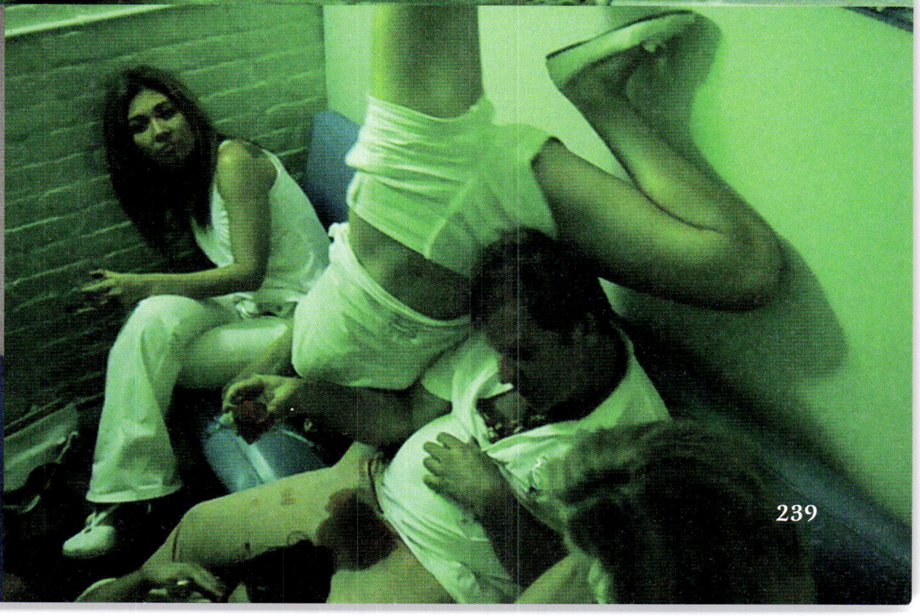

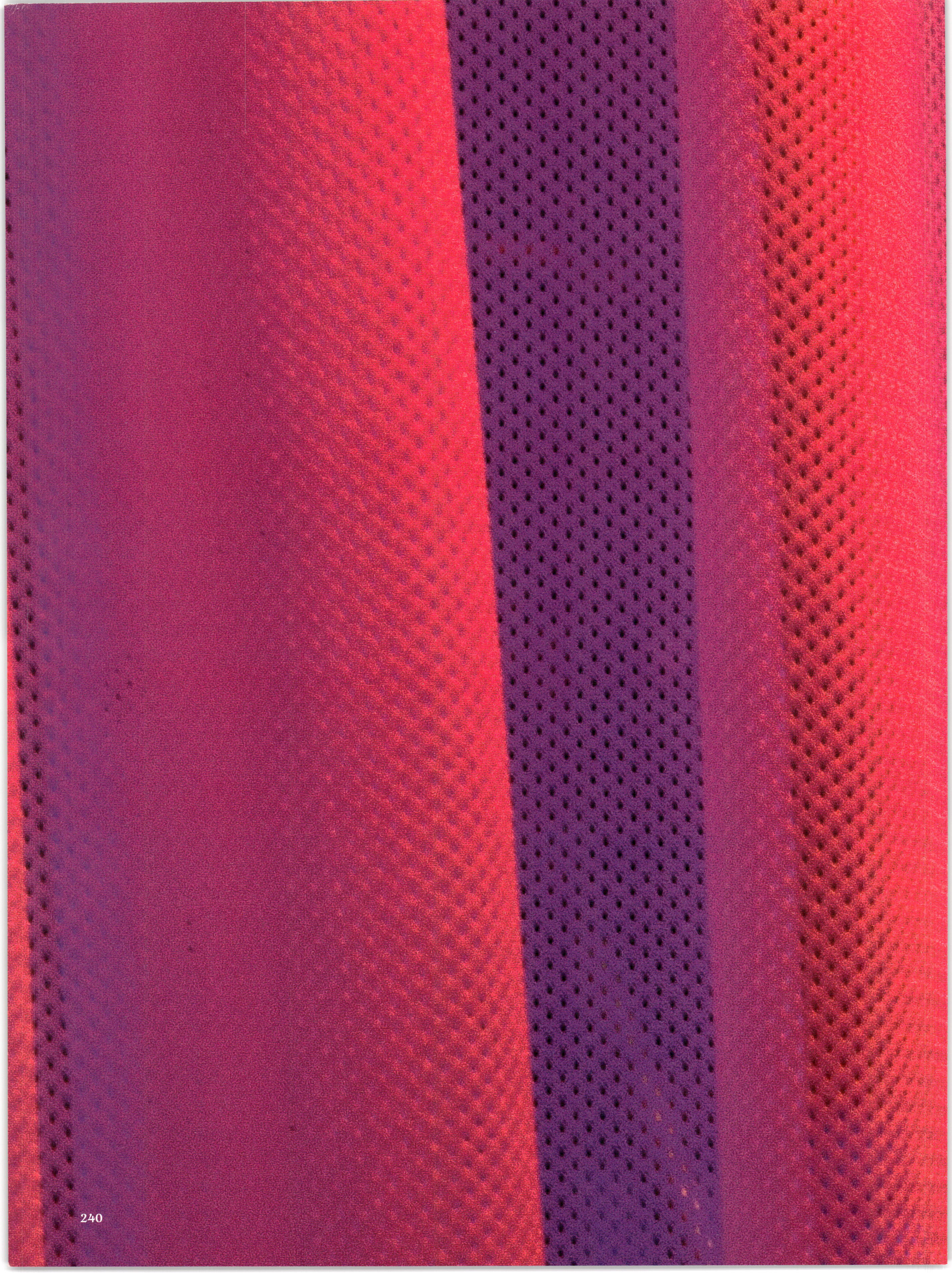

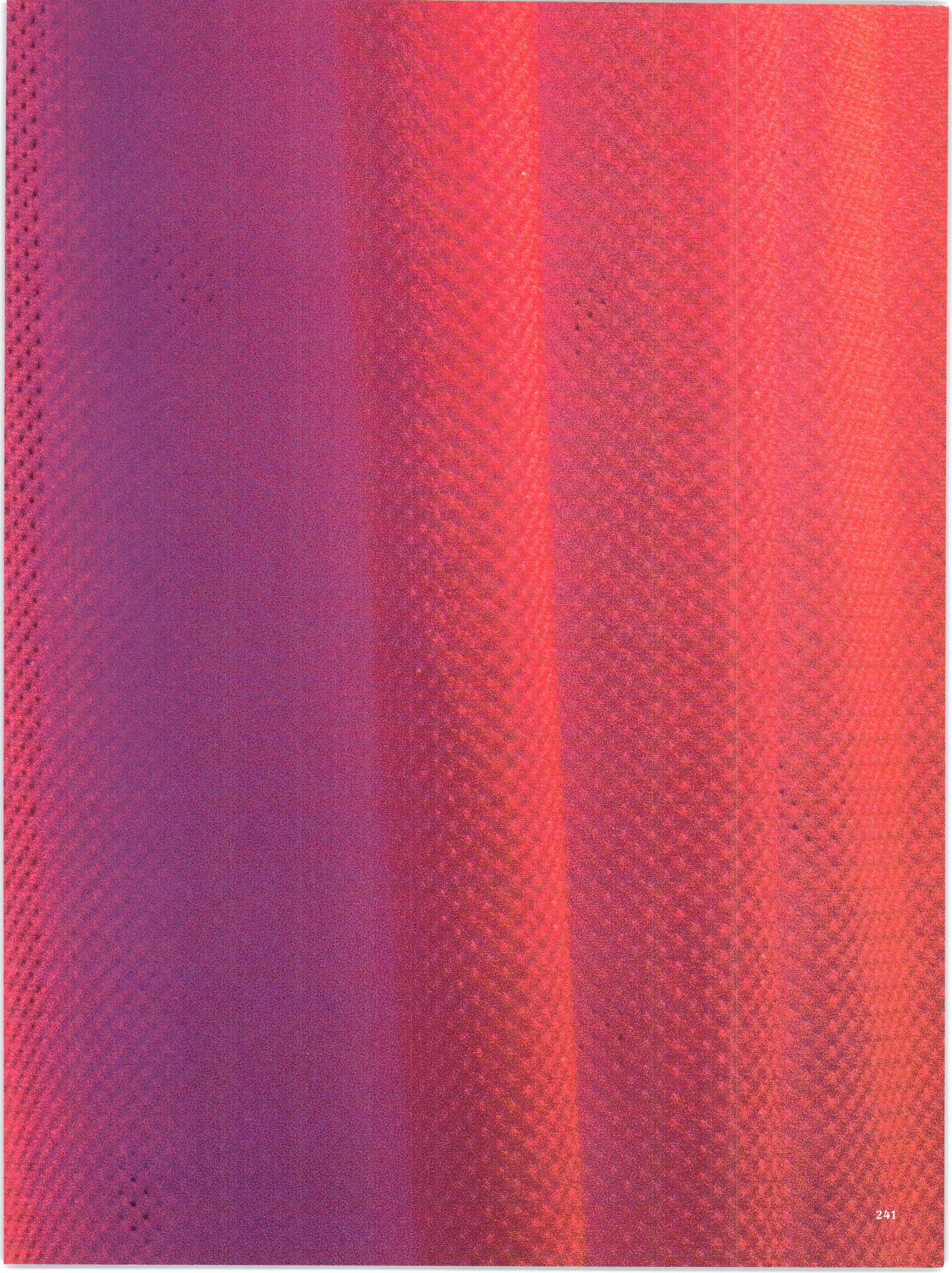

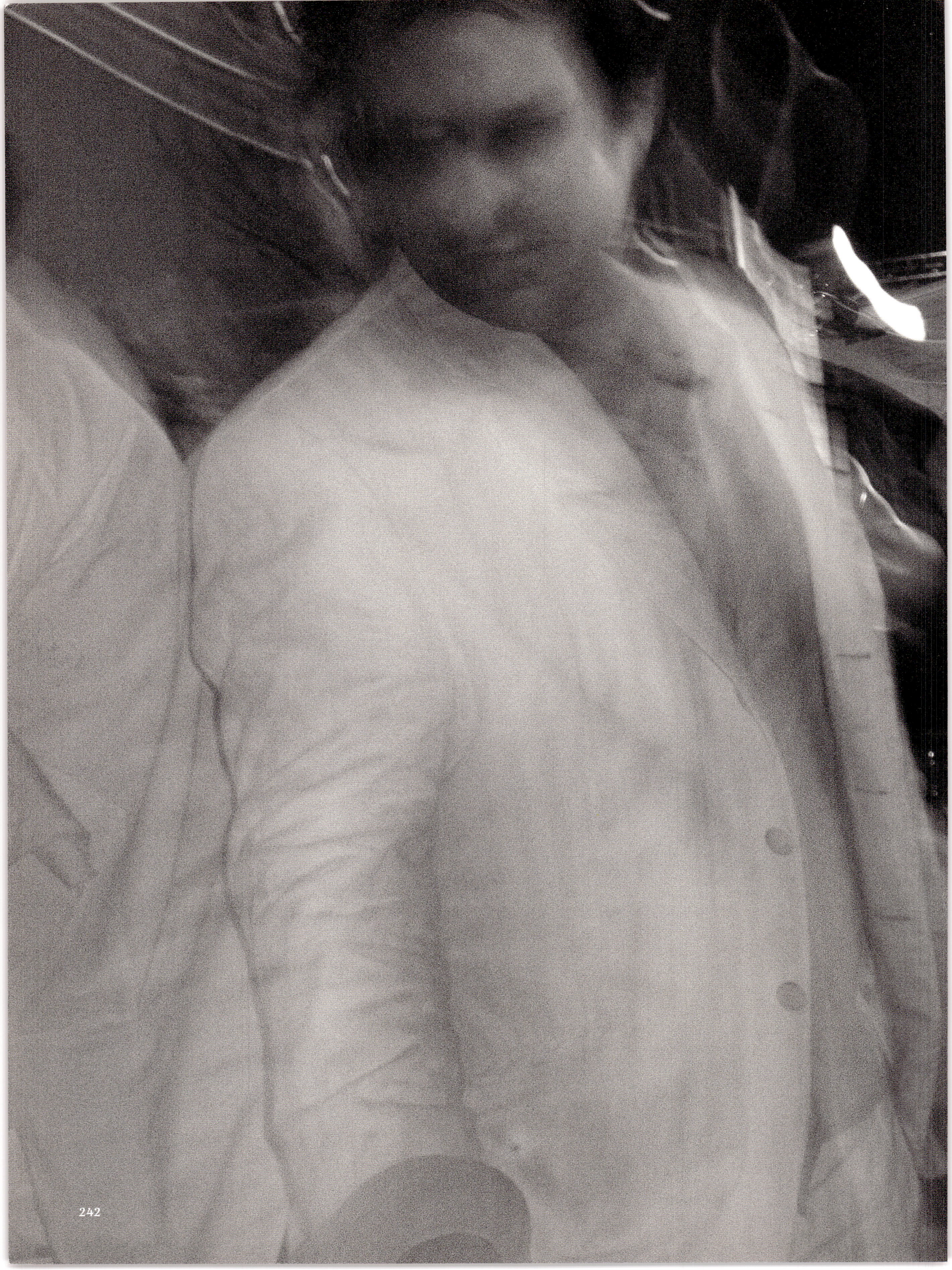

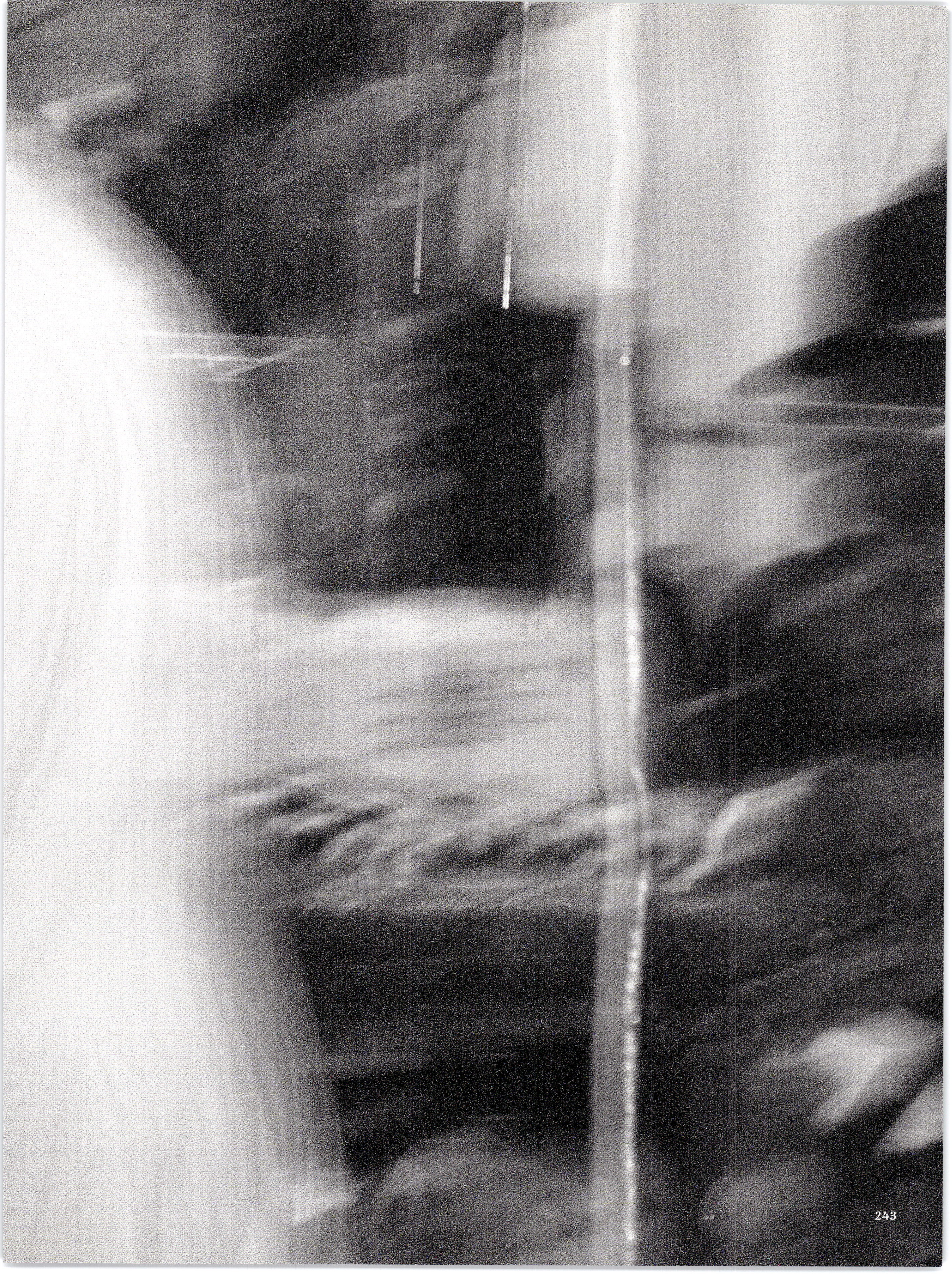

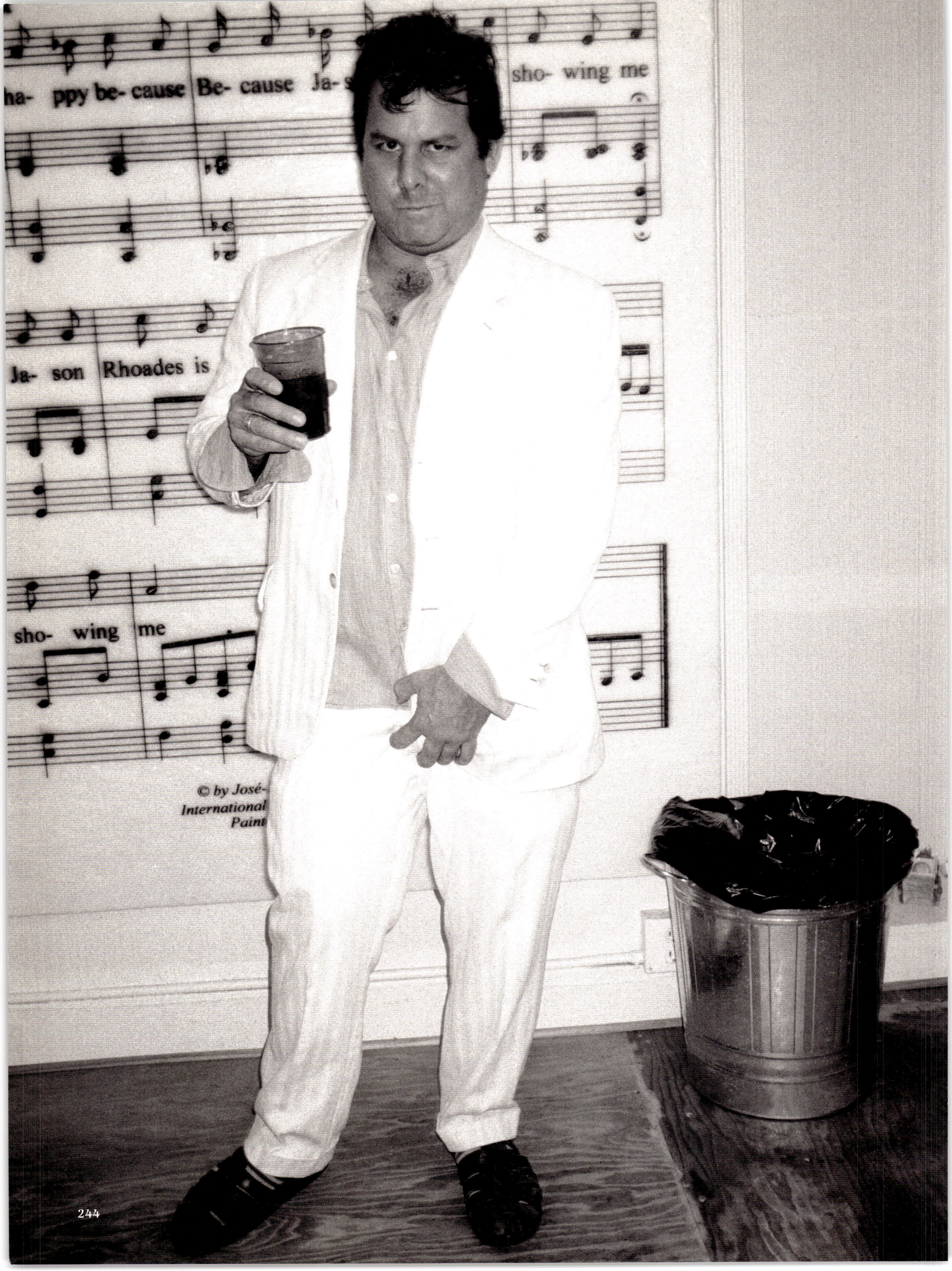
ha- ppy be- cause Be- cause Ja-
sho- wing me
Ja- son Rhoades is
sho- wing me
© by José-
International
Paint

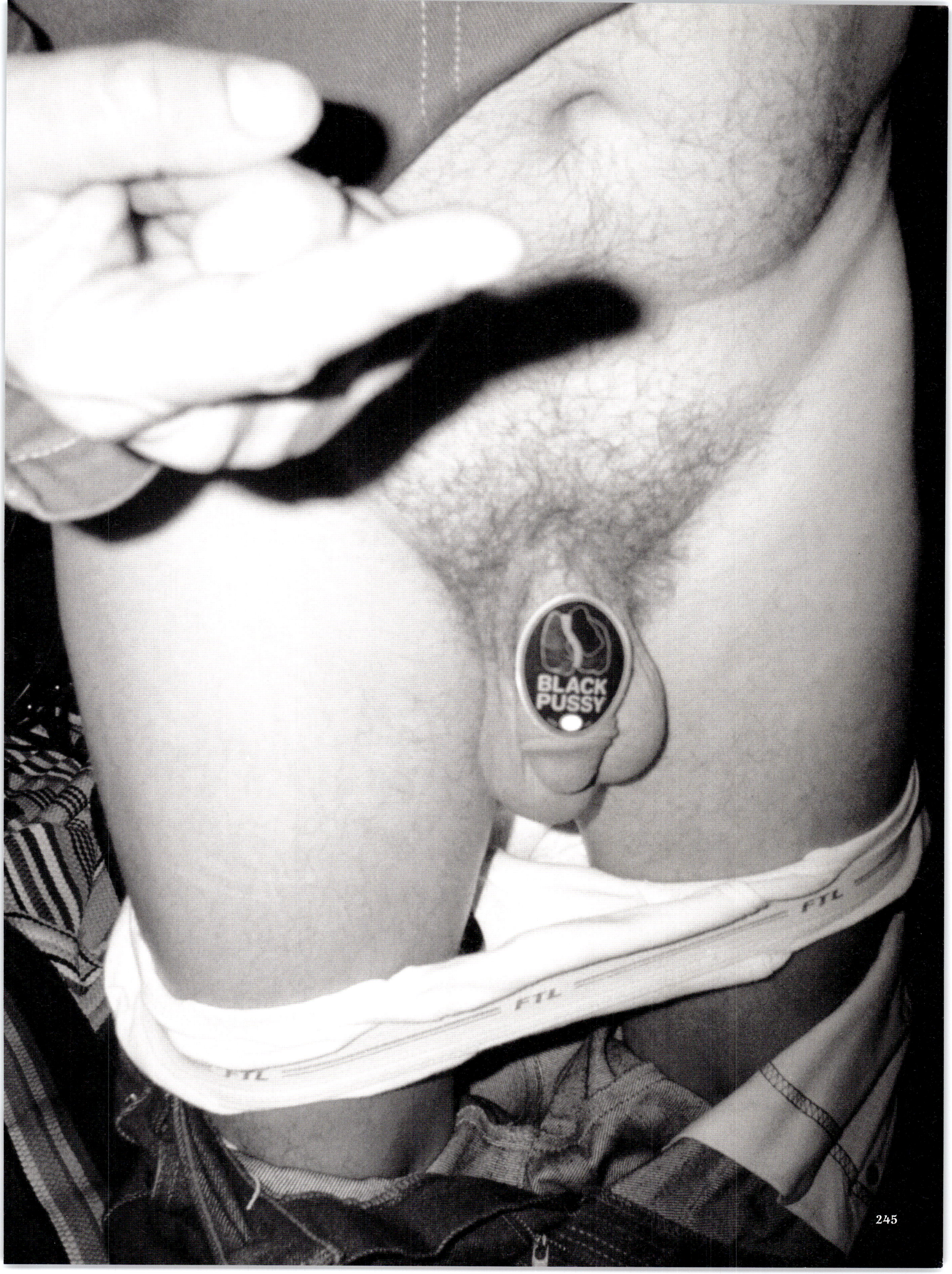
BLACK
PUSSY
FTL
FTL
FTL
FTL

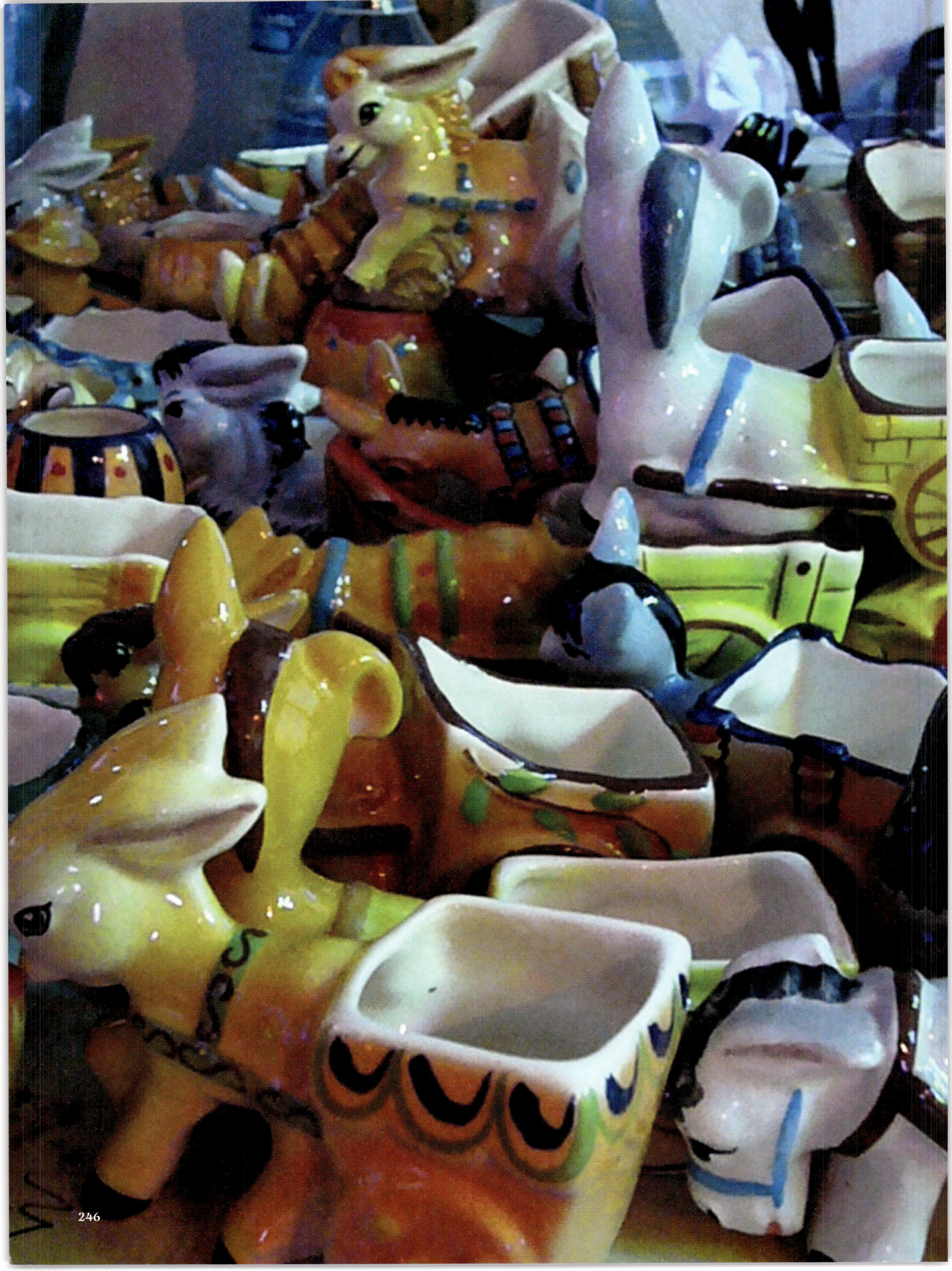

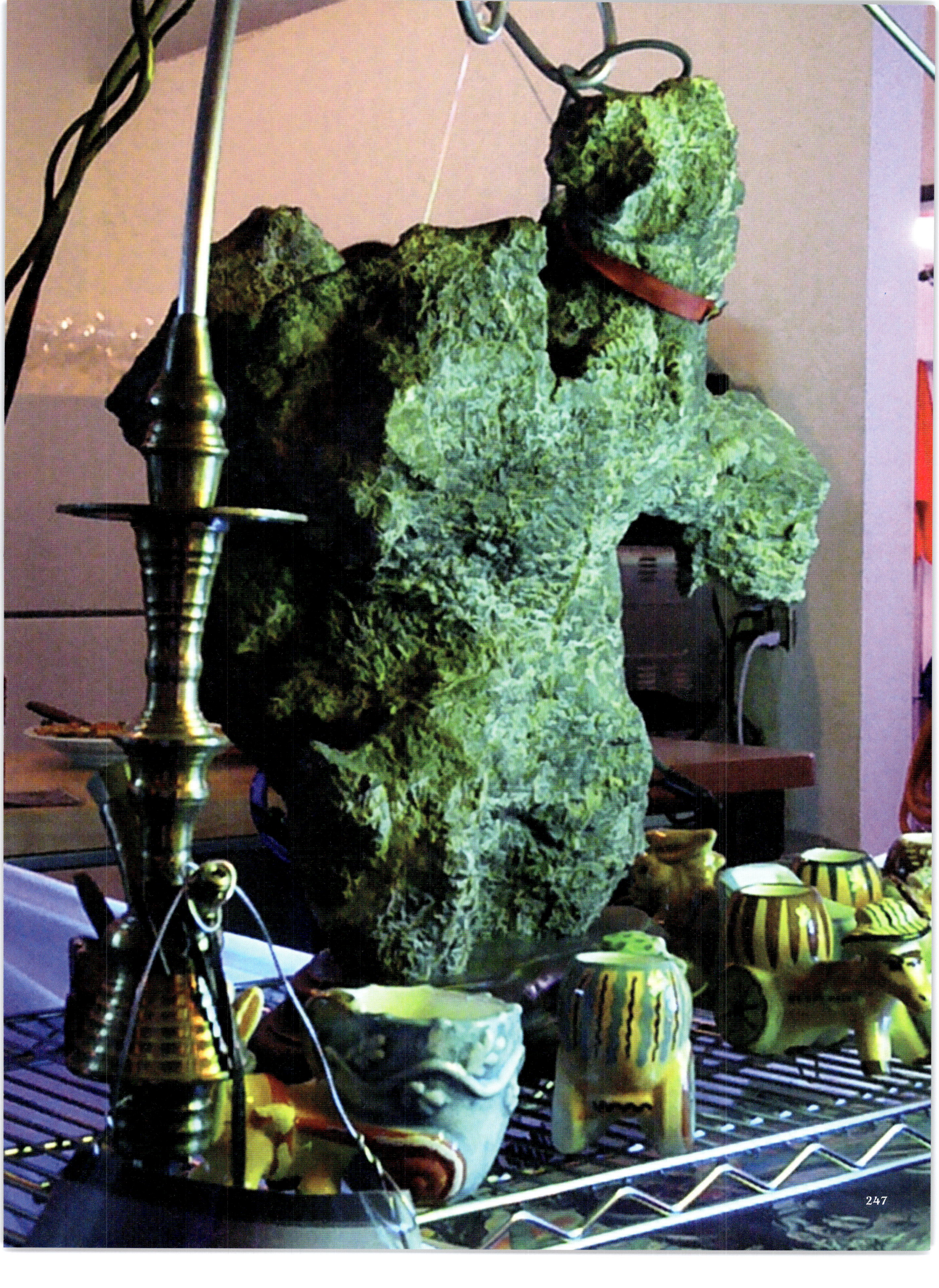

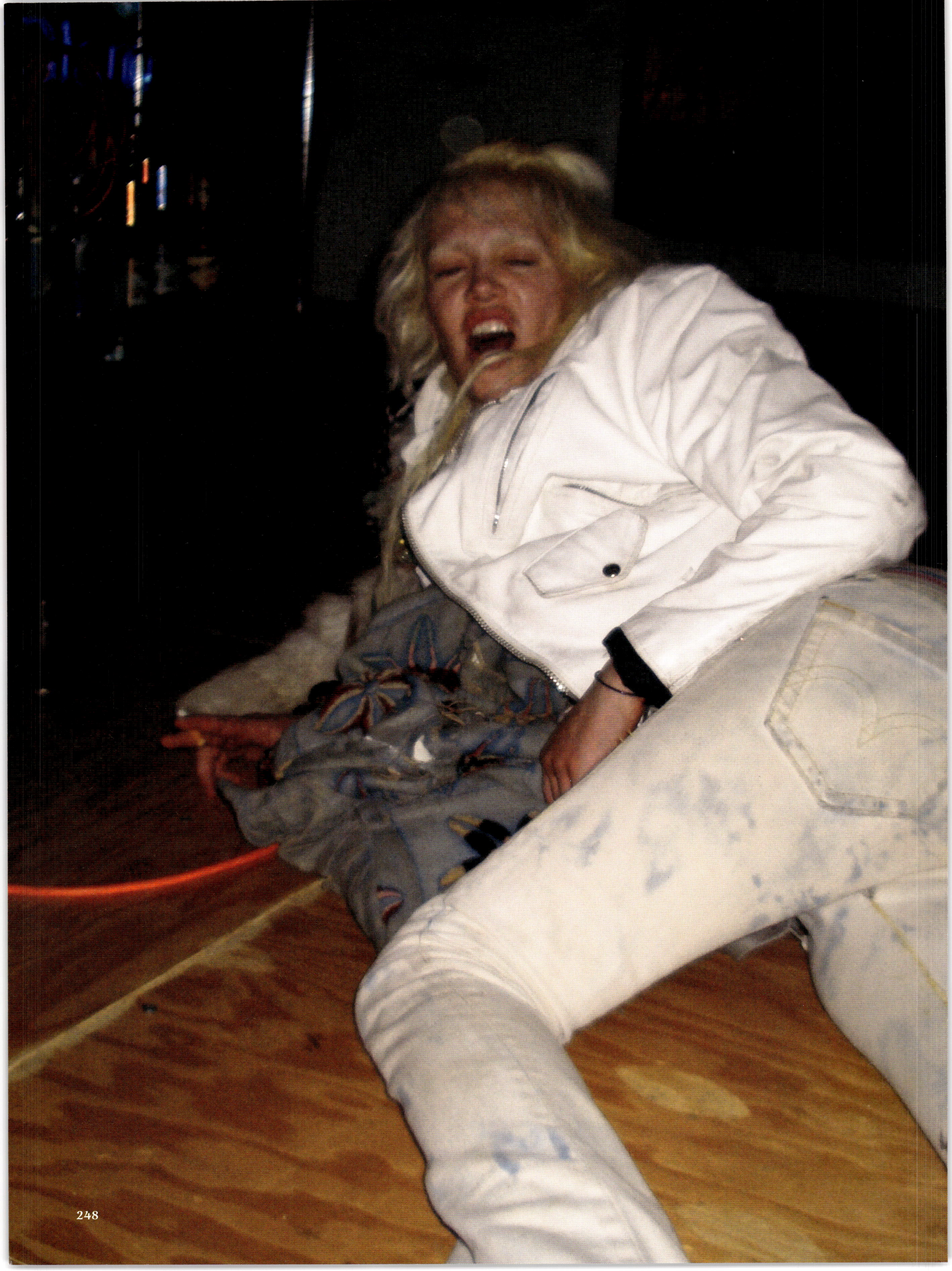

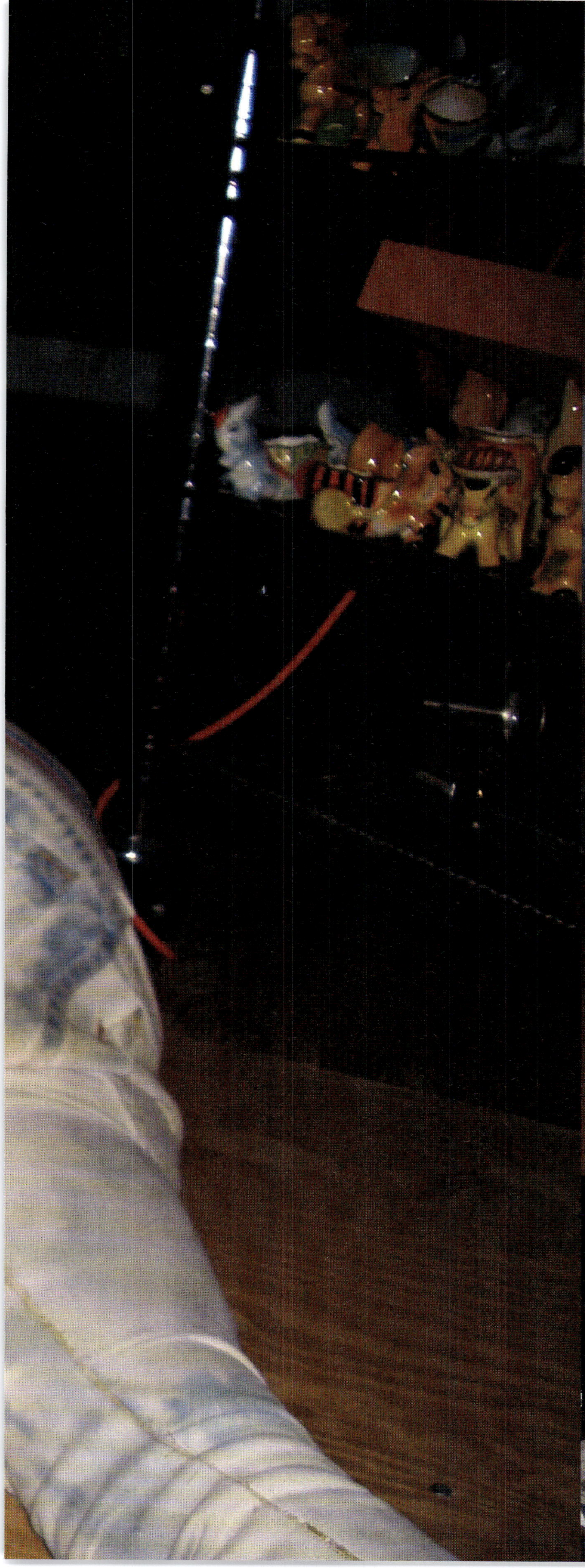

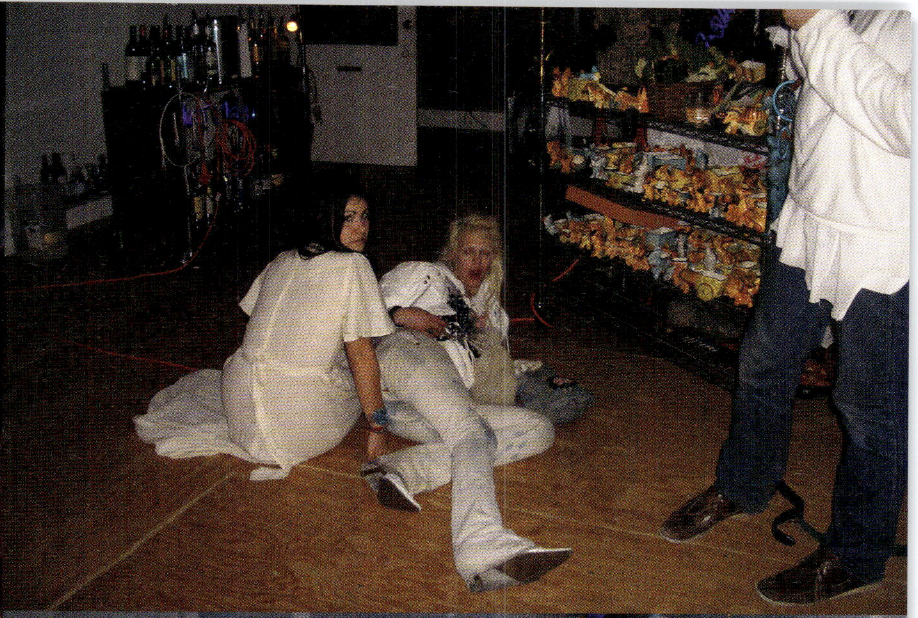

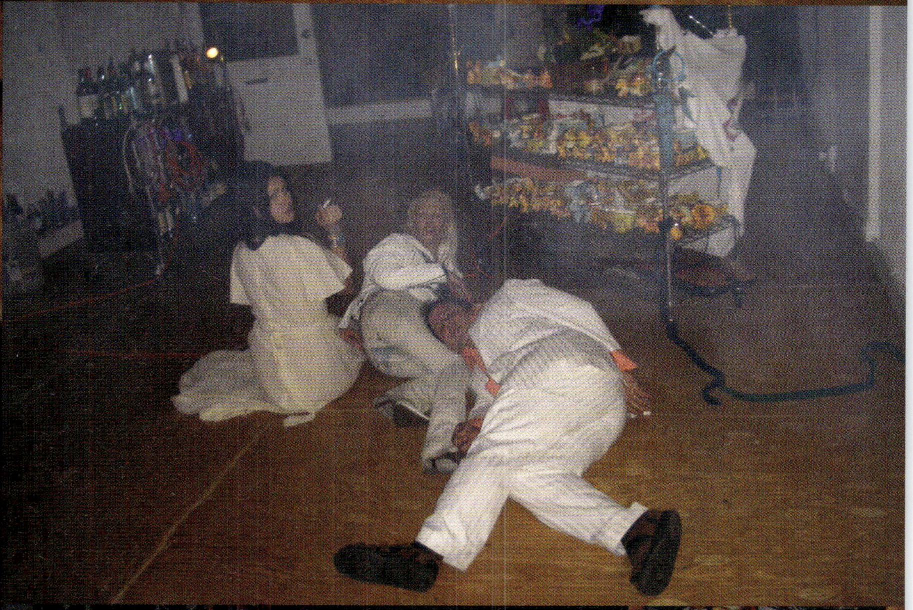

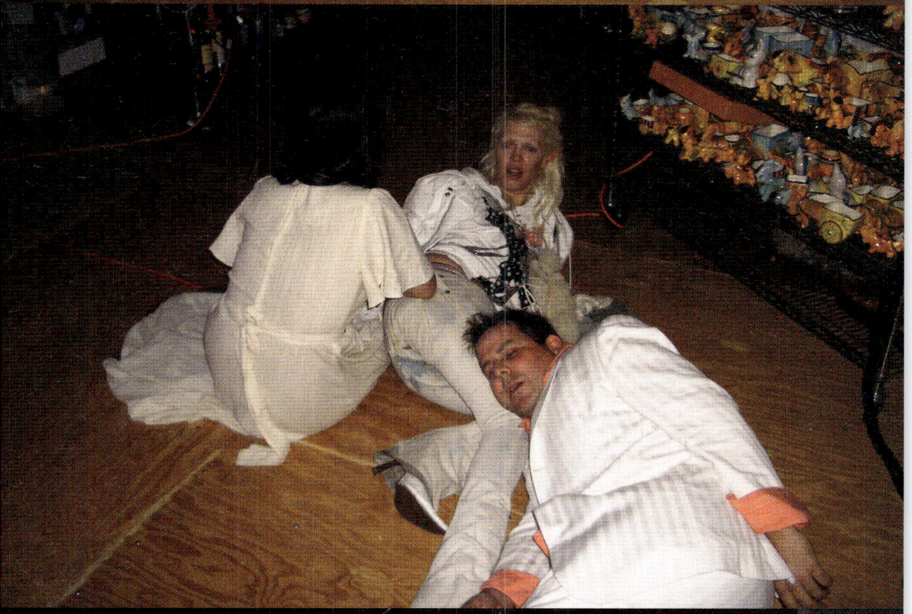

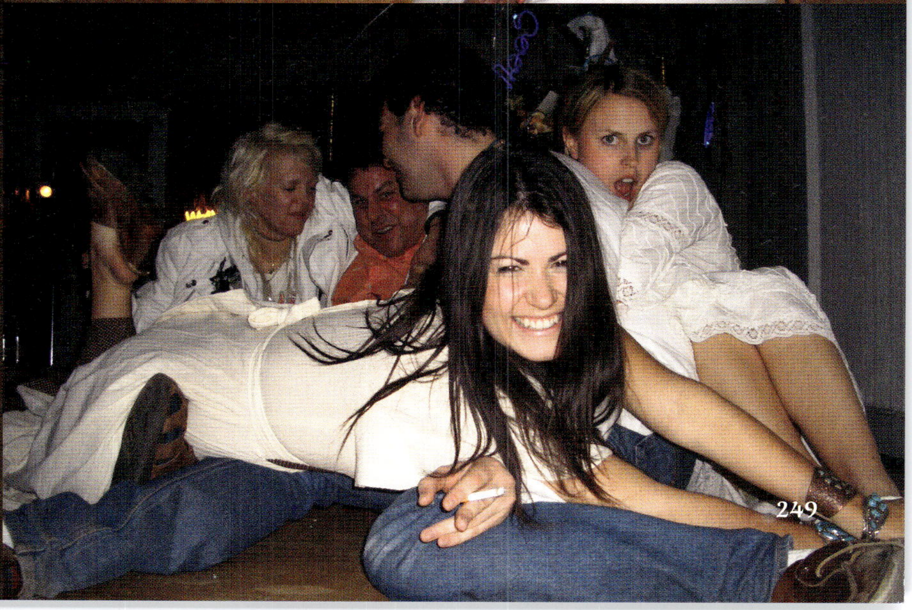

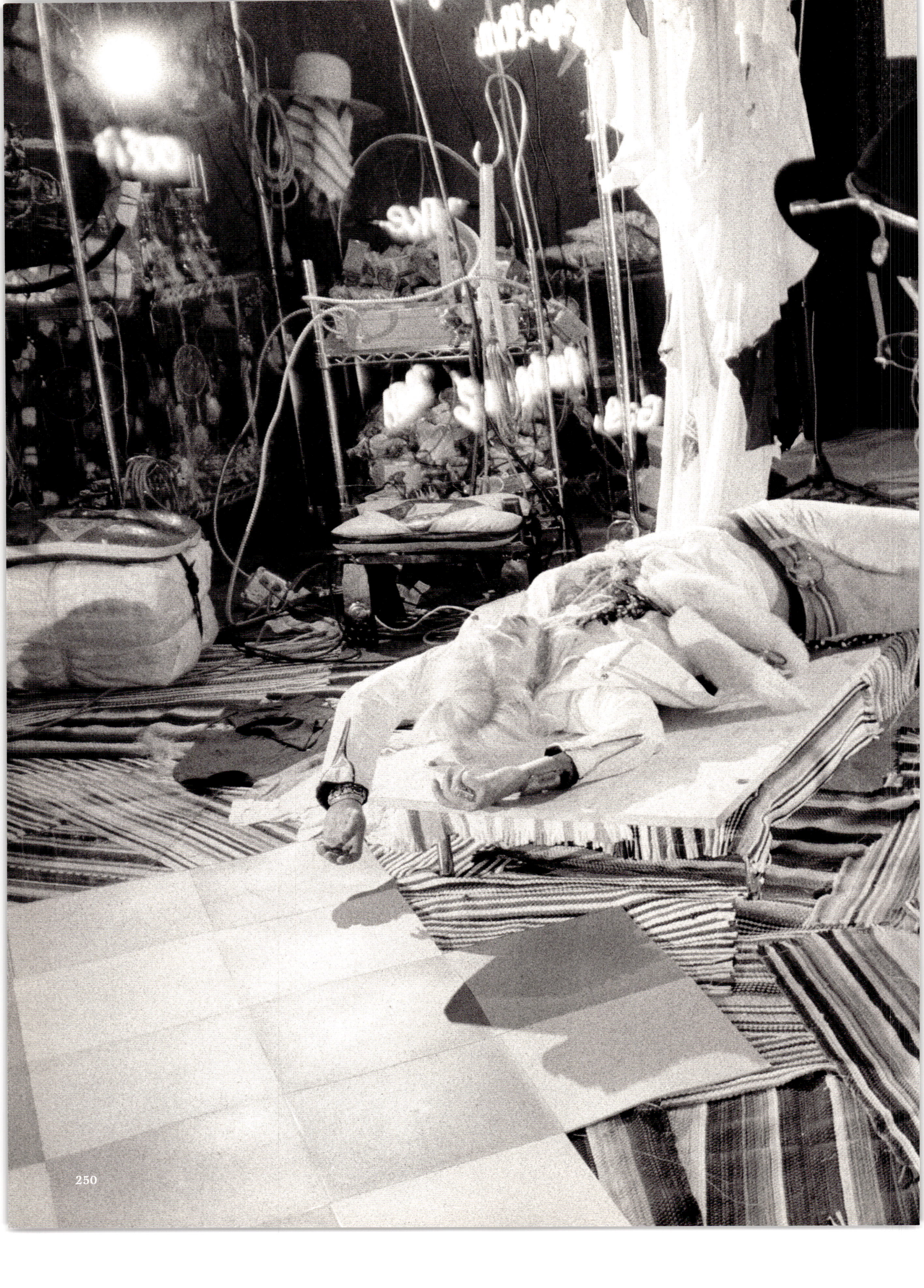

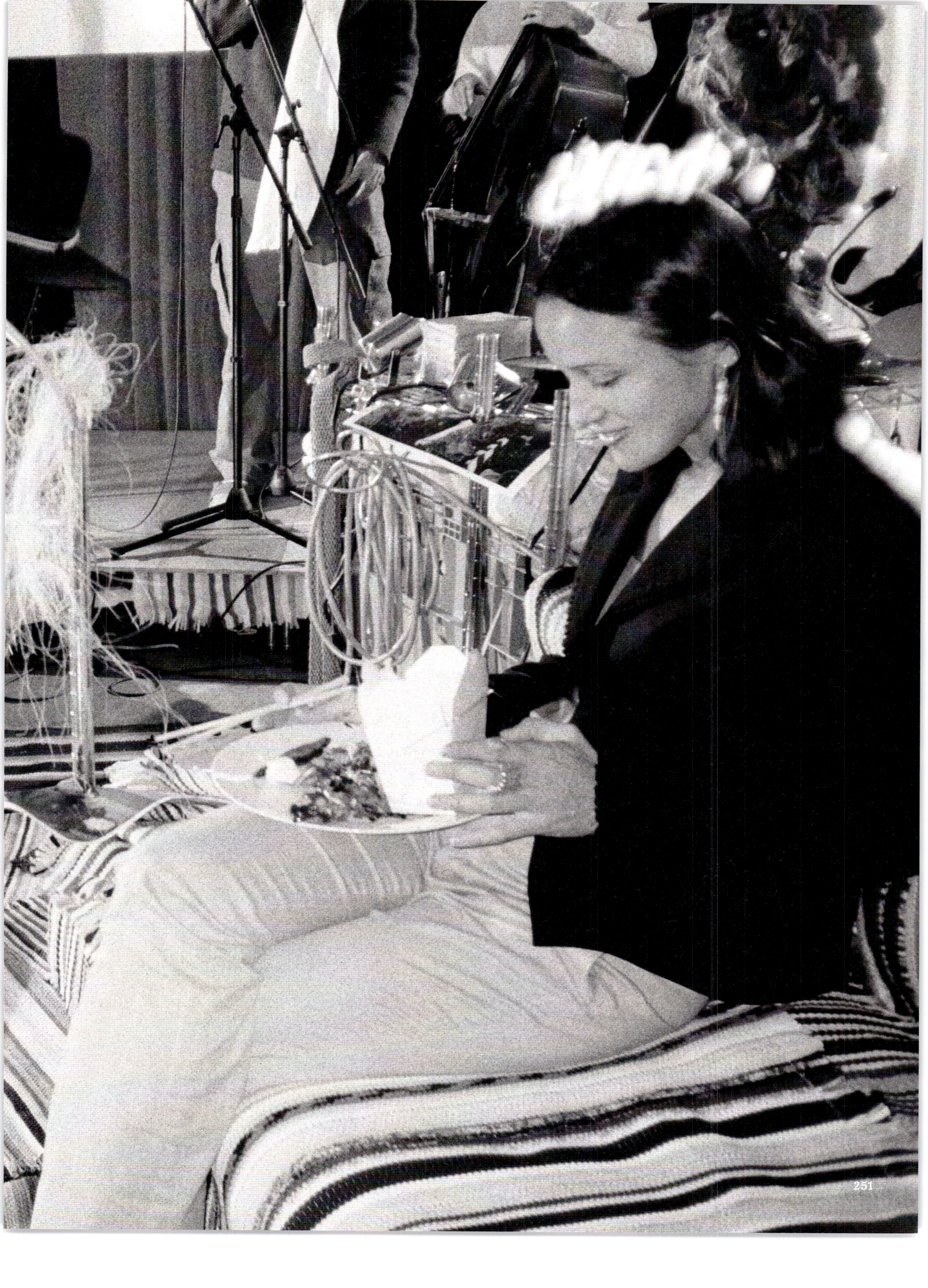

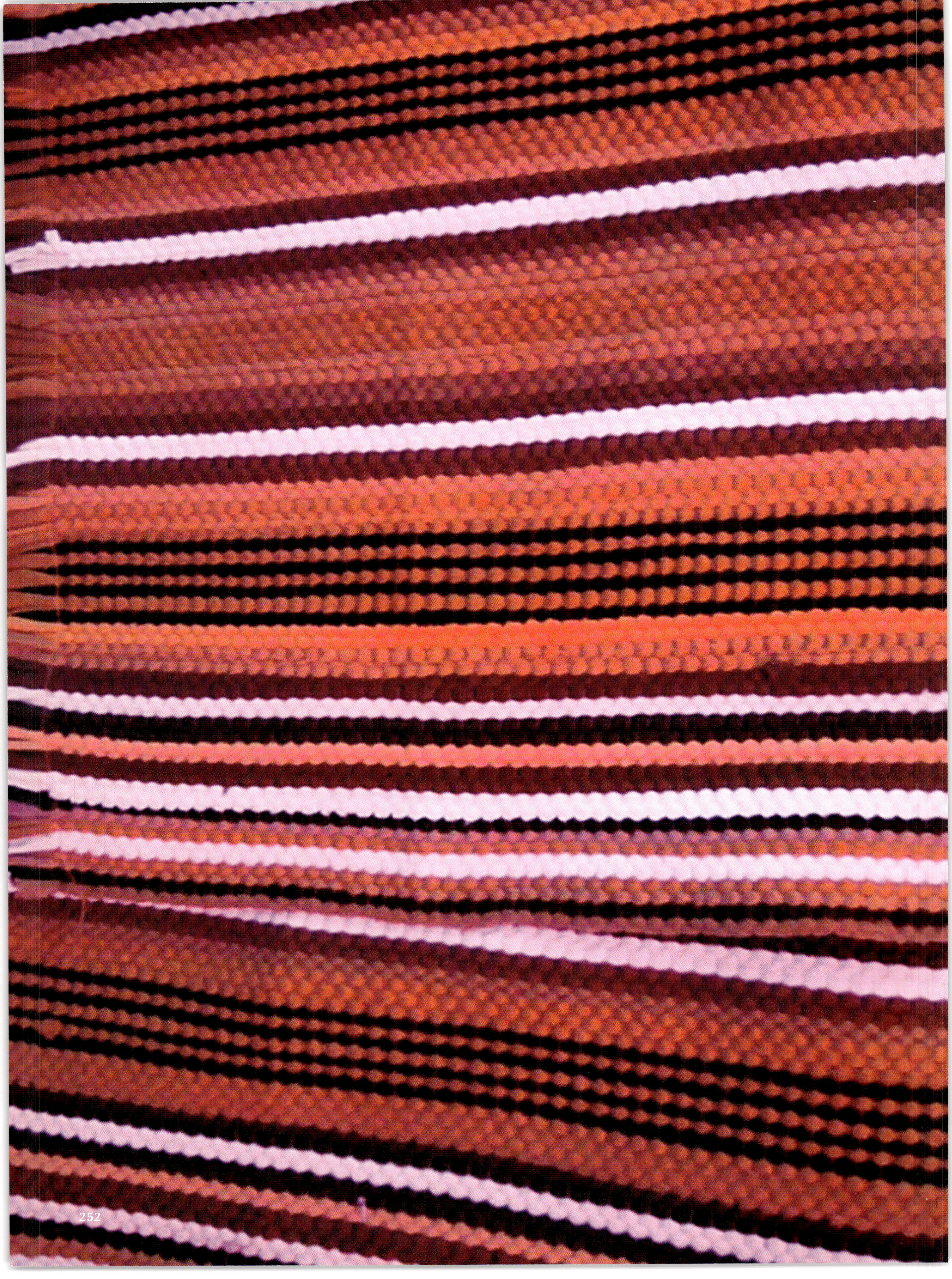

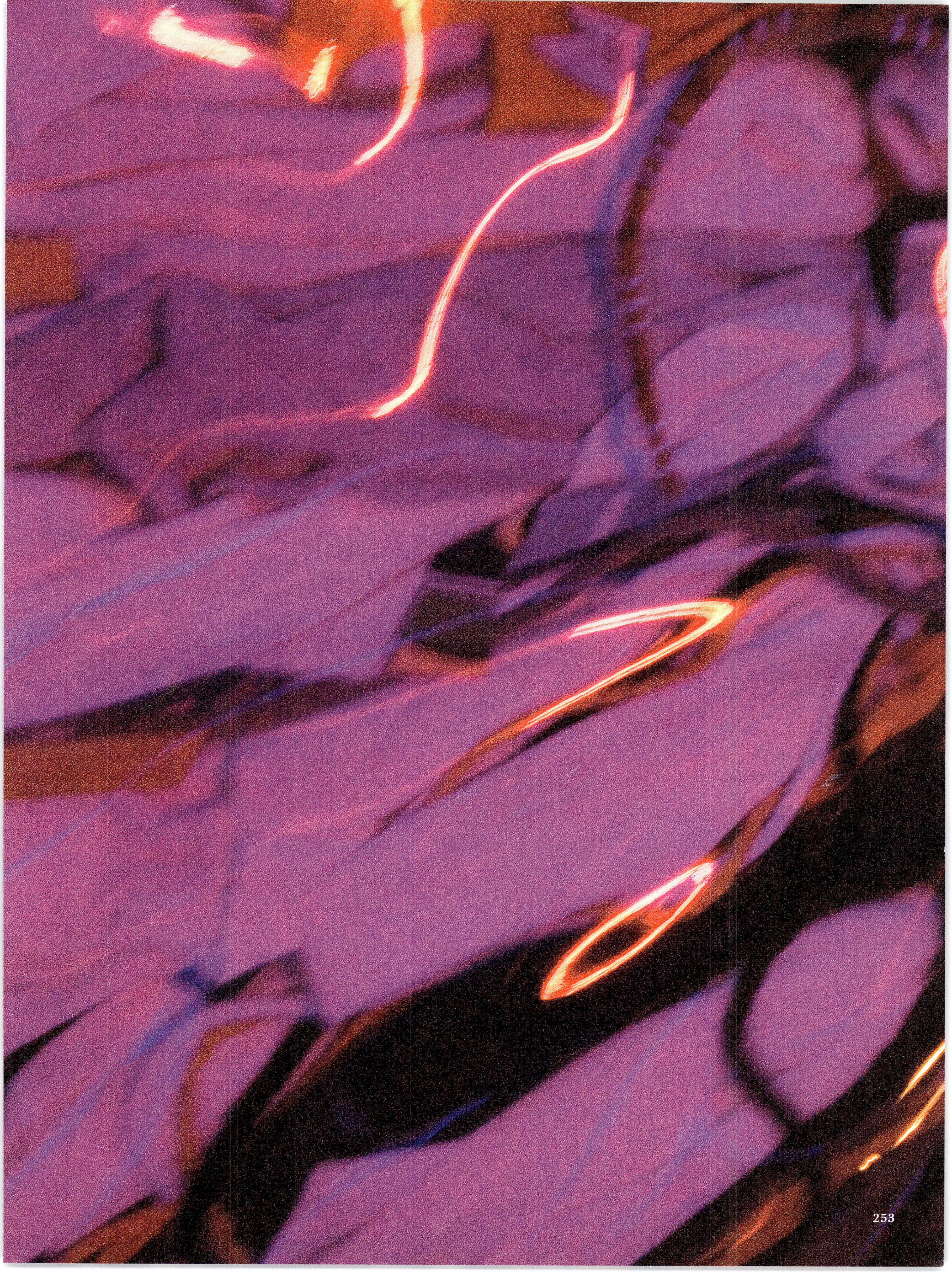

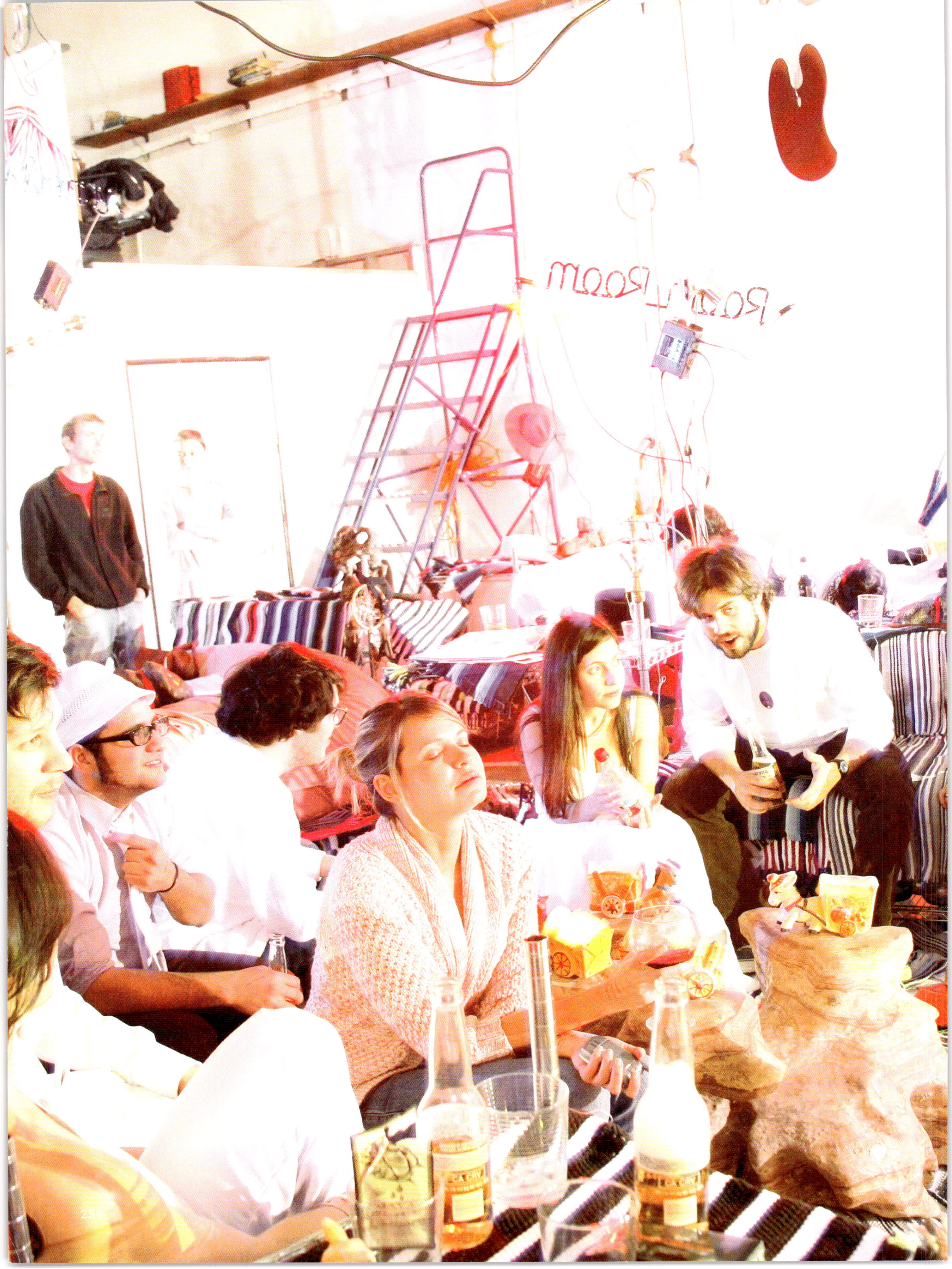

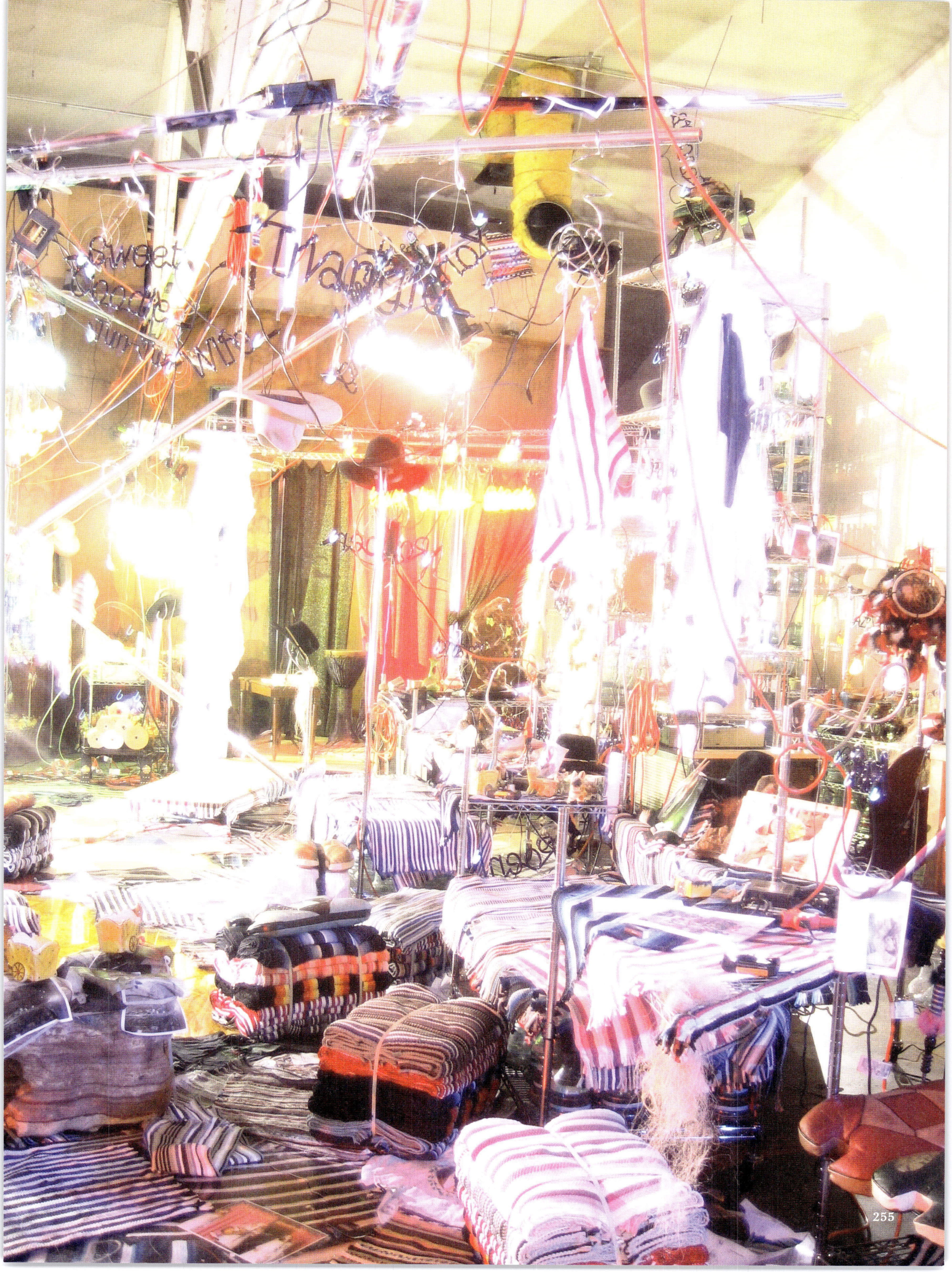
Sweet

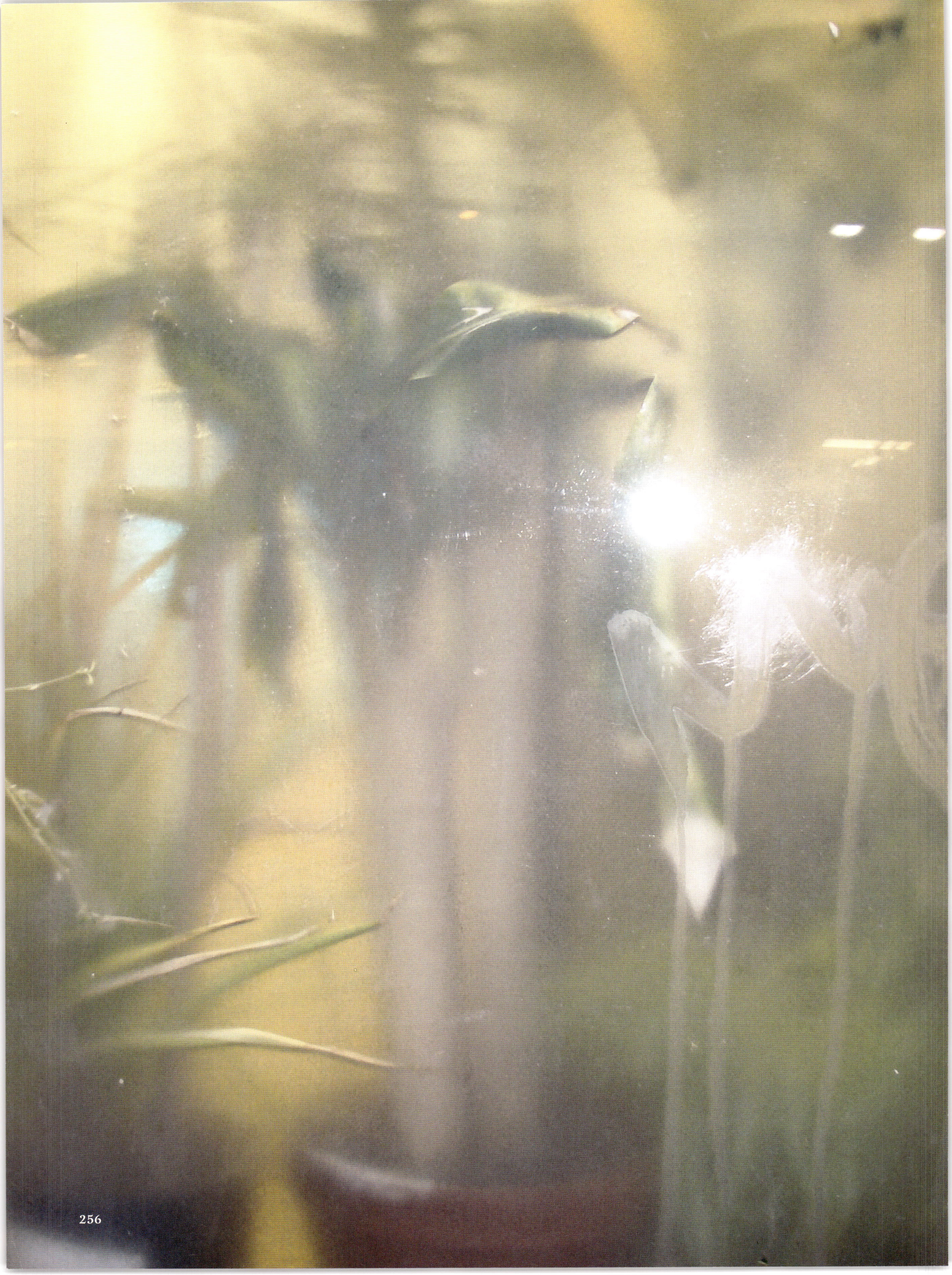

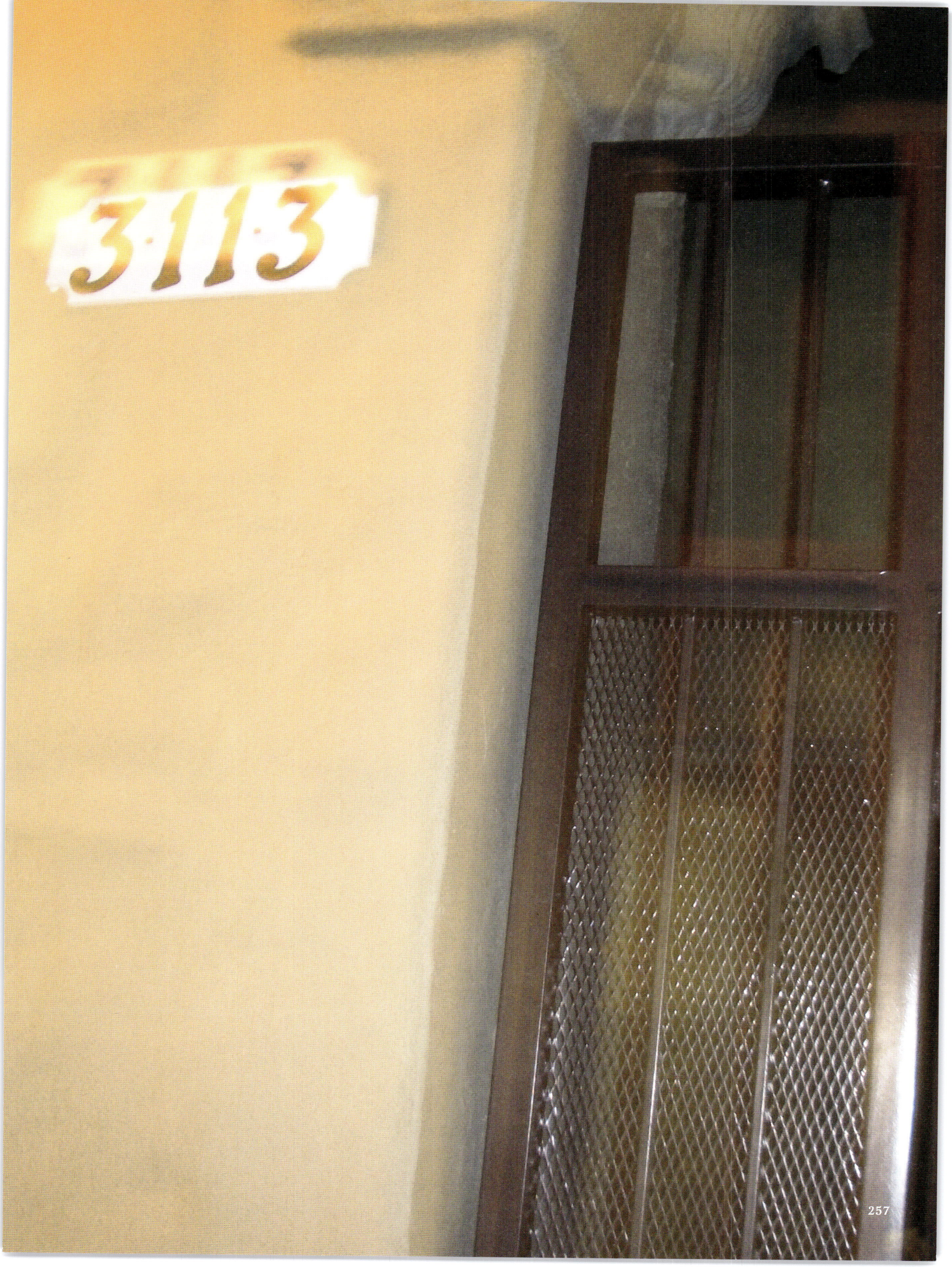
3113

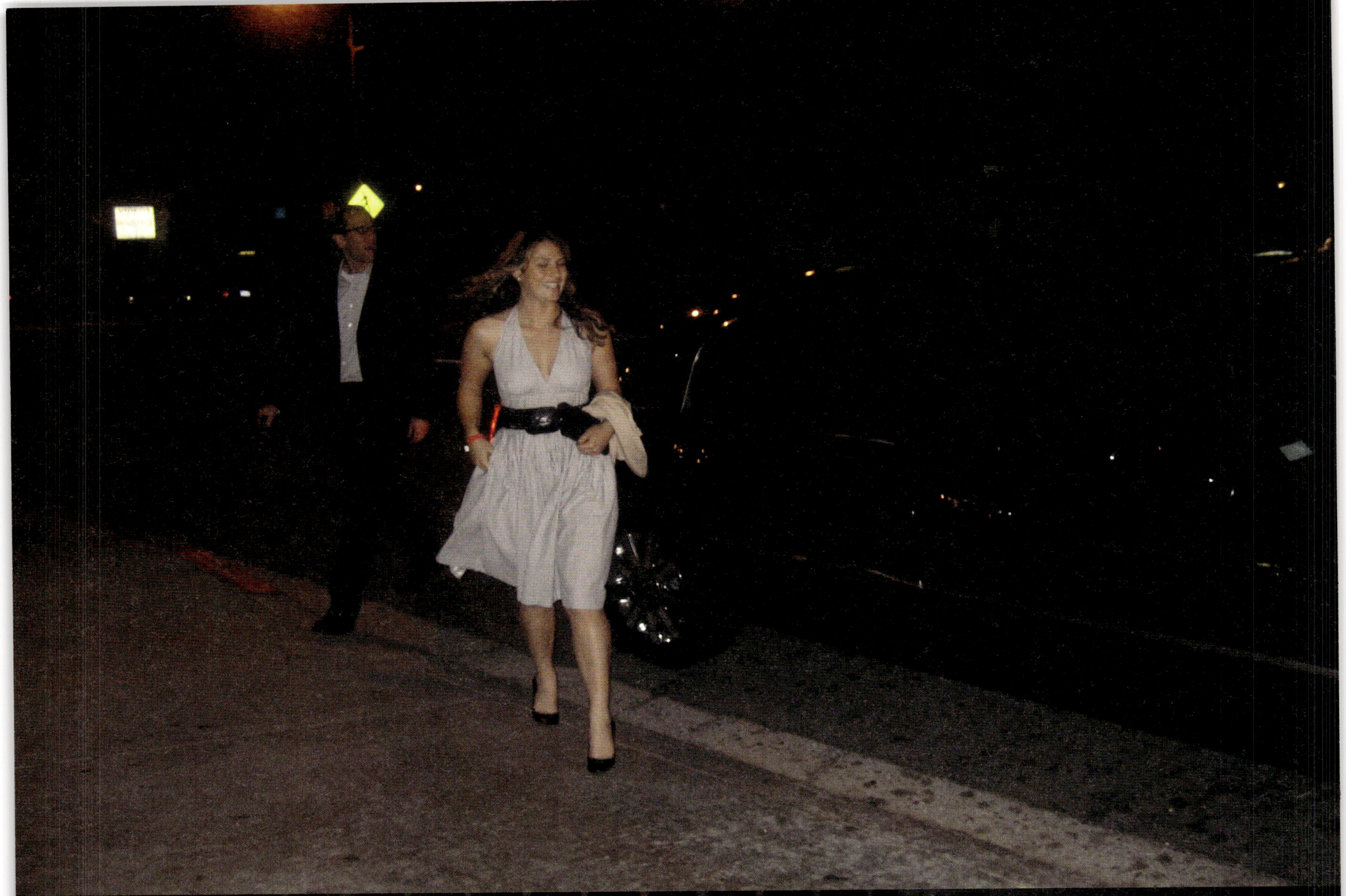

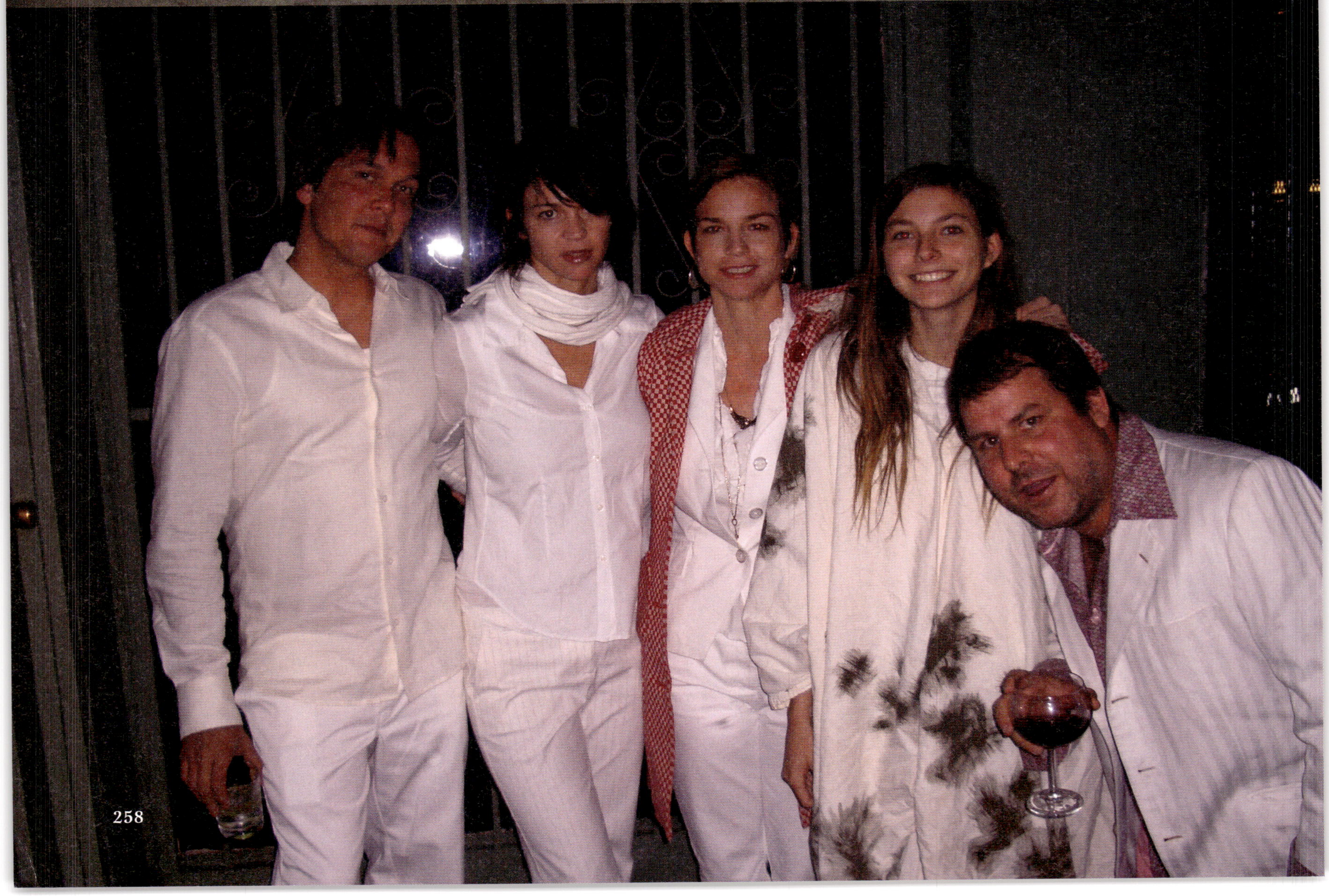

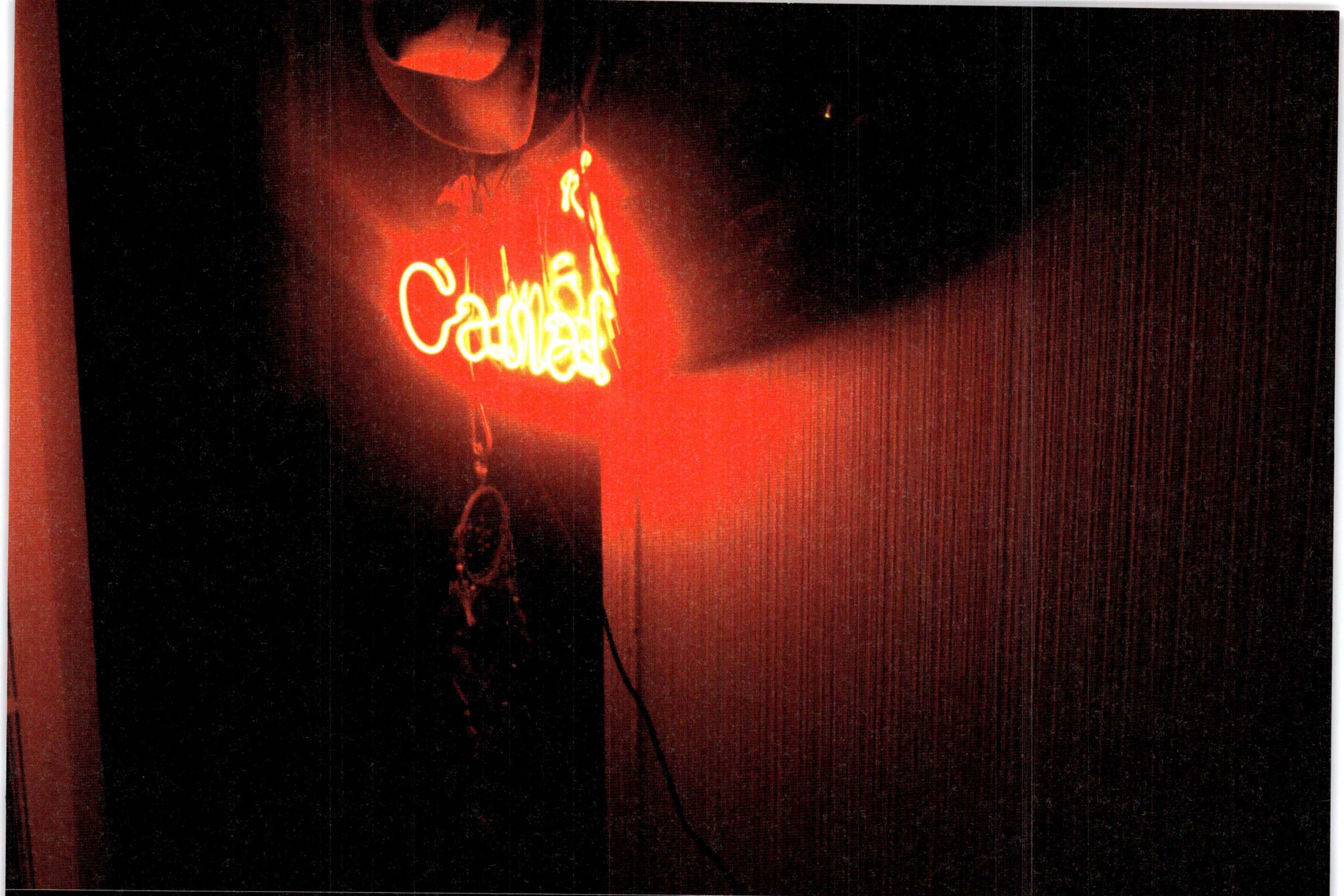

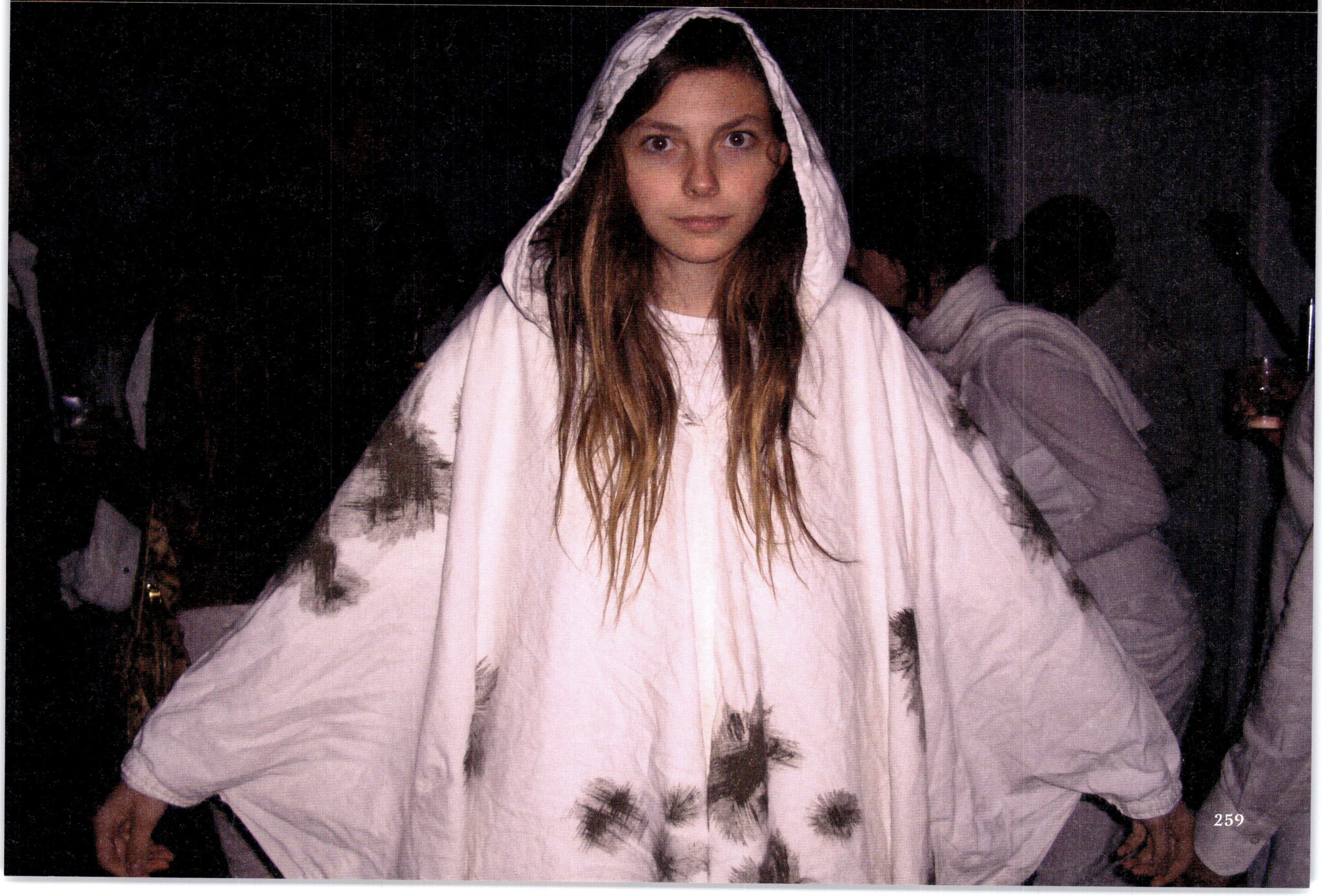

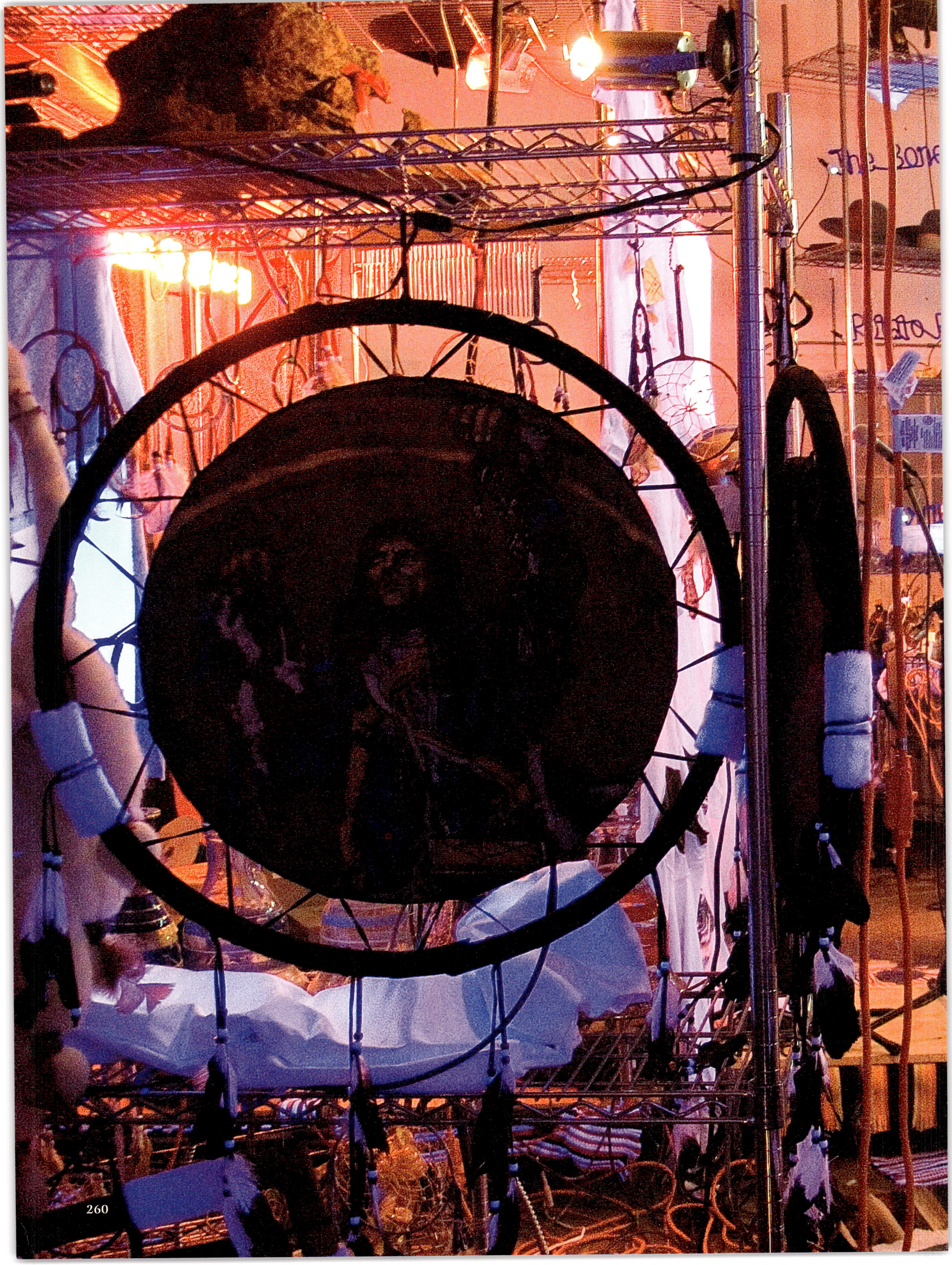

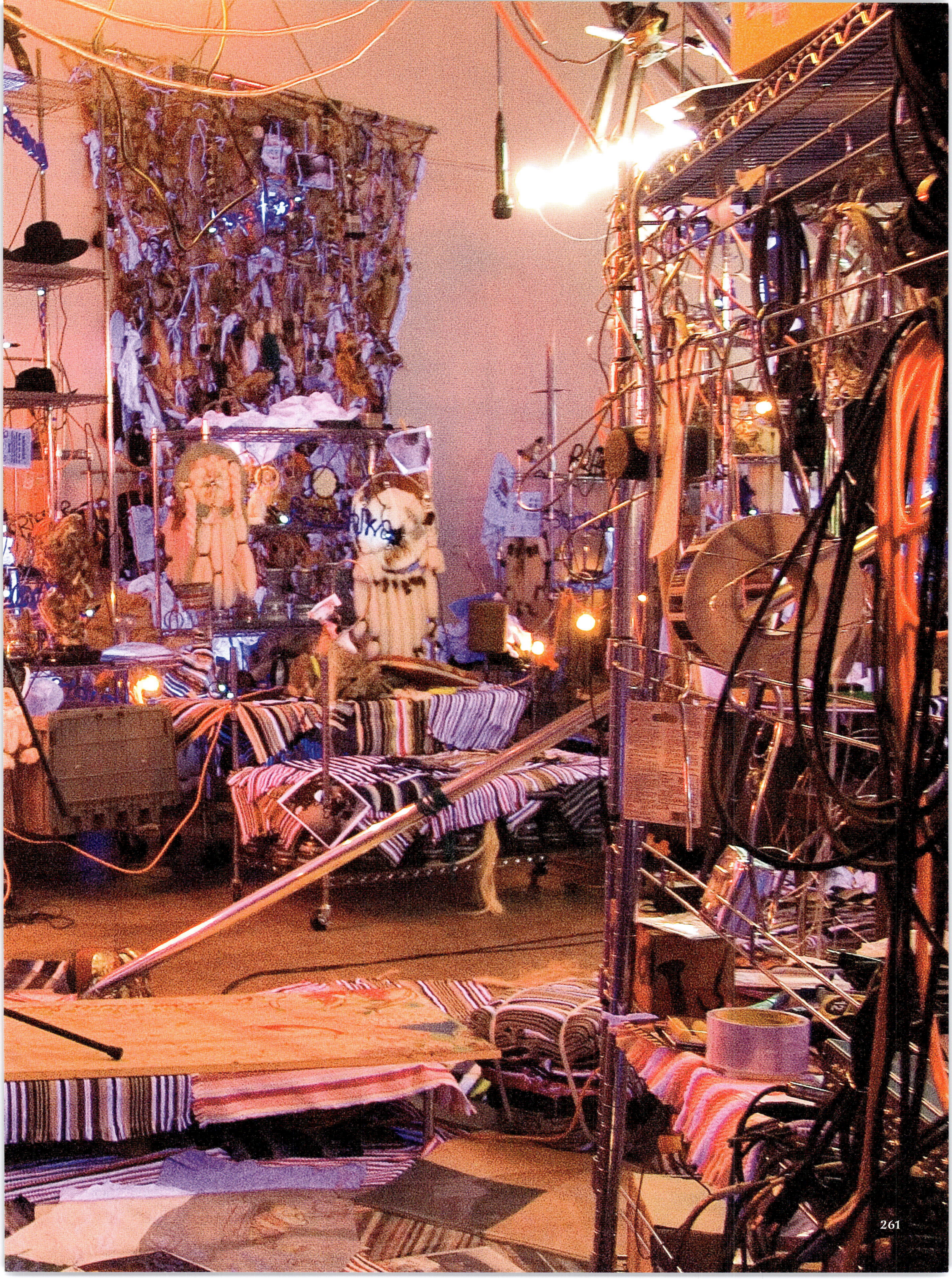

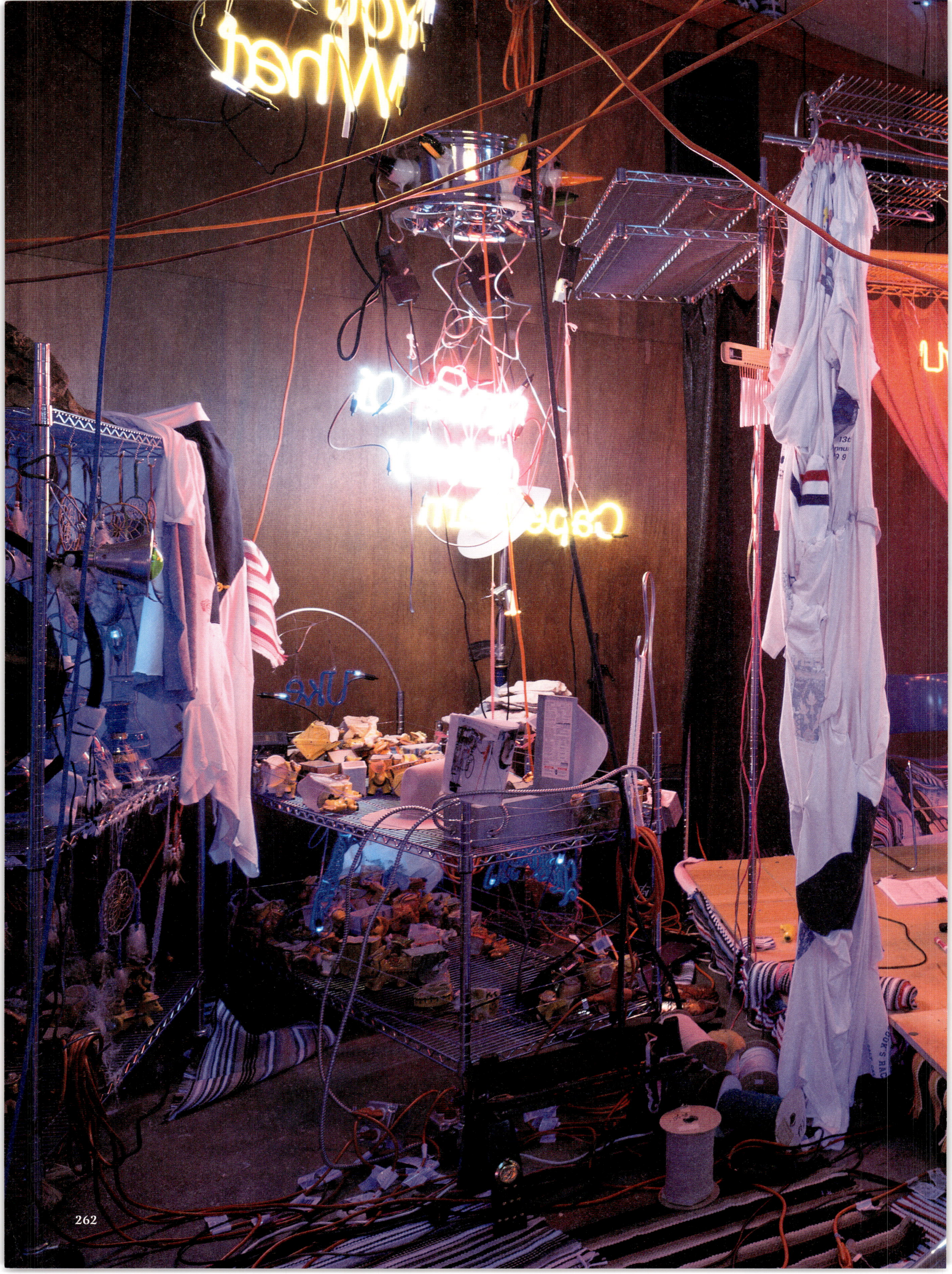

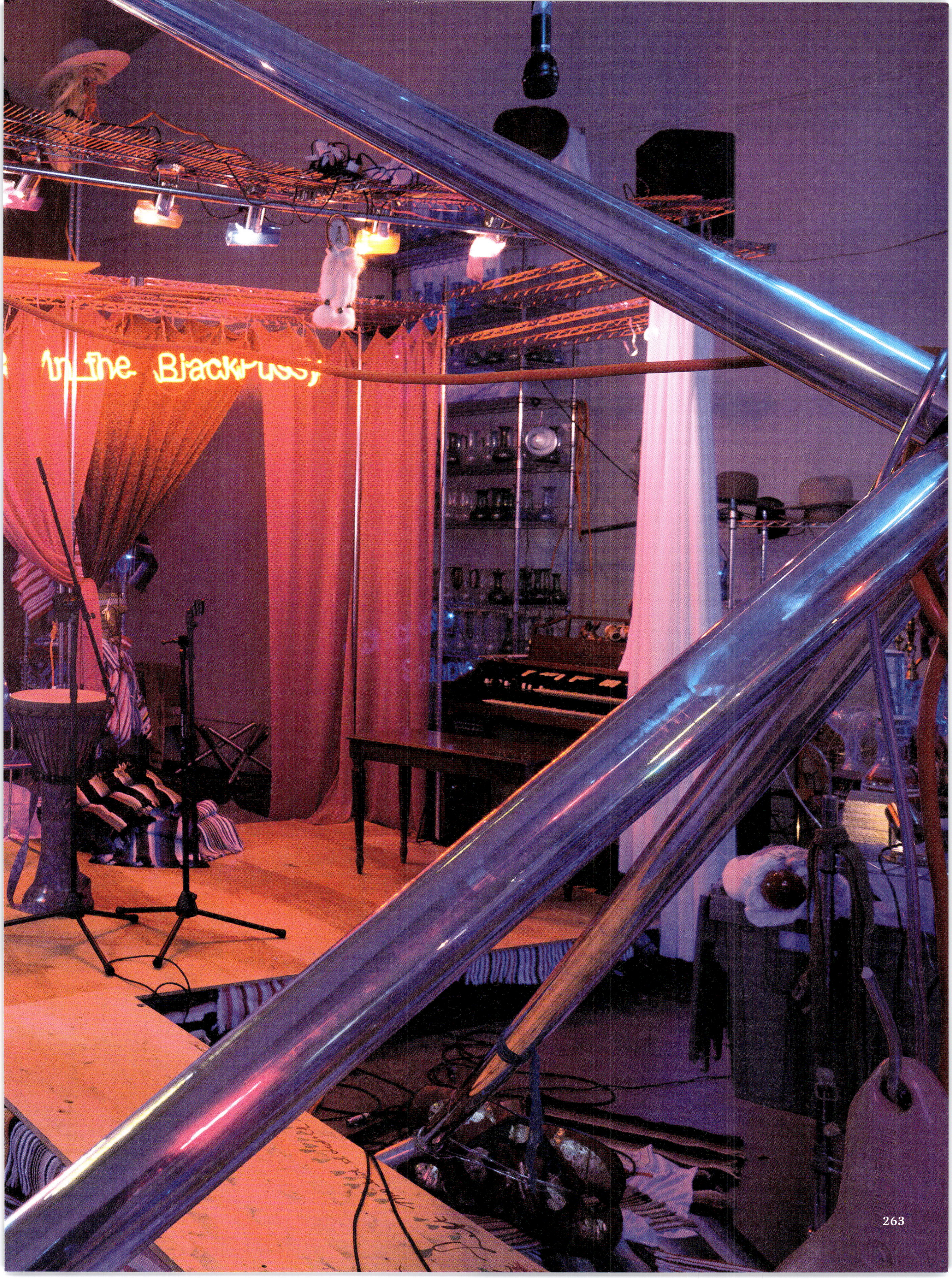

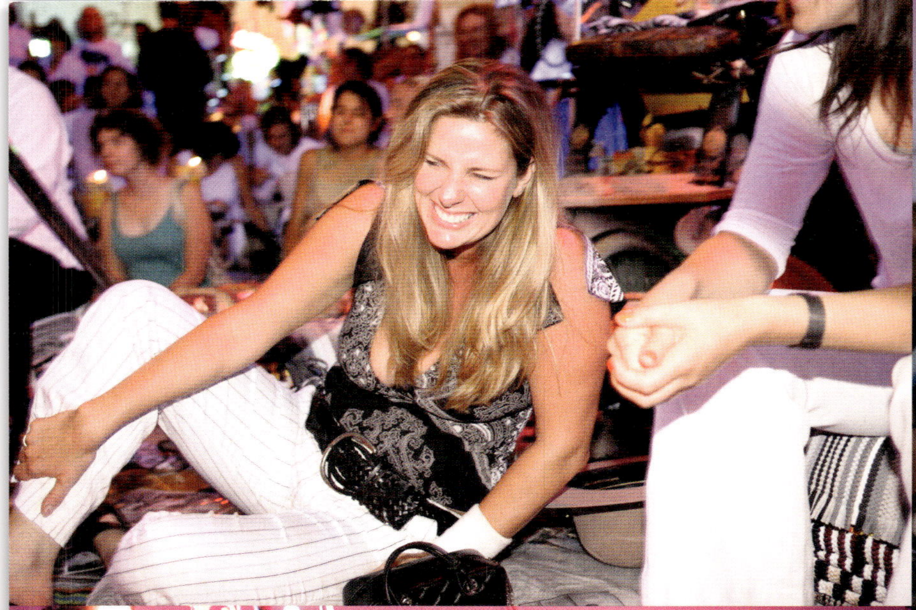
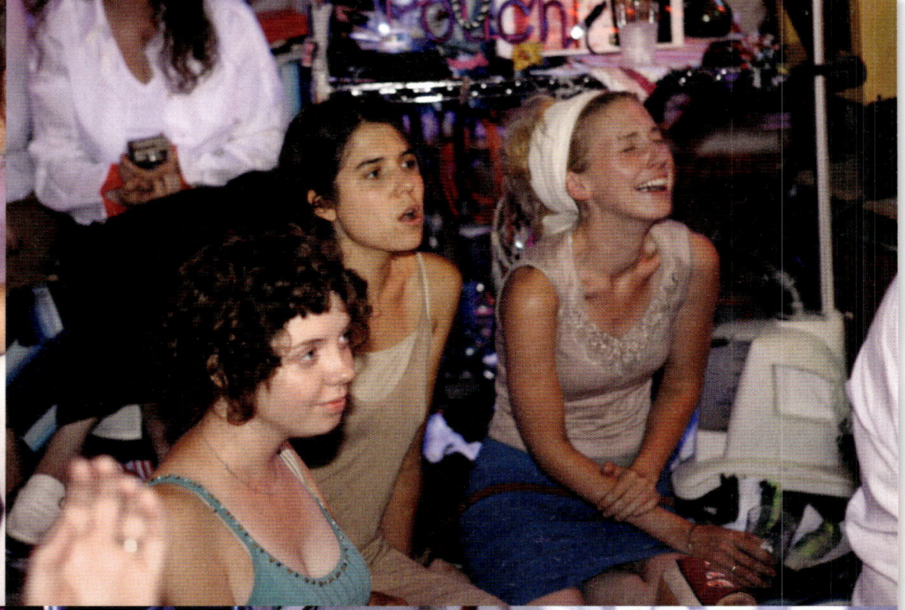
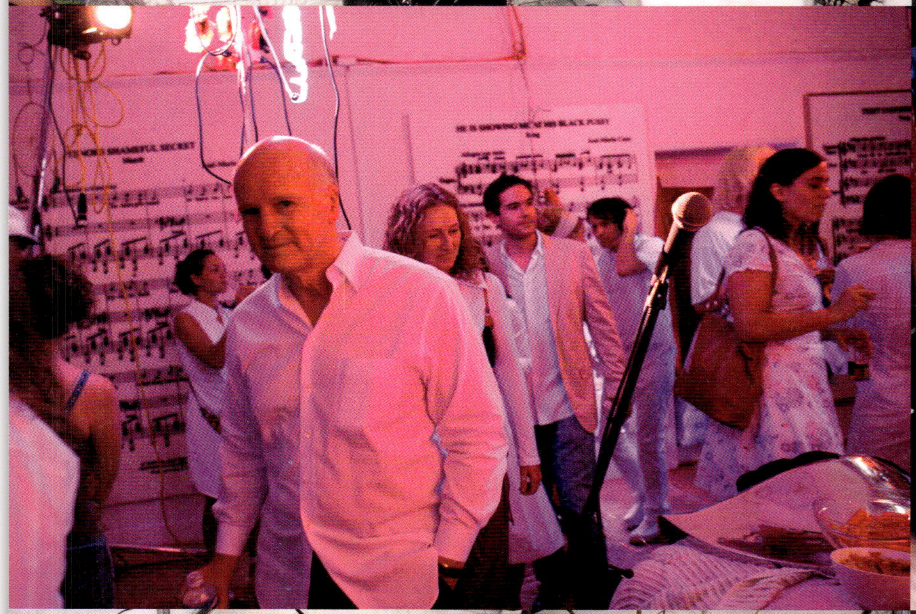
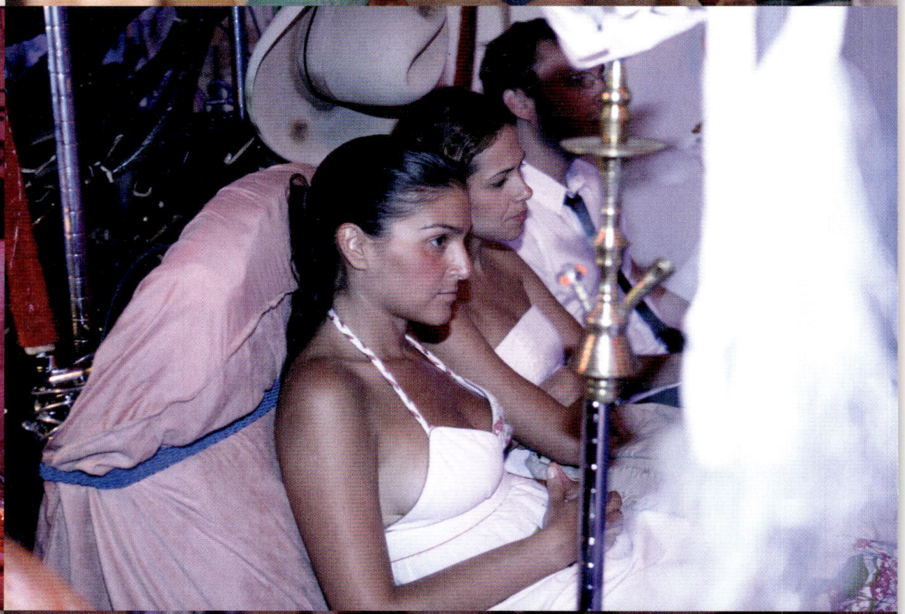
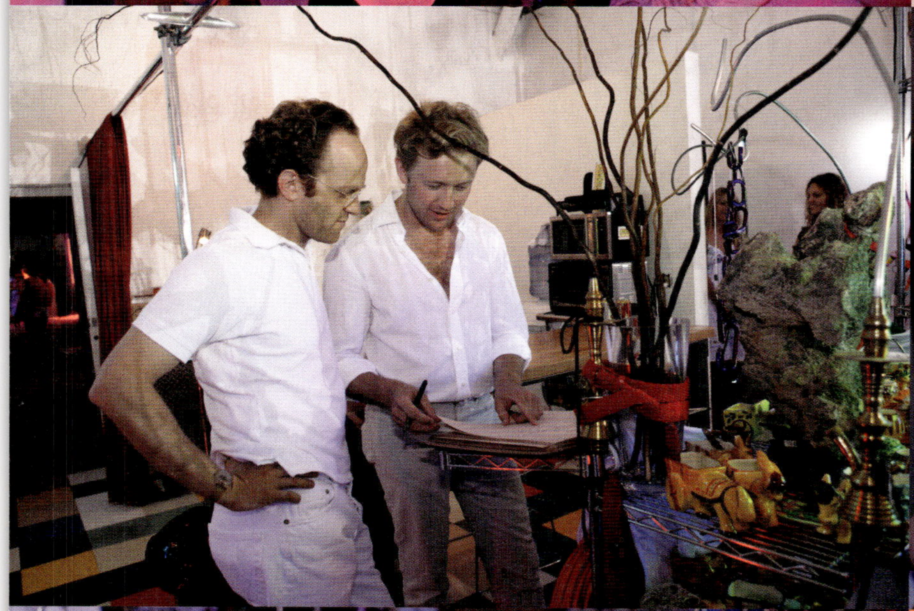
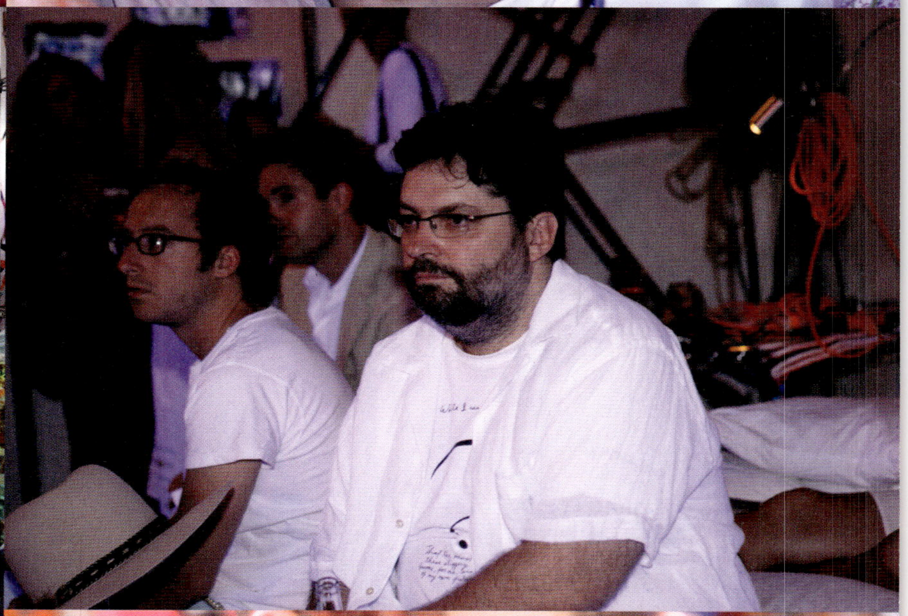
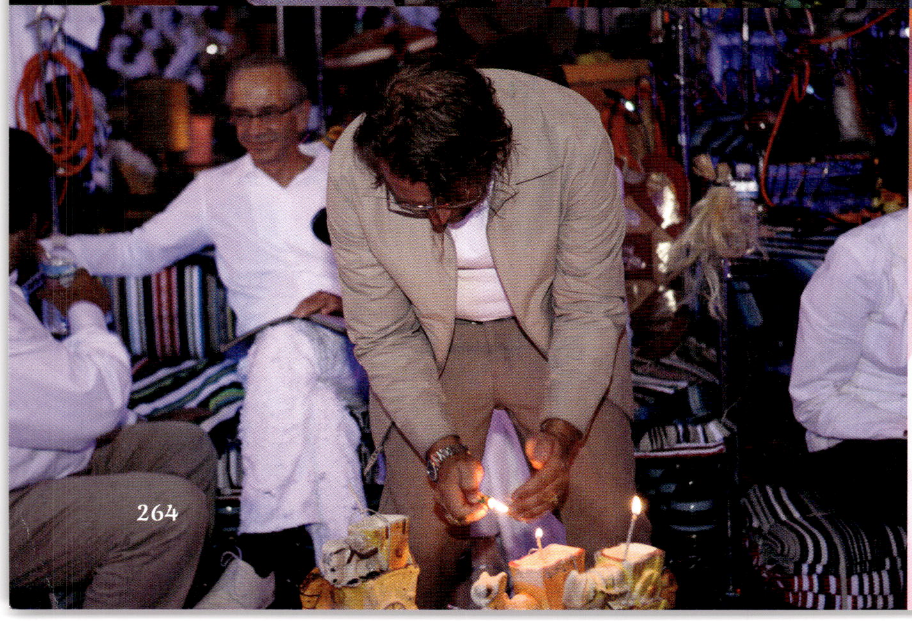
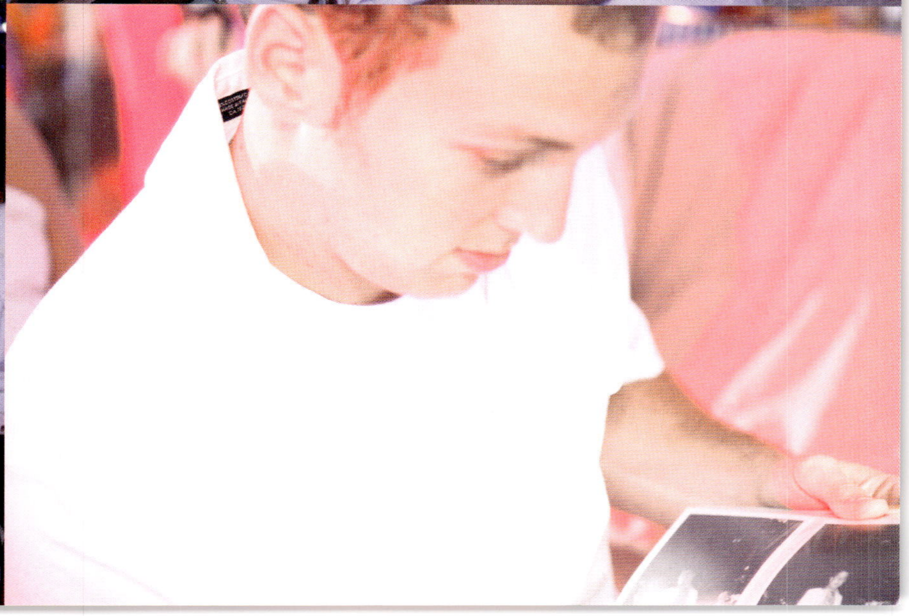

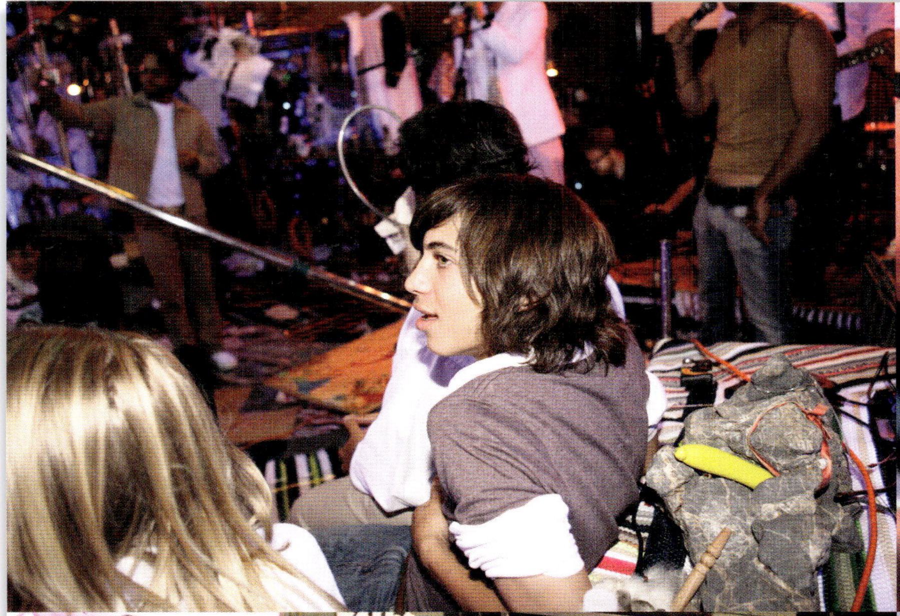
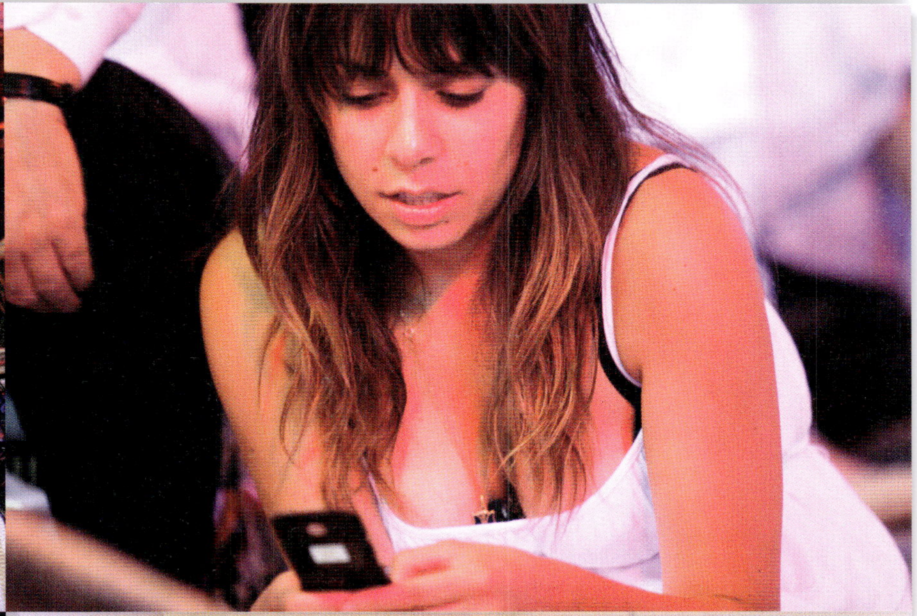
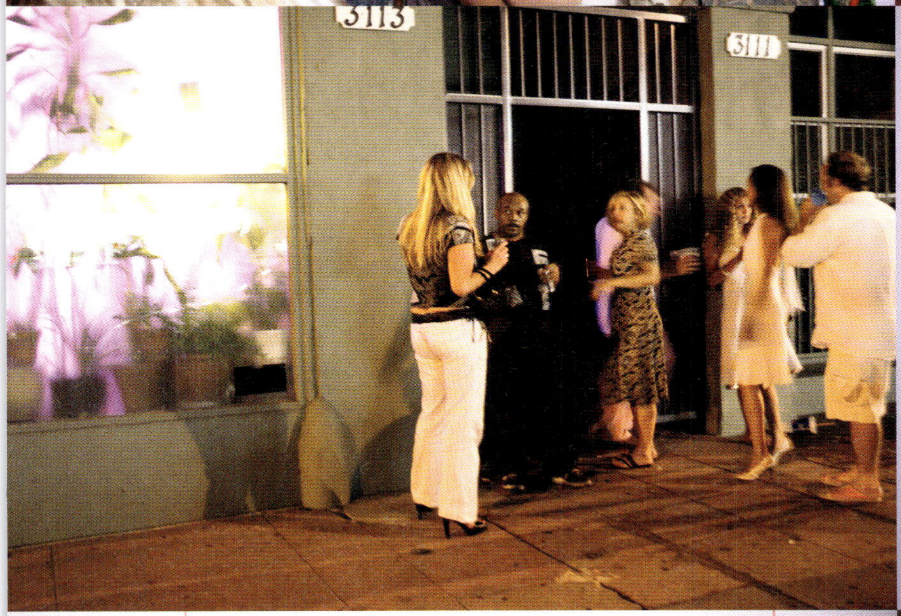
3113
3111
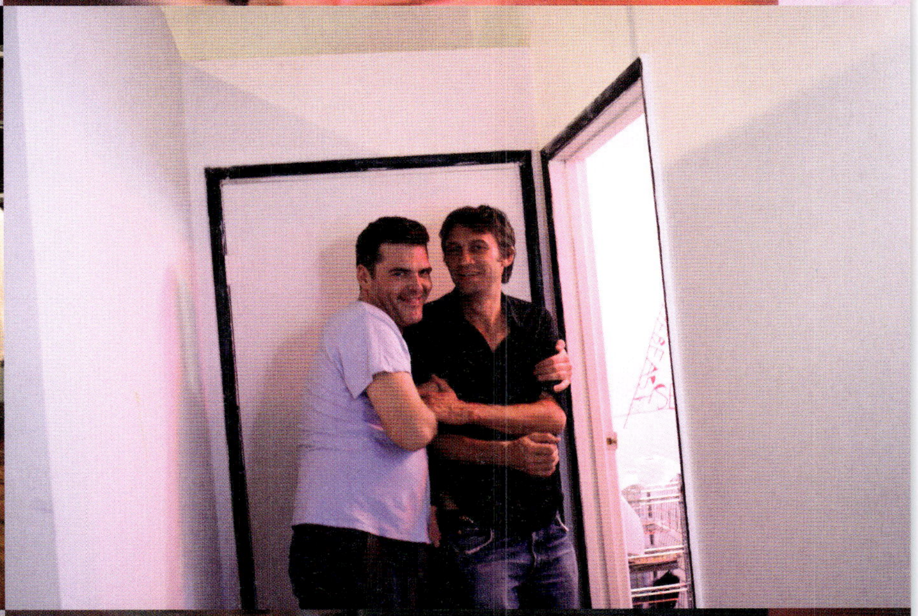
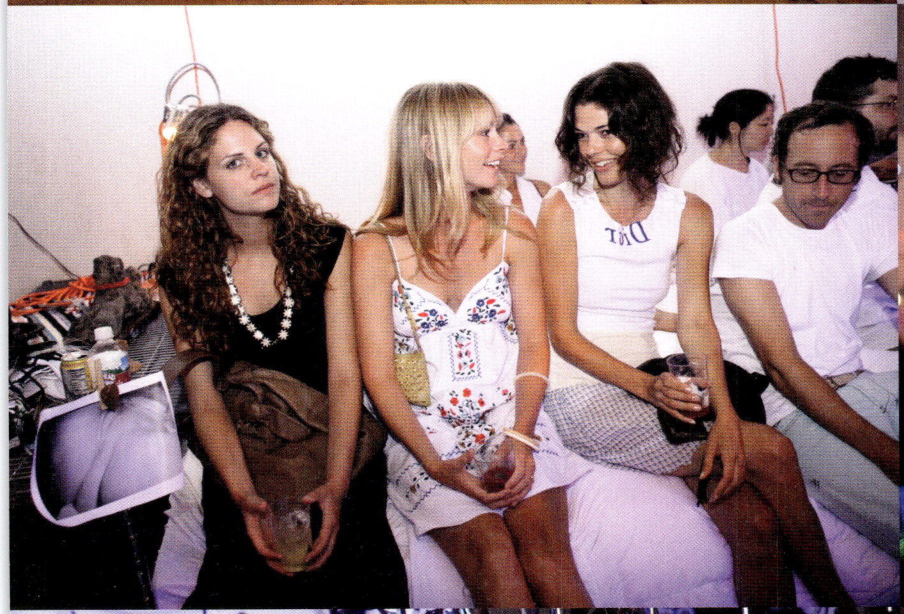
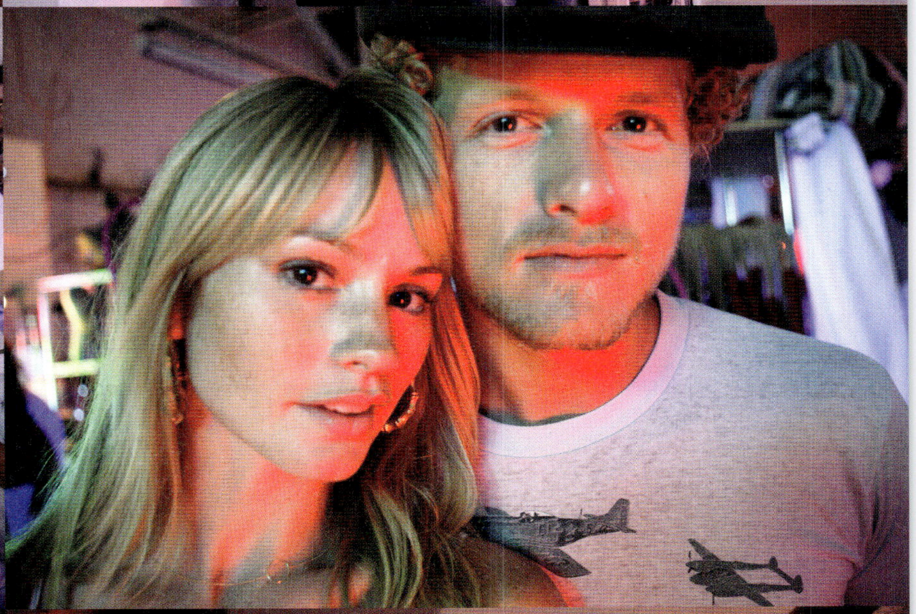
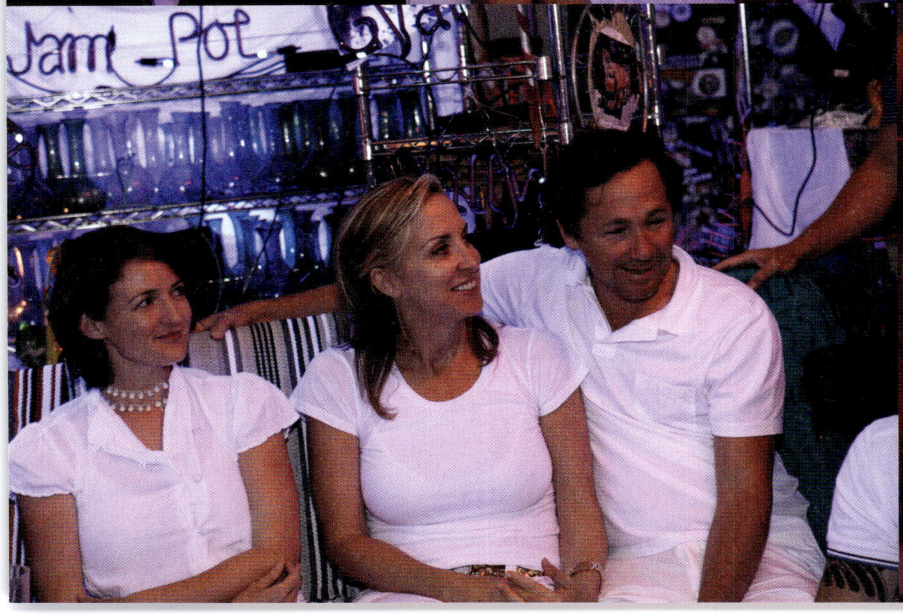
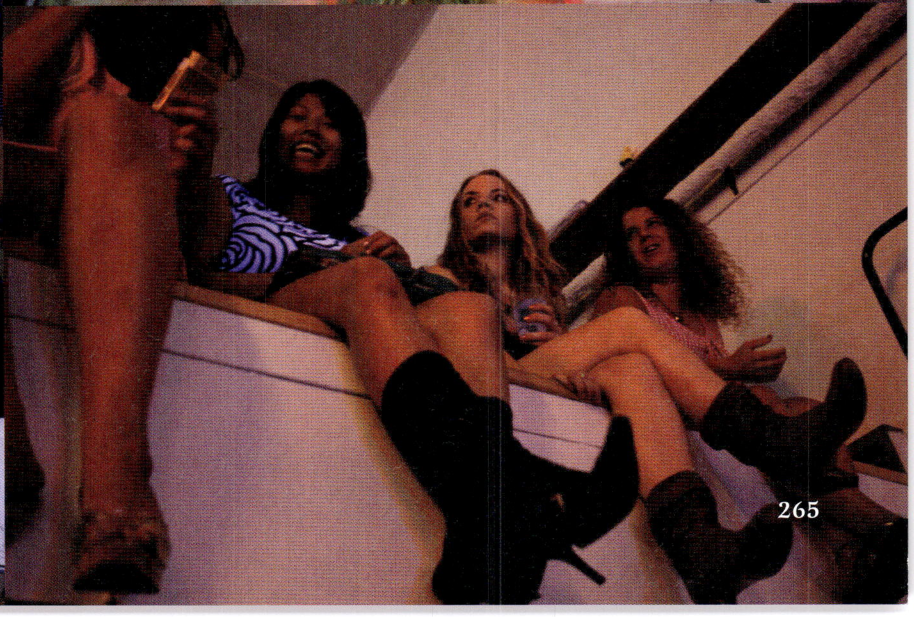

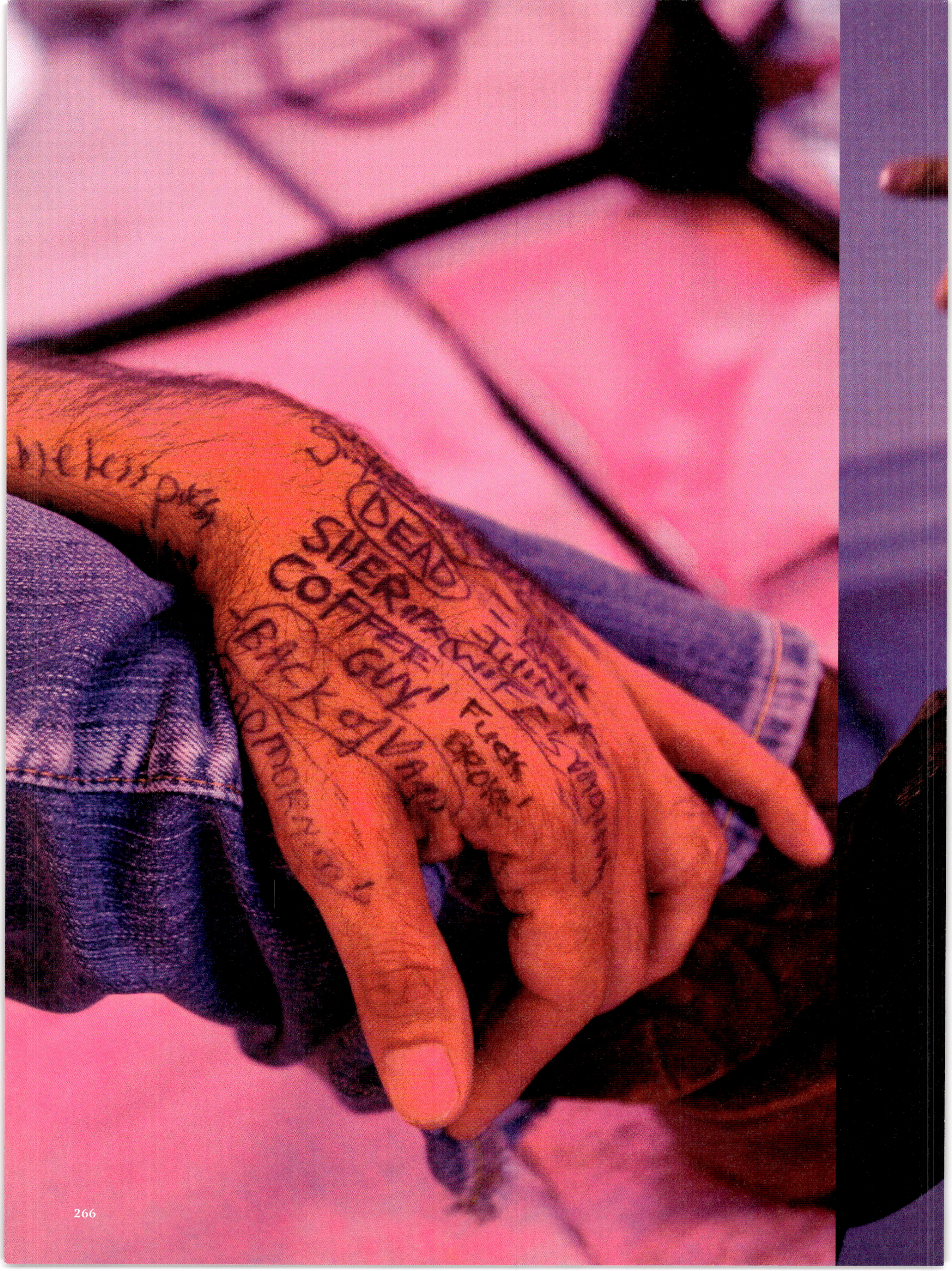
DEAD

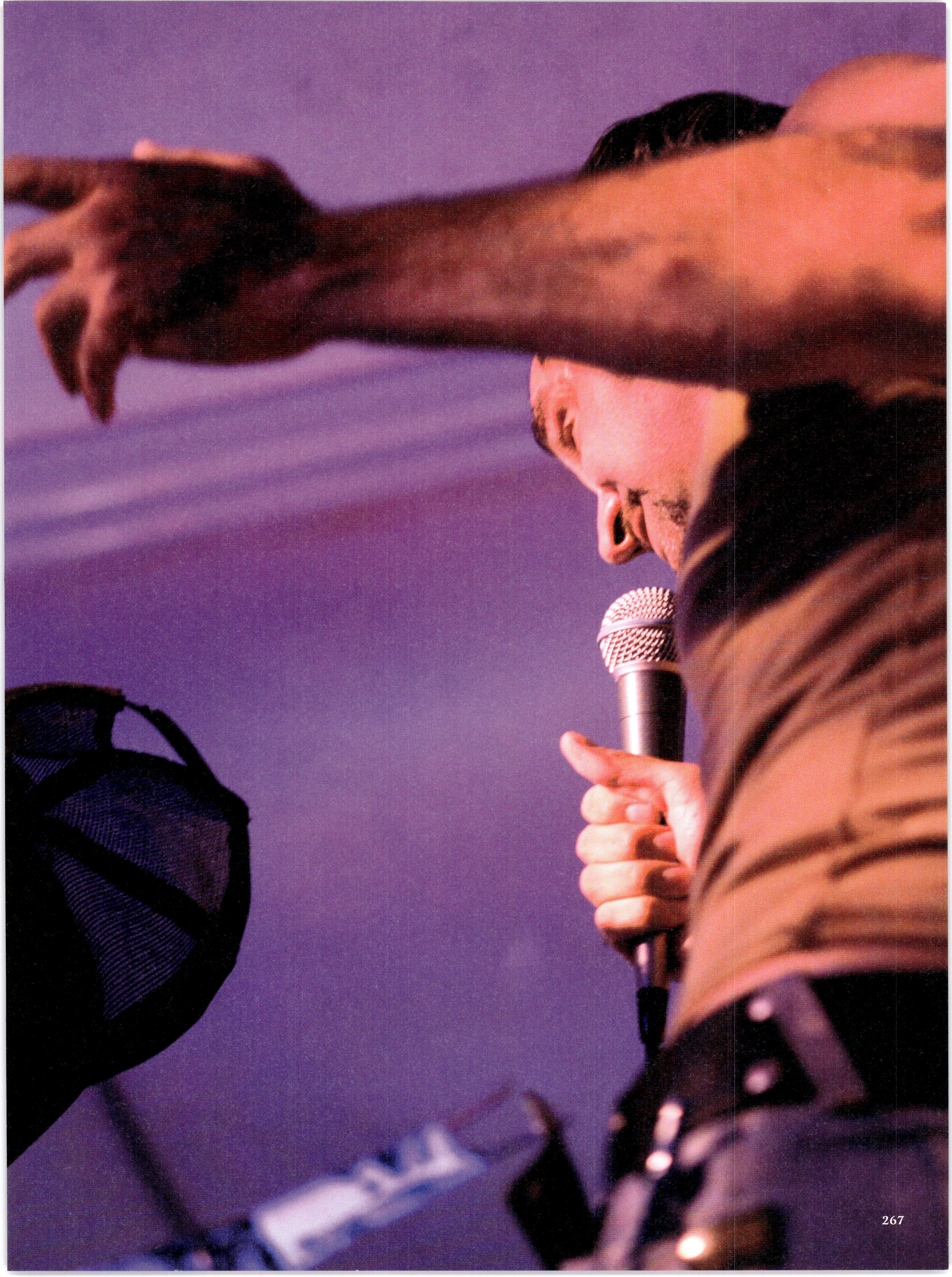

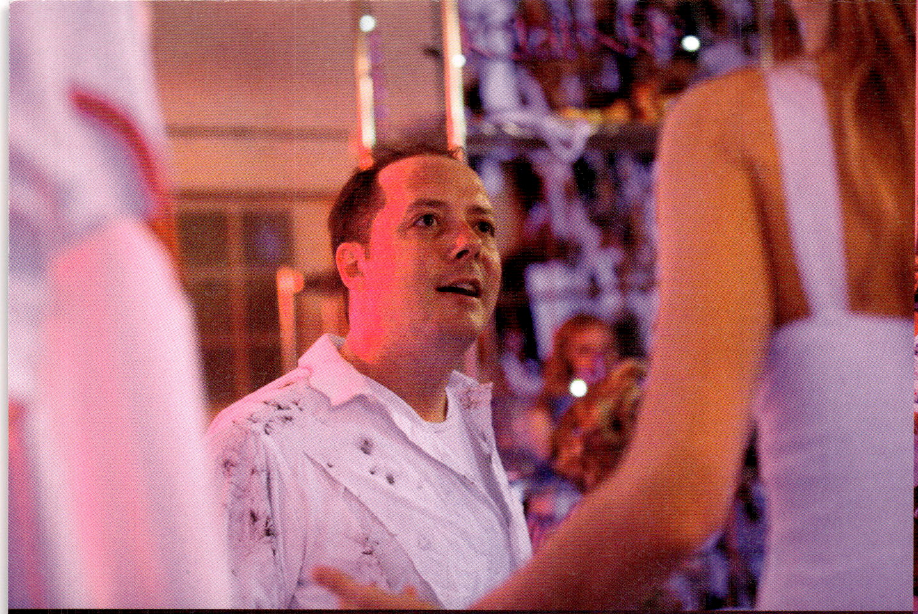

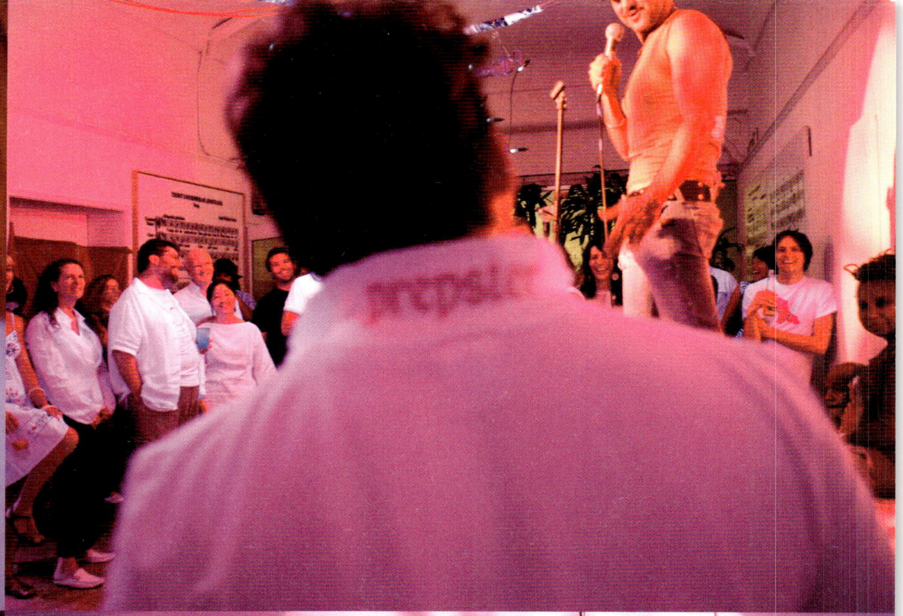
prepster

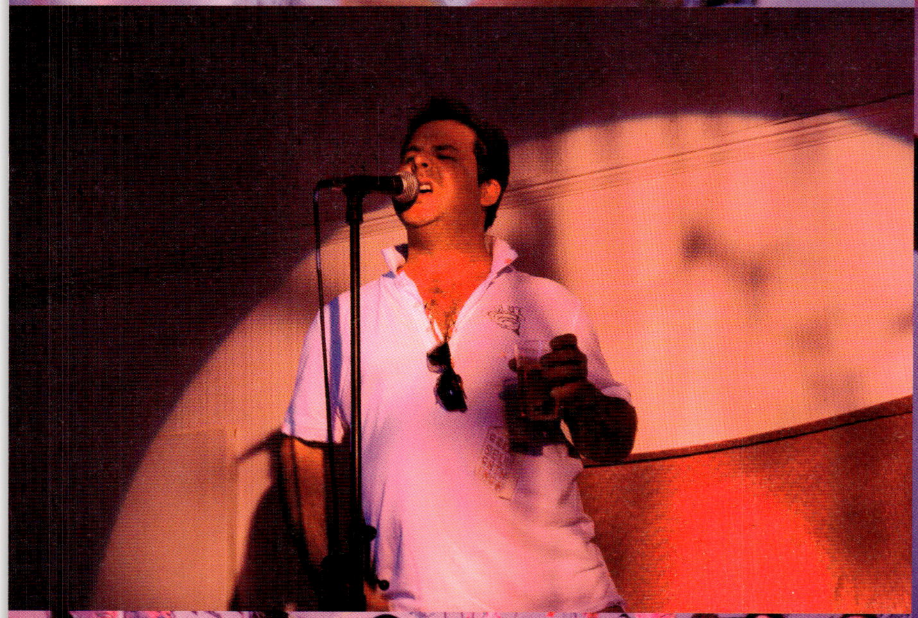

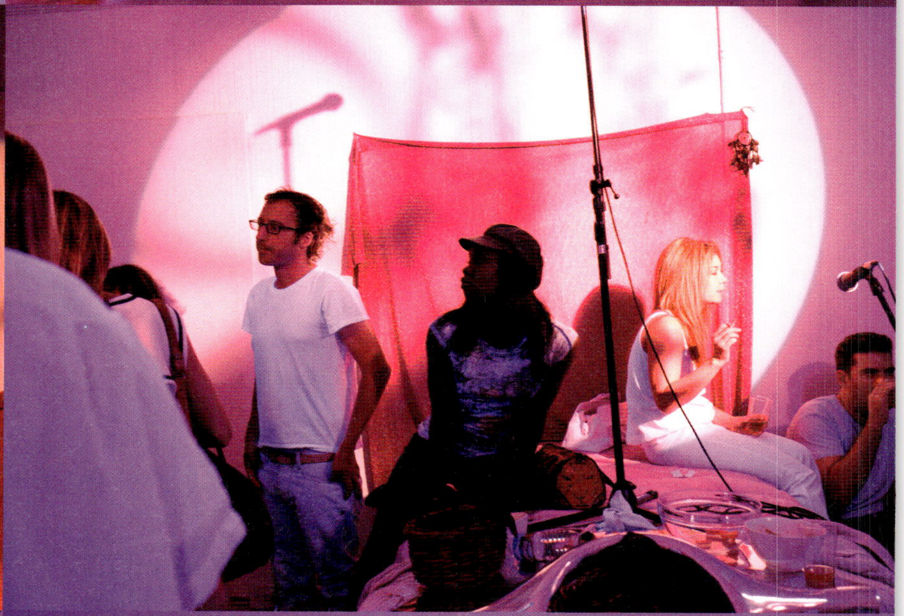

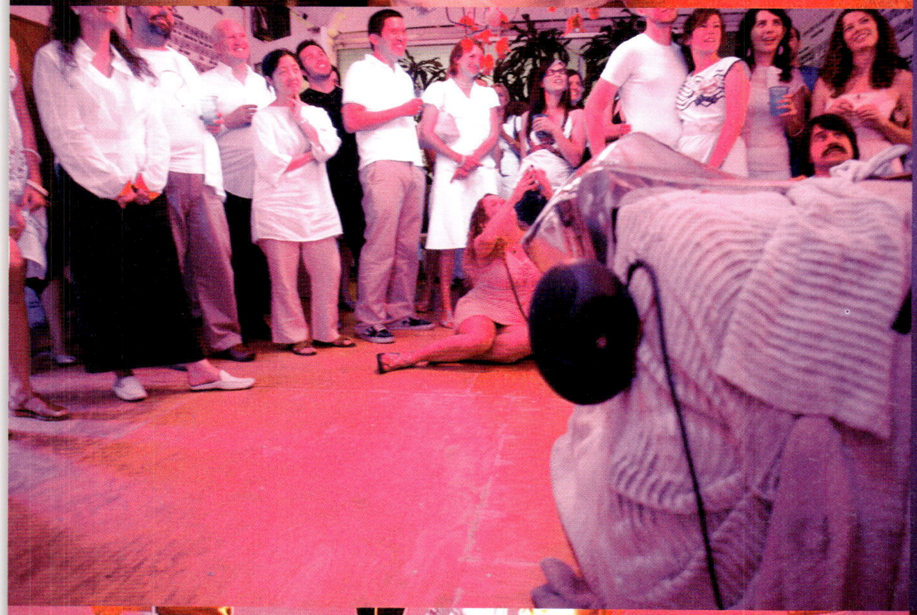

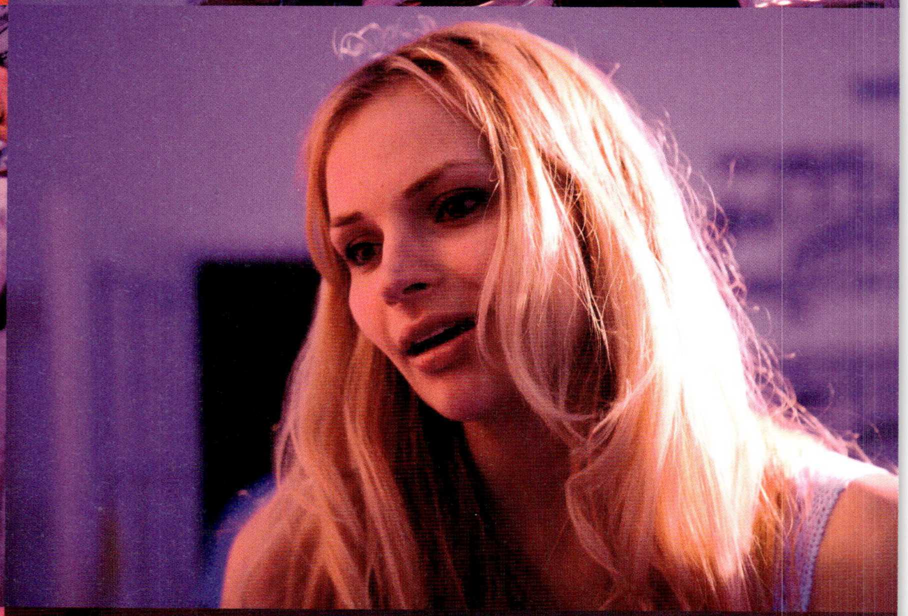

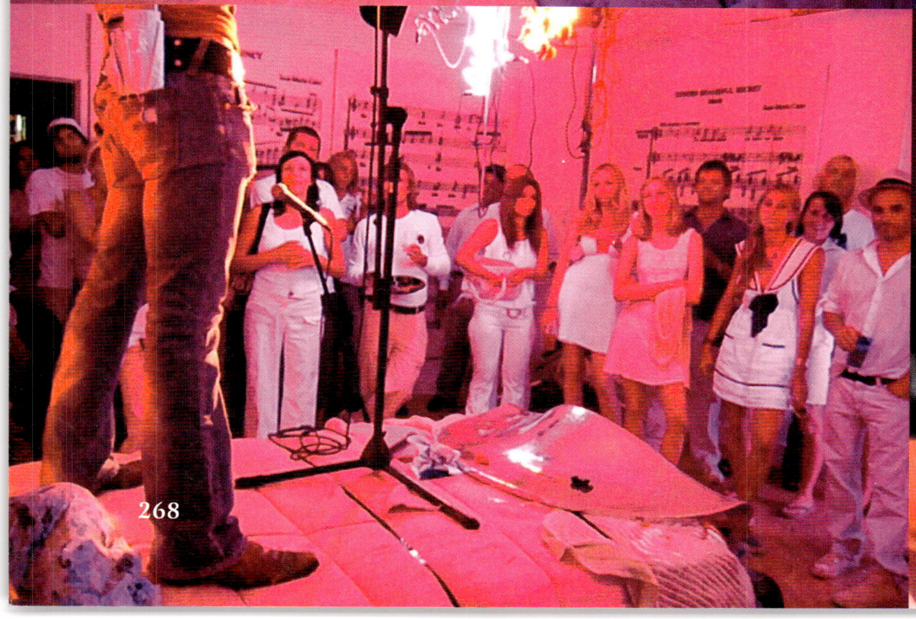

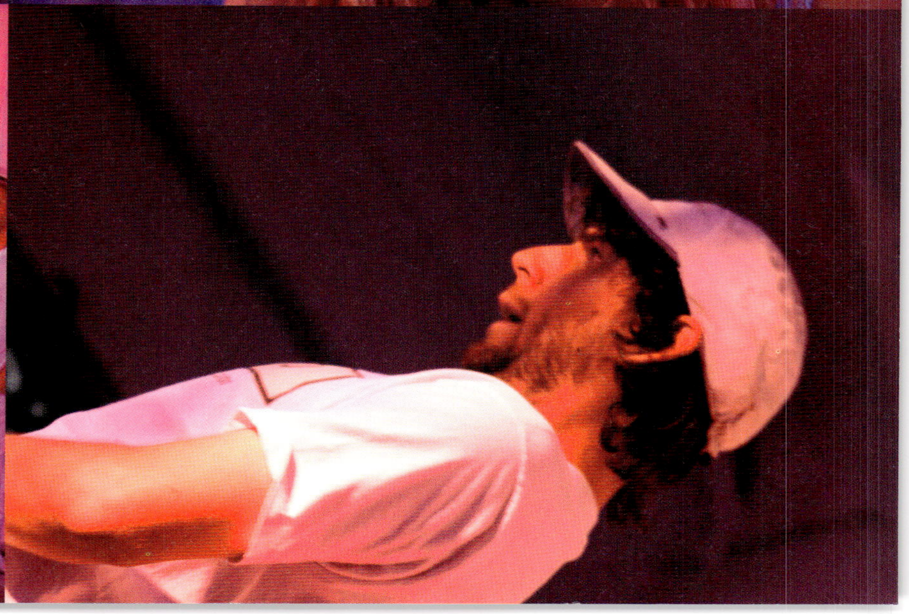

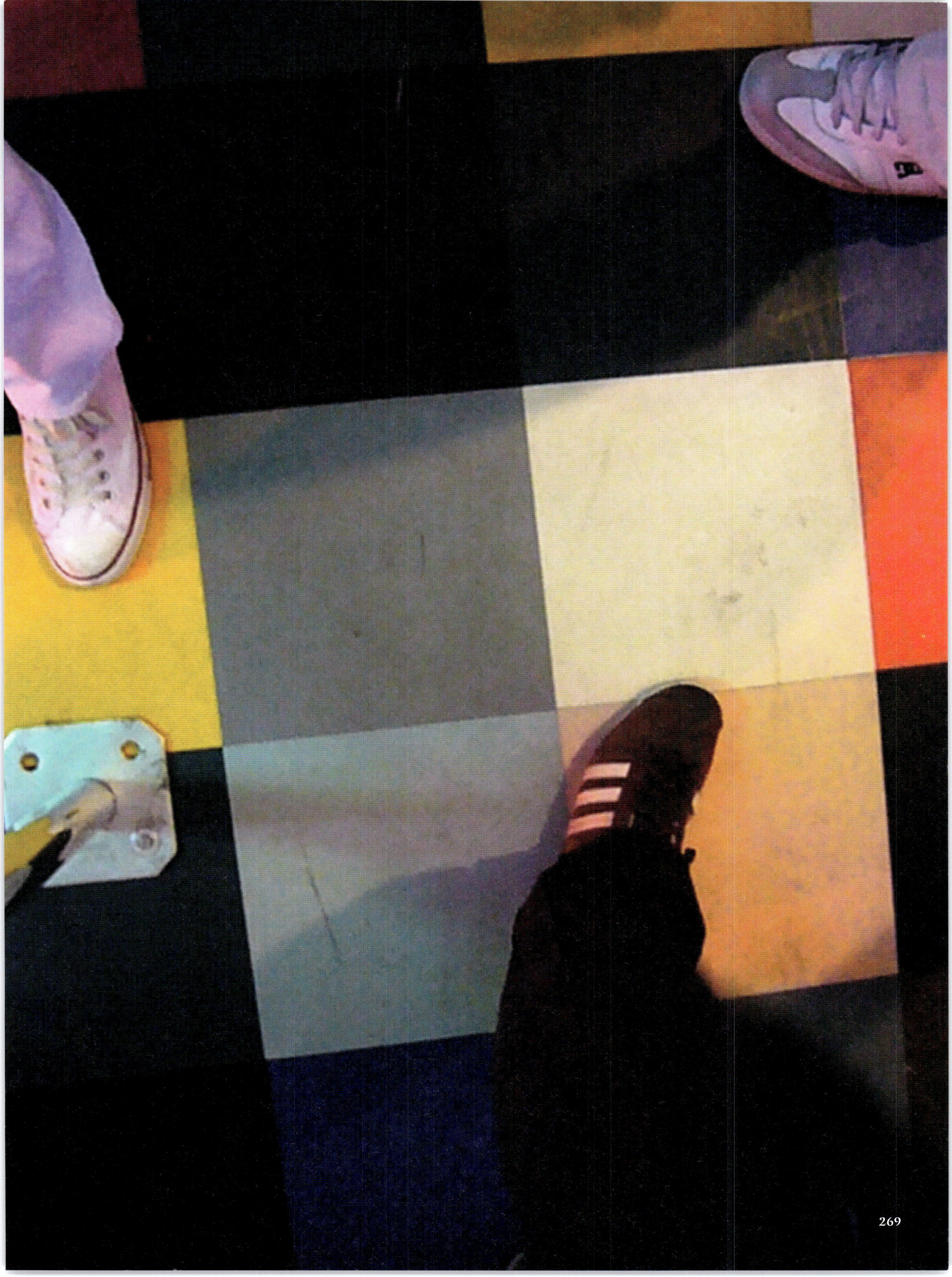

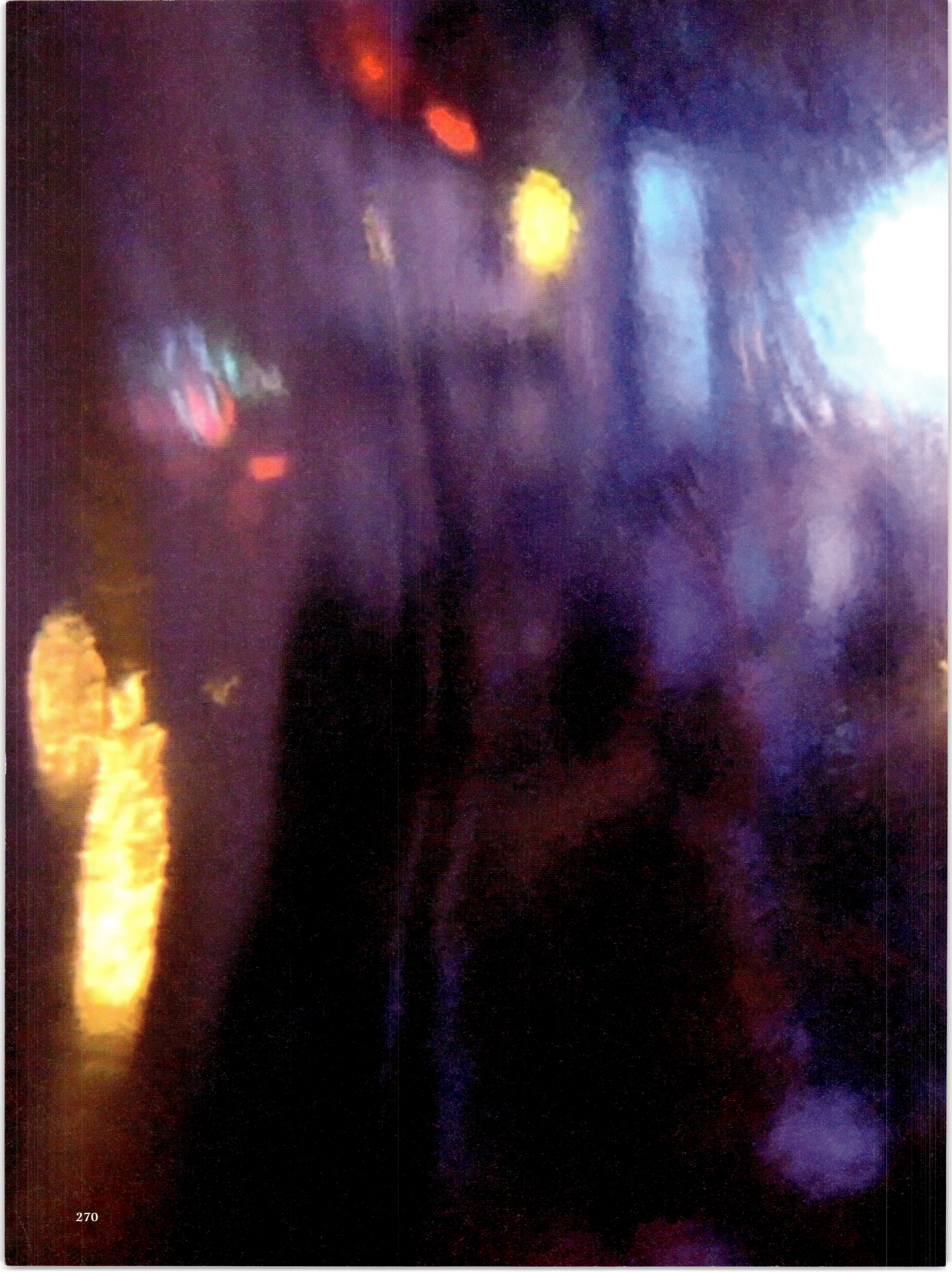

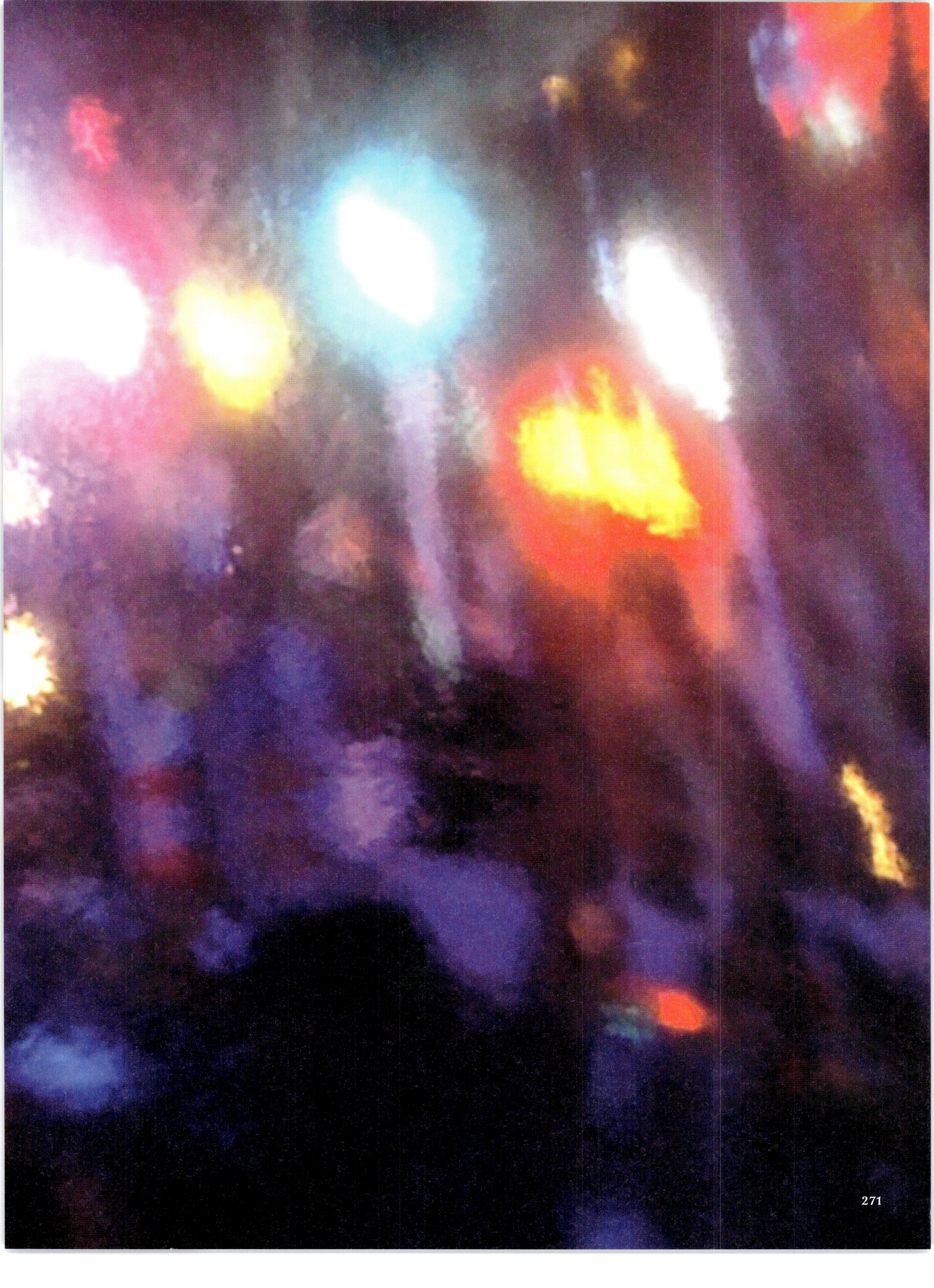

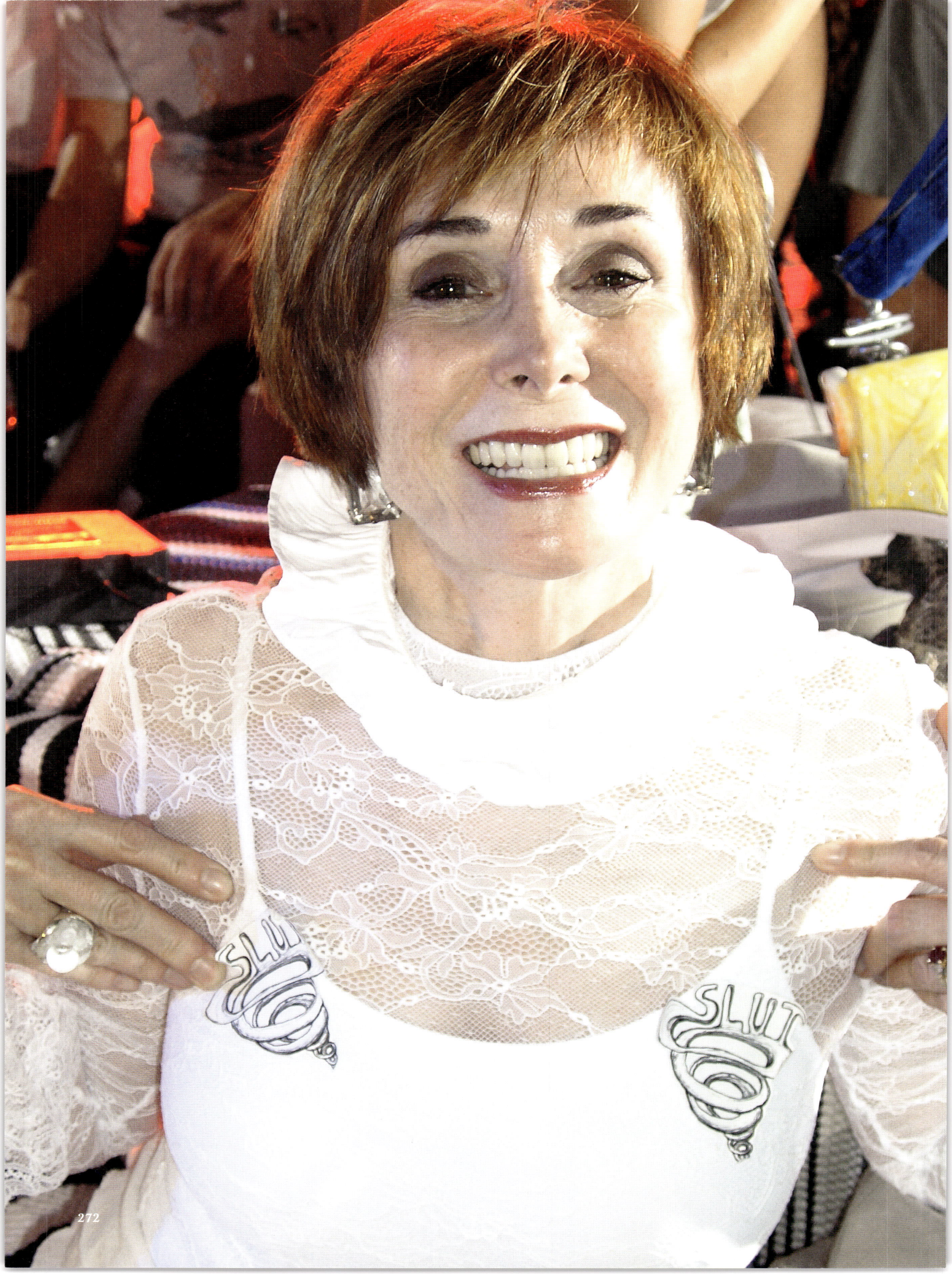
SLUT
SLUT

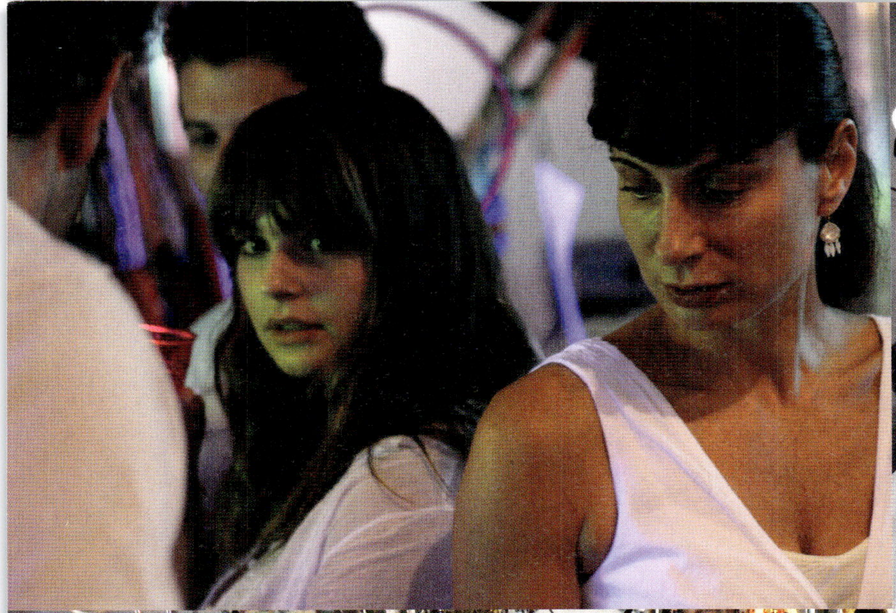

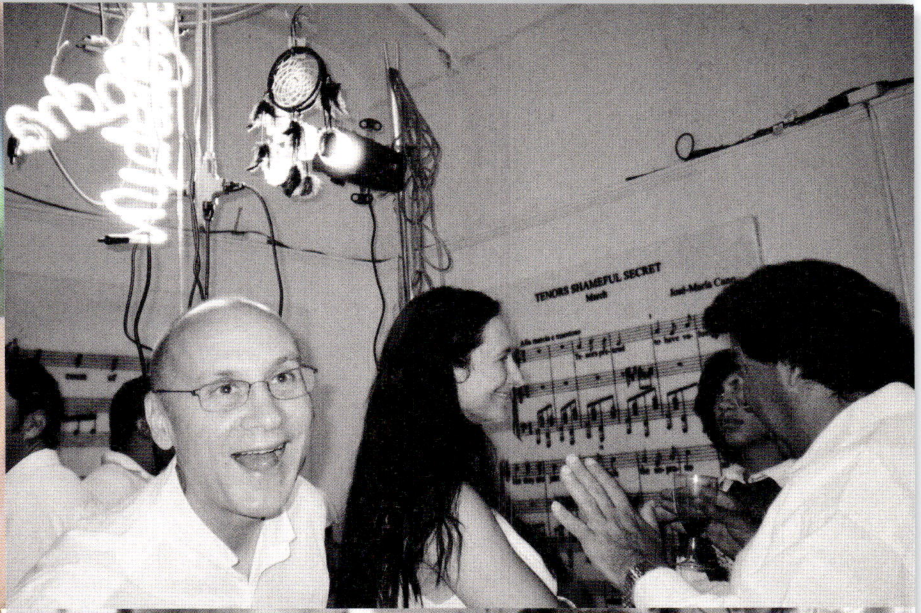
TENORS SHAMEFUL SECRET

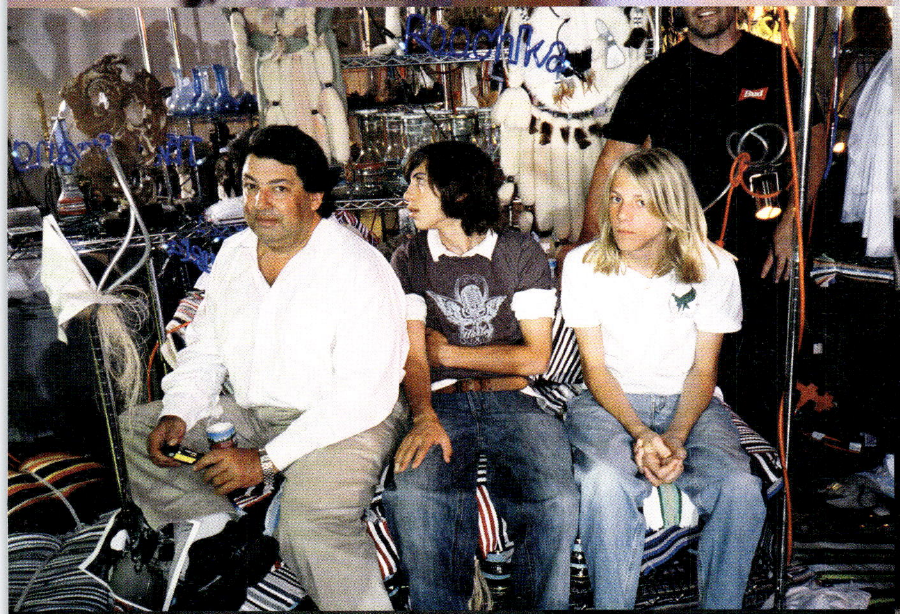

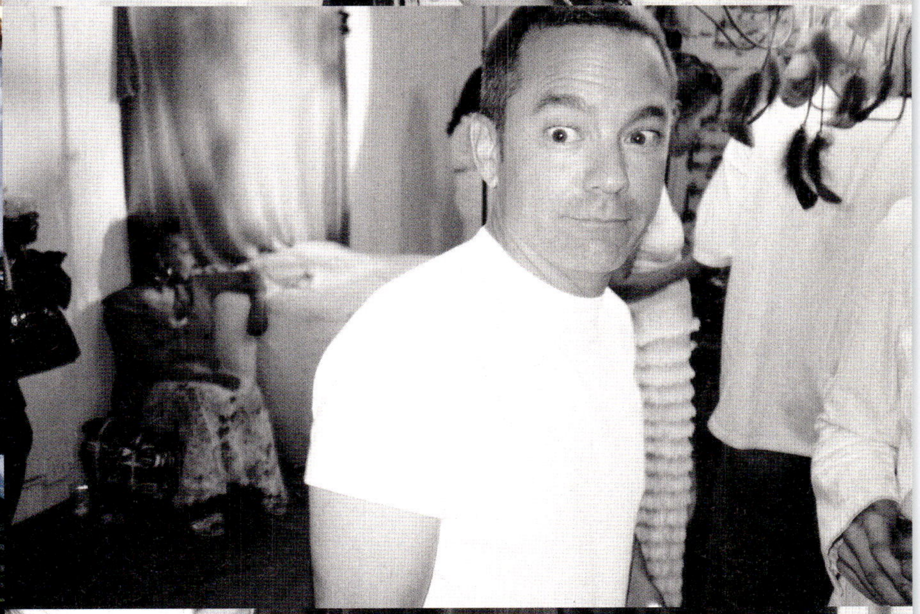

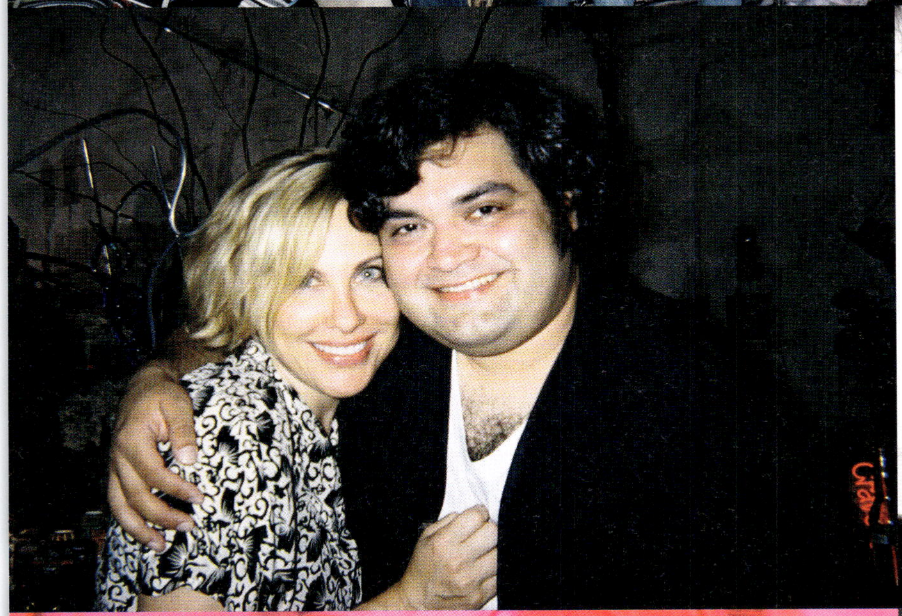

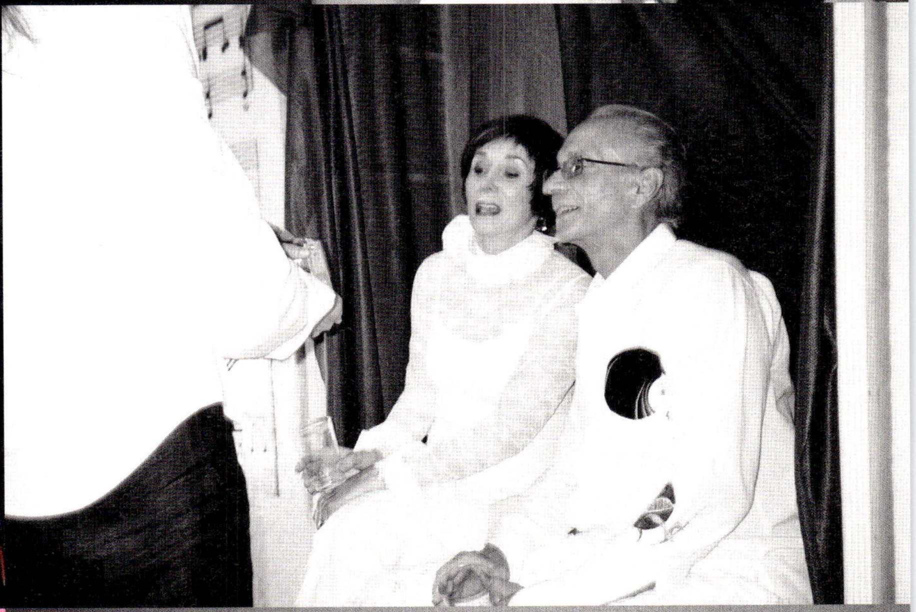

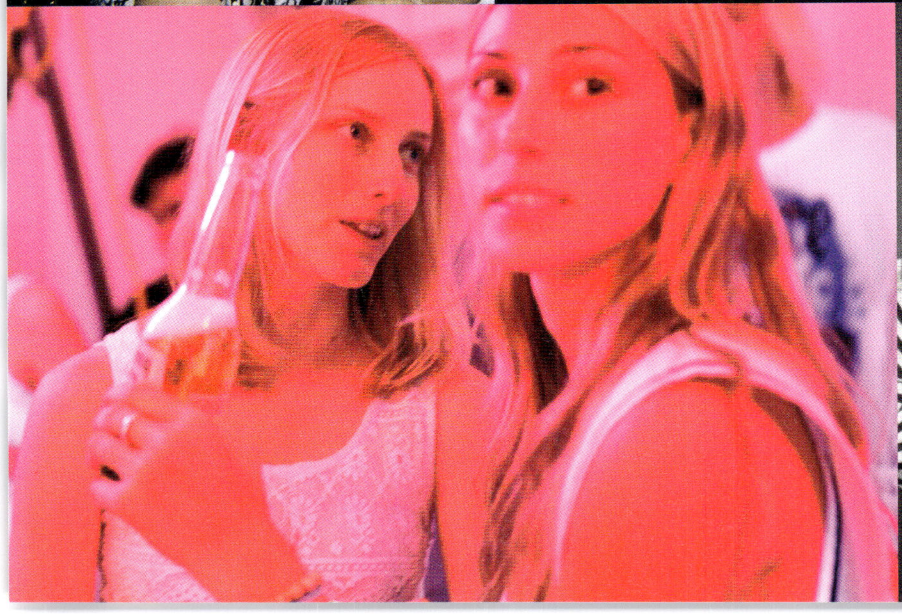

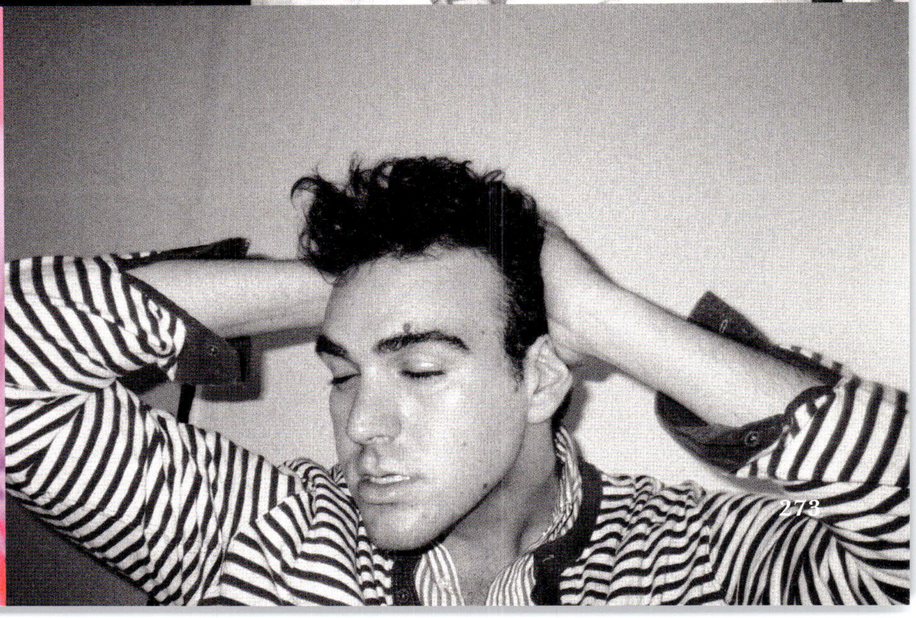

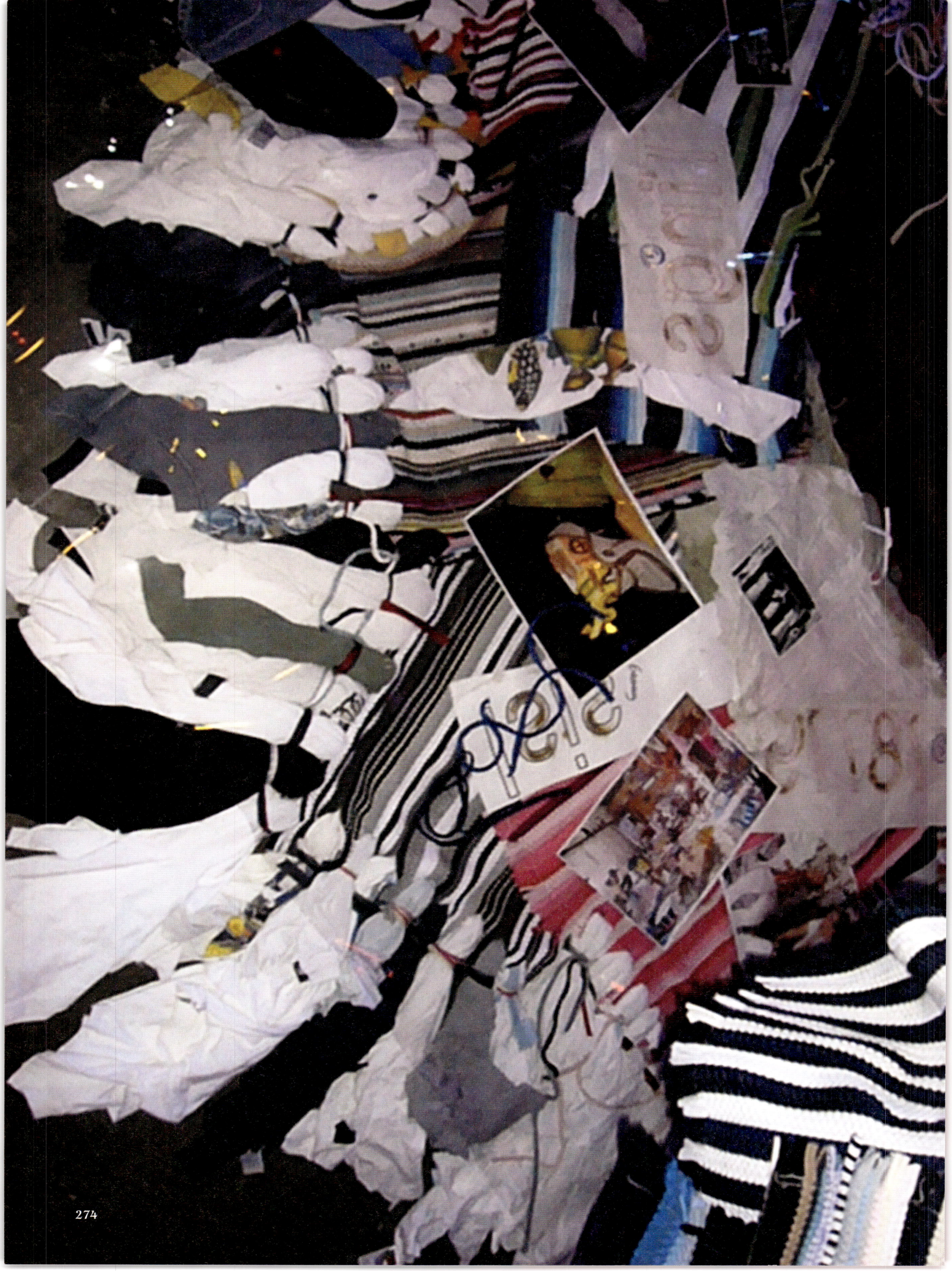

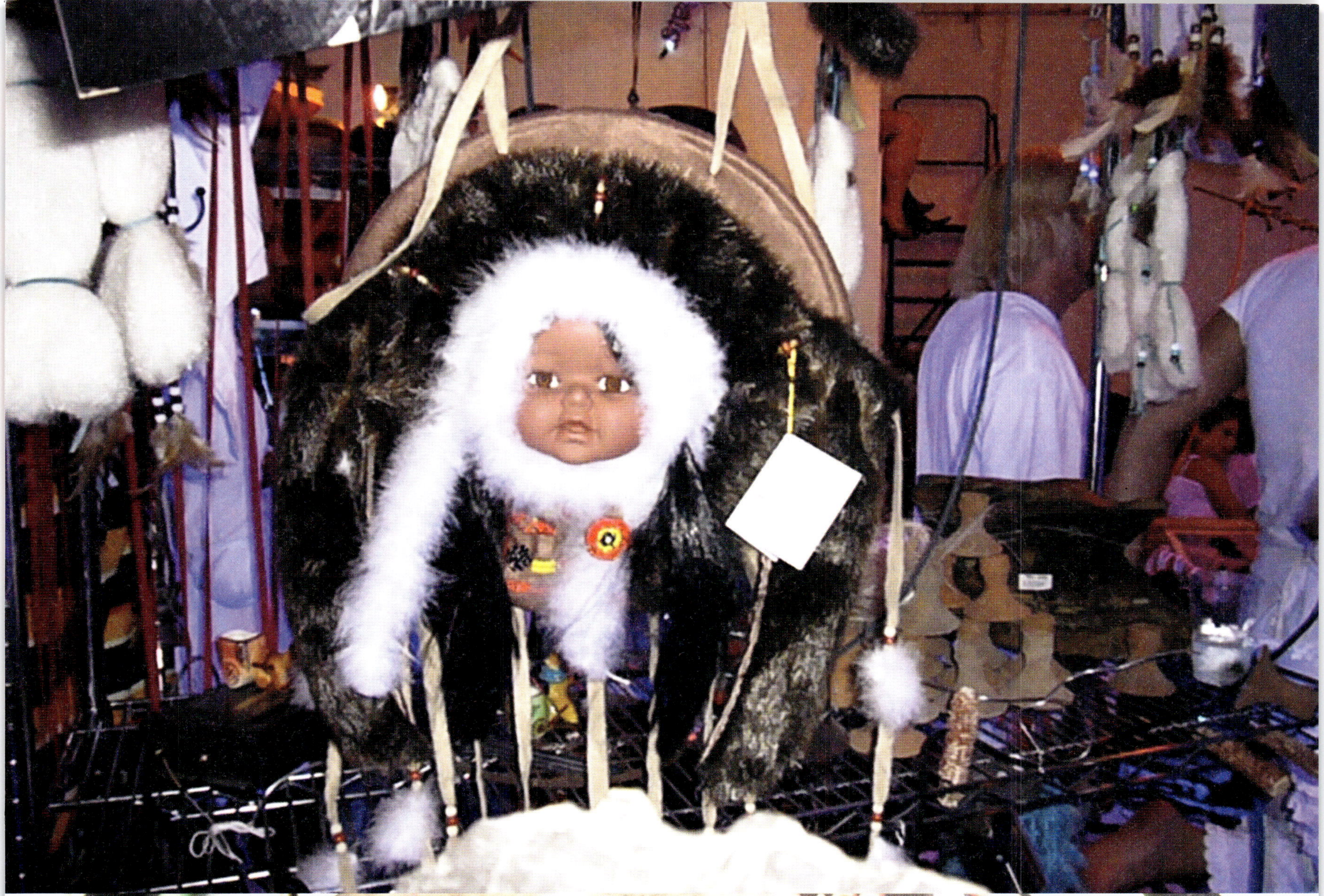

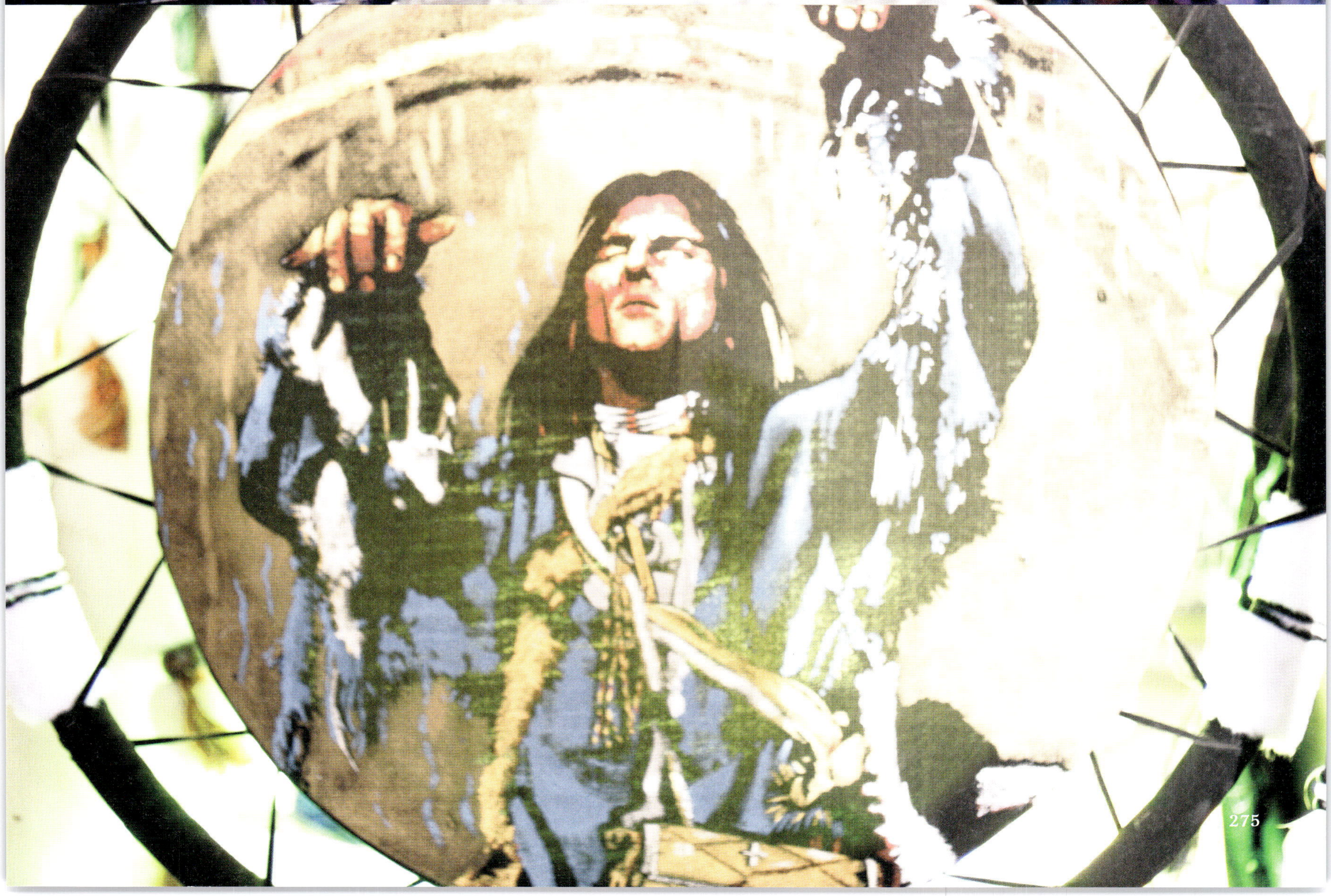

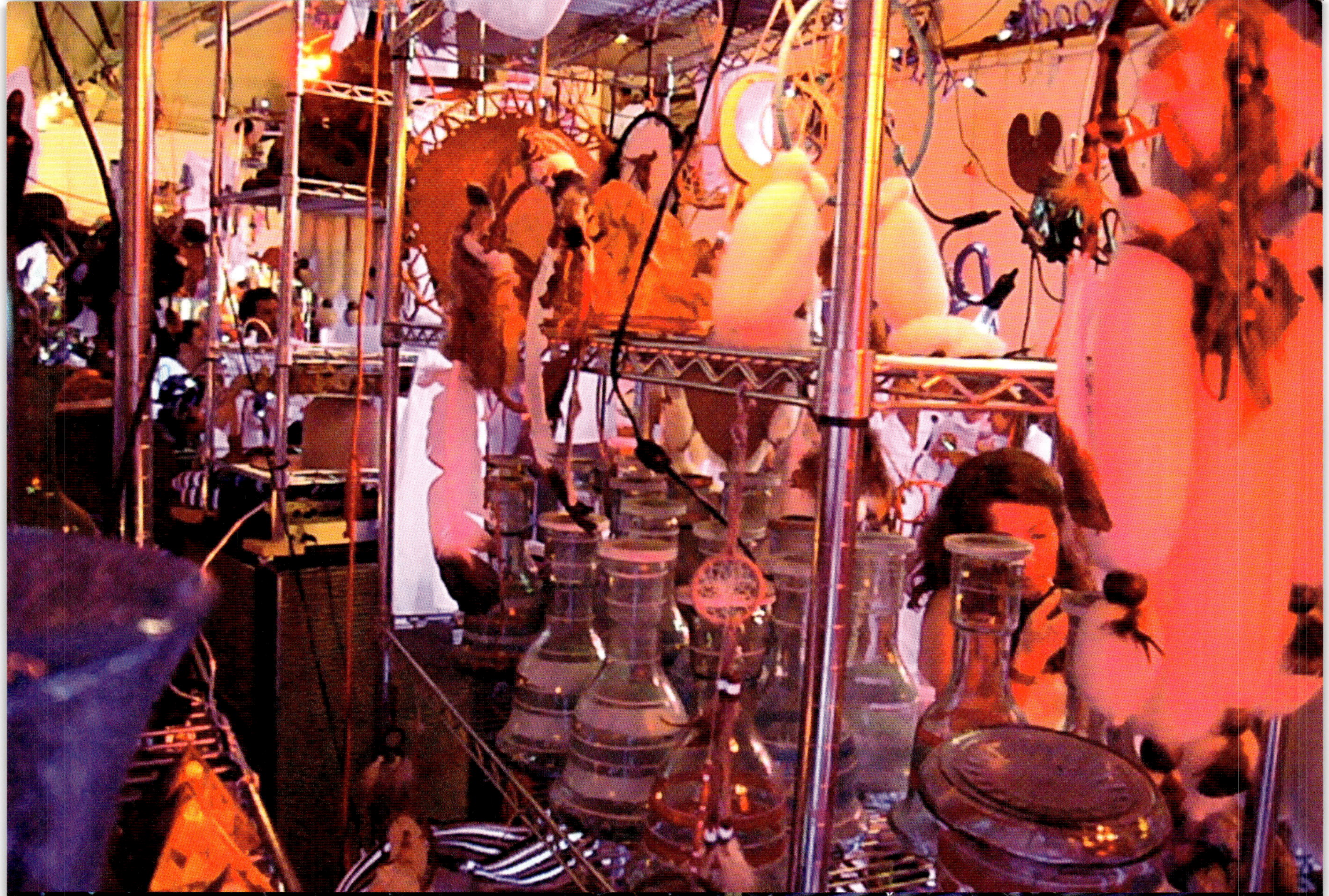

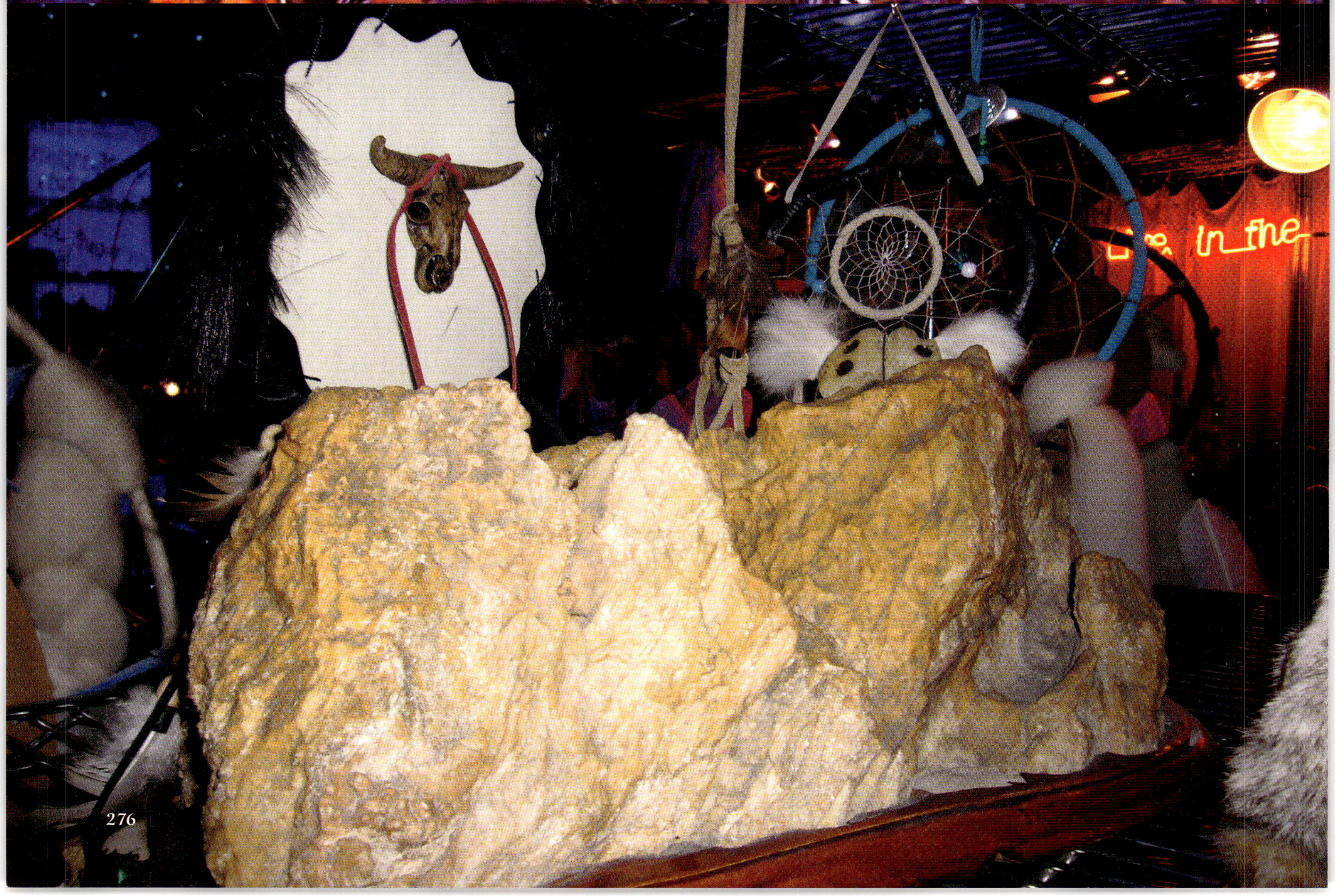
in the

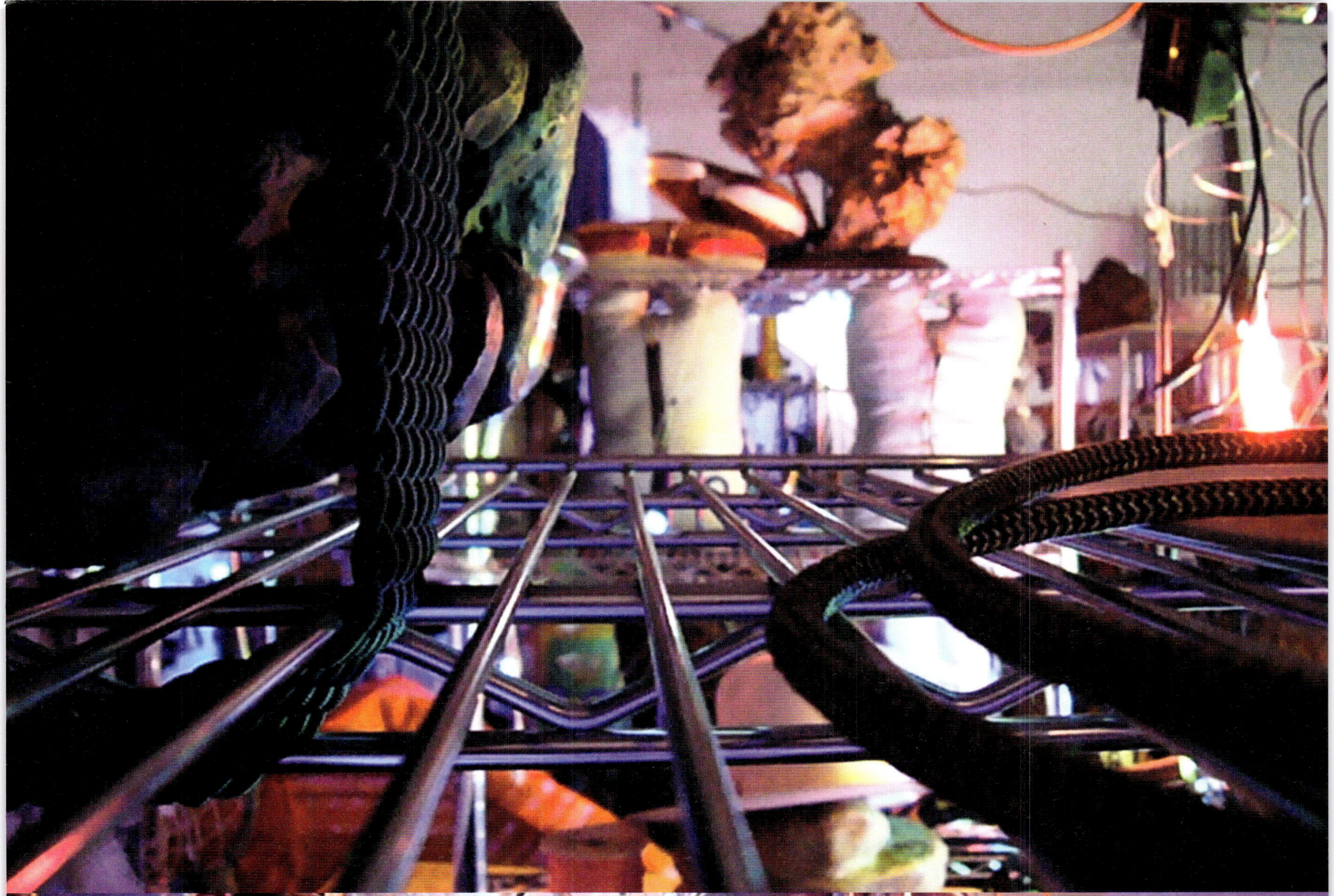

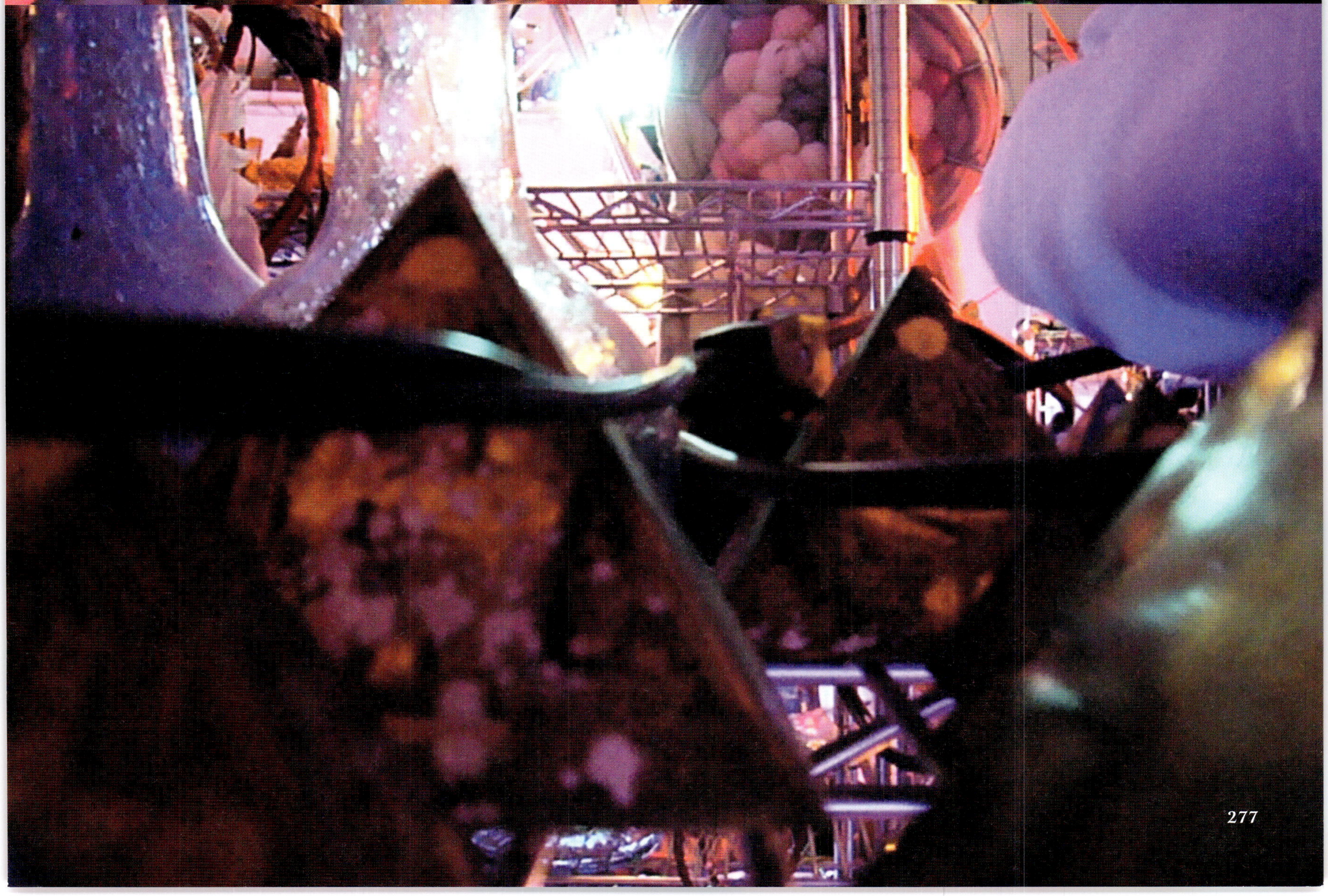

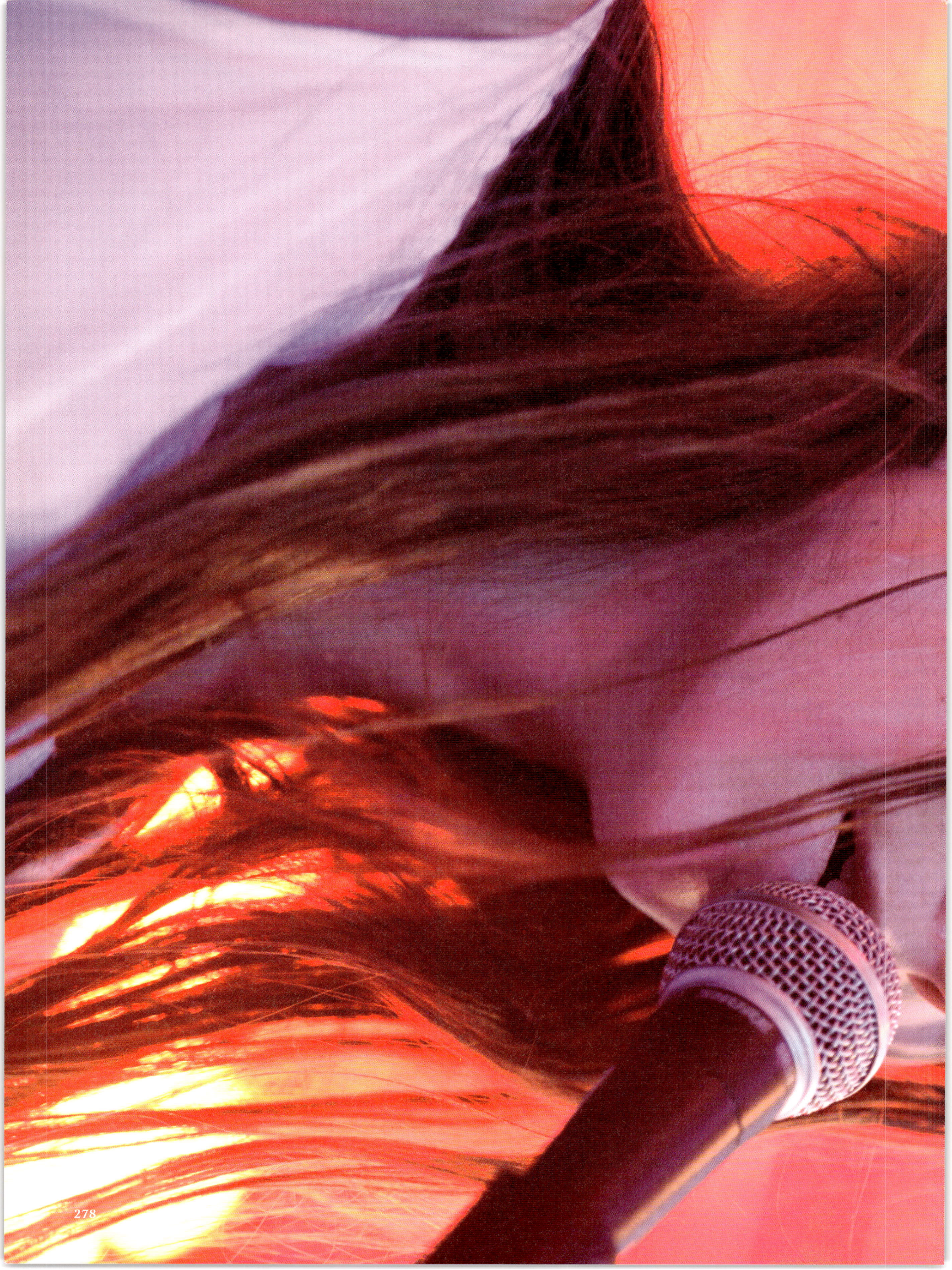

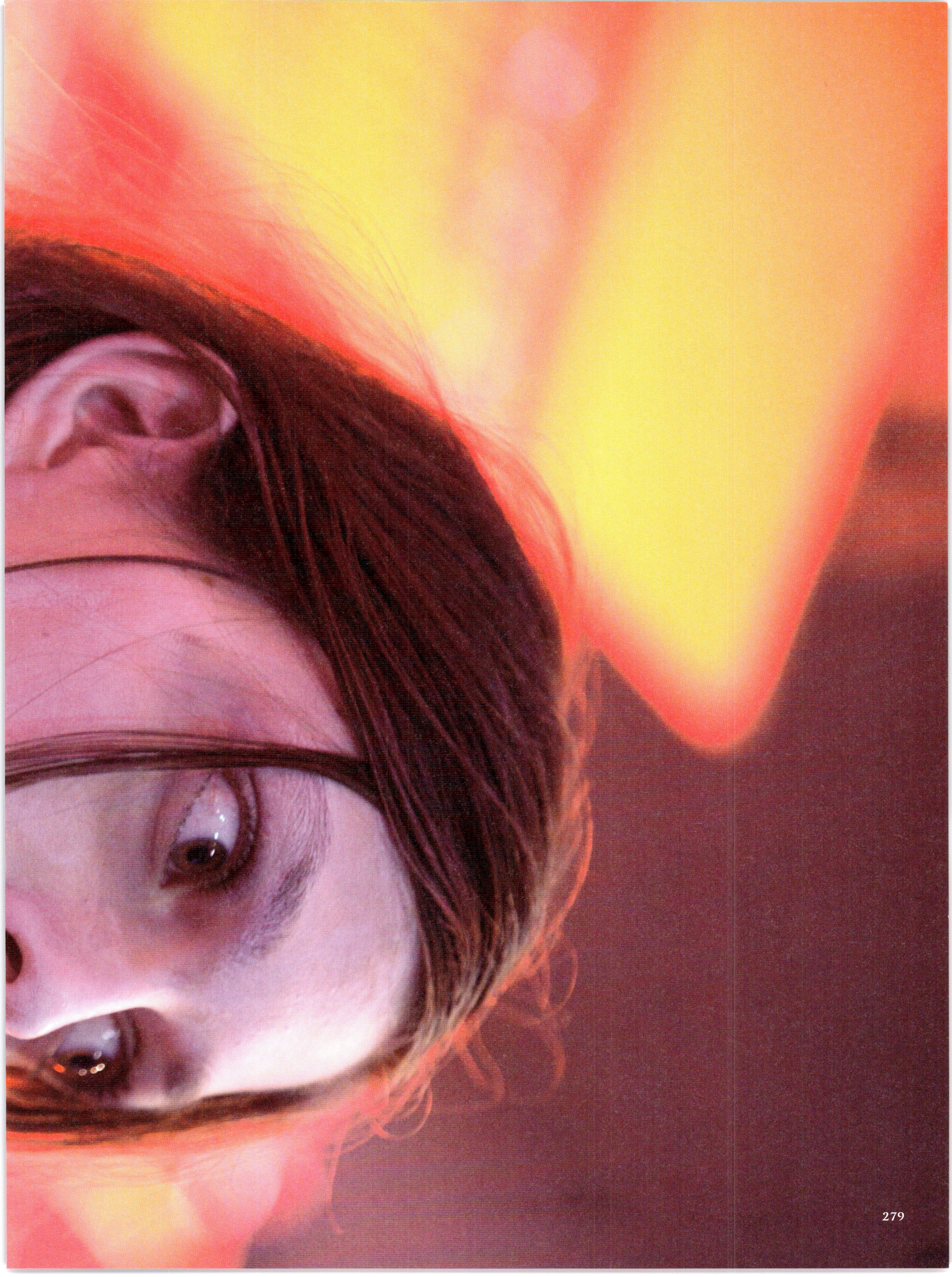

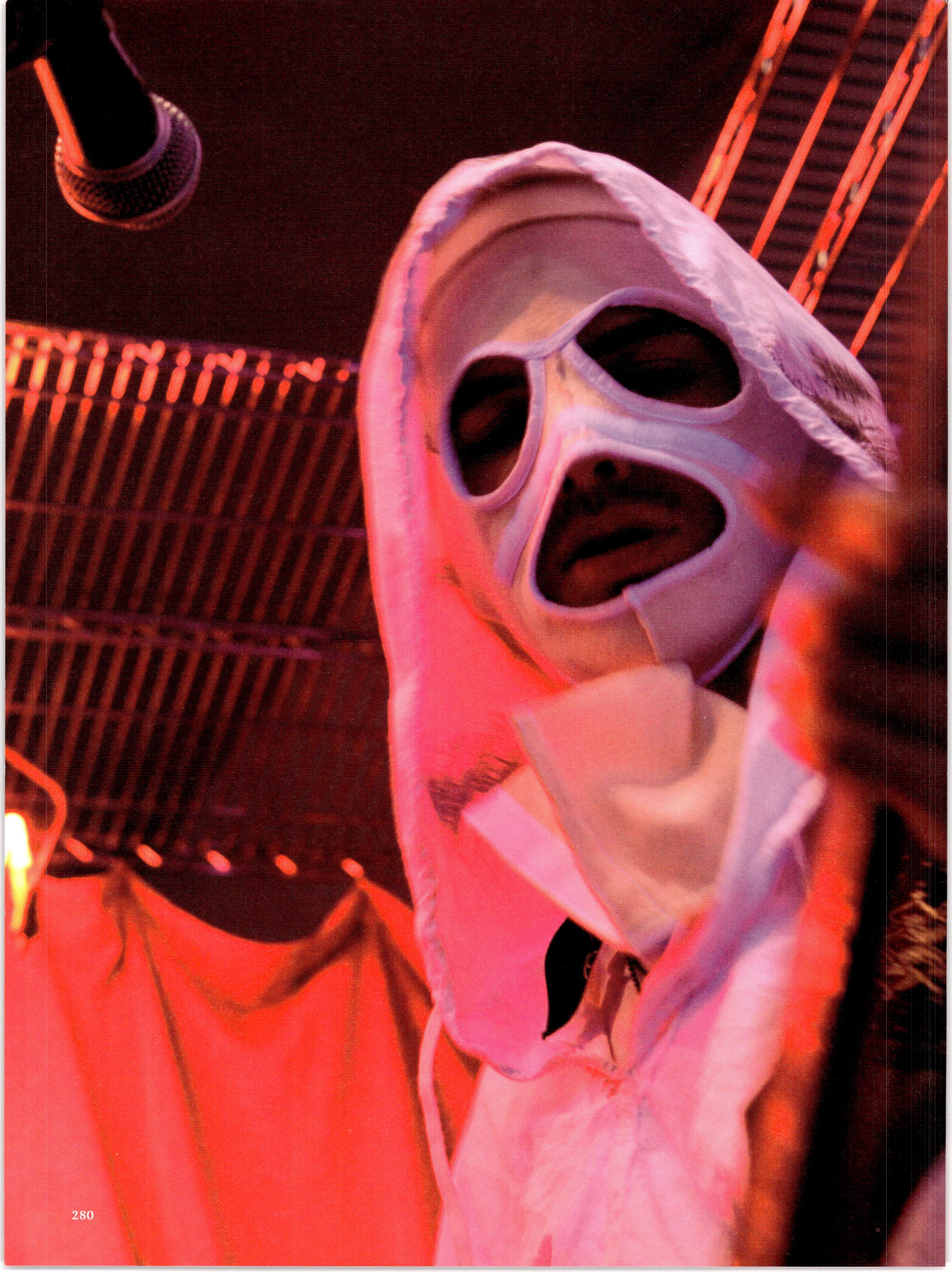

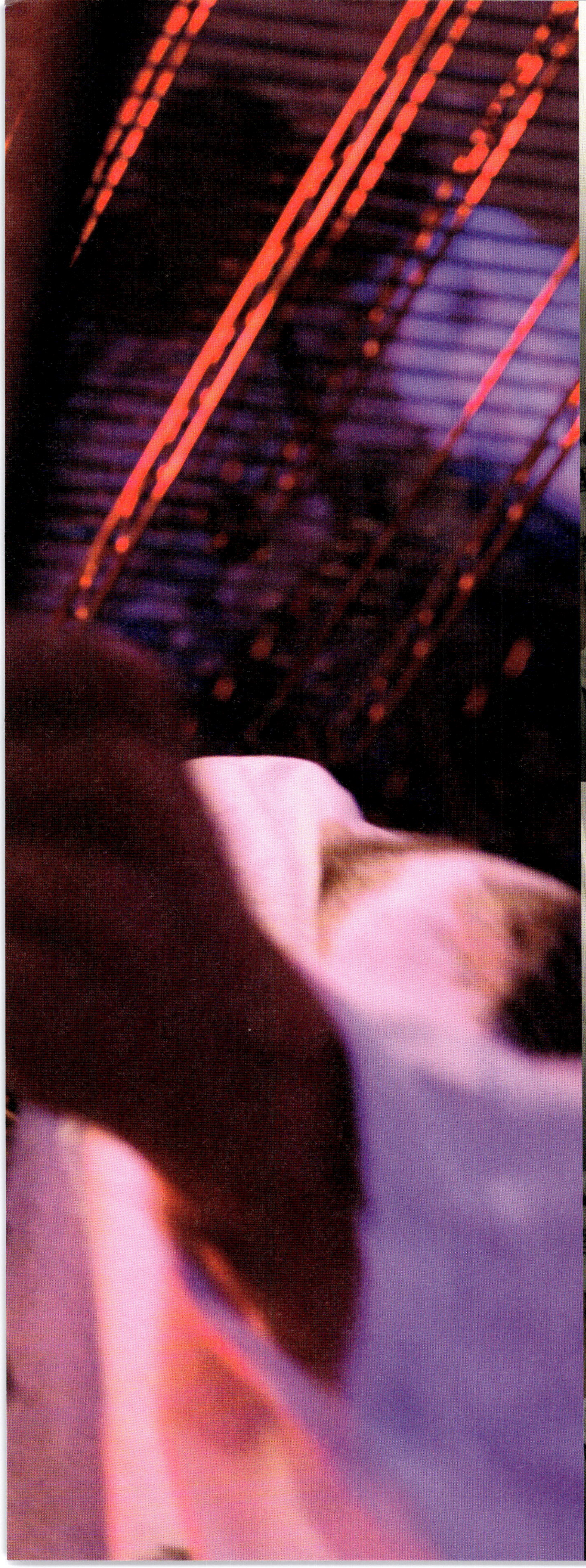

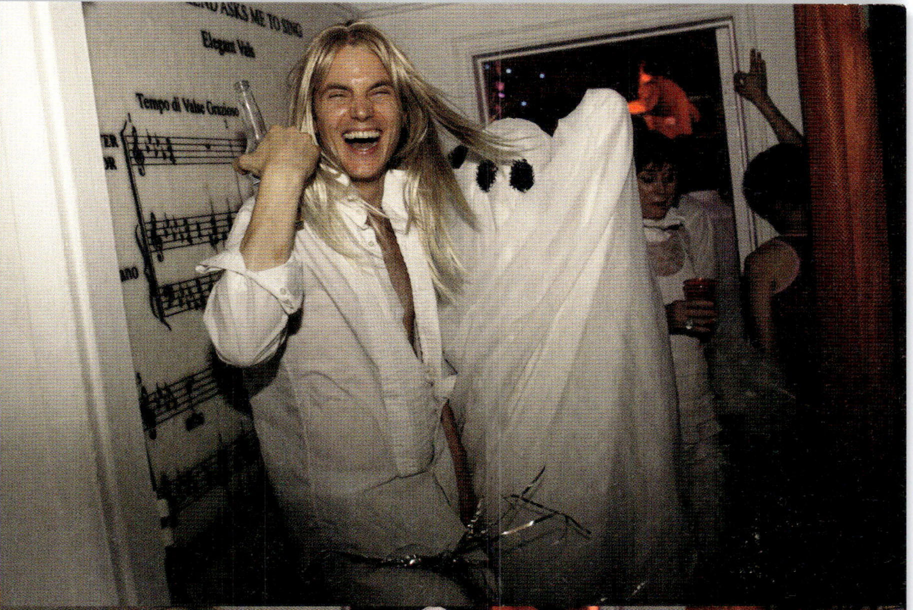
ASKS ME TO SING
Tempo di Valse Grazioso

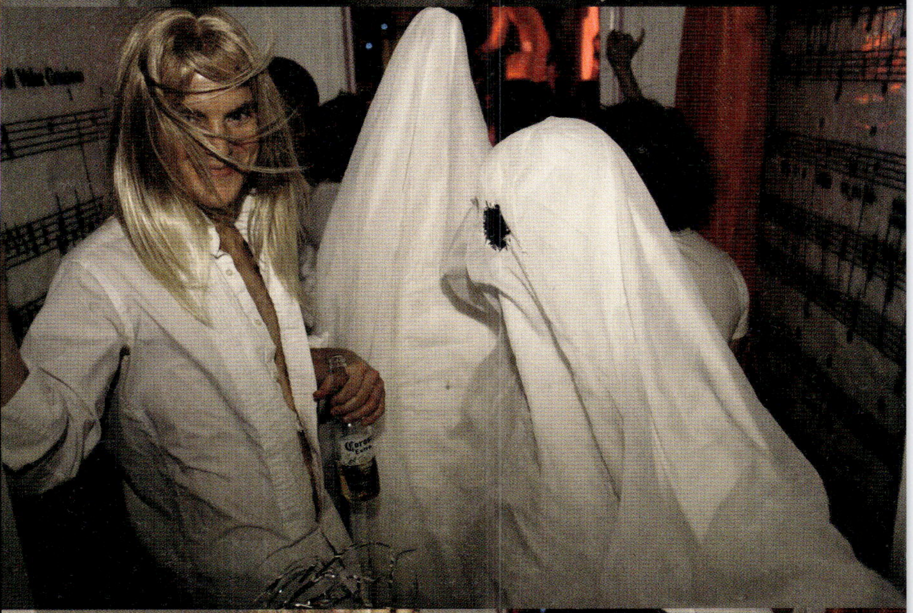

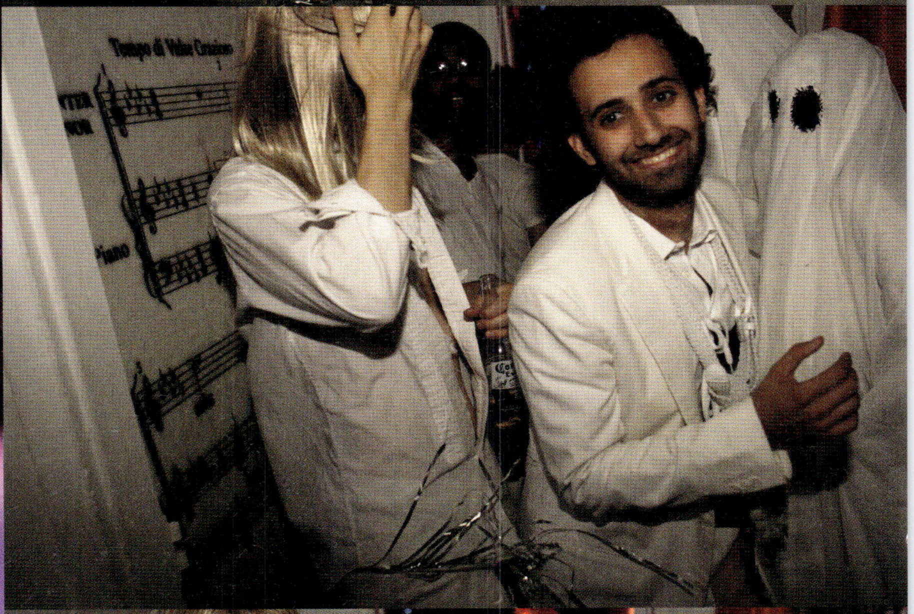

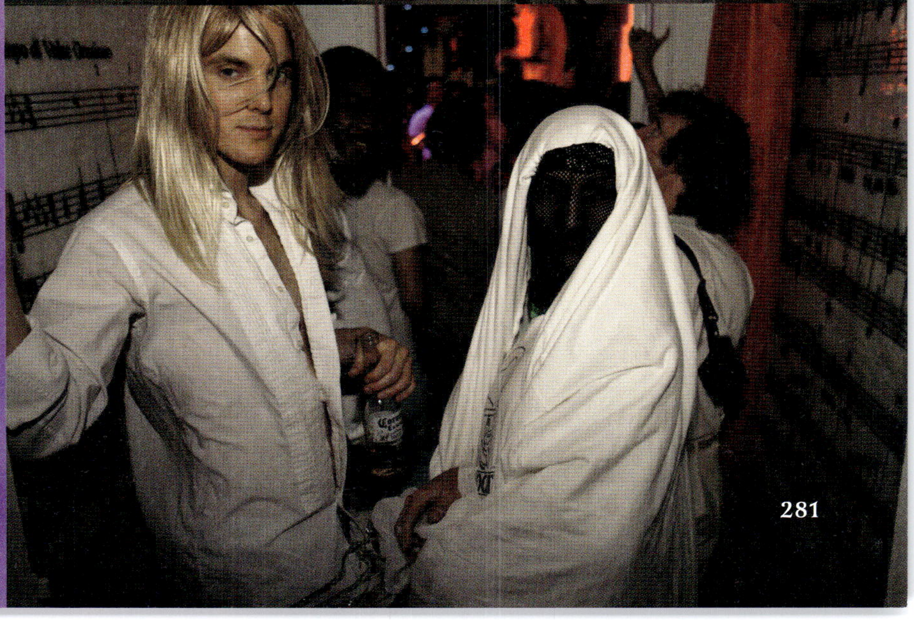

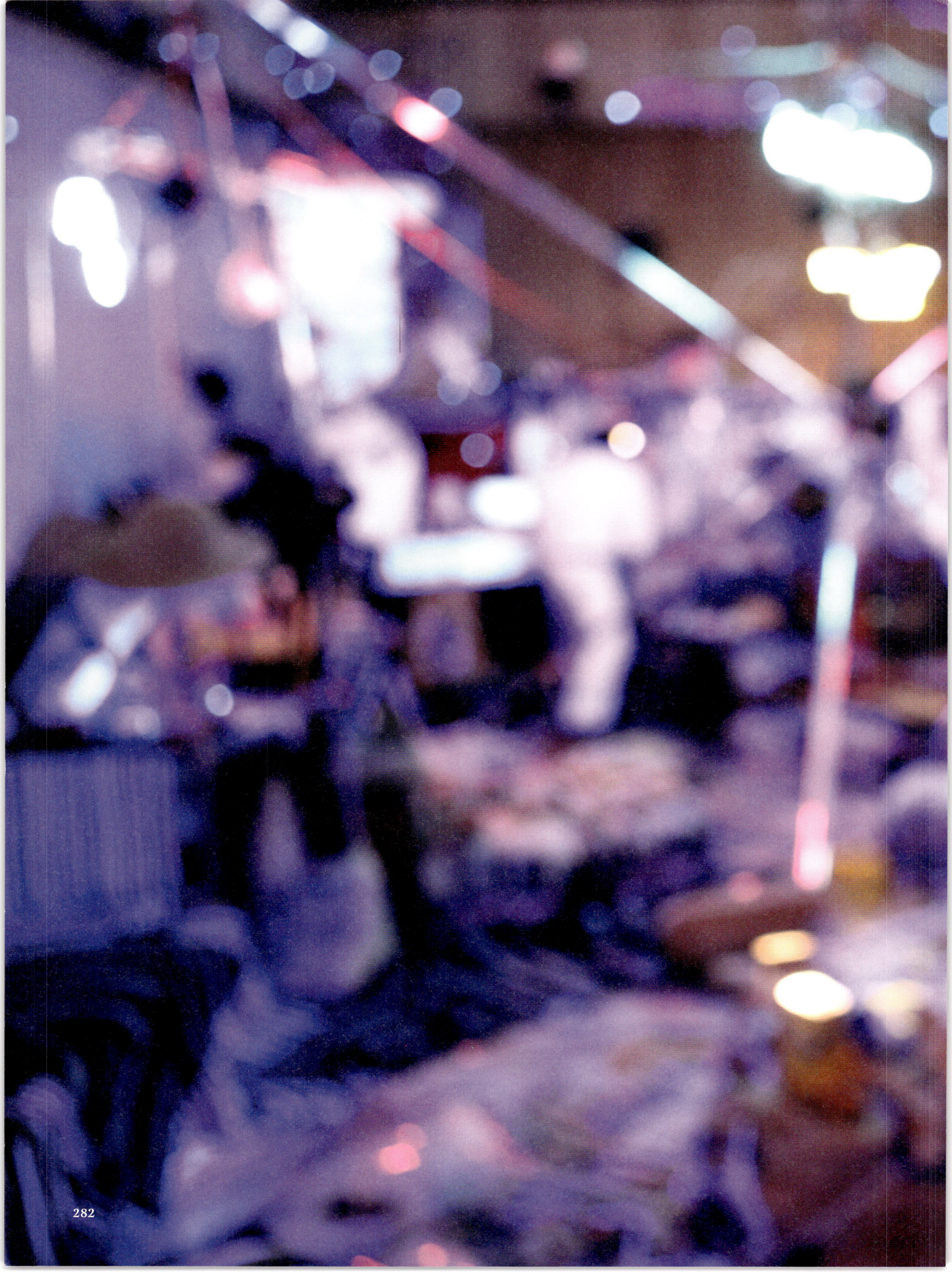

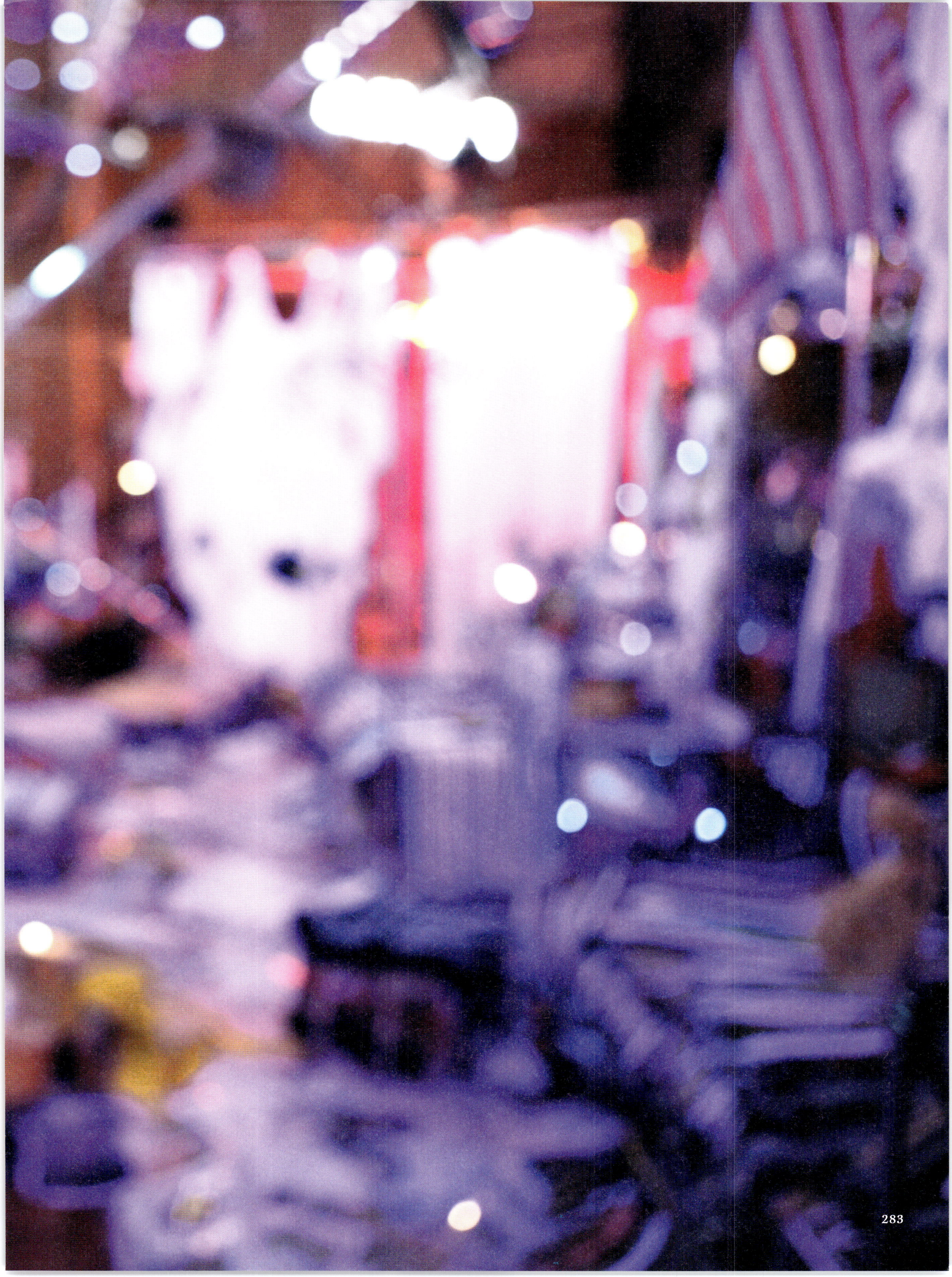

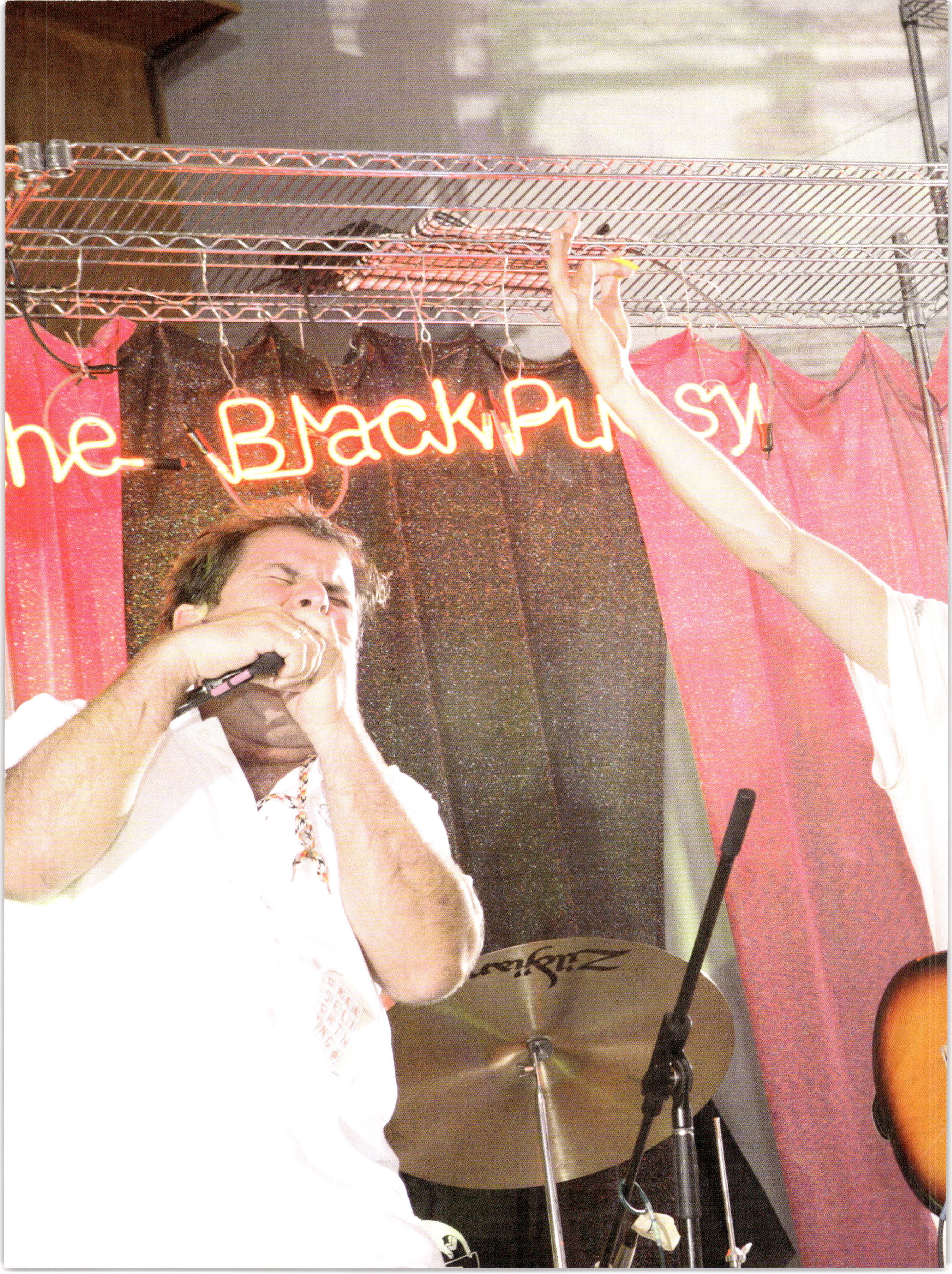

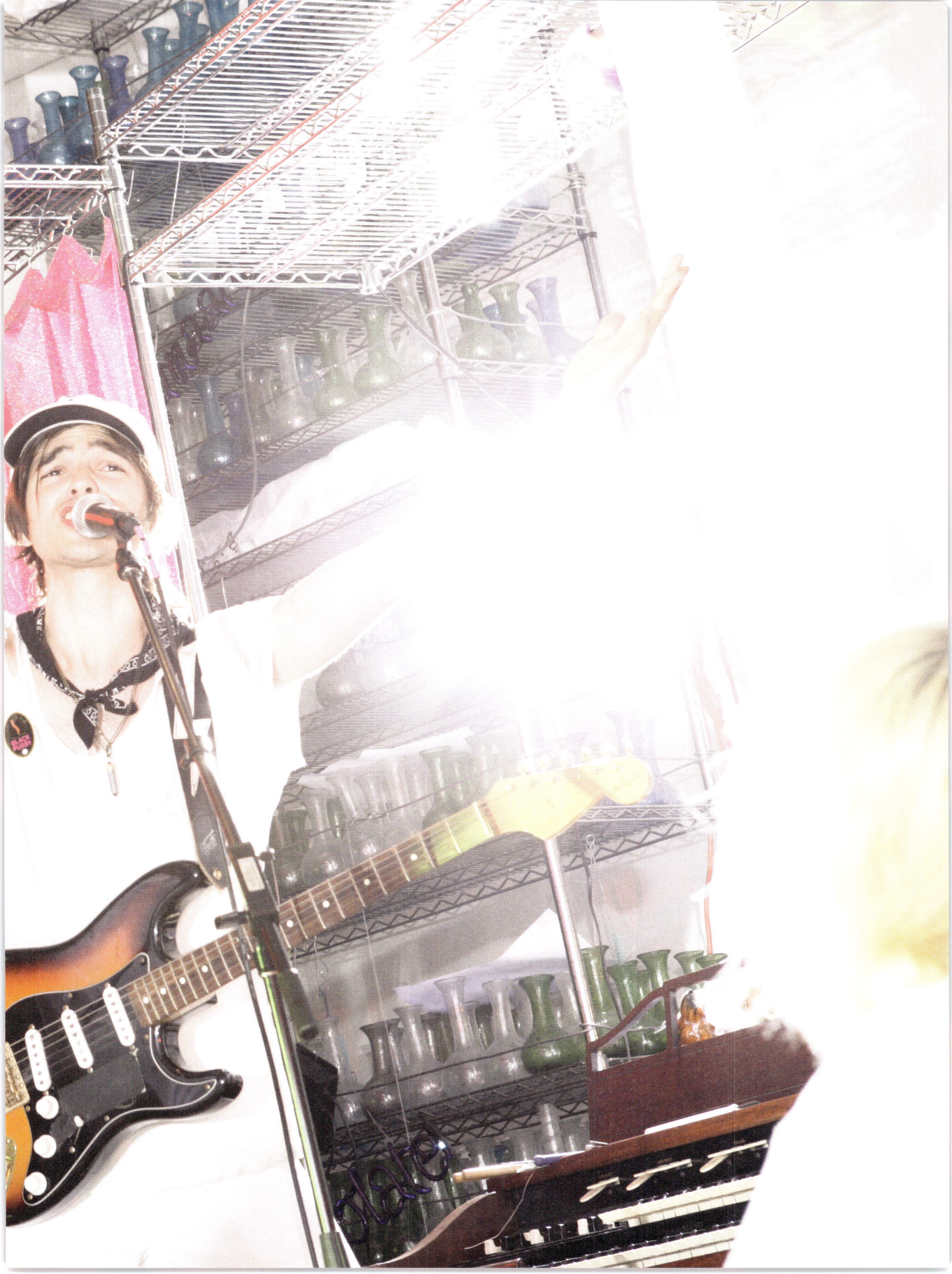

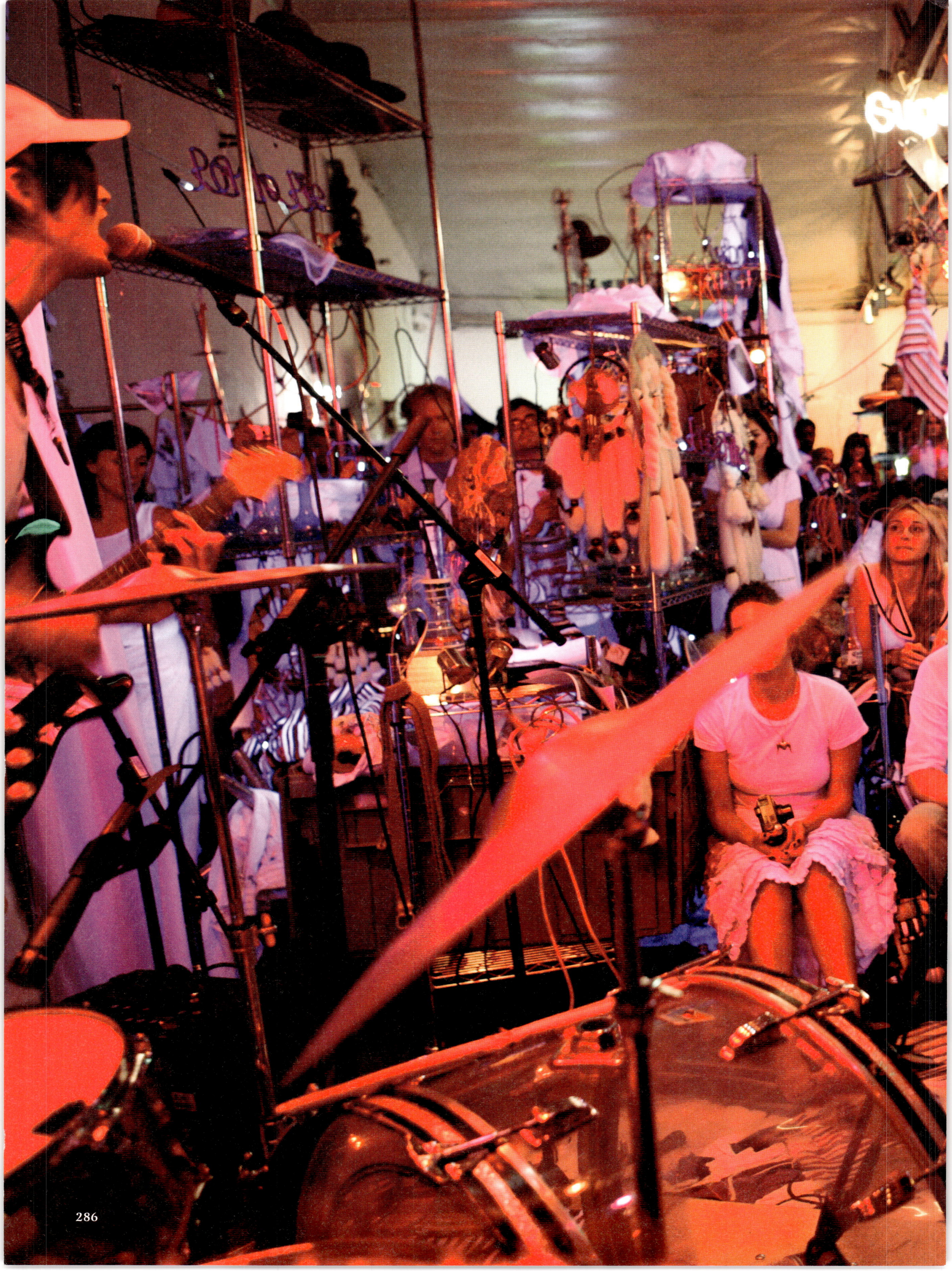

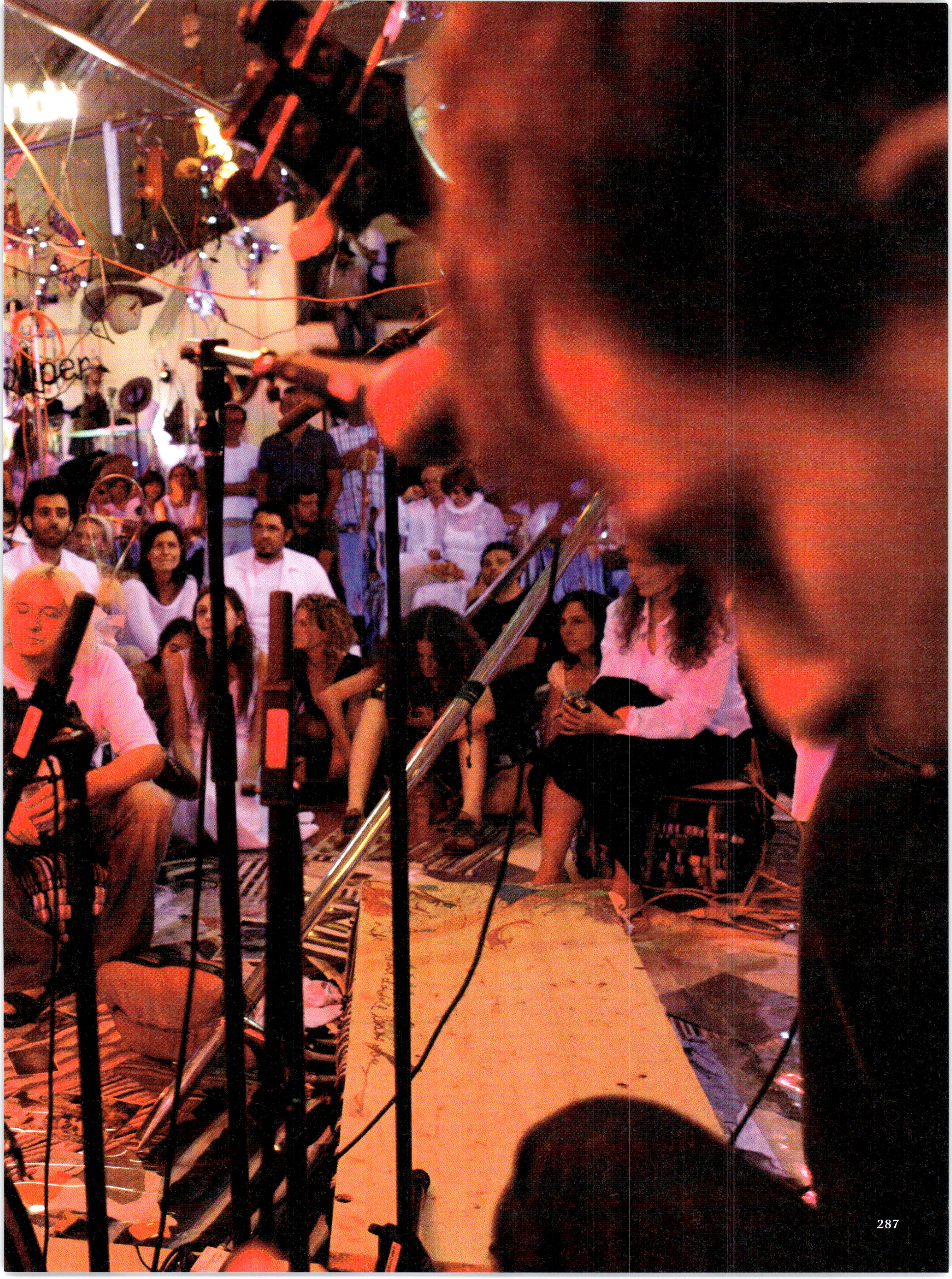

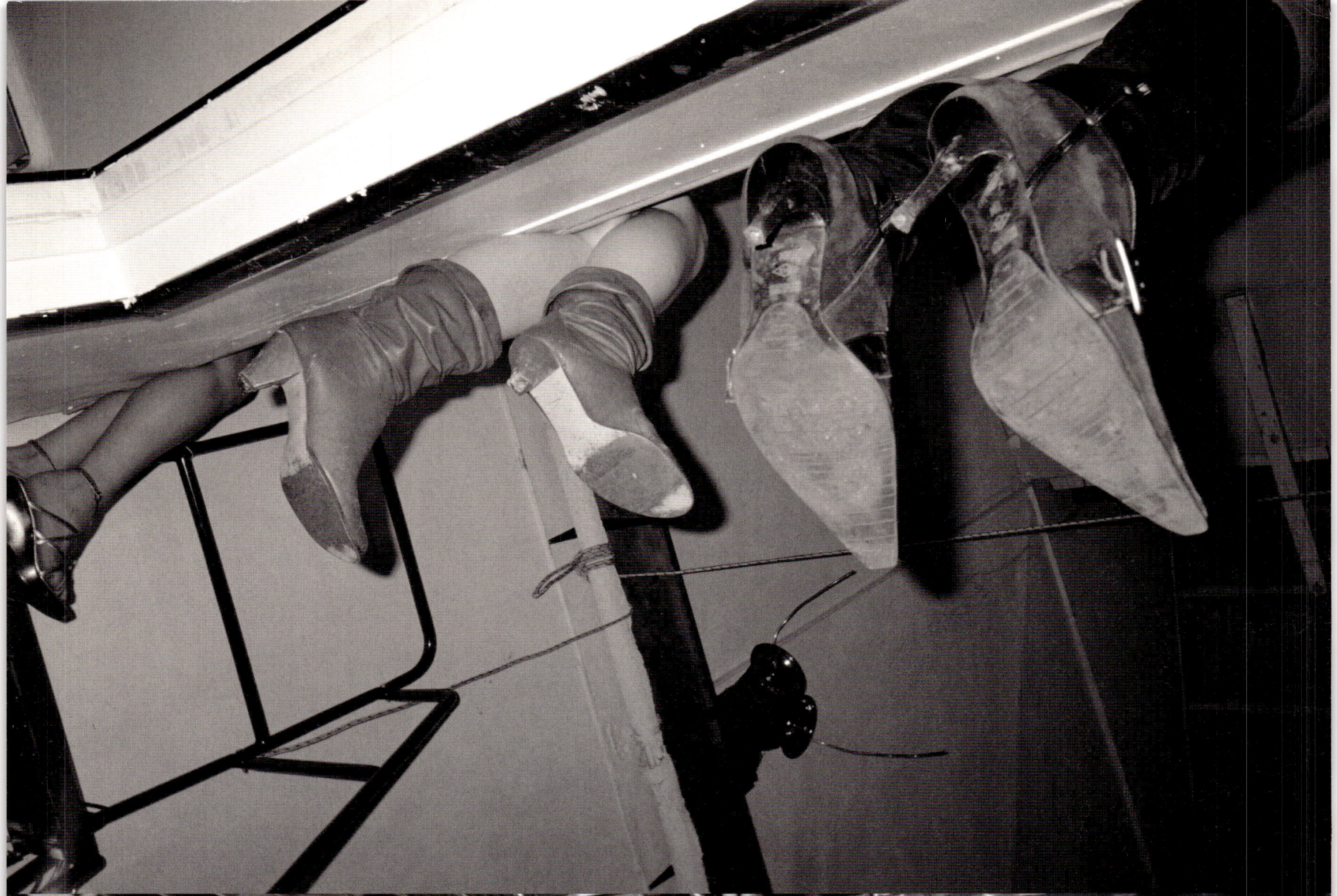

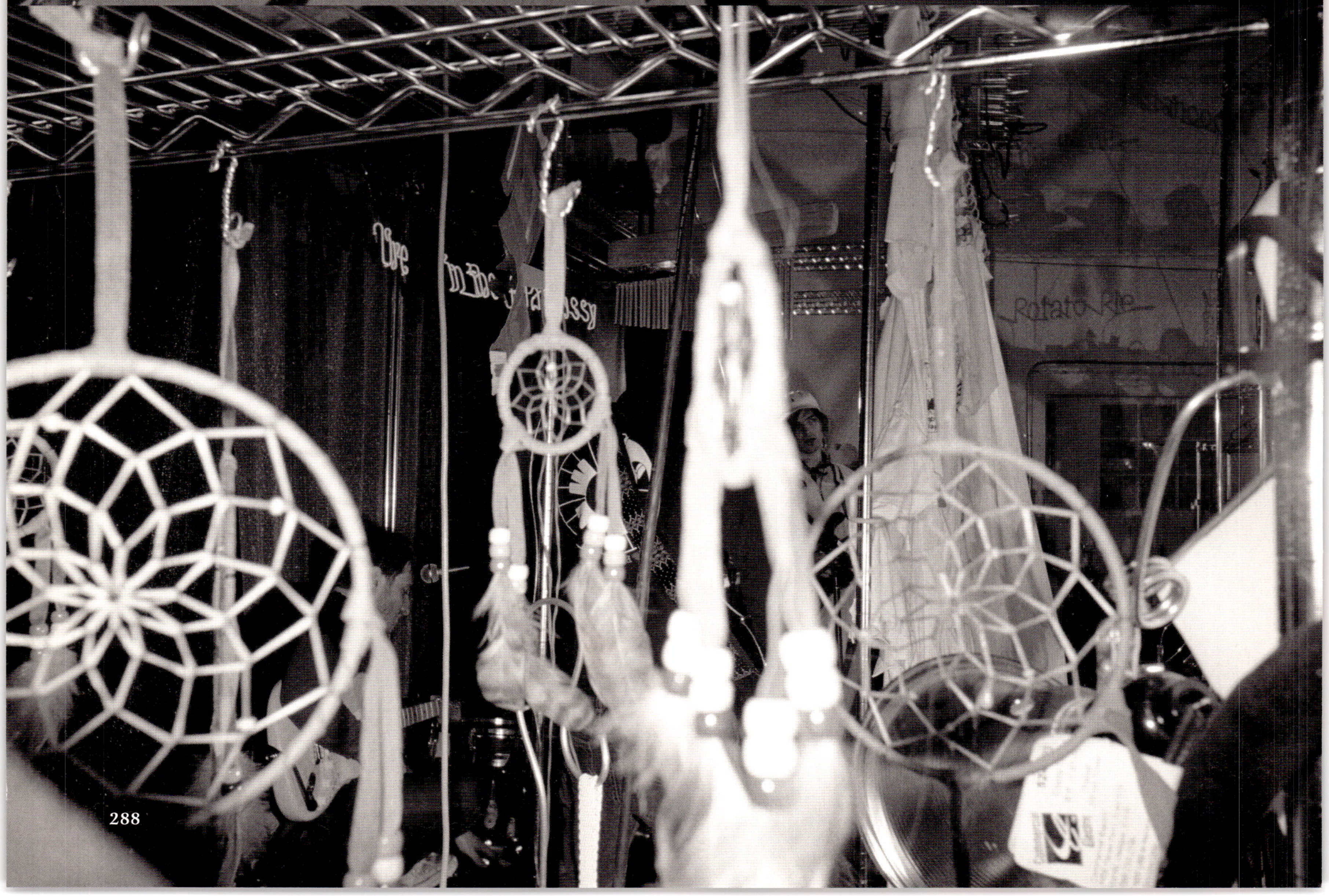

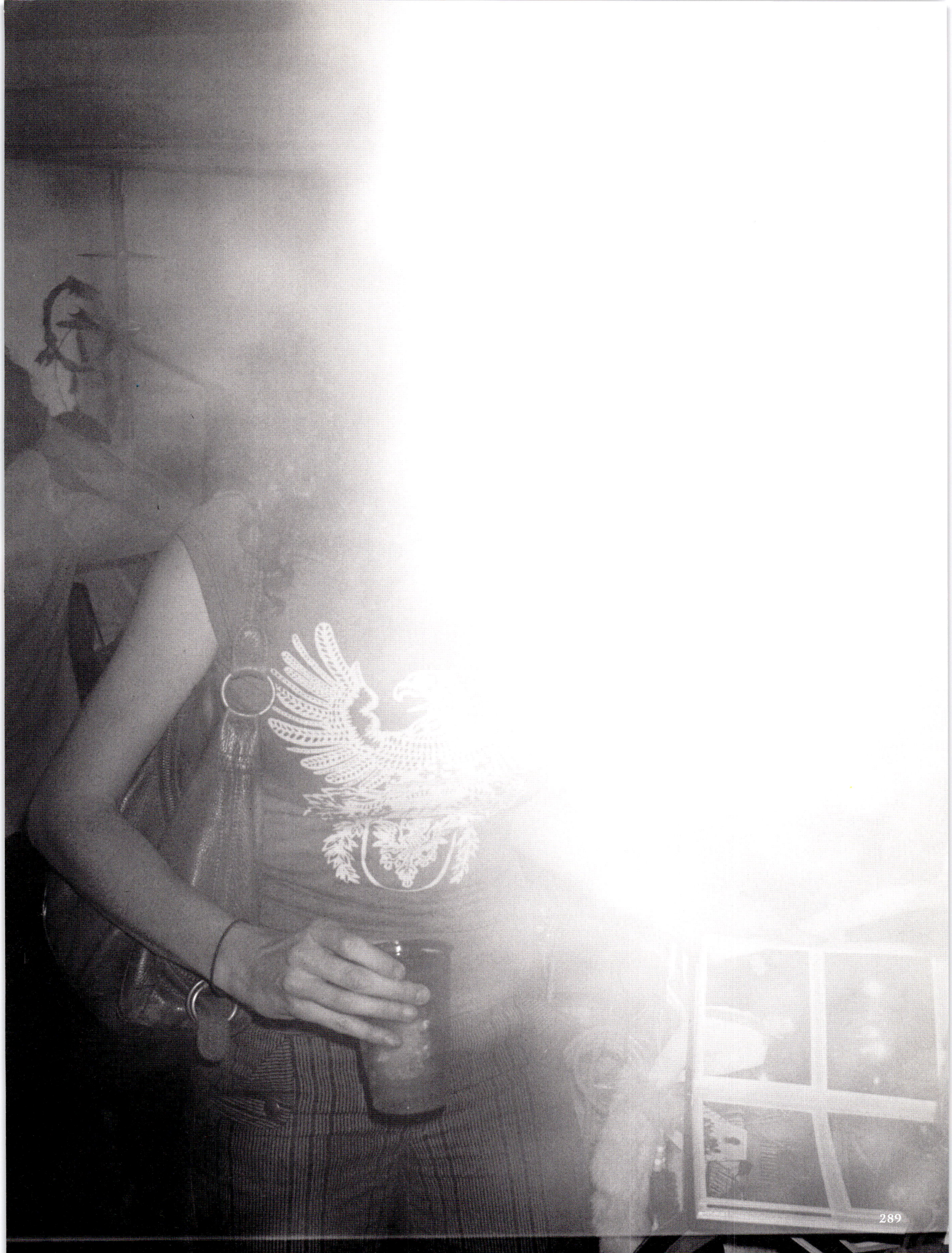

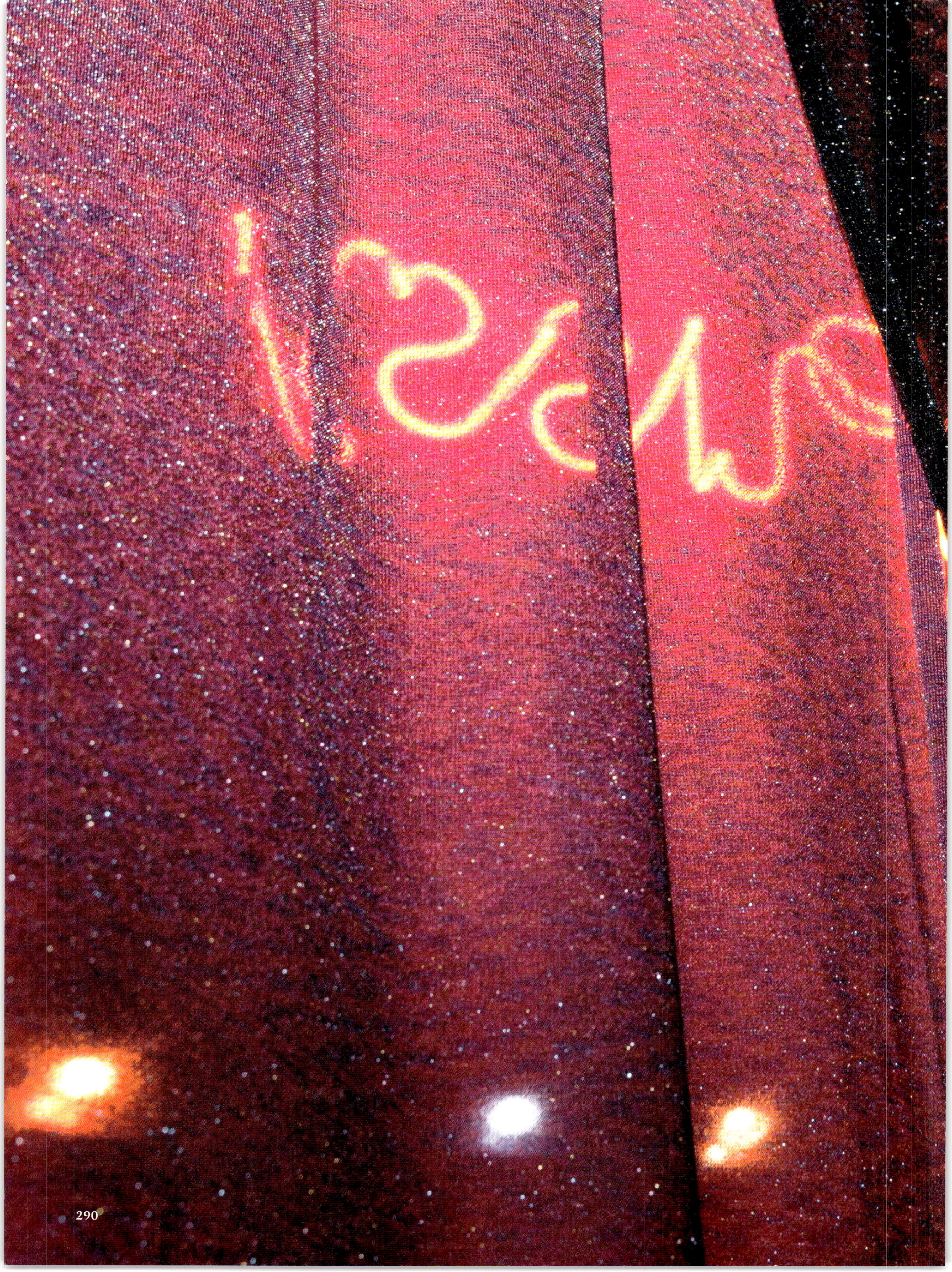

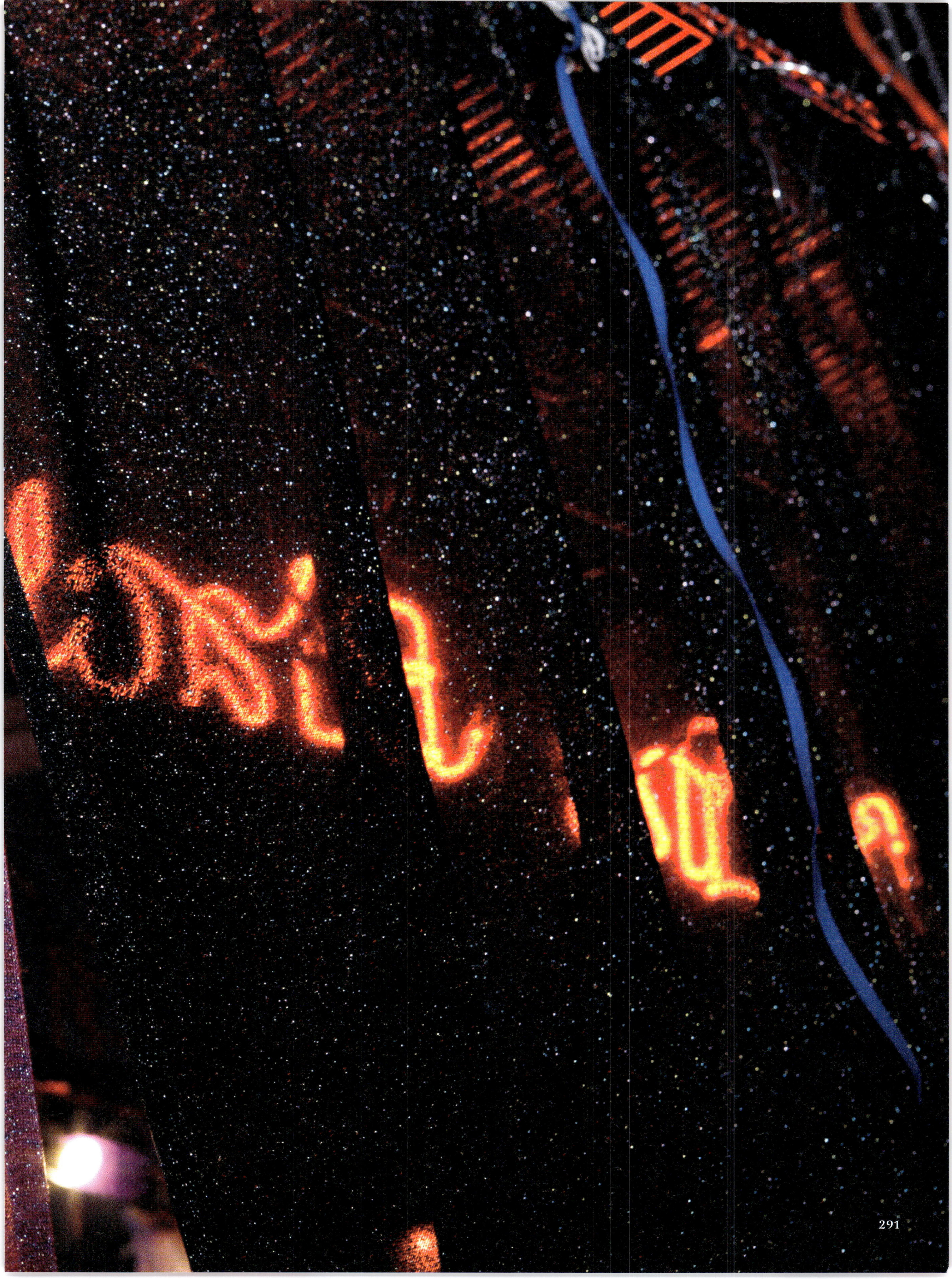

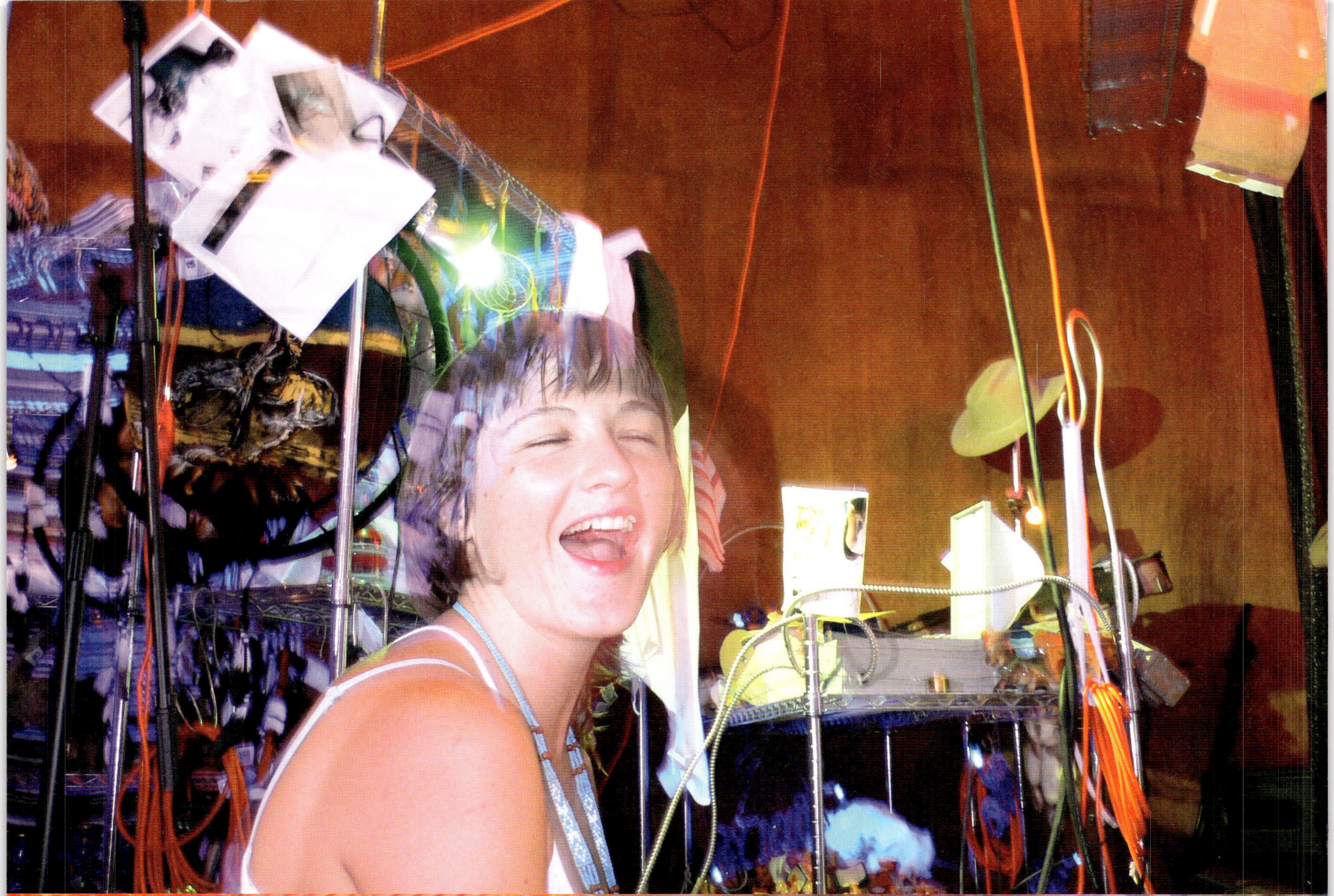

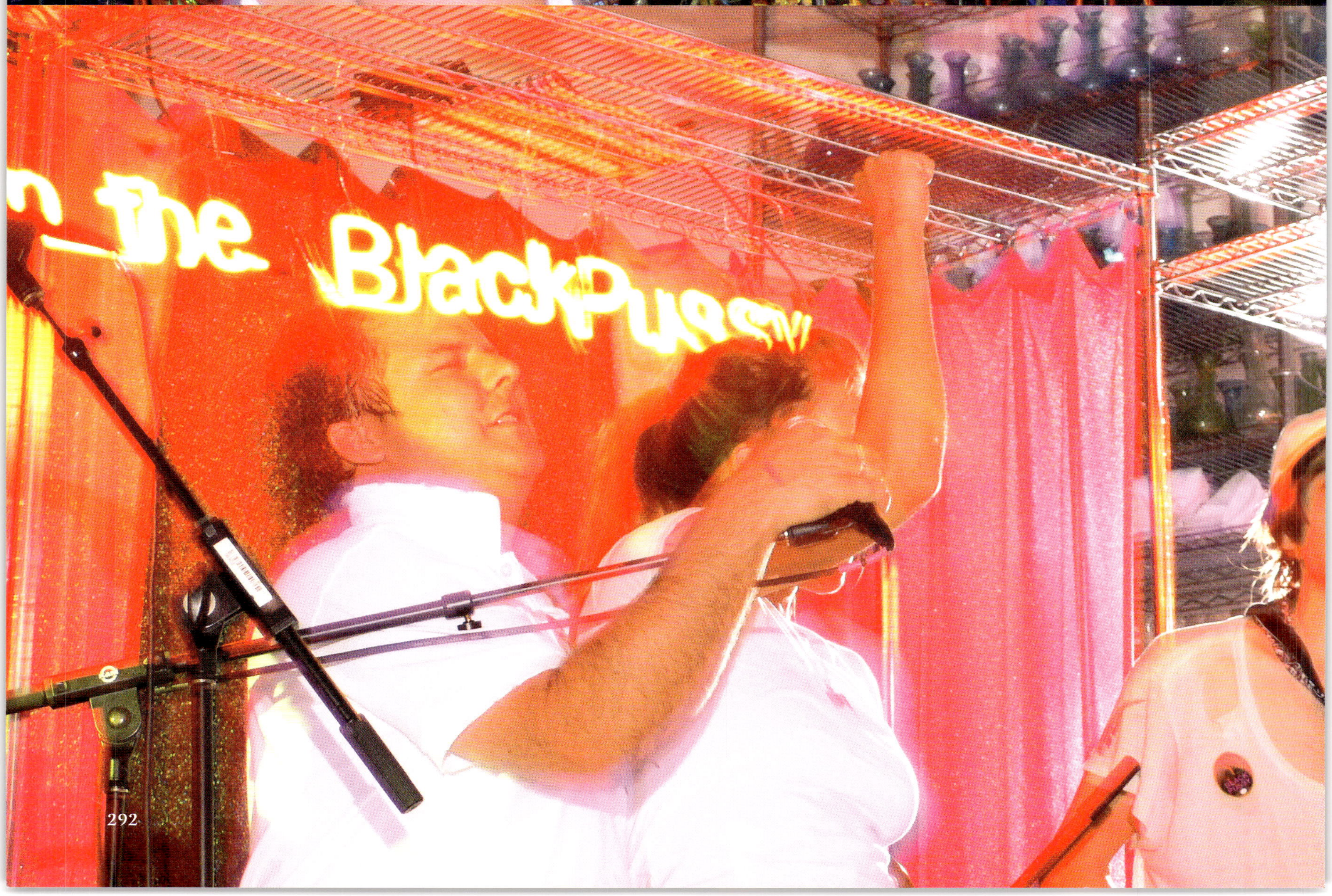
the

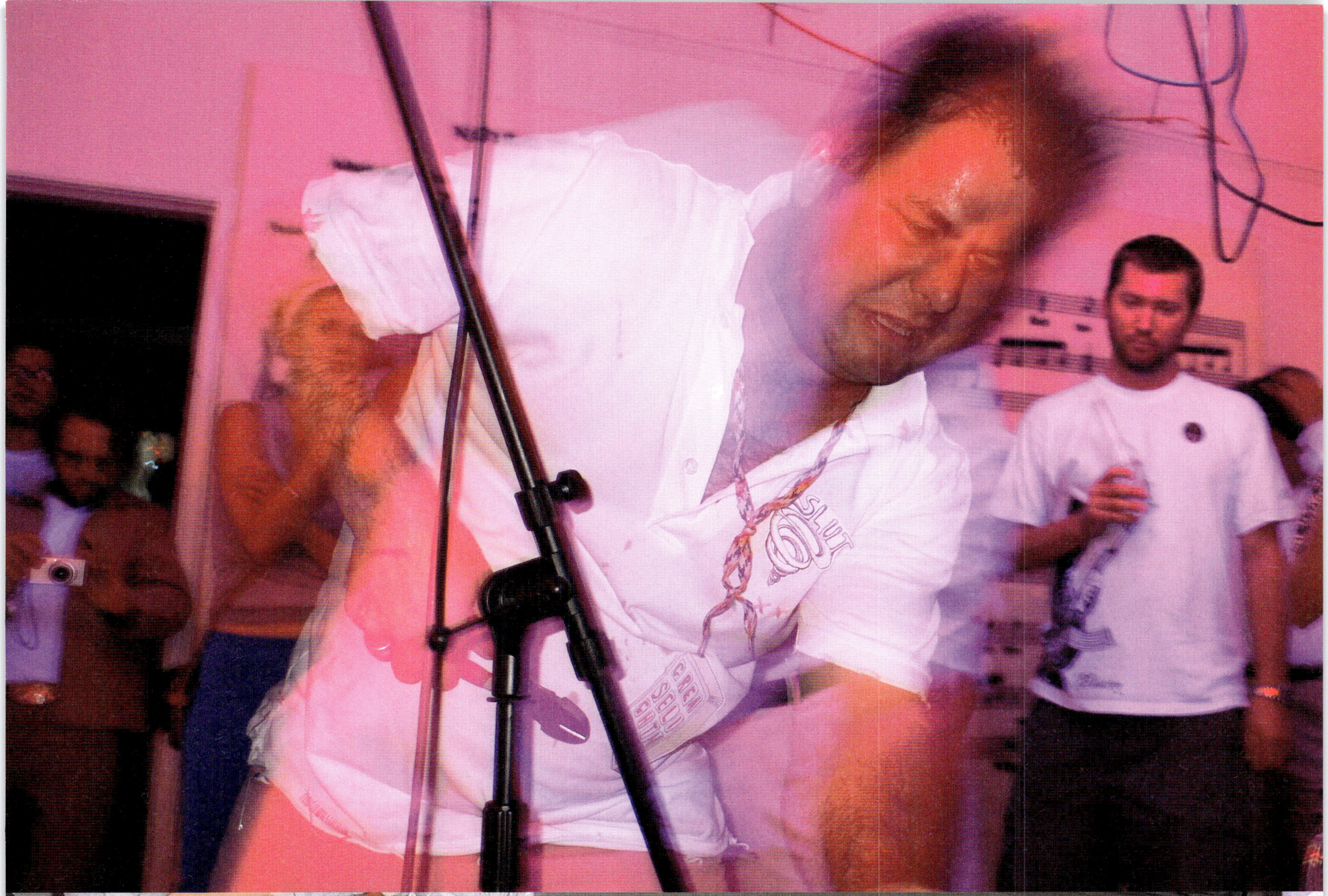
SLUT

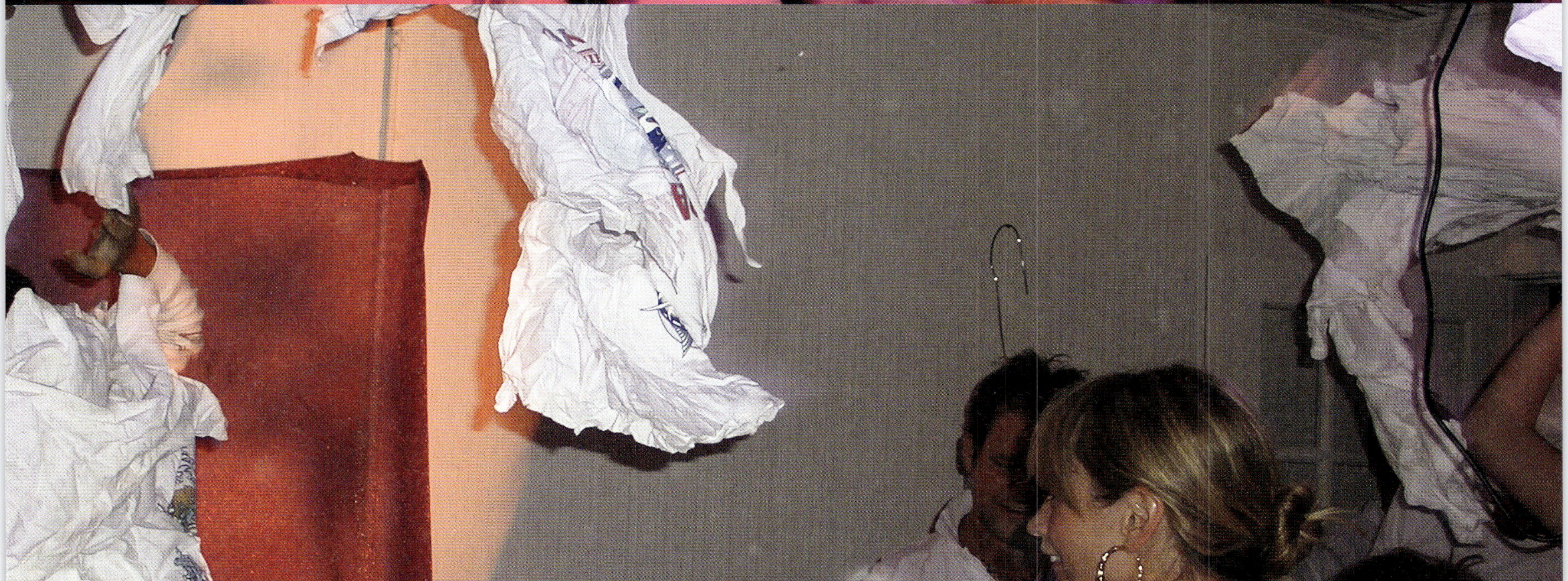

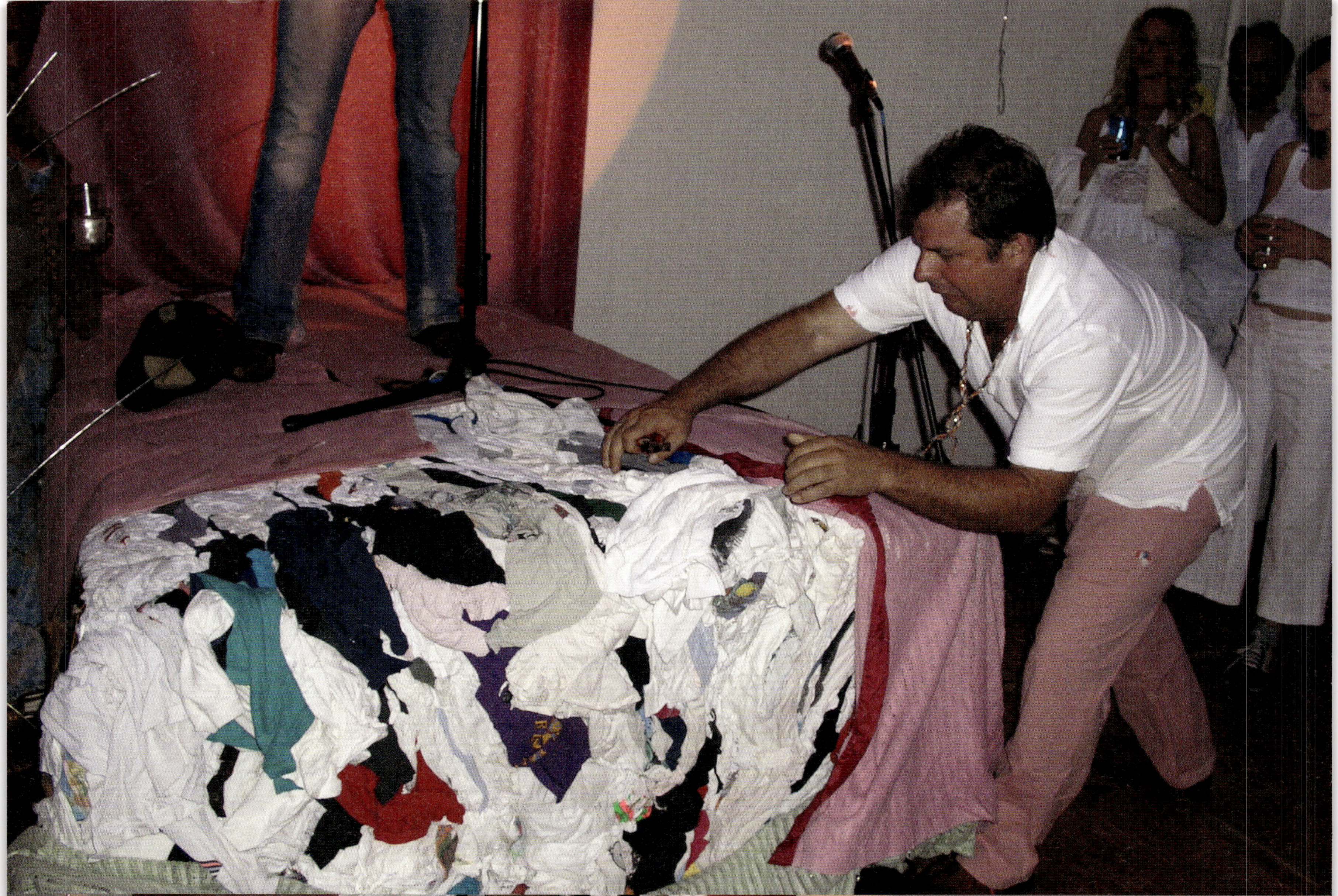

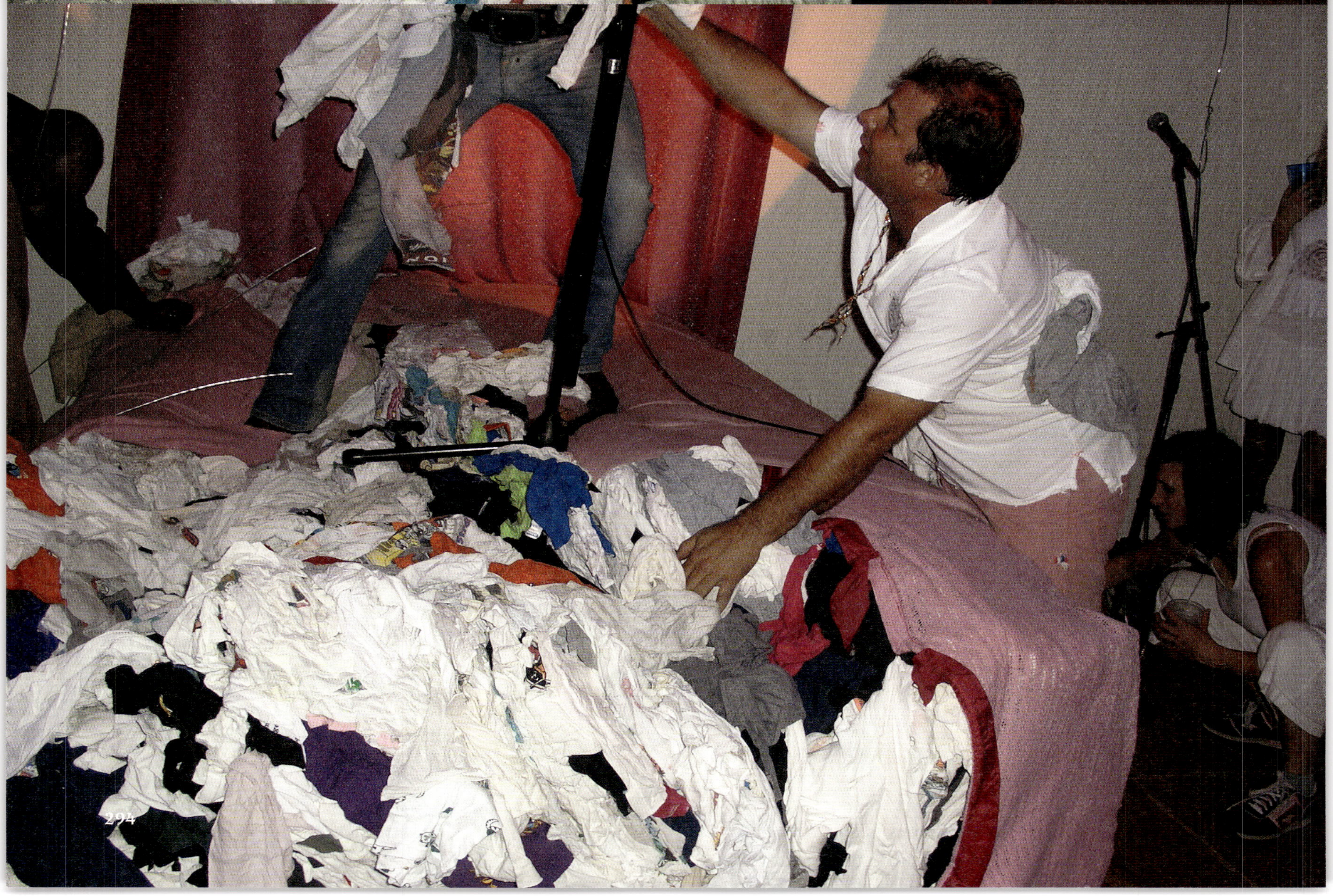

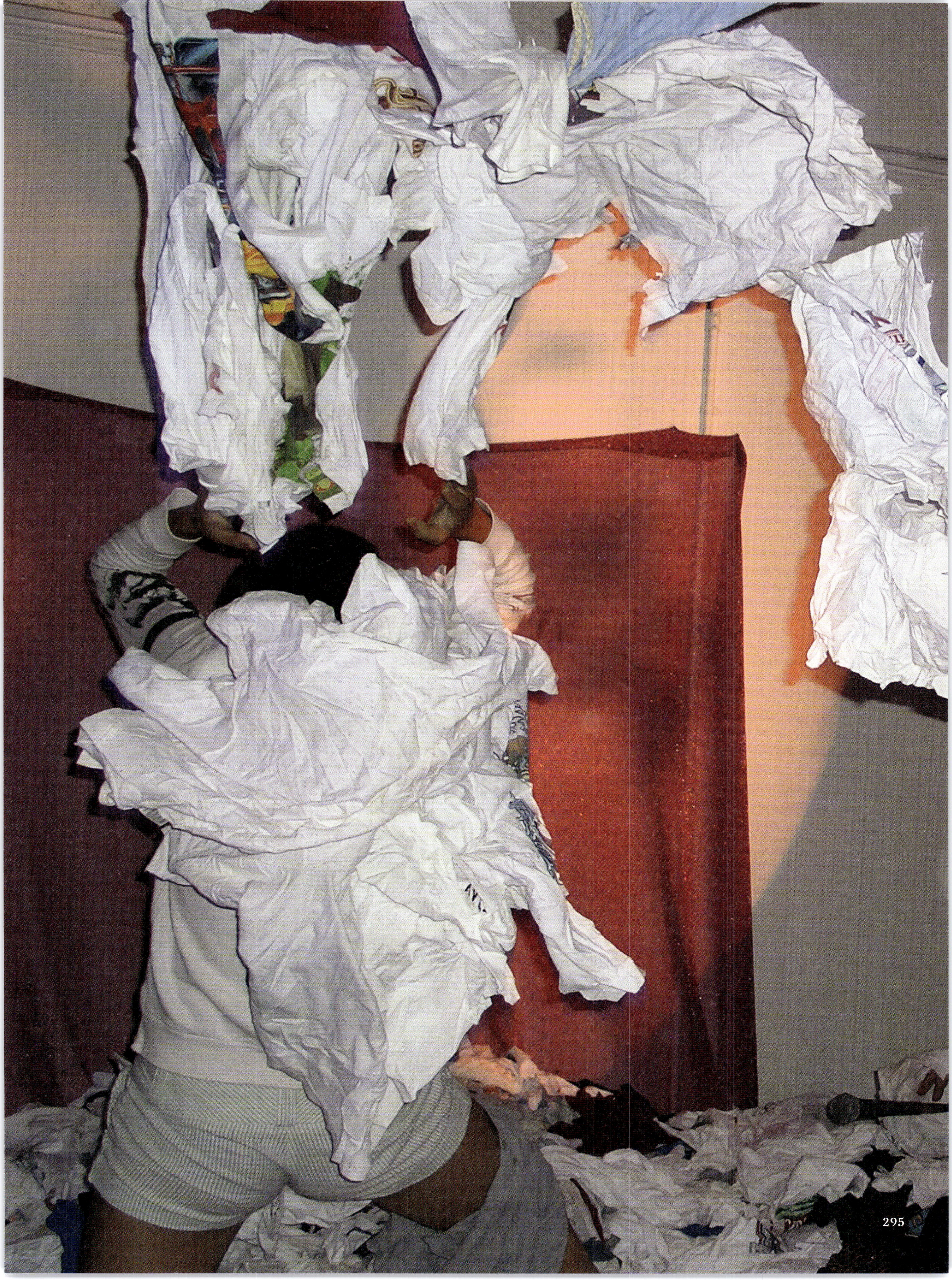

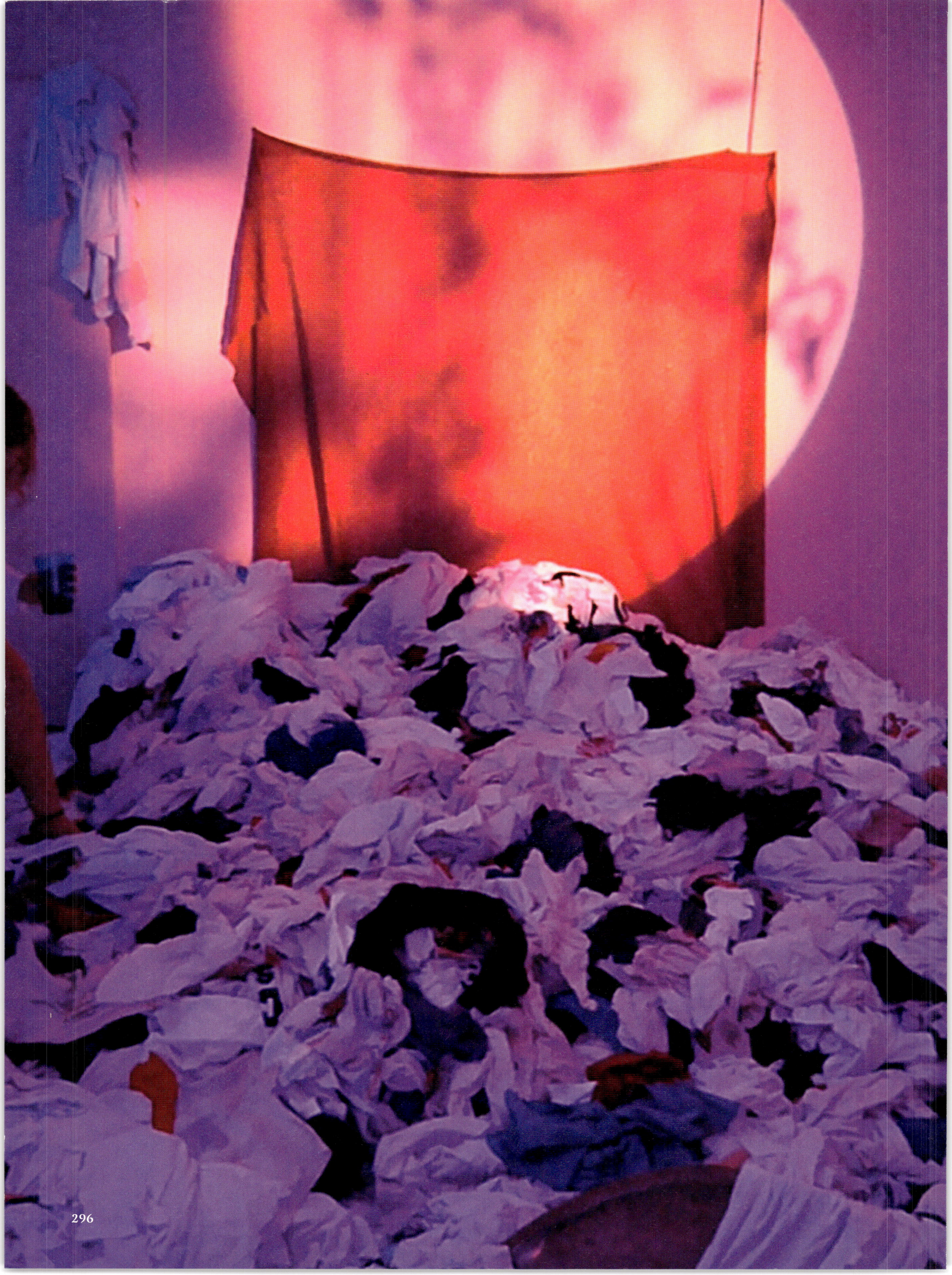

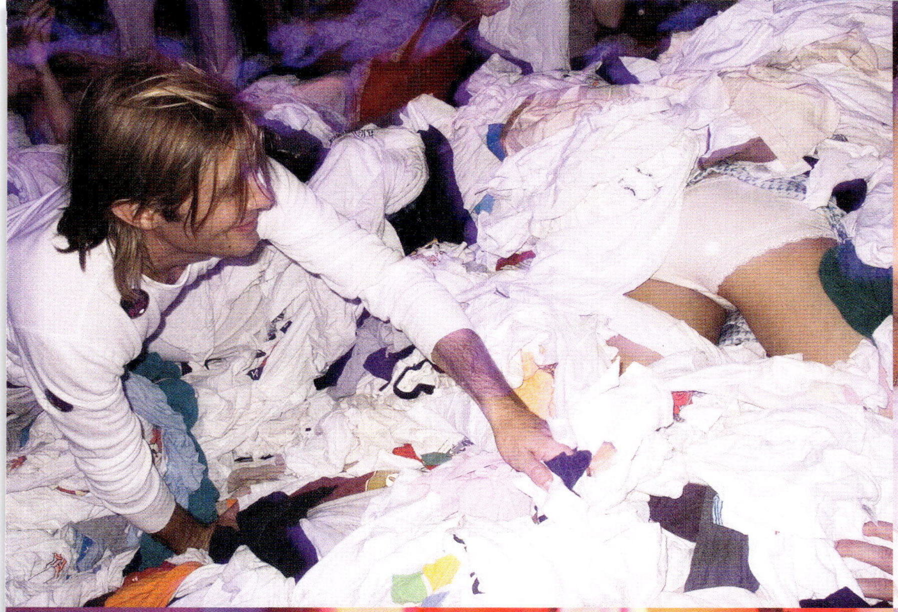
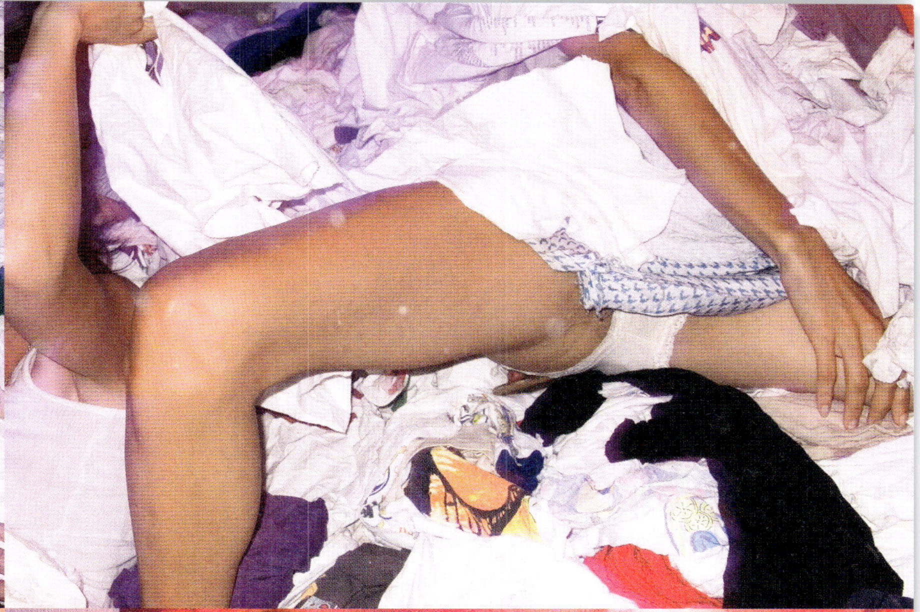
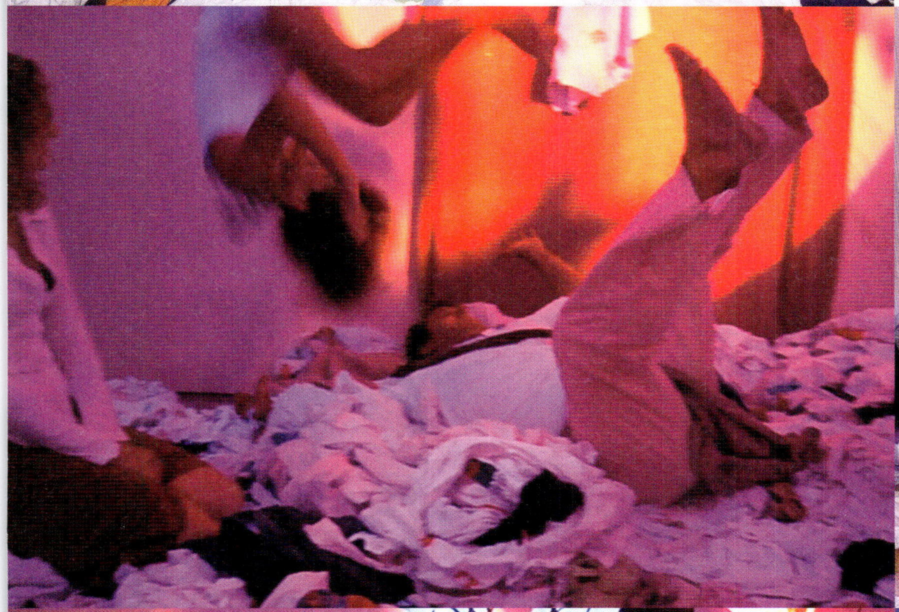
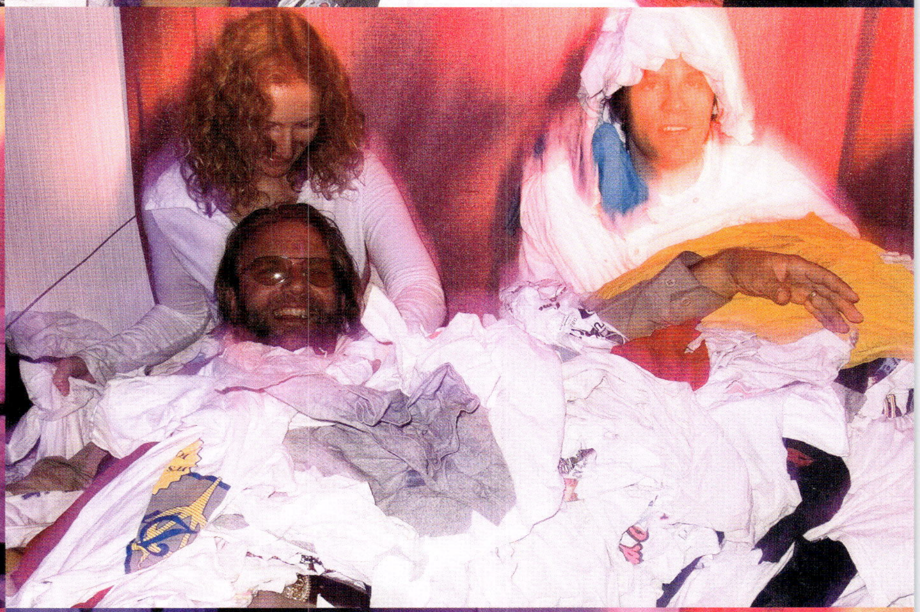
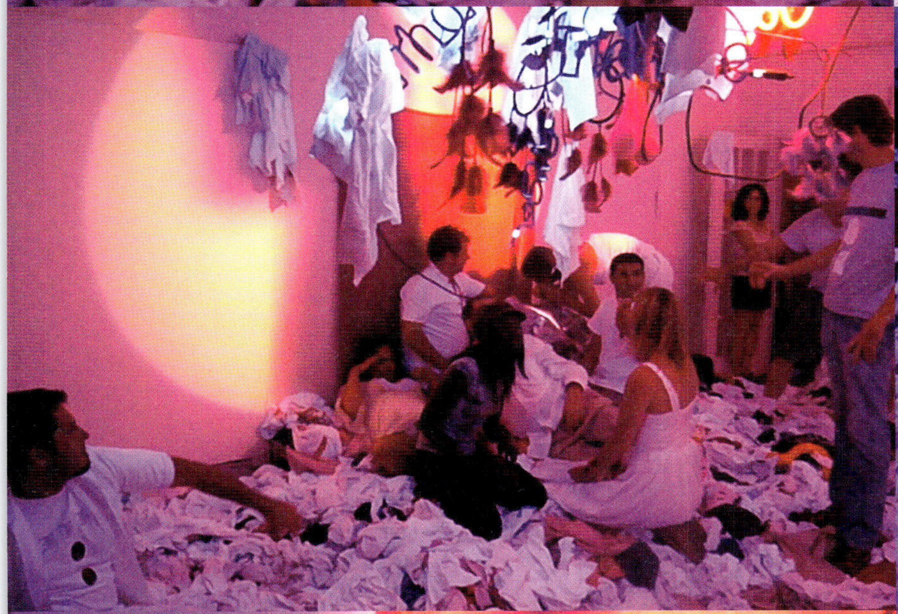
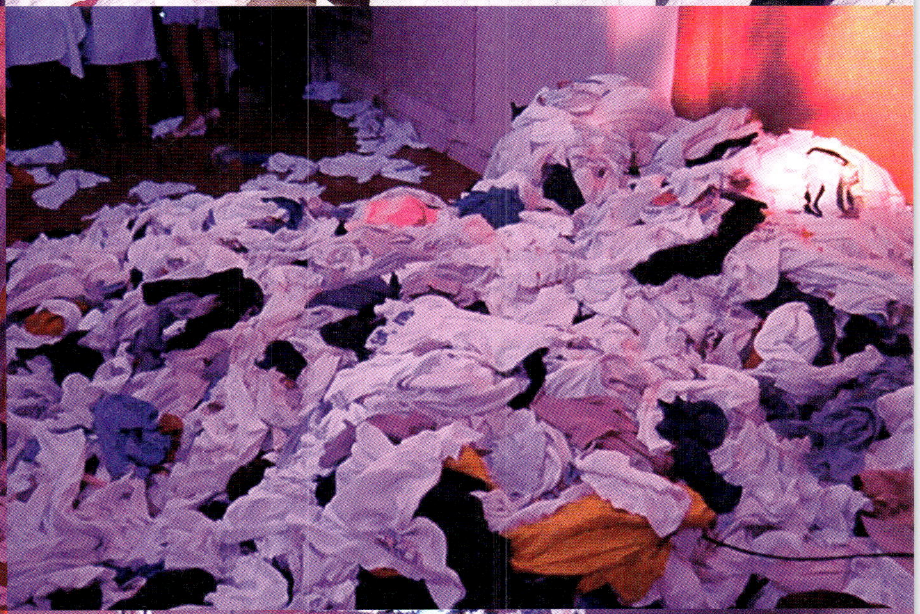
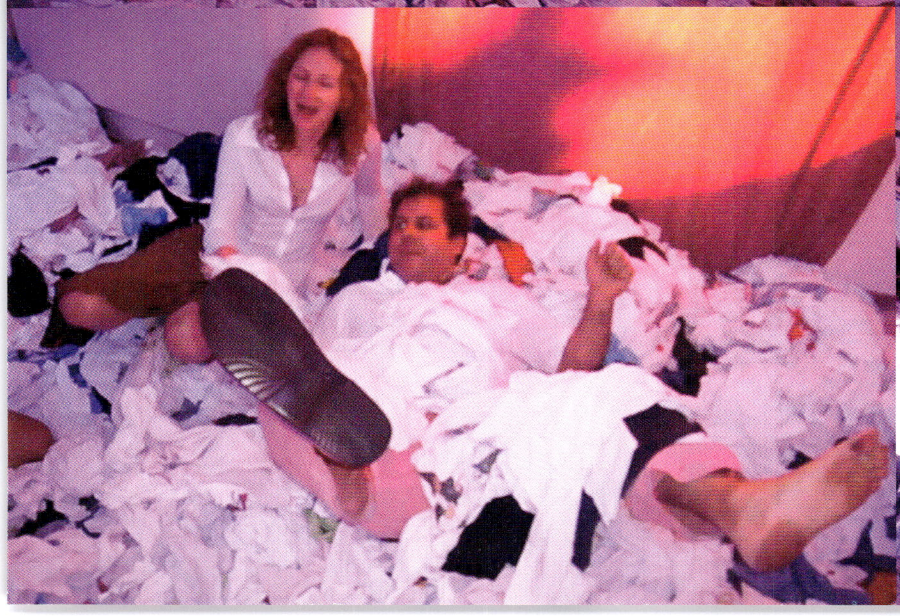
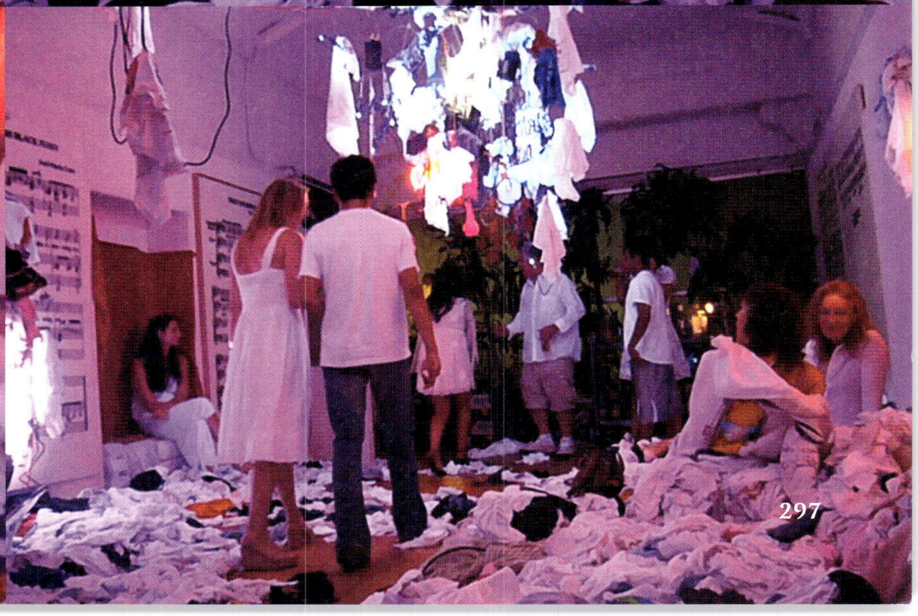

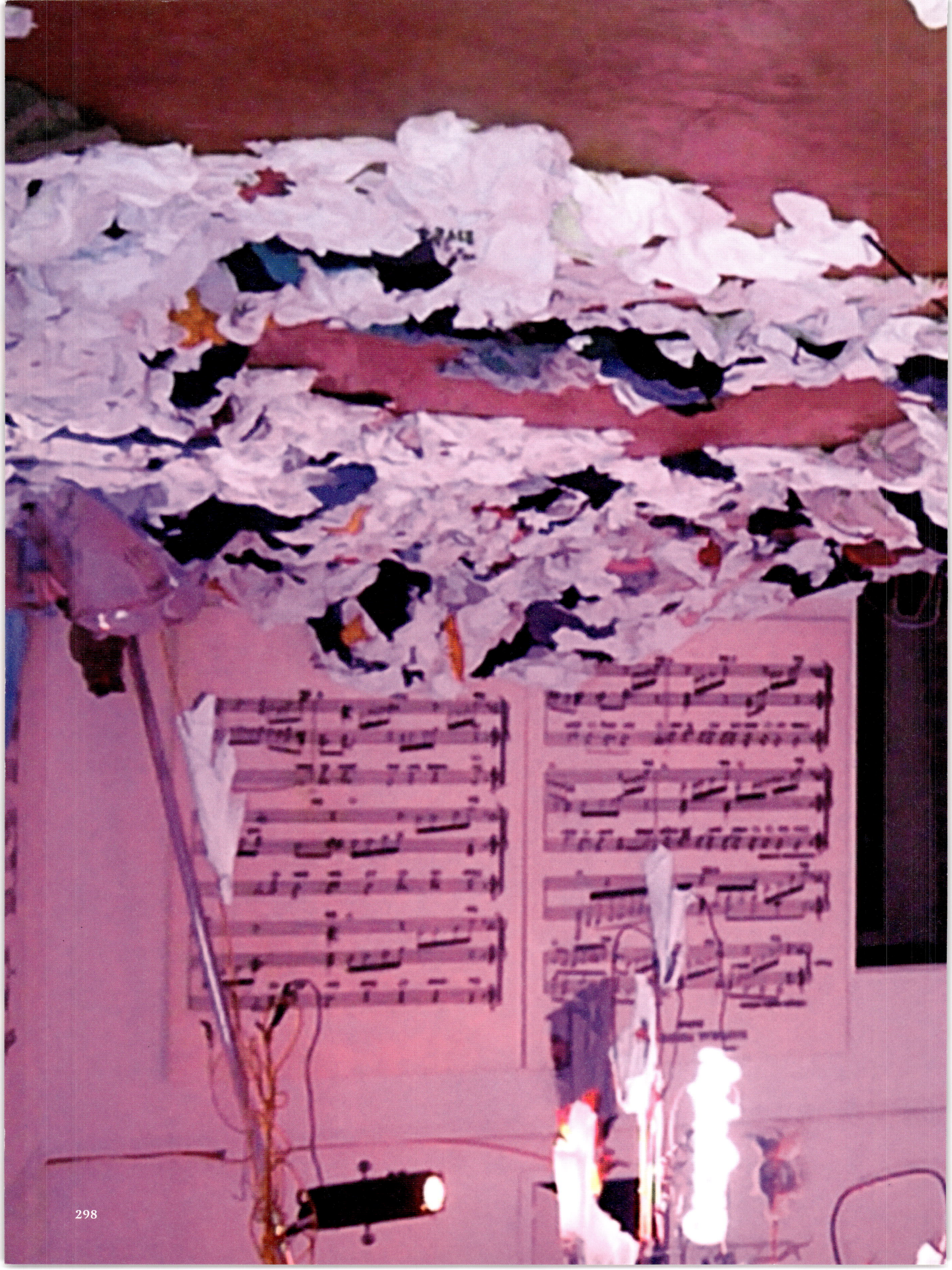

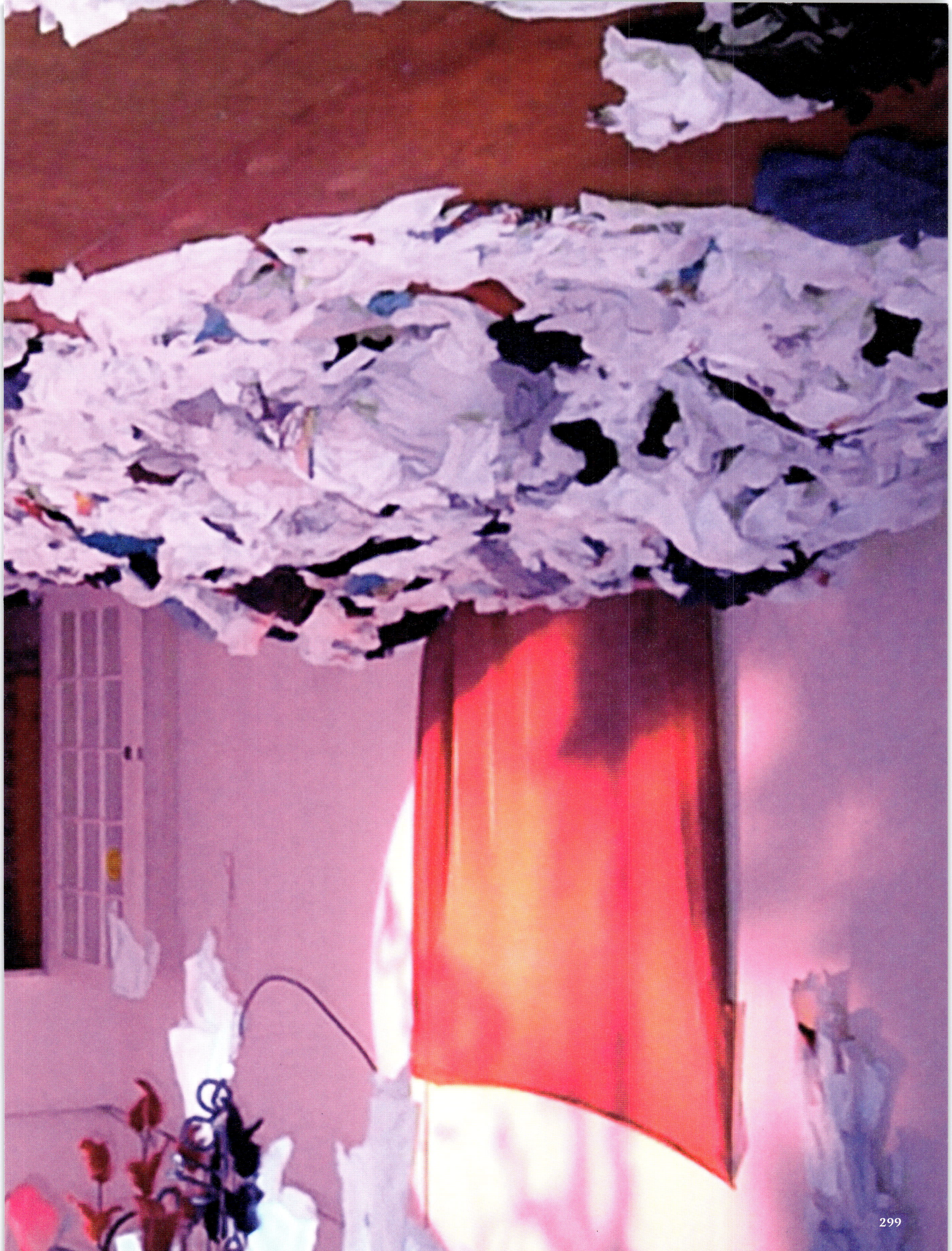

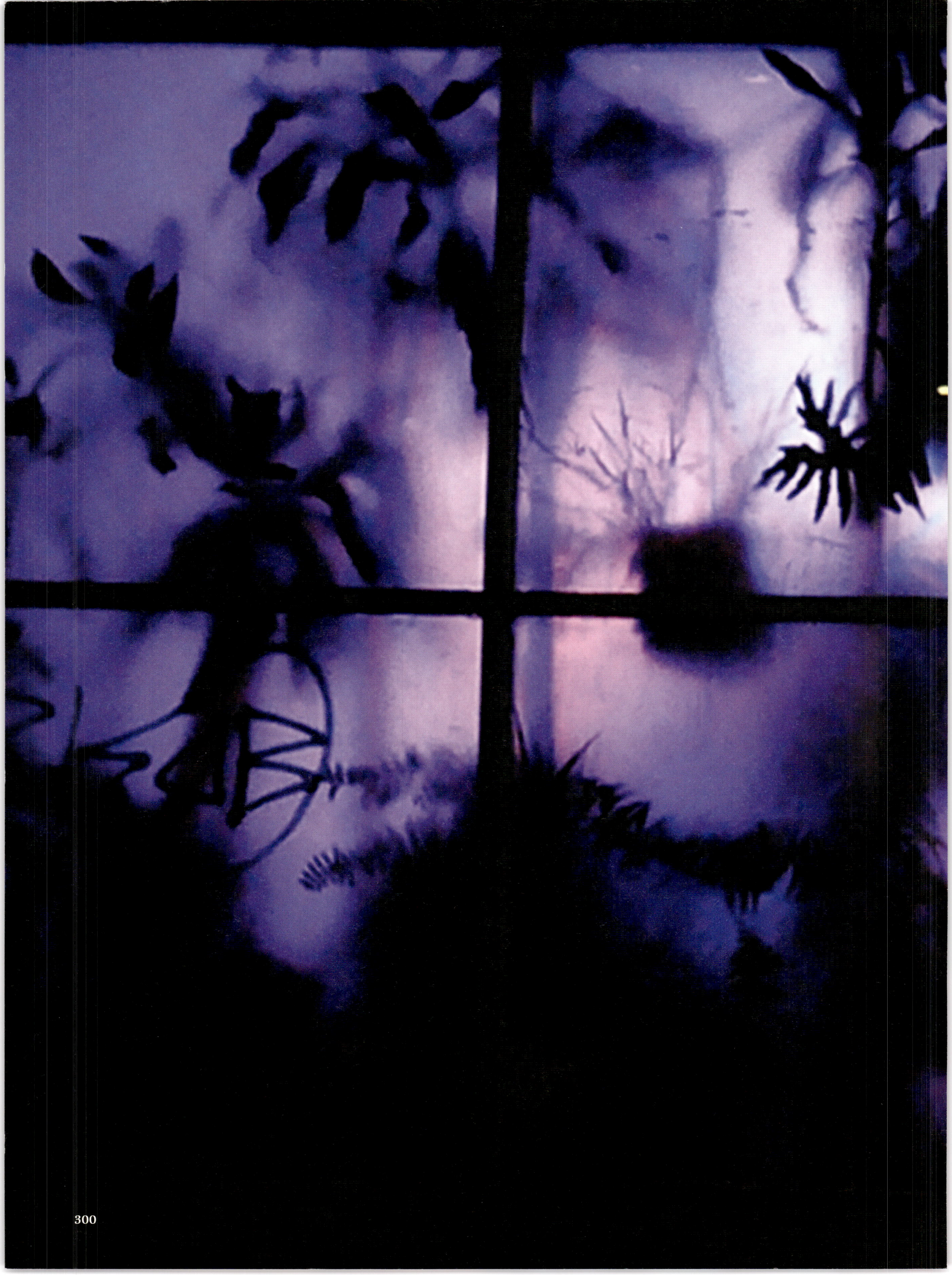

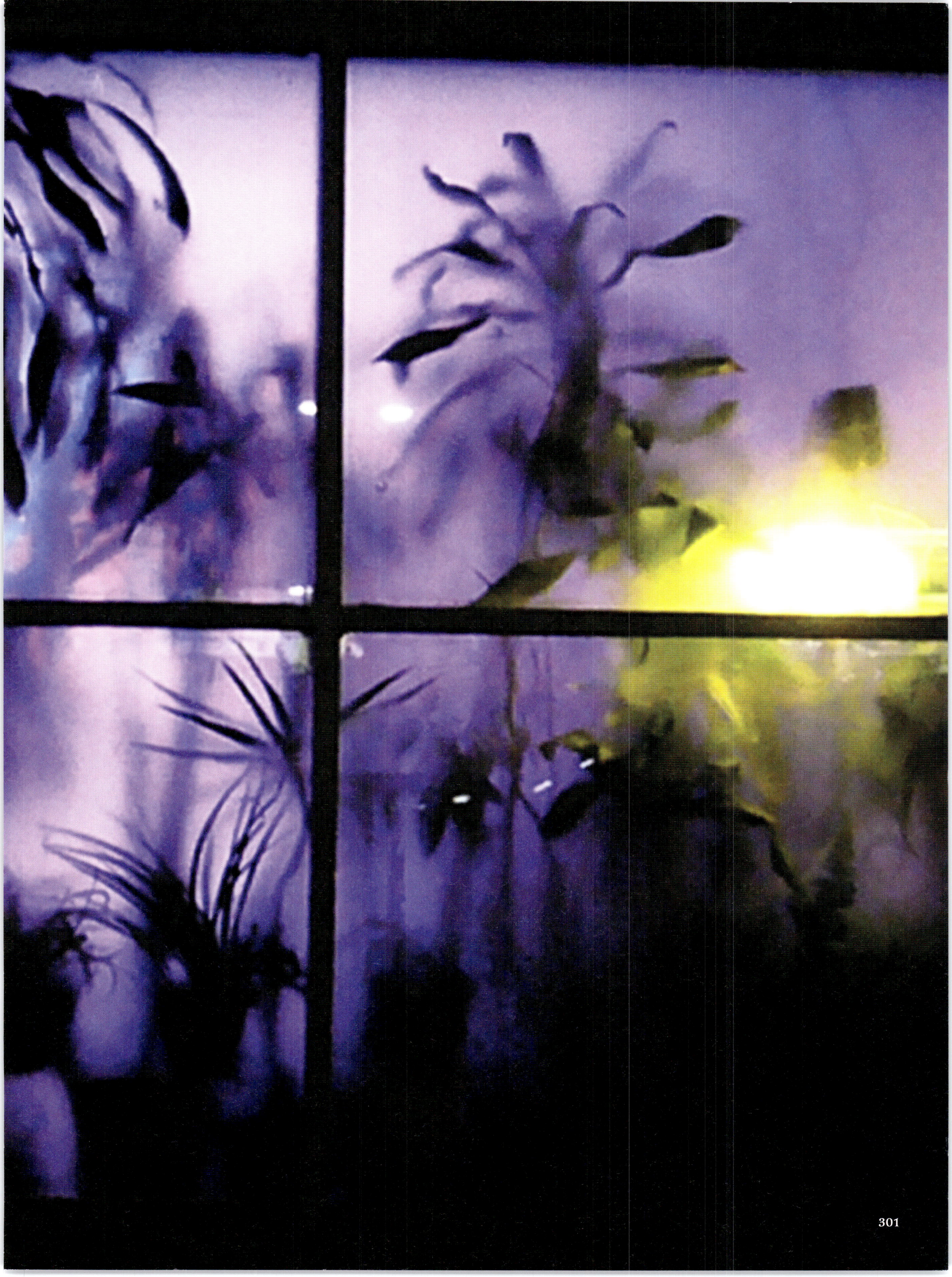

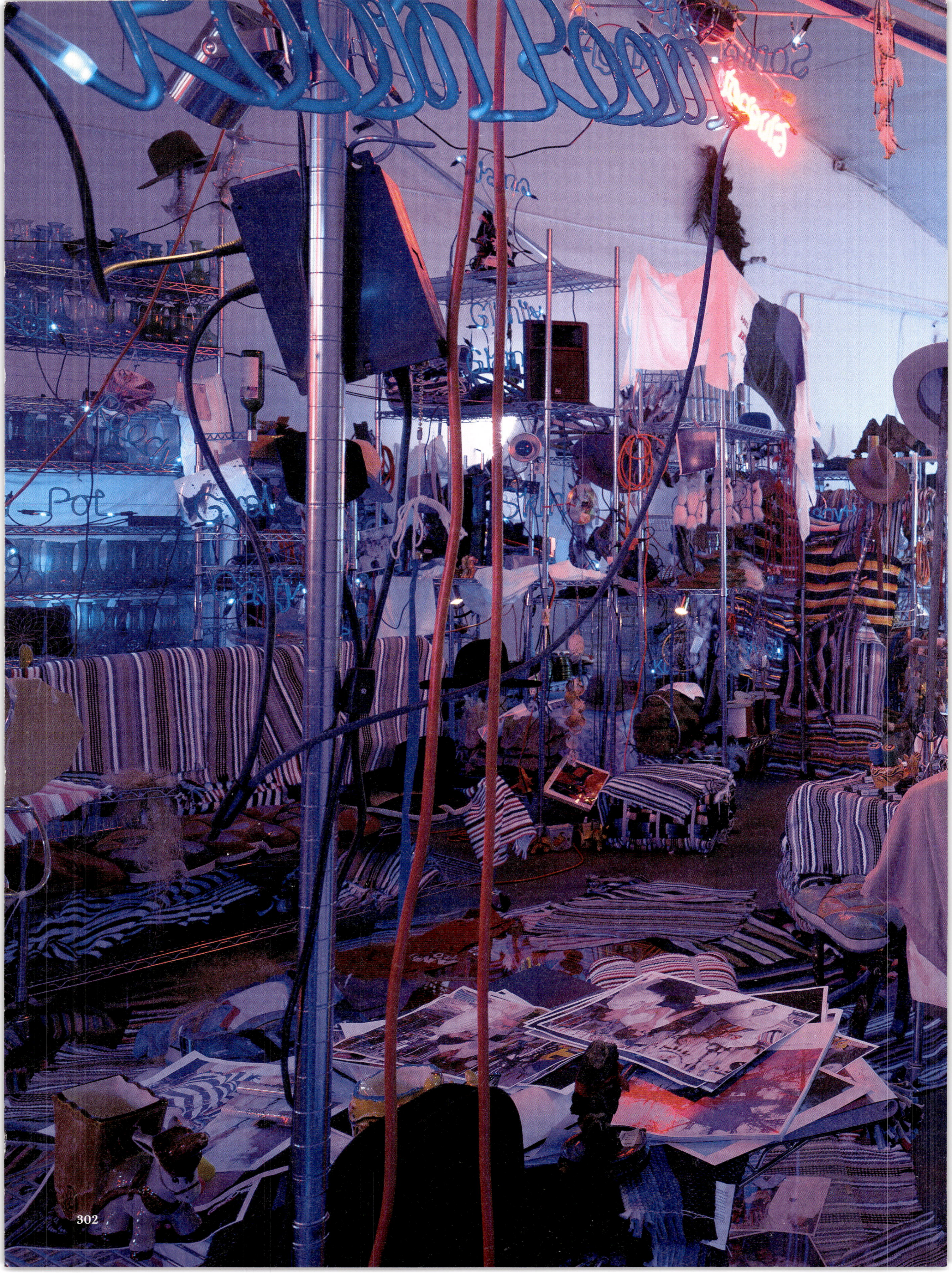

Room Room
Pot
Peach

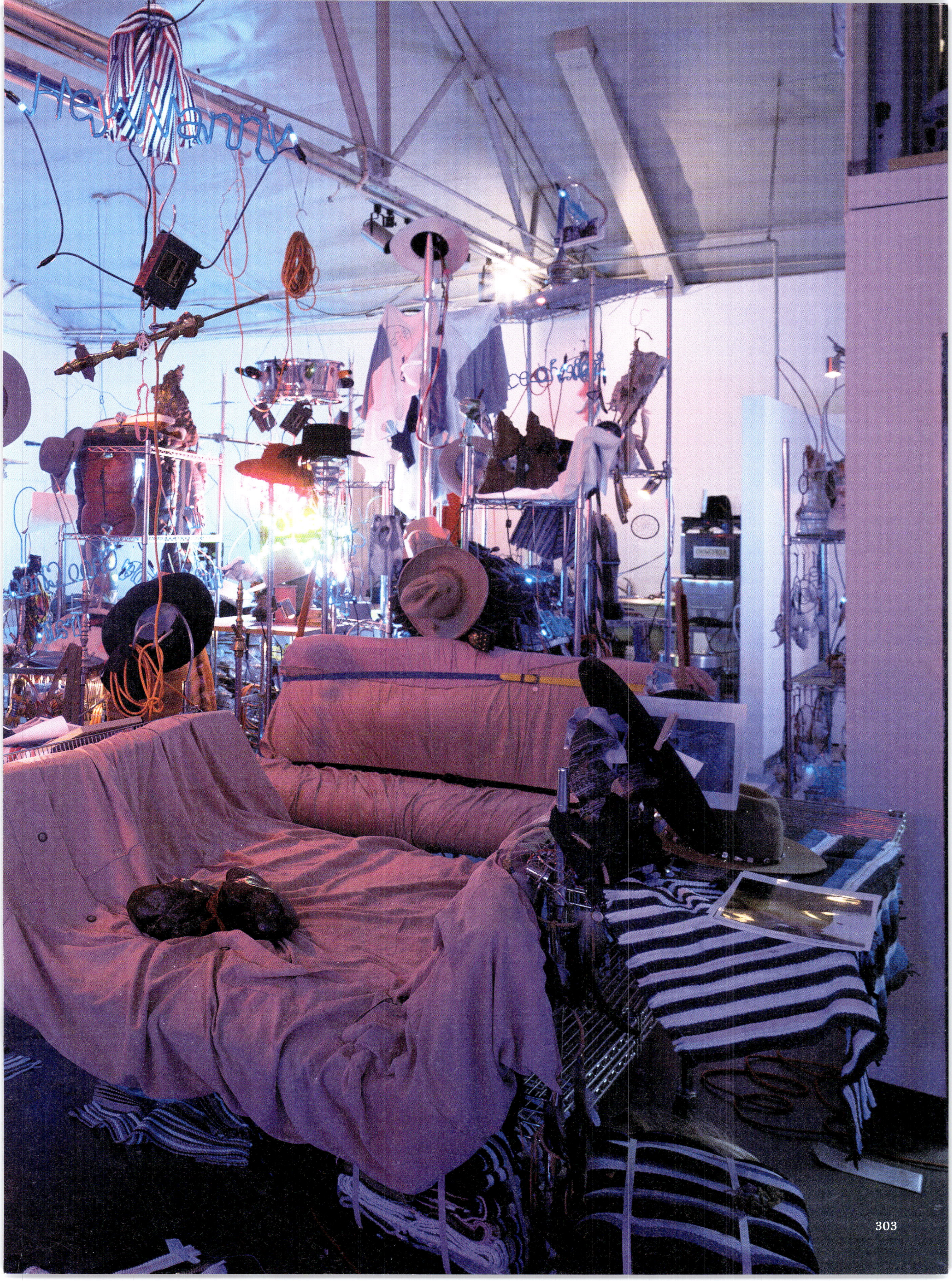
Hey Manny

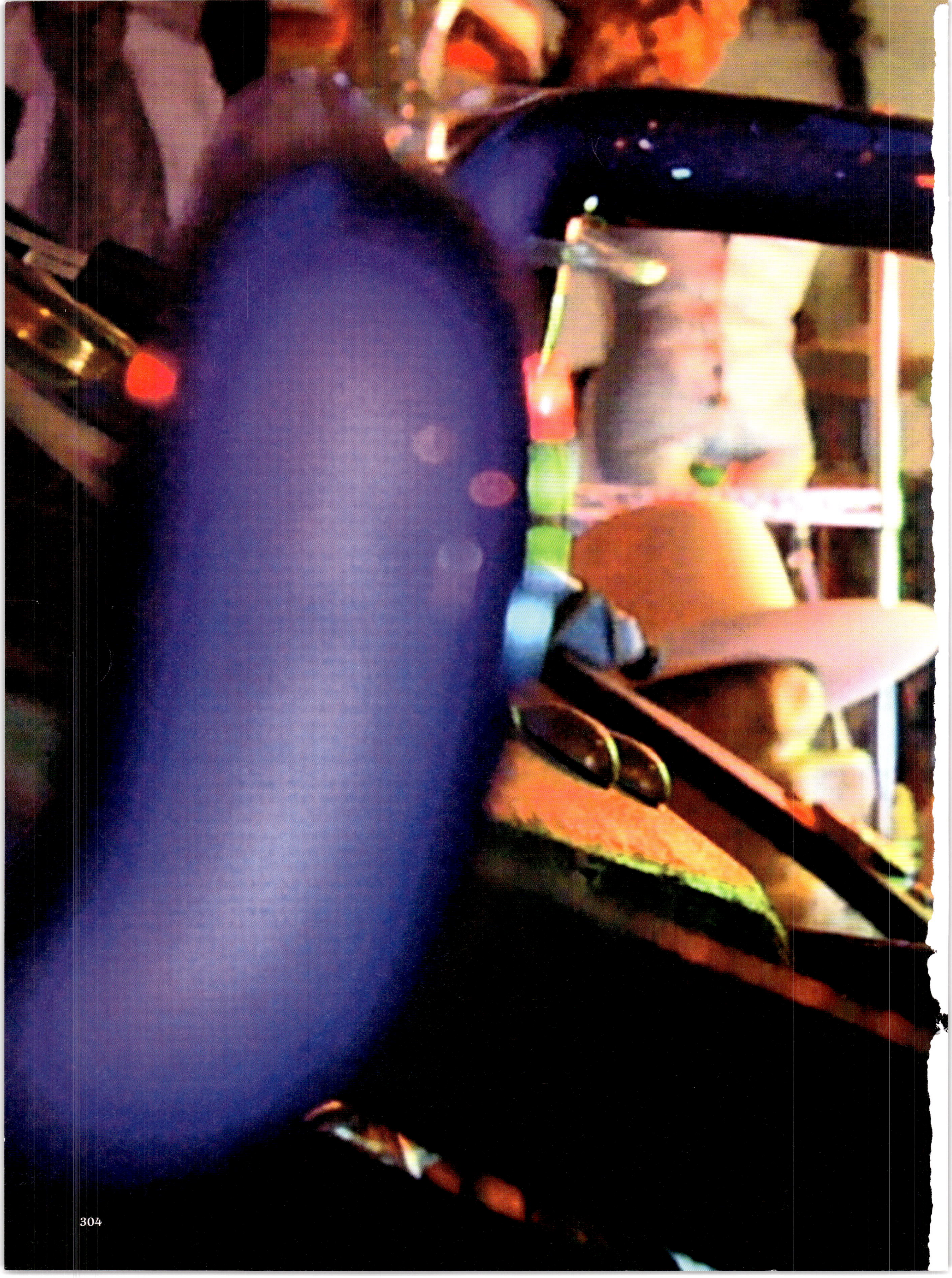

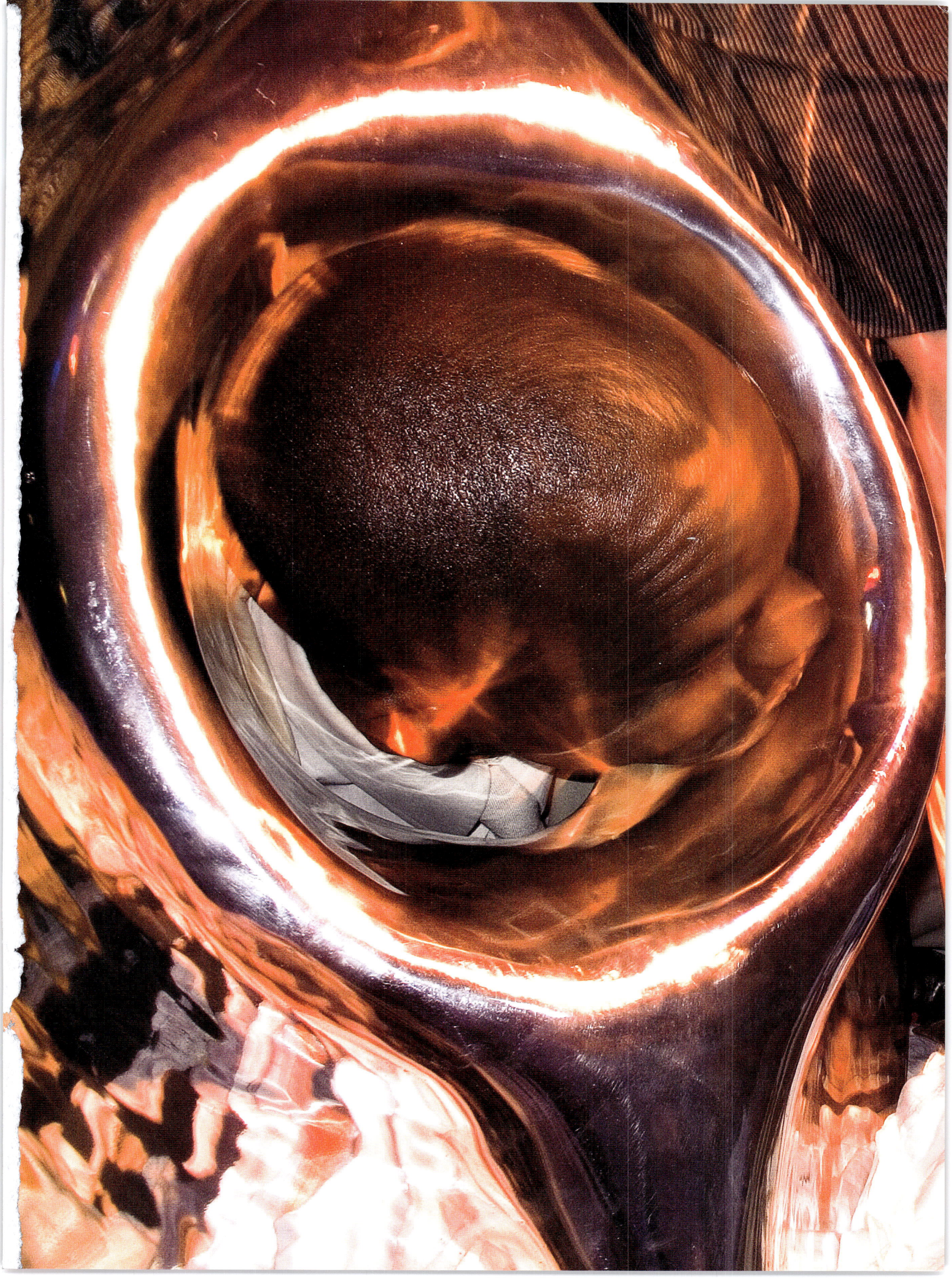

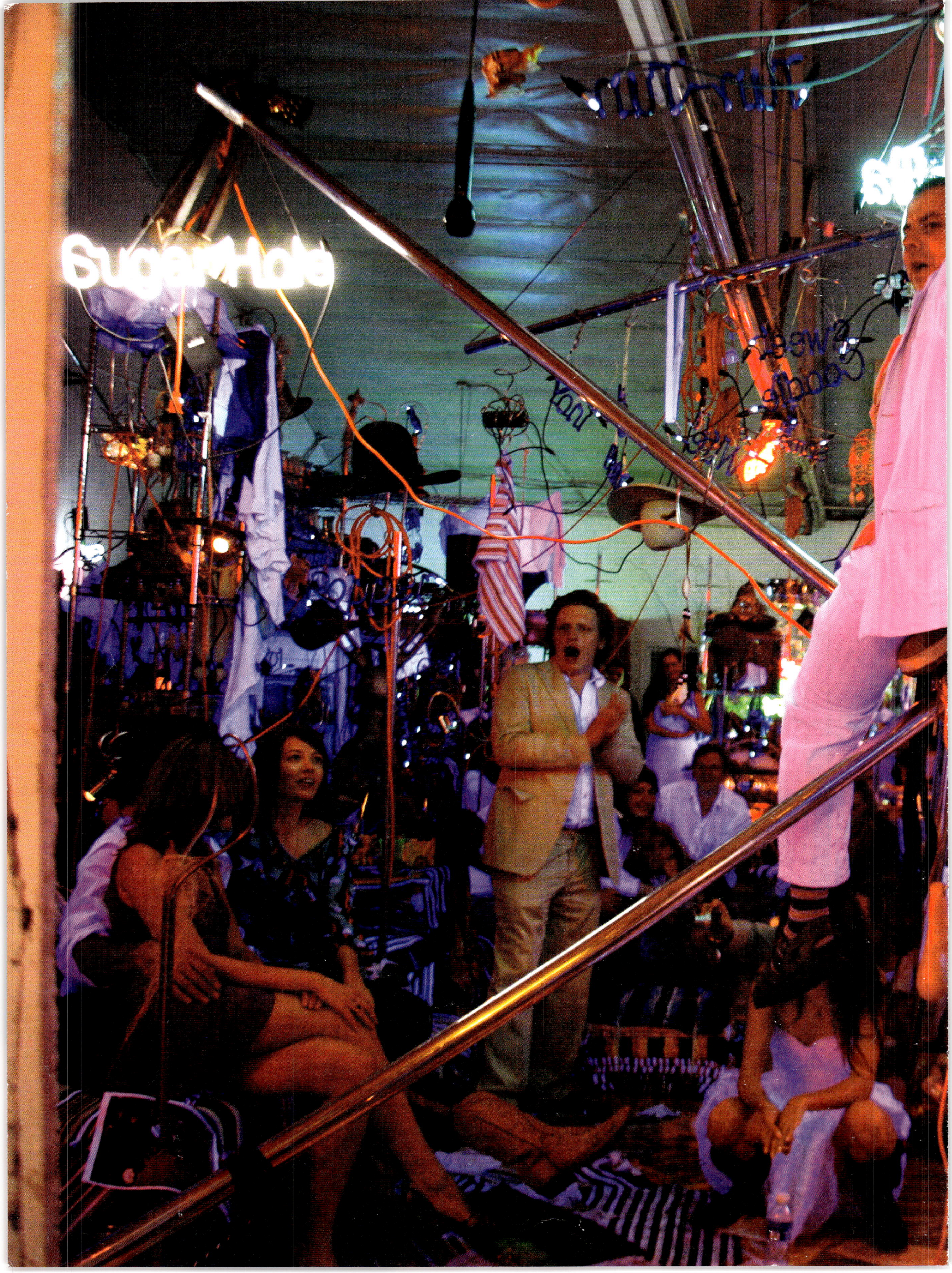